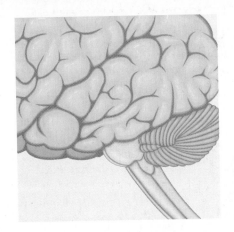

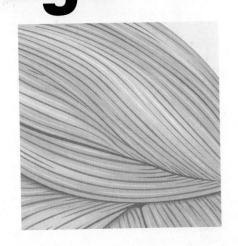

The Medical Language

A Programmed, Body-Systems Approach

DALE **P**IERRE **L**AYMAN, AS, BS, MS, EdS, PhD

Professor
Department of Natural Sciences
Joliet Junior College
Joliet, Illinois

TERESA **E**NGLAND, MSN, RN, *Contributor*

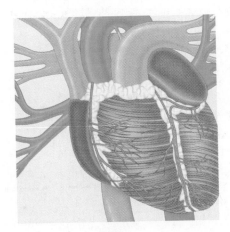

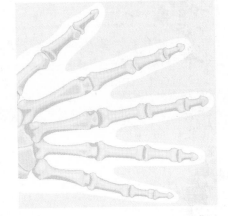

Delmar Publishers Inc.™

An International Thomson Publishing Company

New York • London • Bonn • Boston • Detroit • Madrid • Melbourne • Mexico City
Paris • Singapore • Tokyo • Albany NY • Belmont CA • Cincinnati OH

NOTICE TO THE READER

Cover Design: Precision Graphics
Delmar Staff

Publisher: David C. Gordon
Acquisitions Editor: Adrianne C. Williams
Developmental Editor: Helen V. Yackel
Project Editor: Melissa A. Conan

Production Coordinator: Mary Ellen Black
Art and Design Coordinator: Mary E. Siener
Editorial Assistant: Jill Rembetski
Asst. Marketing Manager: Darryl L. Caron

For more information, contact:
Delmar Publishers Inc.
3 Columbia Circle, Box 15015
Albany, New York 12212-5015

International Thomson Publishing
Berkshire House
168-173 High Holborn
London, WC1V7AA
England

Thomas Nelson Australia
102 Dodds Street
South Melbourne 3205
Victoria, Australia

Nelson Canada
1120 Birchmont Road
Scarborough, Ontario
M1K 5G4, Canada

International Thomson Publishing GmbH
Konigswinterer Str. 418
53227 Bonn
Germany

International Thomson Publishing Asia
221 Henderson Bldg. #05-10
Singapore 0315

International Thomson Publishing Japan
Kyowa Building, 3F
2-2-1 Hirakawa-cho
Chiyoda-ku, Tokyo 102
Japan

COPYRIGHT © 1995 BY DELMAR PUBLISHERS INC.
an International Thomson Publishing Company
The ITP logo is used under license

Printed in the United States of America

1 2 3 4 5 6 7 8 9 10   XXX   01 00 99 98 97 96 95 94

Library of Congress Cataloging-in-Publication Data:
   Layman, Dale Pierre.
      The medical language: a programmed, body-systems approach / Dale Pierre Layman.
         p.   cm.
     Includes index.
     ISBN 0-8273-5612-9
     1. Medicine—Terminology—Programmed instruction.   I. Title.
     [DNLM: 1. Anatomy—programmed instruction.   2. Anatomy—terminology.
     3. Physiology—programmed instruction.   4. Physiology—terminology.
     5. Diagnosis—terminology.   6. Diagnosis—programmed instruction. QS 18 L427m 1994]
   R123.L36 1994
   610'.14—dc20
   DNLM/DLC
    for Library of Congress
                                        93-37629
                                          CIP

DEDICATION

This book is fondly dedicated to my loving wife, Kathleen, and to my wonderful children, Andrew, Alexis, Allison, and Amanda.

CONTENTS

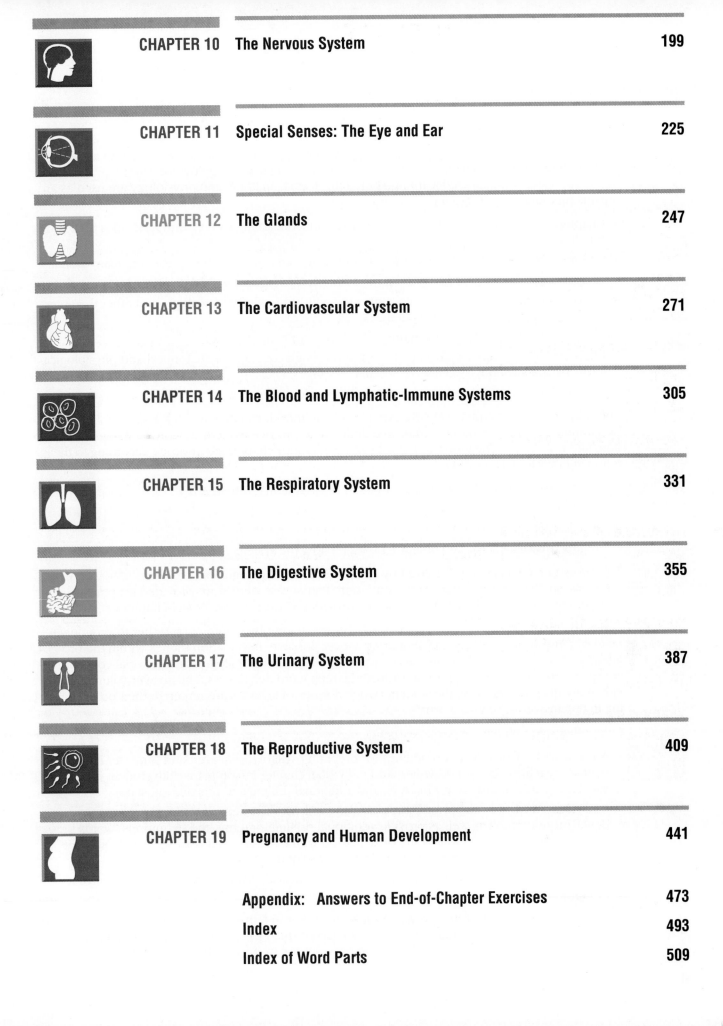

PREFACE

The Medical Language: A Programmed, Body-Systems Approach has been developed to answer the needs of learners and teachers who want to study medical terminology by body systems, through a highly successful programmed learning approach. Normal anatomy and physiology are used as an organizing tool for most chapters.

- Chapter 1 acquaints the student with the programmed learning format and basic rules of word building.
- Chapter 2 brings in the concepts of words and word parts related to the diseases of many systems.
- Chapter 3 presents words and word parts associated with lab tests and diagnoses in general.
- Chapter 4 considers word elements connected with surgery, pharmacology, and other therapies that can be applied to all body systems.
- Chapter 5 focuses on the broad terms of body structure and function.
- Chapters 6–18 present a comprehensive and thorough coverage of anatomical and physiological terms by specific body systems.
- Chapter 19 focuses on pregnancy and human development.

The subject of each chapter is clearly explained in an introductory essay. This essay is followed by programmed learning frames for extensive drilling and practice in medical word building, dissection, and translation. The terms and word parts in a typical chapter are grouped according to the following four topical headings:

1. Normal structure and function of a particular body system (Normal A & P)
2. Diseases affecting the system
3. Lab tests and diagnoses of problems affecting the system
4. Surgery, pharmacology, and other therapies treating the system

This programmed material is followed by exercises for word recognition, meanings, dissection, synthesis, spelling, abbreviations, and translation. Partial case studies are provided for practice in word usage and interpretation. The appendix provides answers to the end-of-chapter exercises.

A special system of phonetic pronunciation helps the learner by guiding him or her to pronounce medical terms using whole simple words whenever possible. Information frames within the programmed sections provide interesting background. Entertaining analogies and pictorial concepts are sprinkled throughout to illustrate Latin and Greek word derivations. The answer columns provide immediate feedback for the student (when a series of answers are required, their order of listing in the answer column may vary).

Comprehensive supplement package:

- An Instructor's Guide includes outlines for preparing syllabi for quarter- and semester-length courses, teaching tips and strategies, and individual chapter lesson plans with student review sheets, activities, transparency masters, and additional drilling and practice questions.
- A package of two 90-minute audiotapes is also available. The tapes are structured to aid students' pronunciation as well as provide additional drilling for terms and definitions. Words presented on the audiotapes follow the presentation within the text and correspond to a student review sheet within each chapter of the Instructor's Guide.
- A computerized bank of 1,000 questions with answers is available. The IBM format easily creates a variety of testing materials.

In summary, this is a complete package for learning medical terminology in a way that is organized and comprehensive—a thorough body-systems-based format. Its unique blend of programmed instruction and background essay information provides a new approach to the subject.

ACKNOWLEDGMENTS

Many thanks go to the editorial and production team at Delmar for their faith and vision in the project. Particular gratitude is expressed to Adrianne Williams, Acquisitions Editor, whose patience and understanding allowed me to complete a huge volume of material after I was seriously injured; Helen Yackel, Developmental Editor, who was there to ensure accuracy and completeness; Jill Rembetski, Editorial Assistant, who handled the many letters, packages, and administrative details involved throughout the project; Melissa Conan, Project Editor, who worked to ensure grammatical accuracy and consistency; Mary Siener, Art and Design Coordinator, who helped create the impressive color illustrations and design; and Mary Ellen Black, Production Coordinator, who saw to the many details of turning all our work into an actual book.

Special thanks go to Teresa England, who contributed additional frames for pronunciation and items for further drilling in the end-of-chapter exercises.

Finally, I would like to thank all my colleagues who reviewed the evolving manuscript and helped shape it into a quality product:

Constance M. Dellinger, BA, MA
Jackson Adult Education Director
Jackson Public Schools
Jackson, MI

Teresa England, MSN, RN
North Montco Vo Tech
Lansdale, PA

Brenda Foster
East Tennessee State University
Elizabethton, TN

Michelle A. Green, MPS, RRA
State University of New York
College of Technology at Alfred
Alfred, NY

Shelli Meador
Professional Court Reporting School
Richardson, TX

Karen Melcher
Northeast Iowa Community College
Calmar, IA

A. Christine Payne
Sarasota Vo-Tech Center
Sarasota, FL

Donald C. Rizzo, PhD
Chairperson: Division of Natural Sciences and
    Mathematics
Marygrove College
Detroit, MI

Molly Savage, BSN, RN
Central Piedmont Community College
Charlotte, NC

Janet Sesser, RMA (AMT), CMA
Bryman School
Phoenix, AZ

HOW TO USE THIS BOOK

The following describes the major text features. By familiarizing yourself with these features, you can use this book effectively to learn the medical language.

The format for this text is called **programmed learning,** which stimulates active student participation by challenging you to supply answers to blanks in a series of frames.

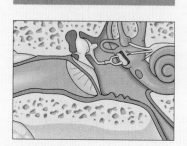

Organized by Body Systems

This book presents a unique combination of medical terminology with human anatomy and physiology in health and disease. Specifically, it presents a broad overview of medical terminology organized by **body systems** and represented by corresponding icon tabs. Medical terms associated with the heart and blood vessels, for instance, are found in the chapter on the cardiovascular system, which is represented by the heart icon.

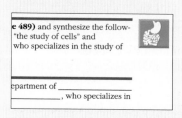

Chapter Icons

Icons associated with chapter material are used as tabs on right-hand chapter pages to assist you in easily locating each chapter. The icons are also listed next to their corresponding chapter titles in the table of contents.

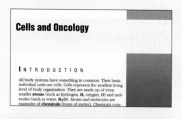

Chapter Introduction

Each chapter has an **Introduction** in regular essay format. It serves to orient you to the material being presented. When the chapter covers a body system, the system's basic elements of structure and function are discussed. Full-color art visually illustrates important concepts covered in the introduction. A colorful sidebar appears on every introduction, making the beginning of each chapter easy to find.

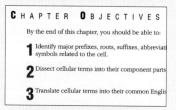

Learning Objectives

Following the introduction is a set of learning objectives. These help you to focus on topics of primary importance and provide you with an outline of study that is revisited and reinforced in the exercises.

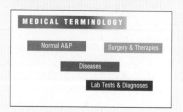

Subdivision of Terms into Four Content Areas

Starting with Chapter 6, the terms in each chapter are subdivided into four separate content areas. These areas are **normal anatomy and physiology (A & P); diseases and abnormalities; lab tests and diagnoses;** and **surgery, pharmacology, and other therapies.** This organization of chapter subdivisions follows the normal progression of the disease process, from health to disease, diagnoses, and treatment. To help you stay organized, and for easy recognition, each area is represented by a bar scheme of a different color—red, purple, blue, and green, respectively.

Term Overview

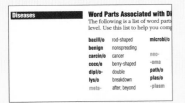

At the start of each chapter subdivision, the relevant terms, word parts, and abbreviations are listed for easy reference.

Programmed Learning and Reinforcement

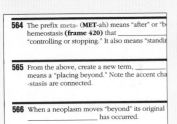

The learning approach utilized in this text is called programmed learning. To encourage active participation in learning, the sequentially numbered frames contain "hints" or "prompts" to help you fill in the blanks. Immediate feedback is provided by simply consulting the left-hand column, which contains the correct answers for the blanks.

Highlighting of New Word Parts and Terms

564 The prefix meta- (**MET**-ah) means "after" or "b hemeostasis (**frame 420**) that "controlling or stopping." It also means "standi

565 From the above, create a new term, _____ means a "placing beyond." Note the accent cha -stasis are connected.

566 When a neoplasm moves "beyond" its original _____ has occurred.

Each new term is highlighted in bold print and defined. Each prefix is found in orange and each **suffix** in light blue. This consistent use of two colors for identifying word parts will help you learn by associating color with the correct word part.

An Easy "Sounds Like" Pronounciation System

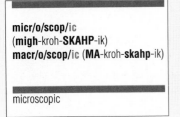

micr/o/scop/ic
(migh-kroh-**SKAHP**-ik)
macr/o/scop/ic (**MA**-kroh-**skahp**-ik)

microscopic

A simple phonetic pronunciation system has been developed to help you pronounce words using standard English letters to create sounds. The portion of the word receiving primary emphasis is printed in **CAPITAL LETTERS** with bold type. Secondary emphasis is indicated by **lowercase letters** with bold type. The whole pronunciation is provided for each new term within parentheses, for instant guidance.

Unique Illustration Program

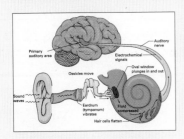

Full-color illustrations of body structures provide valuable reference for terms of normal anatomy and physiology, as well as terms in the other content subdivisions. Supporting these illustrations is a unique pictorialization of some of the actual ancient Greek and Latin word derivations of medical terms. This feature is designed to familiarize you with the romance and adventure of the medical language.

A Variety of Chapter Exercises

Terms and Their Abbreviations
In the list below, when the term is given, write its abbreviation in th corresponding term.

TERM	ABBR
1. endoplasmic reticulum	
2. _____	DPT
3. cancer	
4. _____	ICF
5. _____	DNA
6. extracellular fluid	

In addition to the extensive drilling within the frames, additional exercises are provided at the end of each chapter. These exercises tie back into the chapter objectives and include a variety of testing formats, such as **Meanings of Selected Roots, Word Dissection and Translation, Terms and Their Abbreviations, Word Spelling,** and **New Word Synthesis.** Partial **Case Studies**, with multiple choice questions, challenge you to recall terms used in actual clinical context. The answers to the exercises appear in the appendix.

CHAPTER 1 Programmed Learning: A Way to Master the Medical Language

INTRODUCTION

This book is a unique blend of conventional writing about medical terminology and what is called the **programmed approach** to learning. Please follow the directions and read carefully through this chapter. It establishes the foundations and ground rules for all subsequent work.

CHAPTER OBJECTIVES

By the end of this chapter, you should be able to:

1 Explain the fundamental issues behind programmed learning of medical terminology.

2 Recognize the main sections and elements of a typical chapter in this book.

3 Define and give examples of prefixes, roots, combining vowels, combining forms, and suffixes.

4 Carry out the process of word dissection or analysis.

5 Translate a medical term into its literal English equivalent.

6 Conduct the process of word building or synthesis.

7 Apply the rules of phonetic pronunciation to medical terms.

8 Apply the rules for forming word plurals.

Programmed Learning, Body Systems, and Medical Terminology

1 This book is a **programmed learning** text. With this technique, you are given a small piece of information. You are then asked to use the _____ by filling in a blank. One blank indicates that you write in a single word, two blanks that you write in _____ words.

information
two

2 The above entry labeled **1** is called a **learning frame.** A _____ _____ is a small piece of information, one or more blanks, and an **answer key** in the left margin.

learning frame

3 Each _____ _____ goads or prods you like a stimulus. Your response is to fill in the blanks provided. The _____ _____ located in the left margin provides you with immediate feedback about the correctness of your response.

learning frame

answer key

4 Use a piece of paper to keep the _____ _____ in the left margin covered from now on. After you fill in the blanks, pull the piece of paper down to check your answers.

answer key

5 It is best to fill in blanks using pencil, so that you can erase and correct your mistakes. Resist the temptation to peek ahead at the answer key. This is not a test. Rather, this is an interactive program in which you are free to correct your _____ and learn from them promptly.

mistakes

6 Another benefit of the programmed approach is practice and drilling. Such practice and _____ of previous information is especially valuable in terminology—the "study of terms."

drilling

7 One important aspect of the "study of terms," or _____, is pronunciation. This text has been designed to use **phonetic pronunciations.** The term phonetic derives from ancient Greek. This term can be translated into its literal, or exact, English meaning: "pertaining to the sound of the voice."

terminology

8 The technique called _____ pronunciation is based on the "sound of the voice." Specifically, this system pronounces terms by the way they sound when spoken in common English. The technique is simply to respell the term with letters making sounds that are familiar.

phonetic

9 We can use _____ ("pertaining to sound of the voice") as an example. The pronunciation is set off within parentheses as (**foh-NET**-ik).

phonetic

10 Say the term _____ (**foh-NET**-ik) out loud several times. Hear yourself saying **NET** the loudest. **NET** is the **primary** (most-stressed) accent in this word.

phonetic

primary

11 In this text, the _____ (most-stressed) accent of a term is printed in bold capital letters, as indicated by **NET.** Many terms also contain a **secondary** (less-stressed) **accent.** In phonetic, the secondary accent is **foh.**

secondary
foh

12 In this text, the _____ (less-stressed) accent of a term is indicated by bold lowercase letters, as in _____ for phonetic.

primary
secondary

13 Providing the _____ (most-stressed) and the _____ (less-stressed) accents of a term helps guide you in its pronunciation. Also helpful is the grouping of letters to indicate voice sounds. Consider, for example, **anatomy** (**a-NAT**-oh-mee) and **physiology** (**fih**-zee-**AHL**-oh-jee).

Information Frame

14 Once again, pronounce:

phonetic (**foh-NET**-ik)

anatomy (**a-NAT**-oh-mee)

physiology (**fih**-zee-**AHL**-oh-jee)

Observe the repeated use of certain mouth or voice sounds. For instance, **NAT** is pronounced like the **a** in apple, while **AH** is pronounced as in, "Open your mouth and say, **Ahhhh**!" Note that **mee** and **jee** indicate long **e** sounds, as in, "**Eeeekk**! I **see** a mouse!" In this scheme, the **OH** in **foh** makes the sound of your lips puckering into an "**O**."

Information Frame

15 Pronunciation of terms may vary, however, with the individual instructor or geographic region. When you pronounce a word, you **see** it with one part of your brain, **say** it with another part, and **hear** it with a third.

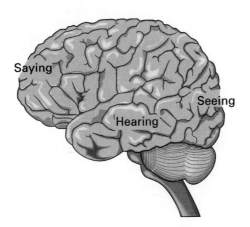

16 On this brain picture, label the areas that function when you **see** words, **say** words, and **hear** words:

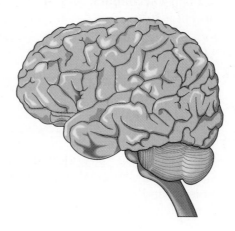

write

17 Programmed learning directs you to **write** words soon after seeing, saying, and hearing about them. As you _____ words, the movement of your hand registers a pattern in your brain.

thinking

18 All of this seeing, saying, hearing, and writing promotes **thinking** about new terms. One reason why programmed learning is so effective is that it promotes greater _____ about terms.

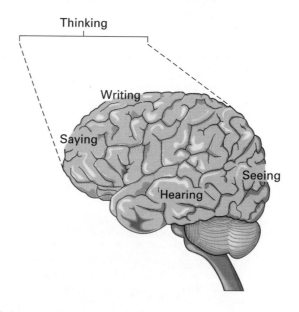

functions
structure

19 Seeing, saying, hearing, writing, and thinking are all body _____ (structures/functions). The brain itself is a body _____ (structure/function).

20 Anatomy is generally defined as "body structure" and "the study of body structures." Physiology is defined as "body function" and "the study of body functions." Therefore, the brain is an example of _____ (anatomy/physiology), while seeing, saying, hearing, thinking, and writing are all examples of _____ (anatomy/physiology).

anatomy
physiology

21 Critical elements in _____ (body structure) and _____ (body function) are the **organs.** Organs are collections of several kinds of tissues that together perform a certain specialized job. The brain, for instance, is an _____ specialized for the function of thinking.

anatomy
physiology

organ

22 The spinal cord, like the brain, is an _____. Part of its _____ (body function) is relaying information back and forth from the brain.

organ
physiology

23 There are levels of anatomy and physiology beyond the _____ level of doing a specialized job. One is called the **organ system** level. An _____ _____ is a collection of related organs that together perform a highly complex job.

organ

organ system

24 The nervous system, for instance, is an _____ _____ including the brain, spinal cord, and nerves as its organs. These organs function together to perform the complex job of communicating and controlling the body's internal environment.

organ system

25 Like the brain, nerves, and spinal cord, most other body organs belong to some particular _____ _____. The skeletal system, for another example, is made up of the bones—organs that attach to one another at their joints.

organ system

26 Most of the terms in this book are organized by chapters that cover particular organ systems. This book is therefore a **programmed** _____ ("study of terms," **frame 6**) that is **systems-based.**

terminology

27 In a typical chapter, normal body structure, or _____, and body function, or _____, of a given organ system are introduced in a separate, nonprogrammed section. Word elements related to this material are then learned within a programmed format.

anatomy
physiology

28 As you know, body structures and functions are not always normal. There are various diseases and abnormalities. Lab tests can help the physician make a **diagnosis** (**digh**-ag-**NOH**-sis) of the problem. A number of therapies can be administered. These include **pharmacology** (**far**-muh-**KAHL**-oh-jee), or treatment with drugs, as well as surgery. Each of these areas has its own set of terms.

---

medical

29 The word **medical** comes from Latin and literally "pertains to healing." Consequently, _____ **terminology** is the "study of terms that pertain to healing."

---

medical
terminology

30 The terminology of "healing" is called _____ _____. It encompasses terms describing diseases and abnormalities, lab tests and **diagnoses** (**digh**-ag-**NOH**-sees), and therapies including pharmacology and surgery.

---

anatomy
physiology
medical terminology

31 This book guides programmed learning of both the terminology of normal body structure, or _____, and of body function, or _____. It also guides the study of the terms of healing, or _____ _____. Separate subsections are provided for each within a typical chapter.

---

medical
phonetic

32 Many of the terms in medical terminology and in the terminology of normal anatomy and physiology ultimately derive from Latin, as in _____ ("pertaining to healing," **frame 29**), or from Greek, as in _____ ("pertaining to the sound of the voice," **frame 7**). The phrase provided in quotation marks after such terms is their literal, or exact, common English translation. You can see that including the identification number of a previous frame containing this meaning helps in the recognition and drilling of terms.

---

word
analysis

33 How does one go about translating medical terms? A good approach is by **dissecting** them—cutting terms into their component word parts. This dissecting process is called **word analysis.** In _____ _____ (term dissection), a new word is treated like a body structure. It is often easiest to understand the brain, a word, or any structure by dissecting it (cutting it apart).

---

dissecting

34 Figure 1.1 shows a series of jointed bones. This illustration can also be seen as a series of joined word parts. One of the best ways to study either jointed bones or joined word parts is by _____, or analyzing, them, that is, cutting them apart.

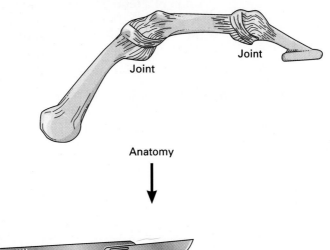

Joint

Joint

Anatomy

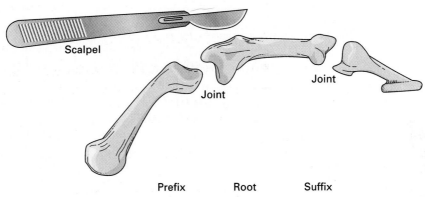

Scalpel

Joint

Joint

Prefix   Root   Suffix

Ana / tom / y

---

phonet
-ic

35 In anatomy, scalpels or knives are used to cut. In terminology, our tool for dissection is the slashmark (/). Take, for instance, the word phonet-ic. This term is analyzed as phonet/**ic**. The slashmark indicates that pho-netic is composed of the two word parts _____ and _____.

---

sound of the voice

36 Phonet is the **root** in phonetic. A **root** is the main idea or concept of a word. Recall (**frame 7**) that phonetic literally means, "pertaining to the _____ _____ _____ _____."

---

root

37 The _____ (main idea or concept) in phonetic means "sound of the voice."

Information Frame

38 What about the rest of phonet/**ic**, which means "pertaining to"? The last part of this dissected word, **-ic**, is a **suffix**. A **suffix** is a letter or letters placed at the end of a word that modify the meaning of the word.

---

root
suffix

39 Every term we will study contains at least one _____ (main idea) and a _____ (word-modifying ending).

-ic

40 The suffix in phonetic is _____. It means "pertaining to" or its equiva-lent, such as "referring to" or "relating to (something)."

-ic
phonet

41 The meaning of the suffix usually comes first in the literal English translation of a term. Phonetic, for example, literally "pertains to (refers to; relates to) the sound of the voice." The meaning of the suffix, _____, precedes the meaning of the root, _____, in the English translation.

medic/**al**
medic
-al
-ic
-al
pertaining to

42 Phonetic is not the only term whose suffix means "pertaining to." In medical the suffix is **-al**, which has the same meaning as **-ic**. Medical is properly subdivided as _____ /_____, where _____ is the root and _____ is the suffix. Two adjectival suffixes you have learned are _____ and _____. They mean "_____ _____."

pertains
to healing

43 Since **medic** means "healing," medic/al literally "_____ _____ _____." Once again, the meaning of the suffix comes first in the term's translation.

suffix

44 Let us now consider anatomy, a term with a different root and suffix. The root here is **tom**, or "cutting." The letter **-y**, being at the very end, must be the term's _____. It means the "action, process, or condition of (something)."

ana/tom/y

45 Anatomy is subdivided as _____ /_____ /_____. You undoubtedly recognize the root and suffix. But what about the word part in front? This is called a **prefix.** A **prefix** is a letter or letters that come before the root, thereby modifying the meaning of a word.

ana-

46 The prefix in anatomy is _____, which means "up" or "apart."

action of cutting
up
apart

47 Looking back through **frames 44–46,** you should be able to translate ana/tom/y as the "_____ _____ _____ (something) _____ or _____." Again, note that the meaning of the suffix comes first.

prefix

ana-
root
-y

48 Not every term contains a _____ (letter or letters before a root). For those that do, the usual sequence of occurrence is prefix-root-suffix. In the word anatomy, the prefix is _____. Tom, which means "to cut," is the _____. The suffix is _____, and it means the "action, process, or condition of."

Information Frame

49 In phonet/**ic**, medic/**al**, and ana/tom/**y**, the suffix following the root is a **vowel** or starts with a vowel. Remember that vowels are the letters **a, e, i, o, u,** and sometimes **y.** A general rule in terminology is: **A vowel is used to hook word parts together.**

vowel

50 Since **-ic,** the suffix in phonetic, begins with a _____, **i,** it can be hooked directly to the end of the root, phonet.

ostearthral (ahs-tee-AHR-thrahl)

51 A similar situation exists for combining roots. Take two roots: oste (**ahs-tee**) or "bone," and arthr (**AHR**-thr), or "joint." Each begins with a vowel, so they can be directly hooked together. Now use the suffix in medical to build a single term that means, "pertaining to bones and joints": _____.

ostearthral

52 The general procedure you used to create _____ ("pertaining to bones and joints") is called word building or word synthesis.

building
synthesis

53 Word _____ or _____ is the process of combining word parts to make a single new term.

compound word

54 Some new terms consist of two or more roots. These are called **compound words.** Because it contains two roots, ostearthral is considered a _____ _____.

oste/arthr/**al**
oste
arthr
compound

55 Ostearthral is properly dissected as _____ / _____ / _____. Its two roots (major concepts) are _____ ("bone") and _____ ("joint"). Therefore, it is a _____ word.

compound

56 It is vital to spell all medical terms (including _____ words with several roots) correctly. Smooth pronunciation of terms makes their spelling much easier.

combining

57 Pronunciation is often helped by a **combining vowel.** A _____ vowel is a vowel (usually an **o**) placed between word parts to make their pronunciation easier.

combining vowel

0

58 If we add a _____ _____ to oste, we obtain **oste/o.** The most common combining vowel used to connect word roots is _____.

form

59 Oste/o is technically called a **combining form.** A combining _____ is the addition of a word root plus a combining vowel.

combining form
oste

0

60 Oste/o is considered a _____ _____ because it consists of the root, _____, plus the combining vowel, _____.

arthr/o
arthr

0

61 The phrase "combining form" derives from the fact that oste/o, in its present "form," often helps in the "combining" of oste with other word parts. Create a combining form for arthr: _____ /_____. In the combining form **arthr/o,** _____ is the root and _____ is the combining vowel. A combining vowel is used between word parts to make pronunciation easier when consonants are being connected.

Information Frame	**62** Combining forms such as oste/o and arthr/o are used for two reasons: (1) to combine a root with a suffix or another root that begins with a **consonant** (some letter other than **a, e, i, o, u,** or **y**). (2) to make the pronunciation of the resulting term easier.
oste/o/arthr/al (**ahs**-tee-oh-**AHR**-thrahl)	**63** Let us consider practical application of the reasons cited in **frame 62**. Using the combining form oste/o, build a single term that means "referring to bones and joints": _____ /_____ /_____ /_____.
2	**64** Pronounce ostearthral and osteoarthral out loud to yourself. Which version seems smoother and easier to say? Refer to **frame 62.** The best reason for using osteoarthral is listed as reason _____ (1/2).
speed/o/meter	**65** Let's create a compound word applying the combining vowel principle. Combine the root **speed** and the word **meter** ("an instrument used to measure"). The result is _____ /_____ /_____, with the word meter now a suffix.
speed/o/meter (spee-**DAH**-meh-ter) 1	**66** A _____ /_____ /_____, not a speedmeter, is literally "an instrument used to measure speed." Again, refer to **frame 62**. Speedometer is used for reason number _____ (1/2). Note that when speed and meter are united with a combining vowel, there is a change in pronunciation.
oste/o/meter (**ahs**-tee-**AH**-meh-ter) **arthr/o/meter** (ahr-**THRAH**-meh-ter)	**67** By similar thinking, build two terms with the following meanings: "an instrument used to measure bones" _____ /_____ /_____ "an instrument used to measure joints" _____ /_____ /_____
-o/logy	**68** Often, a combining vowel will be used in front of a suffix starting with a consonant, and it is used consistently. A good example is **-logy**. This noun suffix means "the study of (something)." Since it begins with **l**, a consonant, the suffix is usually seen with **o** in front of it as in _____ /_____.
termin/o/logy **physi/o/logy**	**69** Several terms cited earlier are built with this combining vowel and suffix. They are _____ /_____ /_____ ("the study of terms," **frame 6**) and _____ /_____ /_____ ("the study of body functions," **frame 20**).
oste/o/logy (**ahs**-tee-**AH**-loh-jee) **arthr/o/logy** (ahr-**TRAHL**-oh-jee)	**70** Similarly, we can synthesize _____ /_____ /_____ ("study of the bones") and _____ /_____ /_____ ("study of the joints"). Pronounce osteology and arthrology several times. Note the accent change when the combining forms oste/o and arthr/o are combined with **logy**. Pronounce the words several times using the pronunciation guide.

Information Frame

71 To summarize word building, we can again make an analogy with jointed bones (Figure 1.2). Certain word parts fit together smoothly and snugly, like jointed bones directly inserted into one another. Here, no combining vowel is required to soften their contact. Other word parts require the placement of combining vowels between them, as do bones with soft **cartilage** (**KAR**-tih-lehj), or "gristle," cushioning their tips.

FIGURE 1.2

"Smooth" versus "Rough" Fitting of Bones and Word Parts

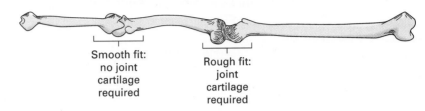

Smooth fit: no joint cartilage required

Rough fit: joint cartilage required

Speed + –meter

Speed / o / meter
"Rough" fit of word parts, a combining vowel required

Oste + –on

Oste / on
"Smooth" fit of word parts, no combining vowel required

Information Frame

72 The end of each chapter in this text contains exercises on the three main processes of terminology: **word building, word dissection,** and **word translation.**

Information Frame

73 Also of great importance are the rules of word pronunciation and the formation of word plurals. Table 1.1 provides some helpful rules for pronunciation.

TABLE 1.1

Some General Rules for Pronunciation

"p" rule	A **p** beginning a word is silent if it is followed by a consonant. Ex: **Pneumonia** is pronounced as **noo-MOHN**-yuh.
"g" rule	A **g** followed by an **i, e,** or **y** is pronounced with a soft "j" sound, while **g** followed by an **a, o, u,** or **consonant** is pronounced with a hard "g" sound. Ex: A soft "j" in **giant,** a hard "g" in **gate.**
"c" rule	A **c** followed by an **i, e,** or **y** is pronounced with a soft "s" sound, while a **c** followed by an **a, o, u,** or **consonant** is usually pronounced with a hard "k" sound. Ex: A soft "s" in **city,** but a hard "k" in **cast.**

k
s
silent
hard g
soft j

74 In applying the pronunciation rules, consider some specific choices:

for **thoracostomy,** the **c** sounds like _____ (s/k)

for **appendicitis,** the **c** sounds like _____ (s/k)

for **pneumothorax,** the **p** is _____ (silent/pronounced)

for **gonads,** the **g** sounds like _____ (soft j/hard g)

for **laryngitis,** the **g** sounds like _____ (soft j/hard g)

Information Frame

75 Another valuable feature are rules for forming word plurals. A list of these is shown in Table 1.2.

TABLE 1.2

Some General Rules for Forming Word Plurals

Terms with Singular Ending in	Have Plural Using	Example
-a	-ae or -as	vertebra: vertebrae or vertebras
-ax	-aces	thorax: thoraces
-ex	-ices	apex: apices
-is	-es	psychosis: psychoses
-ix	-ices	appendix: appendices
-ma	-mata or -mas	sarcoma: sarcomata or sarcomas
-on	-a	mitochondrion: mitochondria
-um	-a	bacterium: bacteria
-us	-i	coccus: cocci

cardia
carcinomata
carcinomas
ganglia
bronchi

76 In applying the rules for forming plurals, make a few specific choices:

for plural of **cardium,** use _____

for plural of **carcinoma,** use _____ or

_____

for plural of **ganglion,** use _____

for plural of **bronchus,** use _____

Information Frame

77 Answers to the end-of-chapter exercises are shown in the **Appendix.**

---

78 You have been introduced to the principles of programmed learning as they apply to medical terminology. If you still don't understand something, go back and review the appropriate frames. Now, it's on to the main chapters! Good luck!

Word Dissection and Translation

Analyze the following terms by dissecting them with slashmarks and identifying their word parts. To the right of each term, write its correct English translation.

Key: R (root), cv (combining vowel), P (prefix), S (suffix)

1. anatomy

_____/_____/_____   _____
  P   R   S

2. physiology

_____/____/_____   _____
      R   cv   S

3. terminology

_____/____/_____   _____
      R   cv   S

4. osteometer

_____/____/_____   _____
      R   cv   S

5. pharmacology

_____/____/_____   _____
      R   cv   S

Fill in the Blanks

1. tom is a word _____.

2. -y is a noun _____.

3. -ic and -al are adjectival _____.

4. physi/o is a combining _____.

5. oste/arthr/al is a _____ word.

6. ana- is a _____.

7. The o in oste/o is a combining _____.

8. -o/logy is a _____.

9. medic is a _____.

10. -meter is a _____.

Singular or Plural

In the list below, identify whether the term is singular or plural. Then reverse the form and rewrite accordingly.

1. vertebrae   (S/P) _____
2. thorax   (S/P) _____
3. psychoses   (S/P) _____
4. sarcomata   (S/P) _____
5. mitochondrion   (S/P) _____
6. apices   (S/P) _____
7. appendix   (S/P) _____
8. cardium   (S/P) _____
9. cocci   (S/P) _____
10. bronchus   (S/P) _____

CHAPTER 2 Words, Word Parts, and Diseases in General

INTRODUCTION

As indicated in Chapter 1, **medical terminology** is a language, mainly Latin and Greek in origin. This language covers four broad subject areas:

1. Normal anatomy and physiology.

Anatomy deals with body structures and the study of body structures. Physiology involves body functions and the study of these body functions. The heart, for instance, is a spade-shaped organ within the chest (anatomy) that stores and pumps the blood (physiology).

2. Diseases and abnormalities.

Body structures and functions are not always normal. During development within the **uterus** (**YOO**-ter-us), or womb, structures may fail to form properly. When normal structures are formed, through the years they may become diseased or injured. For example, the **septum** (**SEP**-tum), or "wall," normally present between the two sides of the heart may fail to develop. Heart disease, the number one killer in the United States today, involves the filling up and blocking of previously normal arteries with thick deposits of fatty material.

3. Lab tests and diagnoses.

How does one know whether particular body structures and functions are normal or diseased? Use of lab tests to measure aspects of body structure and function is critical. These and other **diagnostic** (**digh**-ag-**NAHS**-tik) procedures allow the physician and nurse to make an accurate assessment of the current status of a patient's health.

4. Surgery, pharmacology, and other therapies.

Once a disease or abnormality has been diagnosed, what is to be done about it? Treatment occurs by various therapies, including pharmacology, the use of drugs. The most drastic treatment of all is surgery.

Summary

In conclusion, the world of medical terminology is a collection of Latin and Greek words and word parts. Recall from Chapter 1 that these word parts are roots, suffixes, combining vowels, combining forms, and prefixes. Some of this collection of word parts is general in nature. The rest is used to describe normal anatomy and physiology, diseases and abnormalities, lab tests and diagnoses, and surgery, pharmacology, and other therapies. The total content of this discipline can be represented by color bars.

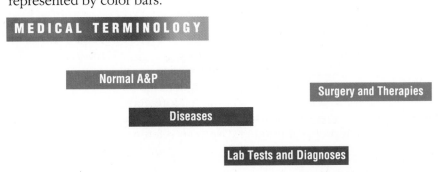

MEDICAL TERMINOLOGY

Normal A&P

Diseases

Surgery and Therapies

Lab Tests and Diagnoses

Abbreviations are also important in terminology. For instance, A & P is an accepted abbreviation for anatomy and physiology.

Chapter 2 will present you with programmed information on general word parts that can be widely applied to all four subject areas in the text. Words and word parts describing disease in general will also be discussed.

C H A P T E R   O B J E C T I V E S

By the end of this chapter, you should be able to:

1 Identify some prefixes, roots, and suffixes that can be generally applied to all areas of medical terminology.

2 Build new medical terms associated with disease in general.

3 Explain the meaning of some prefixes, roots, and suffixes associated with disease conditions in general.

4 Translate disease-related terms into their common English equivalents.

Normal A & P

General Word Parts for Medical Terminology

The following is a list of common prefixes generally used in medical terminology. Use this list to help you complete **frames 79 to 85.**

a-	no; not; without	hemi-	partial; half	pre-	before
an-	without; not	mal-	bad	primi-	first
anti-	against	mono-	single; one	pro-	before; in front of
auto-	self; own	multi-	many	quadri-	four
bi-	two	neo-	new	semi-	partial; half
con-	together; with	normo-	normal	sym-	together; with
contra-	opposite; against	pan-	all	syn-	together; with
demi-	partial; half	poly-	many	tri-	three
di-	two; double	post-	after; behind	uni-	one
eu-	good; normal				

---

prefixes

79 Letters preceding the root in a word are called _____ **(frame 45)**. Some of these word elements tend to be used for almost all the organ systems.

---

uni- (**YOO**-nee)
mono- (**MAH**-noh)
bi- (**BIGH**)
di- (**DIGH**)
tri- (**TRIGH**)
quadri- (**KWAHD**-rih)
multi- (**MUHL**-tee)
poly- (**PAHL**-ee)

80 Note from the preceding list that there are several prefixes indicating **number of things.** For instance, _____ means "one," and _____ indicates "single" or "one." "Two" is represented by either _____ or _____. "Three" is denoted as _____, and "four" is represented as _____. More generally, _____ and _____ mean "many." Now try to name a common term that uses each prefix of number. Use your reference dictionary if necessary.

---

semi- (**SEHM**-ee)
demi- (**DEHM**-ee)
hemi- (**HEHM**-ee)
pan- (**PAN**)
half

81 A second broad group are prefixes of **proportion.** Either _____ or _____ or _____ mean "partial or half." At the most extreme, _____ connotes "all." In the word semi/conscious, the prefix semi- means "_____." Semi- is a qualitative half. Hemi- is a measurable half.

primi- (**PRIGH**-mih)
neo- (**NEE**-oh)
pre- (**PREE**)
pro- (**PROH**)
post- (**POHST**)

82 A third general group of prefixes are those of **time sequence.** For instance, _____ is "first," and _____ is "new." Two prefixes, _____ and _____, indicate "before." The prefix _____, means "after."

con- (**KAHN**)
sym- (**SIHM**)
syn- (**SIHN**)
a-
an-
anti- (**AN**-tee)
contra- (**KAHN**-truh)

83 A fourth prefix group covers **inclusion or exclusion.** Three prefixes (_____, _____, _____) are those of inclusion, indicating "together" or "with." Prefixes of exclusion are _____ and _____ denoting "without." Extreme exclusion, being "against" (_____) or "opposite" (_____) is given by two prefixes.

mal- (**MAL**)
eu- (**YOO**)
normo- (**NOR**-moh)

84 A fifth group are the prefixes of **state of well-being.** While at least one prefix (_____) implies being "bad," two prefixes, _____ and _____, imply being "good" or "normal."

auto- (**AW**-toh)

85 Finally, prefixes of possession include _____, which labels something as "self" or "own."

The following is a list of common word roots with combining vowels generally used in medical terminology. Use this list to help you complete **frames 86 to 89.**

albin/o	white	**erythr/o**	red	**purpur/o**	purple
aut/o	self; own	**heter/o**	difference	**rube/o**	red
chlor/o	green	**home/o**	sameness; constancy	**scler/o**	hard
chrom/o	color			**tom/o**	cut
cirrh/o	yellow	**leuk/o**	white	**troph/o**	nourishment
cyan/o	blue	**melan/o**	black	**xanth/o**	yellow

root

86 Remember (**frame 36**) that each word contains a _____ (main idea or concept).

chrom/o (CROH-moh)
albin/o (AL-bigh-noh)
leuk/o (LOO-koh)
melan/o (MEL-uh-noh)
chlor/o (KLOR-oh)
purpur/o (PUR-pur-oh)
cirrh/o (SIR-oh)
xanth/o (ZAN-thoh)
cyan/o (SIGH-an-oh)
erythr/o (eh-RITH-roh)
rube/o (ROO-bee-oh)

87 Examine the preceding list and observe the combining form for "color": _____ /____. Two color-related combining forms stand for "white": _____ /____ and _____ /____. Their opposite, _____ /____, is the concept of "black." Fill in the blanks indicating the remaining colors:

_____ /____	"green"
_____ /____	"purple"
_____ /____	"yellow"
_____ /____	"yellow"
_____ /____	"blue"
_____ /____	"red"
_____ /____	"red"

auto- (AW-toh)
home/o- (HOH-mee-oh)
heter/o- (HET-er-oh)

88 There are a number of word parts suggesting self or sameness. For instance, _____ indicates "self or own." "Sameness or constancy" is indicated by _____ /____. And the opposite, _____ /____, states a "difference."

scler/o (SKLEH-roh)
tom/o (TOH-moh)
troph/o (TROH-foh)

89 Some miscellaneous roots/combining vowels (cv) are _____ /____ for "hard," _____ /____ for "cut," and _____ /____ for "nourishment."

The following is a list of common suffixes generally used in medical terminology. Use this list to help you complete **frames 90 to 103.**

-a	presence of	-ic	pertaining to	-osis	condition of
-ac	pertaining to	-ical	pertaining to	-ous	pertaining to
-ad	pertaining to	-ion	process of	-stasis	controlling; stopping
-al	pertaining to	-is	presence of	-tic	pertaining to
-ar	pertaining to	-ity	condition of	-tion	process of
-ary	pertaining to	-oid	resembling	-um	presence of
-ate	something that	-ology	study of	-us	presence of
-e	presence of	-opsy	view of	-y	action; process; condition of
-esis	condition of	-or	one that; one who		

suffix

90 Chapter 1 **(frame 38)** explained that a _____ is a letter or group of letters located at the end of a word.

9
-ac (AK)
-ad (AD)
-al (AL)
-ar (AHR)
-ary (AIR-ee)
-ic (IK)
-ical (IK-al)
-ous (US)
-tic (TIK)

91 The foregoing list has a total of ____ (give the number) "pertaining to" suffixes. In alphabetical order, the five that start with **a** are: _____, _____, _____, _____, and _____. The two that begin with **i** are _____ and _____. Finally, _____ starts with **o**, and _____ begins with **t**. These suffixes can equivalently be defined as "referring to" or "relating to," thereby avoiding repetition.

adjectives

-ate (AYT)

92 "Pertaining to" suffixes are used as _____
(nouns/adjectives); that is, they modify the meaning of a person, place,
or thing. The words they help create, such as **anatomical** (**an**-uh-
TAHM-ih-kuhl), cannot stand alone. Closely related to "pertaining to" is
the suffix _____, which usually indicates "something that."

-oid (OYD)

93 Another suffix used as an adjective is the one appearing in **thyroid**
(**THIGH**-royd). This term literally means "resembling a shield (thyr)."
The suffix for "resembling" must therefore be _____.

thyr/oid

94 Forming the front of the voicebox is the _____ / _____ ("shield-
resembling") cartilage.

thyroid cartilage

95 **Galen** (**GAY**-len), an early Roman physician, coined the phrase
_____ _____, or "shieldlike gristle." He
noted that this structure "resembled" a large oblong "shield" used by
early Greek soldiers. (See Figure 2.1.)

FIGURE 2.1   **The Thyroid "Shield-Resembler"**

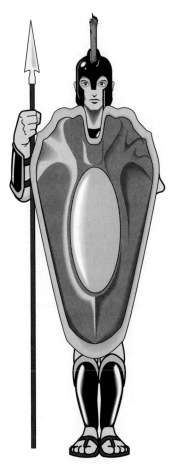

Greek soldier
with shield

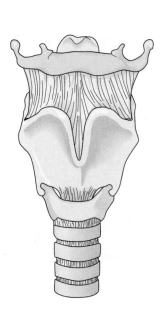

The thyroid
cartilage "shield"

96 Ancient Greek fighters sometimes dislodged wooden doors and used them as shields. The doors were eventually modified into oblong shields with a deep notch at the top for placement of the chin. The shields covered the front of the warriors from their necks down to their legs.

5
-a
-e
-is
-um
-us
nouns

97 Other suffixes, unlike **-oid**, are used to create nouns. (Remember that a noun is a person, place, or thing.) For instance, the list beginning this section has _____ (give the number) "presence of" suffixes. Cited alphabetically, these are _____, _____, _____, _____, and _____. All these suffixes help create _____ (persons, places, or things).

-ion (IGH-on)
-tion (SHUN)
-esis (EE-sis)
-ity (IH-tee)
-o/sis (OH-sis)
-y

98 Closely related to these are the "process of" suffixes, _____ and _____, and the "condition of" suffixes, _____, _____, and _____ /_____. A hybrid member of both suffix groups is the single letter _____ ("action; process; or condition of," as found in anatomy, **frame 44**).

-o/logy
-opsy (AHP-see)
-or
-stasis (STAY-sis)

99 A final group are the **miscellaneous suffixes**. These include _____ /_____ ("study of," **frame 68**), _____ ("view of"), _____ ("one that; one who"), and _____ ("controlling; stopping").

-stasis

100 Pronounce this word: hemostasis (**hee**-moh-**STAY**-sis). Looking back at the previous frame, note that this term ends with the miscellaneous suffix _____, which means "controlling or stopping."

hem/o/stasis
hem (**HEEM**)
combining vowel
combining form

101 The term is subdivided as _____ /_____ /_____. In this case, _____ is the root, while **o** is the _____ _____ (**frame 57**). Together, **hem/o** is the _____ _____.

controlling (stopping) bleeding

102 **Hem** means "blood" or "bleeding." Therefore, **hemostasis** literally means, "_____ _____."

hemostasis

103 The process of _____ ("controlling bleeding") is essential to survival after certain diseases or injuries produce significant blood loss.

104 Individual prefixes, roots, and suffixes, as well as entire words that contain them, will now be considered for diseases in general.

Chapter 2 Words, Word Parts, and Diseases in General

Word Parts Associated with Diseases in General

The following is a list of word parts generally used in connection with diseases. Use this list to help you complete **frames 105 to 160.**

alges/i	sensitivity to pain	-ia	abnormal condition of	**mortal/i**	death
-algia	pain			**necr/o**	death
asthen/i	weakness of	-iasis	abnormal condition of	-o/rrhagia	a bursting forth of
brady-	slow			-o/rrhexis	rupture of
chondr/o	cartilage	-ism	abnormal condition of	**path/o**	disease
chron/o	time			-penia	deficiency of
drom/o	running	-itis	inflammation of	-porosis	condition of pores or holes
-dynia	pain of	**leps/o**	seizure		
dys-	bad; difficult; painful	**lept/o**	seizure	-ptosis	drooping; sagging
		lesion	wound; injury	**pyr/o**	fever; fire
esthes/i	feeling; sensation	**leth/o**	death	**scler/o**	hard
hyper-	above; above normal	**malac/o**	destructive softening	tachy-	fast
				traum/o	wound; injury
hypo-	below; below normal	**megal/o**	large	**traumat/o**	wound; injury
		morbid/o	illness	**troph/o**	nourishment

---

organ

105 Various disease conditions can affect any of the _____ **(frame 23)** systems. Many of the words in this section will appear again.

---

lesion (**LEE**-zhun)
morbid/o (**MOR**-bid-oh)
path/o (**PATH**-oh)
traum/o (**TRAW**-moh) or
traumat/o (**TRAW**-mah-toh)

106 In the preceding list, there is one root and four combining forms meaning "disease," "illness," or "wound or injury." The root is _____. The combining forms are _____ /____, _____ /____, _____ /____, and _____ /____.

---

morbid/ity (mor-**BID**-ih-tee)

107 Lesion itself is also a word. Morbid can be used alone as an entire adjective. Alternatively, **-ity** can be added to create _____ /_____, "a condition of illness."

---

lesion
morbidity

108 If a person suffers some _____ ("wound or injury"), it may well result in _____ ("condition of illness").

---

traum/a
traumat/ic

109 Like lesion, **traum** and **traumat** indicate wounding or injury. Take the terms trauma (**TRAW**-mah) and traumatic (traw-**MAT**-ik). Insert slash-marks (/) into these terms, thereby subdividing them into their component word parts: _____ /____ and _____ /____.

---

trauma
traumatic

110 By looking at the suffix added to traum or traumat, you can see that _____ indicates "presence of injury," while _____ "pertains to an injury."

-pathy	**111** There is a suffix in the list, _____, that includes path within it as a root.
-pathy	**112** The suffix _____ indicates "disease of (something)." It will appear again in later chapters, preceded by an appropriate root for the system suffering the disease.
-ia (**EE**-ah) -iasis (**IGH**-uh-sis) -ism (**IZ**-m)	**113** Three suffixes mean "abnormal condition" or "unhealthy state": _____, _____, and _____.
hypo/chondr/ia hypo/chondr/iasis	**114** Suffixes indicating an abnormal condition can be integrated with various roots and prefixes. The prefix hypo- (**HIGH**-poh), for instance, means "below, below normal, or deficient." The combining form (cf) chondr/o (**KAHN**-droh), denotes "cartilage." Use this information to help you dissect **hypochondria** (high-poh-**KAHN**-dree-ah) as _____ /_____ /_____ and **hypochondriasis** (**high**-poh-kahn-**DRIGH**-uh-sis) as _____ /_____ /_____.
hypochondria hypochondriasis	**115** Both _____ and _____ can be translated as, "an abnormal condition below the cartilage (of the ribs)."
Information Frame	**116** **Hippocrates** (hih-**PAH**-krah-**teez**), the Father of Modern Medicine, was an ancient Greek physician who named many abnormal body conditions. The terms hypochondria and hypochondriasis ultimately derive from his observation that certain people (called **hypochondriacs**) tend to suffer from imaginary pains in the region below the cartilage of the ribs.
morbidity -esthes/ia (es-**THEE**-zee-uh)	**117** Whether a person truly has _____ ("condition of illness") or not, he or she may feel something abnormal or bad. A combining form for "feeling or sensation" is **esthes/i** (es-**THEE**-zee). Adding the ending in hypochondria yields _____ /_____ , a large suffix.
-esthesia	**118** The large suffix _____ translates as "an abnormal condition of feeling or sensation."
hypo/esthesia (**high**-poh-es-**THEE**-zee-uh)	**119** Adding the prefix in hypochondria yields _____ /_____.
hypoesthesia	**120** Just as -esthesia denotes "an abnormal condition of sensation," _____ denotes "an abnormal condition of deficient sensation."

hyper/esthesia
(**high**-per-es-**THEE**-zee-uh)

121 The exact opposite of hypo- is hyper-, which indicates something "above normal or excessive." Knowing this fact should allow you to build _____ /_____, "an abnormal condition of excessive sensation."

hypoesthesia
hyperesthesia

122 Either _____, too little sensitivity, or _____, too much sensitivity, is a disease state.

Information Frame

123 A clinical **symptom** is something a patient feels or notices. A clinical **sign** is something that a health professional measures or notices about a patient.

syn/drom/e (**SIHN**-drohm)

124 Some signs and symptoms "run (**drom**) with" a disease, occurring at the same time. The large suffix -**drom/e** (**DROHM**) means "a running," and syn- (**frame 83**) is a prefix for "with." Build a single term that means "a running with": _____ /_____ /_____.

pro/drom/e (**PROH**-drohm)

125 The prefix pro- (**frame 82**) means "before." Consequently, _____ /_____ /_____ translates as "a running before."

prodrome

syndrome

126 A _____ (prodrome/syndrome) is a collection of signs and symptoms that comes before an actual disease, as sniffles before a cold. Conversely, a _____ (prodrome/syndrome) is a collection of signs and symptoms that "run with," or occur together with, an illness. An example is a fever during a head cold.

Information Frame

127 Syndromes or prodromes are often associated with pain. Two suffixes on the list, -**algia** (**AL**-juh) and -**dynia** (**DIGHN**-ee-uh), represent "pain." A closely related root, **alges** (al-**JEEZ**), denotes a "sensitivity to pain."

-**algesia** (al-**JEE**-zee-uh)

128 Just as -esthesia was built from *esthes* (**frame 117**), we can build _____ from alges.

-esthesia
-algesia

129 Be sure to distinguish _____ ("an abnormal condition of sensation") from _____ ("an abnormal condition of sensitivity to pain"). It is important to realize that pain is just one of many different bodily sensations.

hypo/algesia
hyper/algesia

130 Two terms involving pain sensitivity are **hypoalgesia** (**high**-poh-al-**JEE**-zee-uh) and **hyperalgesia** (**high**-per-al-**JEE**-zee-uh). The first term is dissected as _____ /_____, the second as _____ /_____.

hypoalgesia
hyperalgesia

131 Following a pattern like that for words containing -esthesia, _____ is "an abnormal condition of deficient sensitivity to pain," while _____ is "an abnormal condition of excessive sensitivity to pain."

hypoalgesia hyperalgesia	**132** A person suffering from _____ might not withdraw in time from a serious, tissue-damaging situation. The below-normal sensitivity to pain would probably not serve as an effective warning signal. A person afflicted with _____, on the other hand, might be driven to madness by overreacting to even the slightest hint of pain. The prefix dys- **(DIHS)**, in general, indicates something "bad, difficult, or painful," towards which a person might overreact.
-e acut/e -ic chron/ic	**133** Pain can be described as either **acute** (ah-**KYOOT**) or **chronic** (**KRAH**-nik) in nature. Acute contains the suffix _____ ("presence of," **frame 97**). Therefore, acute is analyzed as _____ /_____. Chronic includes the suffix _____, the same one found in traumatic (**frame 109**). Consequently, chronic is analyzed as _____ /_____ .
acut (ah-**KYOOT**) **chron** (**KRAHN**)	**134** The root in acute is _____. It means "sudden." The root in chronic is _____, meaning "time."
acute chronic	**135** A person suffering a "sudden" heart attack would be in _____ pain. A person suffering from prolonged cancer would probably be experiencing _____ pain, lasting for a long "time."
Information Frame	**136** The word parts dealing with sensations and pain are shown in the summary diagram in Figure 2.2.

FIGURE 2.2   **Summary Diagram of Sensations and Pain**

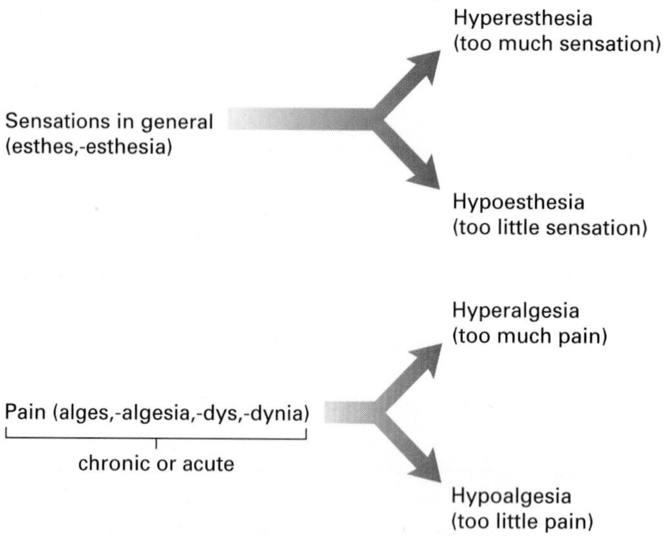

Sensations in general
(esthes,-esthesia)
→ Hyperesthesia
(too much sensation)
→ Hypoesthesia
(too little sensation)

Pain (alges,-algesia,-dys,-dynia)
chronic or acute
→ Hyperalgesia
(too much pain)
→ Hypoalgesia
(too little pain)

Information Frame	**137** Pain, whether chronic or acute, can be due to a variety of causes. One is **edema** (eh-**DEE**-mah), or "a swelling" that pushes on a nerve. Another is some type of -**megaly** (**MEHG**-ah-lee), or "condition of enlargement."

edema **-megaly** **megal** (MEHG-al)	**138** An _____ ("swelling") can result in a painful enlargement of the affected body area. The large suffix _____ ("condition of enlargement") contains a root, _____, plus a smaller suffix, **-y**.
hyper/troph/y troph	**139** The term **hypertrophy** (high-**PER**-truh-**fee**) means "a process of excessive nourishment." This term is subdivided as _____ / _____ / ____, where the prefix is that in hyperesthesia, and the suffix, **-y**, is the same ending as in **-megaly**. The root, _____ **(frame 89)**, denotes "nourishment."
hypertrophy	**140** The excessive nourishment or stimulation of _____ can lead to tissue overdevelopment and an unusually large size. In muscle weight training in males, such enlargement is normal.
a/troph/y a-	**141** The exact opposite of hypertrophy is **atrophy** (**AHT**-roh-fee). This term is dissected as ____ / _____ / ____. It has the same root and suffix as hypertrophy. Only its prefix, ____ (meaning "without") differs.
without atrophy	**142** You may remember **(frame 83)** that a- means "no, not, or _____." Therefore, _____ translates as "a condition without nourishment." This is a process of tissue shrinkage and wasting due to lack of adequate stimulation or nourishment.
-penia	**143** Two suffixes related to atrophy are **-asthenia** (**as-THEE**-nee-uh) and **-penia** (**PEE-nee**-uh). One of these suffixes derives from the Greek term penia, meaning "poverty." The suffix _____, then, implies a "deficiency of" something, as poverty implies a deficiency of money.
-asthenia	**144** The other suffix in **frame 143**, _____, indicates a "weakness of" body parts affected by atrophy.
condition of seizure	**145** Whether weakened or not, a person's limbs may be affected by seizures (violent contractions). Both **leps** (LEPS) and **lept** are roots for "seizure." Just as **-megaly (frame 138)** is a "condition of enlargement," **-lepsy** (**LEP**-see) is a "_____ ____ _____."
leps -y	**146** The root within **-lepsy** is _____, with ____ as the smaller suffix.
Information Frame	**147** Other suffixes for general disease-associated conditions are: **-porosis** (**por-OH**-sis) abnormal condition of pores or holes **-ptosis** (**TOH**-sis) abnormal condition of drooping or sagging **-sclerosis** (**skleh-ROH**-sis) abnormal condition of hardening **-malacia** (mah-**LAY**-shuh) abnormal condition of destructive softening **-o/rrhagia** (or-**AY-juh**) a bursting forth **-o/rrhexis** (or-**EKS**-is) a rupture

148 See if you can apply the facts provided in the previous frame:

-porosis

People suffering from **osteoporosis** (**ahs**-tee-oh-por-**OH**-sis) have abnormally large "holes" in their "bones." The suffix in osteoporosis is _____.

-malacia

A pregnant woman with an inadequate diet may acquire **osteomalacia** (**ahs**-tee-oh-mah-**LAY**-shuh), a destructive "softening" of the "bones." The suffix in osteomalacia is _____.

-sclerosis

Too much fat in the diet may contribute to **arteriosclerosis** (ahr-**tee**-rih-oh-skleh-**ROH**-sis), a "hardening" of the "arteries." The suffix in arteriosclerosis is _____.

-ptosis

Nerve damage to the face may result in **blepharoptosis** (**blef**-ah-roh-**TOH**-sis), a "drooping" of the "eyelid." The suffix in blepharoptosis is _____.

-o/rrhagia

Metrorrhagia (**met**-ror-**AY**-juh) is a "bursting forth" of fluid from the "uterus." The suffix in metrorrhagia is _____ /_____.

-o/rrhexis

Cardiorrhexis (**kar**-dee-or-**EKS**-is) is a "rupture" of the "heart" wall. The suffix in cardiorrhexis is _____ /_____.

Information Frame

149 When body processes occur too "slowly," indicated by the prefix brady- (**BRAHD**-ih), or when they happen too "fast," denoted by the prefix tachy- (**TAK**-ih), disease may also be present.

---

tachycardia
bradycardia

brady/card/ia
tachy/card/ia
suffix

150 Consider two terms, **bradycardia** (brahd-ih-**KAR**-dee-uh) and **tachycardia** (tak-ih-**KAR**-dee-uh). Of these, _____ must indicate an excessively fast heartbeat, _____ an excessively slow heartbeat. Bradycardia may be dissected as _____ /_____ /_____. Tachycardia may be dissected as _____ /_____ /_____. Brady- and tachy- are prefixes, while -ia is a _____.

Information Frame

151 A common disease condition is "inflammation of" a body part, indicated by the suffix -itis (**IGH**-tis).

---

card/itis
-itis

152 For example, carditis (**kar**-**DIGH**-tis) is an "inflammation of the heart." This term is subdivided as _____ /_____. Its suffix is _____.

Information Frame

153 A typical sign of widespread inflammation is "fever," denoted by **pyr/o** (**PIGH**-roh) and **pyret** (**PIGH**-ret).

---

pyret/ic (**pigh-RET**-ik)

154 Using the root ending in **t**, we have _____ /_____, "pertaining to fever," if the suffix in chronic (**frame 133**) is adopted.

---

pyretic

155 A _____ ("feverish") state may be bad enough to cause death.

Chapter 2 Words, Word Parts, and Diseases in General

156 Three combining forms on the list mean "death": These are:
leth/o (**LEETH**-oh)
mortal/i (**MOR**-tal-ee)
necr/o (**NEK**-roh)

---

mortal/ity (mor-TAL-ih-tee)

157 Following the same pattern as morbidity **(frame 107)**, build
_____ /_____, a "condition of death."

---

mortality

158 Morbidity, if left unchecked, may result in _____
("condition of death").

---

necr/o/tic
leth/al

159 Dissecting **necrotic** (**neh-KRAH**-tik) results in _____ /_____ /_____.
Analyzing **lethal** (**LEETH**-uhl) yields _____ /_____. Both of these
terms "pertain to death."

---

necrotic
lethal

160 Necrotic is generally employed to describe dead cells or tissues. Lethal
is often applied to the deadly consequences of particular drugs or
actions. For instance, we can say that the heart muscle was
_____ after its circulation was shut down by injection of
a _____ drug.

---

161 If various disease states are detected soon enough, severe morbidity or
mortality may be prevented. Lab tests and diagnoses play this role. They
have a terminology of their own.

Multiple Choice

1. The prefix meaning new is
   a. normo-   b. neo-   c. primi-   d. auto-

2. The word root for yellow is
   a. chlor/o   b. chrom   c. xanth   d. leuk

3. The prefix for "self" is
   a. uni-   b. mono-   c. di-   d. auto-

4. Which of these prefixes does not belong?
   a. semi-   b. quadri-   c. hemi-   d. demi-

5. Another prefix like normo- is
   a. eu-   b. primi-   c. syn-   d. mal-

6. Troph/o means
   a. difference   b. nourishment   c. constancy   d. hard

Meanings of Selected Roots

Add the correct combining vowel (cv) after each root. Then write the definition of each root in the space provided.

ROOT/CV	DEFINITION
1. chron/_____	_____
2. path/_____	_____
3. alges/_____	_____
4. albin/_____	_____
5. troph/_____	_____
6. pyret/_____	_____
7. traum/_____	_____
8. chondr/_____	_____
9. necr/_____	_____
10. xanth/_____	_____

Word Dissection and Translation

Analyze the following terms by dissecting them with slashmarks and identifying their word parts. To the right of each term, write its correct English translation.

Key: R (root), cv (combining vowel), P (prefix), S (suffix)

1. hyperalgesia

_____/_____
   P   S

_____

2. morbidity

_____/_____
   R   S

_____

3. syndrome

_____/_____/_____
   P   R   S

_____

4. traumatic

_____/_____
   R   S

_____

5. hypoalgesia

_____/_____
   P   S

_____

6. chronic

_____/_____
   R   S

_____

7. osteomalacia

_____/_____/_____
   R   cv   S

_____

8. lethal

_____/_____
   R   S

_____

9. necrotic

_____/_____/_____
   R   cv   S

_____

10. osteoporosis

_____/_____/_____
   R   cv   S

_____

11. hypertrophy

_____/_____/_____
   P   R   S

_____

12. pyretic

_____/_____
   R   S

_____

Word Spelling

Look at each of the terms listed below. Identify those that are misspelled by circling Y for "Yes." Write the correct spelling in the blank.

WORD	MISSPELLED?	CORRECT SPELLING
1. hyperalgesia	Y/N	_____
2. tackycardia	Y/N	_____
3. prodrome	Y/N	_____
4. bradycardia	Y/N	_____
5. hypoasthesia	Y/N	_____
6. hypocondriasis	Y/N	_____
7. acute	Y/N	_____
8. atrophy	Y/N	_____
9. adema	Y/N	_____
10. lesion	Y/N	_____
11. lethal	Y/N	_____
12. cronic	Y/N	_____
13. morbid	Y/N	_____
14. tramatic	Y/N	_____

New Word Synthesis

Using word parts that appear in this chapter, build new terms with the following meanings:

1. _____ controlling sensitivity to pain

2. _____ pertaining to three colors

3. _____ condition of deficient nourishment (or stimulation)

4. _____ resembling (something) sudden

5. _____ a process of self-wasting

6. _____ an abnormal condition of no sensation

7. _____ disease of fever

8. _____ referring to excessive time

9. _____ a yellow wound

10. _____ study of slow death

11. _____ abnormal condition of fast sensation

12. _____ condition of being black

CASE STUDY

Read through the following partial patient history. Note the terms in bold print. A series of multiple choice questions probes your knowledge of these terms.

PATIENT HISTORY

The patient, a 35-year-old female, was admitted for observation after she reported experiencing **hyperesthesia** and **hyperalgesia** in a very severe form. "It was just driving my crazy!" she complained. An examination, however, revealed no **morbid** conditions. Previous history showed physician determination of **hypochondria**. Patient was discharged without treatment.

Case Study Questions

1. **Hyperesthesia** suggests that the patient

   (a) felt numb.

   (b) was paralyzed from the neck down.

   (c) had extreme sensitivity to all stimuli.

   (d) suffered from a very high body temperature.

2. **Hyperalgesia** implies that the patient

   (a) had no sensation to pain.

   (b) experienced extreme sensitivity to pain.

   (c) felt all body sensations very strongly.

   (d) suffered trauma and tissue necrosis.

3. No **morbid** condition tells you that the patient

   (a) was not physically ill.

   (b) may have been partially paralyzed.

   (c) was probably dying.

   (d) was suffering from a lethal disease.

4. Physician determination of **hypochondria** hints that

   (a) potent medication was probably prescribed.

   (b) imaginary pains may have been reported.

   (c) liver damage had occurred.

   (d) hemostasis was interrupted.

CHAPTER 3 Lab Tests and Diagnoses in General

INTRODUCTION

There is a whole set of words, word parts, and abbreviations that deal specifically with lab tests and diagnoses of diseases. The lab tests provide objective, measurable quantities that the physician can use to make an intelligent diagnosis of what is bothering the patient. This chapter focuses on diagnostic terminology that can be applied generally to all the organ systems in the body.

CHAPTER OBJECTIVES

By the end of this chapter, you should be able to:

1 Identify some prefixes, roots, suffixes, and abbreviations describing lab tests and diagnoses in general.

2 Dissect diagnostic terms into their component parts.

3 Translate diagnostic terms into their common English equivalents.

4 Build new medical terms associated with lab tests and diagnoses in general.

Word Parts and Abbreviations Associated with Lab Tests and Diagnoses in General

The following is a list of word parts and abbreviations generally associated with lab tests and diagnoses. Use this list to help you complete **frames 162 to 233.**

auscult/a	listen	**eti/o**	cause	**nucle/o**	kernel
CAT	computed axial tomography	**fluor/o**	luminous	**P & A**	percussion and auscultation
		gnos/o	knowledge		
cine	movies	-gram	record of	**palp/a**	touch
CT	computed tomography	-graph	instrument for recording	**percuss/o**	to beat; tap
				radi/o	rays (x-rays)
dia-	across; through	-graphy	process of recording	**roentgen/o**	x-ray
diagnos/o	knowledge of current status of a disease	**idi/o**	unknown	**scinti/**	spark
		-ist	one who specializes in (something)	**scop/o**	examine
diagnost/o	knowledge of current status of a disease	**lamin/a**	flat plate	**son/o**	sound
		-metry	process of measuring	**steth/o**	chest
		NMR	nuclear magnetic resonance	**therm/o**	heat
electr/o	electrical current			ultra-	beyond; excess
endo-	inner; within				

---

pro-
dia-

162 Perhaps the first thing we should do is distinguish between diagnosis and **prognosis (prahg-NOH-sis)**. The prefix in pro/gnosis is _____, or " before." The prefix in dia/gnosis is _____, "across" or "through." The combining form, **gnos/o (NOHS-oh)**, indicates "knowledge."

---

diagnosis

prognosis

163 A _____ (diagnosis/prognosis) is thus a statement of the nature of a disease, one that the patient is currently going "through" in the course of illness. A _____ (diagnosis/prognosis), however, is a prediction or forecast of the eventual outcome of a disease, "before" this outcome has actually occurred.

---

diagnost/ic (digh-ag-NAHS-tik)

164 An alternate root for *diagnos* is **diagnost (digh-ag-NAHST)**. To build a word meaning "pertaining to diagnosis," use the word root **diagnost** and the suffix in traumat/**ic (frame 109)**. The adjectival form of diagnosis is, therefore, _____ /____.

---

diagnostic

165 Various _____ procedures help determine the exact nature of a particular patient's disease.

---

diagnostic

166 An important _____ technique is simply listening to the patient. **Auscult (AWS-kult)** is a root for "listen."

---

auscult/a/tion
combining vowel

167 Dissect **auscultation** (**aws**-kul-**TAY**-shun) by inserting slashmarks: _____. You were correct if you identified **-tion** as the suffix and **a** as a _____ _____ in this instance.

auscultation

168 Listening to sounds coming from within the body is called _____.

process of listening

169 The suffix **-tion** (**frame 98**) means "process of." Therefore, auscultation literally means a "_____ ____ _____."

Information Frame

170 Other sounds can be produced by gently beating or tapping the body surface. A root for "beat or tap" is **percuss** (per-**KUS**). Touching the body surface with the fingers is also an important means of diagnosis. **Palp** (**PALP**) means "touch."

palp/a/tion (pal-**PAY**-shun)
percuss/ion (per-**KUH**-shun)

171 Just as auscult/a/**tion** is a "process of listening," _____ /____ /_____ is a "process of touching." Similarly, _____ /_____ is a "process of beating or tapping," where **-ion** is the "process of" suffix.

palpation

172 By _____, or gentle touching and probing with the fingers, a physician may be able to detect swollen glands through the skin of the neck.

percussion

173 By _____, or gentle tapping of the skin, a physician may be able to detect abnormal stiffness of the underlying body structures.

percussion
auscultation

174 The process of _____ (tapping) the chest is often accompanied by _____ (listening) of the resulting echo. The echo sounds produced may give the physician or nurse clues to aid in diagnosis.

P & A

175 The diagnostic technique that involves percussion and auscultation is often abbreviated as ____ ____ ____.

P & A

176 A person working in medical records should be able to recognize ____ ____ ____ as an abbreviation for percussion and auscultation in diagnostic reports.

steth/o/scop/e (STETH-oh-skohp)

177 A body location often listened to is the steth (**steth**, a root for "chest"). The combining vowel for steth is **o**. A scop/**e** in general is "an instrument used to examine." The **e** after the root **scop** suggests the instrument. A _____ /_____ /_____ /_____ in particular is "an instrument used to examine the chest."

---

stethoscope

178 A _____ is probably the most-used tool for auscultation.

Information Frame

179 Even in the early days of Hippocrates, auscultation was widely practiced. The ear was directly placed against the chest wall to hear the beating of the heart and the expansion of the lungs. This diagnostic procedure is technically called **direct auscultation** (Figure 3.1A). In 1816 a clever French physician, **Rene Laennec** (lah-**NAY**), invented the procedure called **indirect auscultation.** In this technique, the ear hears body sounds indirectly, through a stethoscope or other instrument (Figure 3.1B). Laennec invented a long, wooden, cylindrical stethoscope based on his observations of young children at play. He noted how the children could clearly hear a pin scratching the end of a solid wooden beam when they placed their ears at the other end.

F I G U R E   3 . 1   **Auscultation**

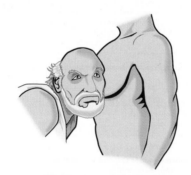

(A) Direct auscultation

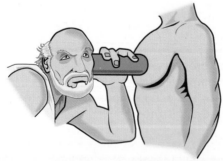

(B) Indirect auscultation

---

180 The stethoscope can be used to hear many inner body sounds—not just those coming from the chest. A prefix for "inner" or "within," is **endo-** (**EN**-doh). The suffix **-o/scopy** (**AHS**-koh-**pee**) is a "process of examining." Two terms can be built from this information:
_____ /_____ /_____, literally "an instrument used to examine the interior" of the body, and _____ /_____ /_____ , the "process of examining the interior" of the body.

endo/**scop**/e (EN-doh-skohp)
end/o/**scopy** (EN-dahs-koh-**pee**)

endoscopy

endoscope

181 The process of _____ uses an instrument inserted into the body through a natural or man-made opening. The instrument is generally called an _____.

endoscope

182 An _____ is usually a flexible tube with a **cold-lighted** tip. This tip allows internal structures to be lit up and viewed without risk of burning them. Figure 3.2 depicts such an instrument examining the interior of the urinary bladder.

F I G U R E   3 . 2   **Endoscopy of the Urinary Bladder**

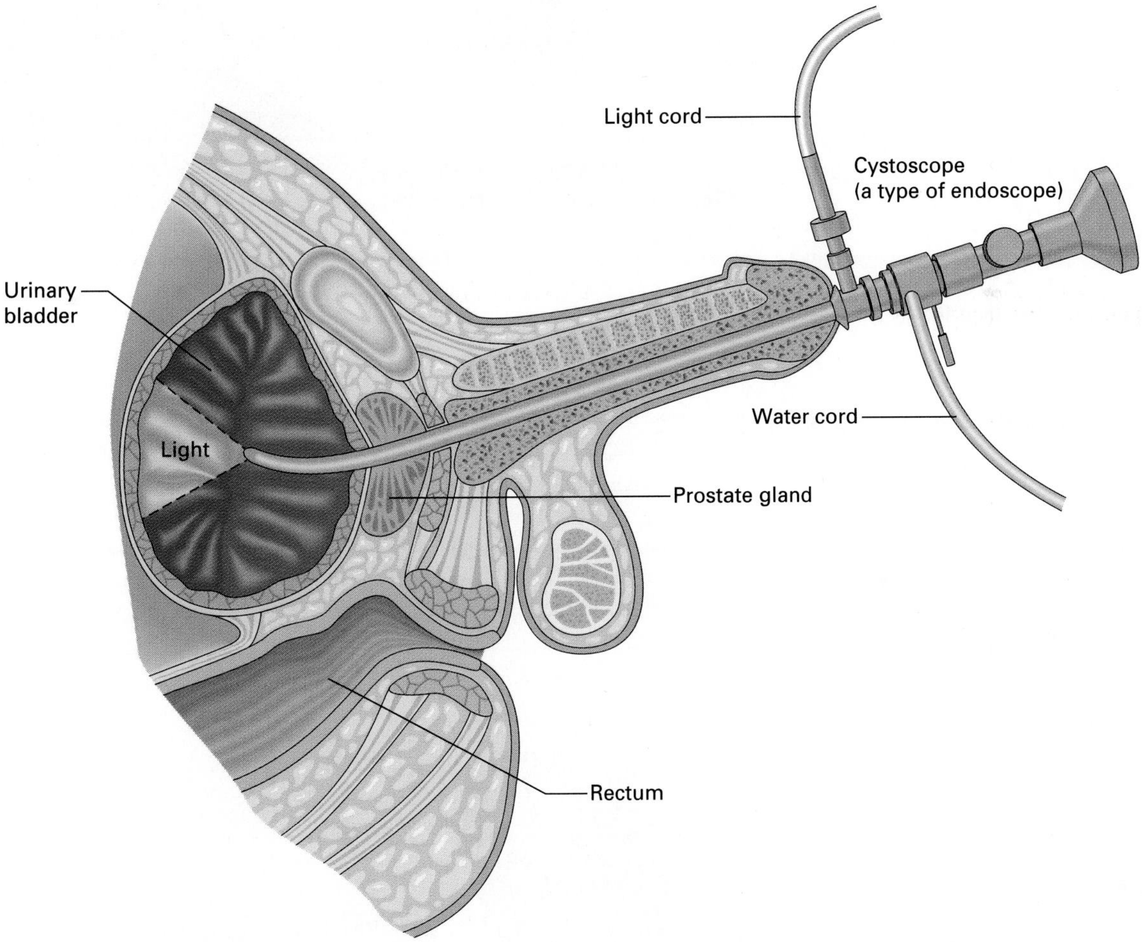

Labels: Light cord — Cystoscope (a type of endoscope) — Urinary bladder — Light — Water cord — Prostate gland — Rectum

fluor/o/scop/e (**FLOO**-roh-**skohp**)

183 A root for "luminous (lighting up)" is **fluor (FLOOR)**. Thus a _____ /_____ /_____ /_____ is "an instrument used to examine (something) by lighting it up."

fluoroscope

184 In actual practice, the _____ is used to take luminous x-ray pictures. Such a device is shown in Figure 3.3.

FIGURE 3.3

Taking X-rays with the Fluoroscope (Photo by Marcia Butterfield, courtesy of W. A. Foote Memorial Hospital, Jackson, MI)

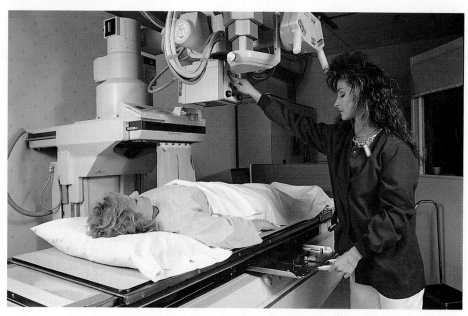

fluor/o/scopy (floo-**RAHS**-koh-**pee**)

185 In a word-building pattern like that in endoscopy, build _____ /_____ /_____ , the "process of examining" objects by taking "luminous" x-ray pictures.

fluoroscopy

186 An x-ray technician might say to a patient, "We're taking you downstairs for _____ , Mrs. Nelson."

Roentgen

187 "X-rays" or "rays" are represented by two different roots: **radi** (**RAY**-dee) and **roentgen** (**RENT**-gun). The second root is named in honor of the discoverer of x-rays, W. K. _____ .

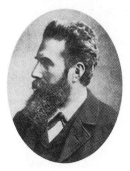

W. K. Roentgen (Photograph courtesy of the Historical Collections of the Library, College of Physicians of Philadelphia)

radi/o/active (**ray**-dee-oh-**AK**-tiv)

188 Use the first root in **frame 187** plus -active to create a new term, _____ /_____ /_____ , or "ray-active."

radioactive

189 X-rays are produced by the continuous decay of _____ ("ray-active") substances, such as radium or uranium.

Information Frame

190 Rays or other forms of energy may be seen on a -gram, or "record" of some kind, by means of a -graph, or "instrument used for recording." The suffix -y, within -graphy (**GRAH**-fee), indicates the "process of."

radi/o/gram (**RAY**-dee-**oh**-gram)
roentgen/o/gram
(**rent-GEHN**-oh-gram)

191 Using both roots for "x-rays" **(frame 187)** plus -gram, build
_____ /_____ /_____ and
_____ /_____ /_____ for "an x-ray record" of some
object.

---

radiogram
roentgenogram

192 A worker in the Medical Records Department of a hospital should be
able to interpret either _____ or
_____ as "an x-ray record." A **radiograph** (**RAY**-dee-
oh-graf) is an alternate name for such a record.

---

radi/o/graph
-graph

193 Radiograph is dissected as _____ /_____ /_____. Even
though **frame 190** said its suffix, _____, was an "instrument
used for recording," radiograph nevertheless has come to mean an x-ray
record itself. A sample radiograph is shown in Figure 3.4 below.

FIGURE 3.4   **A Sample Radiograph**

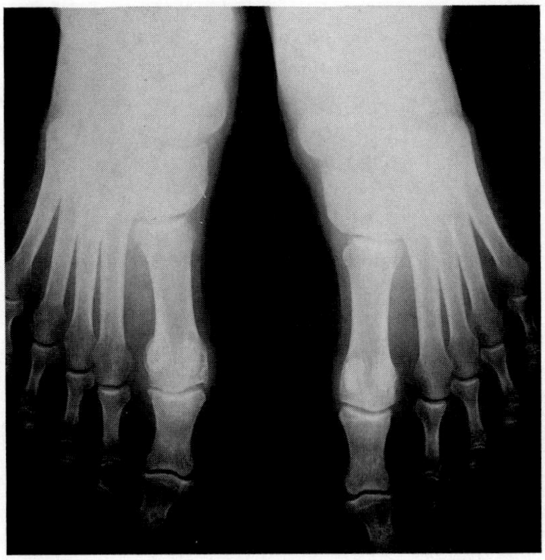

---

radi/o/graphy (ray-dee-**AH**-grah-fee)

194 Using -graphy plus the root in radiograph, build a new term that means
"the process of recording x-rays": _____ /_____ /_____.

---

radiography

195 The recording of x-rays on photographic plates is called
_____.

---

tom/o

196 Other x-ray-related roots/cv include **lamin/a** for "flat plate" and
_____ /_____, for "cut" **(frame 89)**.

---

lamin/a/gram (**LAH**-min- **ah**-gram)
tom/o/gram (**TOH**-moh- gram)

197 Adopting the suffix in roentgenogram, build the following pair of terms:
_____ /_____ /_____ a "flat plate"-like "x-ray record"
_____ /_____ /_____ a thin "cut"-like "x-ray record"

---

laminagram

198 A _____ is obtained when the physician wants to view
only a thin, platelike cross section through a particular part of the body.
The x-ray technician blurs out the area above and below the thin cross
section so that only the strip of interest is readily seen.

tomogram

199 A _____ is obtained when the fluoroscope is rotated such that the x-ray cuts across only a given level of the body.

tom/o/graphy (toh-MAH-grah-fee)

200 Just as radiograms in general are produced by radiography, tomograms are produced by _____ / ____ / _____ , "the process of recording (thin x-ray) cuts" through a given level of the body.

CAT
CT

201 A recent high-tech adaptation of tomography is **computed axial (AKS-ee-ul) tomography (toh-MAH**-grah-fee), also called **computed tomography.** The abbreviation for the first phrase is ____ ____ ____; for the second it is ____ ____. A large fluoroscope is rotated on an axis around the patient, such that an x-ray of a thin cross section all the way through the body can be made. An attached computer generates the x-ray image. Figure 3.5 shows such a **CAT (CT) scanner** in operation.

F I G U R E   3 . 5   **A CAT Scanner** (Photograph courtesy of GE Medical Systems)

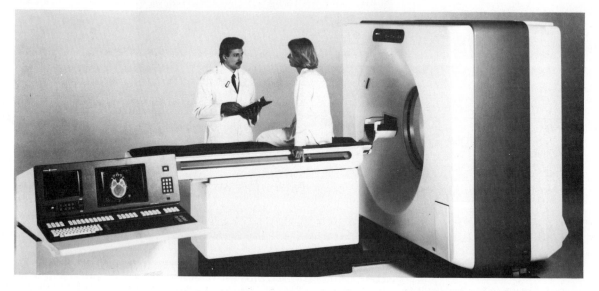

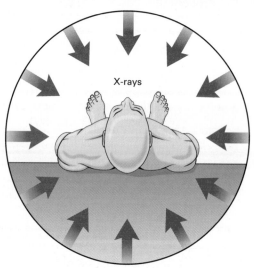

cine/radi/o/graphy (**sin**-ee-**ray**-dee-**AH**-grah-fee)	**202** **Cine** (**SIN**-ee) is a root for "movies." Adding this root to radiography creates _____ / _____ / _____ / _____.
cineradiography	**203** The "process of (taking) x-ray movies" of various body structures in action is called _____.
scinti/grams (**SIN**-tih-**grams**)	**204** Other radiation techniques are employed in **radionuclide** (**ray**-dee-oh-**NOO**-klighd) **imaging,** or **nuclear** (**NOO**-klee-ar) **medicine.** This technique uses radioactive chemicals for diagnosis. **Scinti** (**SIN**-tih), for instance, means "spark." Therefore, _____ / _____ are literally "spark records," just as radiograms are "ray records."
scintigrams	**205** When radioactive material is injected into the body, grid displays, or _____, of the "sparks" (particles and rays emitted) can be produced.
nucle/ar referring to a kernel	**206** **Nucle** (**NOO**-klee) is a root for "kernel." Consequently, nuclear is subdivided as _____ / _____. It means "_____ ____ ____ _____," where **-ar** is the "referring to" suffix.
scintigrams	**207** Nuclear medicine involves radioactive **nuclei** (**NOO**-klee-**igh**), tiny "kernel"-like structures within atoms. The disintegration of such nuclei produces _____ ("spark-records").
-o/logy	**208** Nuclear medicine is a specialty. The suffix, **-ist**, means "one who specializes in (something)." Specializing in something requires great study of the field. You may remember that _____ / _____ **(frame 68)** is a suffix for "study of (something)."
-o/logist (**AHL**-oh-jist)	**209** Extracting the **-y** from **-o/logy** and connecting the resulting fragment to **-ist**, results in a new larger suffix, _____ / _____.
-o/logist	**210** The large suffix _____ / _____ literally means "one who specializes in the study of (something)."
radi/o/logist (**ray**-dee-**AHL**-oh-jist)	**211** Using **radi** as a root for "ray" or "radiation," make a new term that means "one who specializes in the study of rays or radiation": _____ / _____ / _____.
radiologist	**212** After a technician x-rays a patient, the radiographs (radiograms, roentgenograms) are usually handed over to a _____ for in-depth study and examination.

radi/o/logy (ray-dee-AHL-oh-jee)

213 Both x-ray technicians and radiologists work in a hospital's department of _____ / ____ / _____, where "x-ray (images)" are "studied."

---

radiology

NMR

nuclei

214 Related to _____ ("ray-study") and nuclear medicine is **nuclear magnetic resonance (REH-soh-nants)**, abbreviated as ____ ____ ____. This technique produces vertical and cross-sectional images from radio waves released by the movements of hydrogen _____ ("kernels") in a strong magnetic field.

---

nuclear magnetic resonance

215 NMR, or _____ _____ _____, is valuable for producing images showing activity of different parts of the brain.

Information Frame

216 Various other forms of energy can be used for diagnostic imaging. We have, for instance, these energy-related combining forms:

electr/o (ee-**LEK**-troh)   "electrical current"
son/o (**SOH**-noh)   "sound"
therm/o (**THER**-moh)   "heat"

---

son/o/graphy (so-NAH-grah-fee)

217 Just as radi/o/**graphy** involves the production of x-ray images, _____ / ____ / _____ is the "process of recording sound (waves)."

**ultra/son/o/graphy
(uhl-trah-so-NAH-grah-fee)**

218 **Ultra-** is a prefix for "beyond or excess." So _____ / _____ / ____ / _____ is the "process of recording sound (waves) beyond" the usual frequency.

---

ultrasonography

219 In _____, extremely high frequency sound waves are bounced off interior body structures and recorded as images. This technique is very useful for visualizing the unborn child within its mother's uterus.

---

therm/o/graphy

220 In similar fashion, **thermography** (ther-**MAH**-grah-fee) can be subdivided as _____ / ____ / _____.

---

process of
recording heat (waves)

221 Thermography literally means the "_____ ____ _____ _____."

---

thermography

222 The diagnostic imaging technique of _____ "records heat" waves emitted from the body surface. Areas with breast cancer, for example, are generally hotter than the surrounding noncancerous areas.

---

therm/o/gram (THER-moh-gram)

223 Just as a breast tumor might be detected on a radiogram, it might also be found on a _____ / ____ / _____, or "heat record" of breast tissue.

---

thermograms

224 "Heat records," or _____, can be produced in color as well as in black and white.

-meter

225 Besides recording, diagnosis and lab tests include measuring. **Metr** is a root for "measure." Recall **(frame 65)** that _____ is a word or suffix meaning "an instrument used to measure." Similarly, **-metry** (**MET**-ree) indicates the "process of measuring" because the **-y** suffix means "process of."

therm/o/meter
therm/o/metr/y
(ther-MAH-meh-tree)

226 Build two terms that use the information in the preceding frame:
_____ / ____ / _____ "an instrument used to measure heat"
_____ / ____ / _____ / ____ "the process of measuring heat"

thermometer

thermometry

227 A nurse or nurse's aide sticks a _____ under a patient's tongue to gauge body heat or temperature. Technically, the nurse is carrying out _____, the process of measuring heat or temperature in the body.

228 Many diagnostic terms are descriptive, rather than indicating something measured. Observe some abbreviations for a number of descriptive diagnostic terms, along with their meanings, in the list below.

Abbreviation	Meaning
CD	childhood disease
DOA	dead on arrival
DRGs	diagnostic related groups
Dx	diagnosis
exam	examination
FOD	free of disease
FUO	fever of unknown origin
H & P	history and physical
Hx	history
L	left
lab	laboratory
MRI	magnetic resonance imaging
OC	office call
PE	physical examination
PET	positron emission tomography
Pt	patient
R	right
Sx	symptoms
Xr	x-ray

229 Other diagnostic and laboratory terms are closely identified with measurements and units. Some measurement-related diagnostic terms are shown in the list below.

Abbreviation	Meaning
cc (cm³)	cubic centimeter
C	degrees Celsius
c, Ci	curie
C, kcal	Calorie
cm	centimeter
F	degrees Fahrenheit
ht	height
I & O	intake and output
L	liter
ml	milliliter
mm	millimeter
T	temperature
U	units

eti (EE-tee)

230 Measuring, examining, and recording are important aspects of **etiology** (**ee**-tee-**AHL**-oh-jee). When this term is subdivided its root is found to be _____, meaning "cause."

etiology

231 The "study of causes" of various diseases and injuries is called

_____.

path/ic (PATH-ik)
idi/o/path/ic (ih-dee-oh-PATH-ik)

232 The cause of a disease may be known or may remain "unknown," **idi/o** (**IH**-dee-oh). Using **path** for "disease" and the "pertaining to" suffix of pyret/ic **(frame 154)**, build a term that "pertains to disease": _____ /_____. Now extend this thinking to create _____ /_____ /_____ /_____, "pertaining to a disease of unknown (cause)."

etiology
idiopathic

233 Whatever the exact _____ ("cause") of a disease—known or _____ ("unknown")—it still requires treatment.

Multiple Choice

1. The word root for "knowledge" is

a. log   b. gnos   c. path   d. graph

2. A prefix for "inner" or "within" is

a. syn-   b. dia-   c. endo-   d. cine-

3. The combining form for "flat plate" is

a. son/o   b. roentgen/o   c. fluor/o   d. lamin/a

4. A prefix for "before" is

a. dia-   b. pro-   c. syn-   d. endo-

5. The combining form for "cause" is

a. eti/o   b. idi/o   c. gnos/o   d. log/o

6. Which of these suffixes means "one who specializes in (something)"?

a. -gram   b. -ist   c. -metry   d. -graphy

Meanings of Selected Roots

Add the correct combining vowel (cv) after each root. Then write the definition of each root in the space provided.

ROOT/CV   DEFINITION

1. fluor/_____   _____

2. steth/_____   _____

3. auscult/_____   _____

4. electr/_____   _____

5. radi/_____   _____

6. therm/_____   _____

7. son/_____   _____

8. percuss/_____   _____

9. nucle/_____   _____

10. idi/_____   _____

Word Dissection and Translation

Analyze the following terms by dissecting them with slashmarks and identifying their word parts. To the right of each term, write its correct English translation.

Key: R (root), cv (combining vowel), P (prefix), S (suffix)

1. stethoscope

_____/_____/_____/_____   _____
R   cv   R   S

2. radiogram

_____/_____/_____   _____
R   cv   S

3. nuclear

_____/_____   _____
R   S

4. cineradiography

_____/_____/_____/_____   _____
R   R   cv   S

5. radiologist

_____/_____/_____   _____
R   cv   S

6. sonography

_____/_____/_____   _____
R   cv   S

7. thermometer

_____/_____/_____   _____
R   cv   S

8. etiology

_____/_____/_____   _____
R   cv   S

9. idiopathic

_____/_____/_____/_____   _____
R   cv   R   S

10. diagnostic

_____/_____/_____   _____
P   R   S

Terms and Their Abbreviations

In the list below, when the term is given, write its abbreviation in the space provided. When the abbreviation is given, write its corresponding term.

TERM	ABBREVIATION
1. intake and output	_____
2. _____	ml
3. computed axial tomography	_____
4. _____	NMR
5. _____	P & A
6. free of disease	_____
7. symptoms	_____
8. _____	FUO

Word Spelling

Look at each of the terms listed below. Identify those that are misspelled by circling Y for "Yes." Write the correct spelling in the blank.

WORD	MISSPELLED?	CORRECT SPELLING
1. askultation	Y/N	_____
2. scintigrams	Y/N	_____
3. sinradiografer	Y/N	_____
4. radiologist	Y/N	_____
5. ultrasonography	Y/N	_____
6. thermography	Y/N	_____
7. ediology	Y/N	_____
8. endoscopy	Y/N	_____
9. percusion	Y/N	_____
10. rentginogram	Y/N	_____
11. neuclear	Y/N	_____
12. idiopathic	Y/N	_____
13. palpation	Y/N	_____
14. flouroscopy	Y/N	_____

New Word Synthesis

Using word parts that appear in this and previous chapters, build new terms with the following meanings:

1. _____ referring to the chest

2. _____ an instrument used to examine sparks

3. _____ the process of recording sound and x-rays

4. _____ study of luminous (objects)

5. _____ one who studies (the characteristics) of listening

6. _____ pertaining to knowledge before

7. _____ a record of kernels (kernel-like portions of atoms)

8. _____ an x-ray image of electrical current

9. _____ one who specializes in (determining) causes

10. _____ process of measuring a flat plate

11. _____ abnormal softening of the shield resembler

12. _____ abnormal condition below the cartilage

C A S E   S T U D Y

Read through the following radiology report. Note the terms in bold print. A series of multiple choice questions probes your knowledge of these terms.

RADIOLOGY REPORT

Pt: male, age 37

Dx: complete fracture and migration of distal end of R clavicle

Mr. I. M. Strong suffered a severe fall from a moving bicycle, landing on the palm of his extended R hand. **Roentgenography** of the shoulder area revealed complete fracture through the distal end of the R clavicle, with migration of the broken bone fragments under the trapezius muscle. The fracture line, for **idiopathic** reasons, ran horizontally and measured approximately 6 **cm** in length.

Case Study Questions

1. The abbreviation **Dx** means

    (a) prognosis.

    (b) diagnosis.

    (c) prescription.

    (d) treatment.

2. **Roentgenography** of the shoulder implies

    (a) x-ray records.

    (b) auscultation charts.

    (c) radiation records.

    (d) heat charts.

3. **Idiopathic** reasons suggest no known

    (a) diagnosis.

    (b) prognosis.

    (c) treatment.

    (d) cause.

4. The abbreviation **cm** means

    (a) cubic meters.

    (b) centimeter.

    (c) computed measure.

    (d) curie.

CHAPTER 4 Surgery, Pharmacology, and Therapy in General

INTRODUCTION

Various treatments or therapies are available to combat body diseases and injuries. Prominent among these are surgery and applied branches of pharmacology. This chapter features those terms of therapy that could be used for almost any organ system.

CHAPTER OBJECTIVES

By the end of this chapter, you should be able to:

1 Identify some prefixes, roots, suffixes, and abbreviations describing surgery and therapies.

2 Dissect terms of surgery and therapy into their component parts.

3 Translate terms of surgery and therapy into their common English equivalents.

4 Build new medical terms associated with surgery and therapy in general.

Word Parts and Abbreviations Associated with Surgery, Pharmacology, and Other Therapies in General

The following is a list of word parts generally associated with surgery, pharmacology, and other therapies. Use this list to help you complete **frames 234 to 310.**

-amine	nitrogen-containing compound	-in, -ine	a substance	pharmac/o	drug
aque/o	water	ionto	ion (charged particle)	pharmaceut/o	drug
bi/o	life	narc/o	sleep; numbness	-phoresis	carrying; transmission of
-centesis	surgical puncture and tapping of	-o/rrhaphy	suturing of	physi/o	relationship to nature
chem/o	chemical	-o/stomy	forming a permanent opening in		
-desis	binding together of			-plasty	surgical repair
-dot/o	something given	-o/tomy	making an incision into	therapeut/o	treatment
-ectomy	removal of			-therapy	treatment with; treatment of
enter/o	intestine	par-	other than, besides		
hydr/o	water	-pexy	surgical fixation of	-tics	pertaining to
hypn/o	sleep				

---

treatment
-therapy

234 According to the word list, both **therap/o** (**THEHR**-ah-poh) and **therapeut/o** (thehr-ah-**PYOO**-toh) are combining forms for "_____" in general. The suffix _____ means "treatment with" or "treatment of."

---

therapeut/ic (thehr-ah-**PYOO**-tik)

235 Use the second root in **frame 234** plus the suffix in idiopathic **(frame 232)** to build _____ /_____, "relating to treatment."

---

therapies
therapeutic

236 There are many types of "treatments," or _____. A wide variety of _____ techniques are related to such treatments.

---

chem/o (**KEE**-moh)

chem/o/therapy
(**kee**-moh-**THEHR**-ah-pee)

237 Note from the word list that _____ /_____ is a root/cv for "chemical." Use this root/cv to help you build _____ /_____ /_____, that is, "treatment with chemicals."

---

chemotherapy

238 Dangerous cancers are often attacked using _____. Potent drugs target the cancerous cells.

Information Frame

239 Both **pharmac/o** (**FAR**-mah-koh) and **pharmaceut/o** (far-mah-**SOO**-toh) are combining forms for "drug."

---

pharmaceut/ical
(**far**-mah-**SOO**-tih-kal)

240 The second root for "drug" in the preceding frame generally takes -ical **(frame 91)** as its "pertaining to" suffix. This information allows you to build _____ /_____, or "pertaining to drugs."

Chapter 4 Surgery, Pharmacology, and Therapy in General

pharmaceutical	**241** Most of our modern drugs our developed by _____ companies.
pharmac/ist	**242** A pharmacist (**FAR**-mah-sist) mixes and dispenses drugs. This term is subdivided as _____ /_____.
one who specializes in drugs	**243** Containing the suffix, -**ist (frame 208)**, pharmacist literally means "_____ _____ _____ ____ _____."
pharmac pharmac/o/logy (**far**-mah-**KAHL**-oh-jee)	**244** The root in pharmacist, _____, can also be added to the suffix in etiology **(frame 230)**. The new term created, _____ /_____ /_____, means the "study of drugs."
pharmacology	**245** A pharmacist has to enroll in coursework in _____ in order to qualify for the profession.
pharmac/o/logist (**far**-mah-**KAHL**-oh-jist)	**246** Somewhat different from a pharmacist is a _____ /_____ /_____, "one who specializes in the study of drugs."
pharmacist pharmacologist	**247** One would be likely to find a _____ (pharmacologist/pharmacist) working behind the counter in a **pharmacy,** or drugstore. A _____ (pharmacologist/pharmacist) works in a lab, testing drugs in a pharmaceutical company.
chemotherapy	**248** Pharmacology includes _____ (therapy with drugs) as one of its most important subjects. It involves the administration or consumption of various "substances" (-**in** or -**ine**).
-amine (ah-**MEEN**) barbiturate	**249** Some specific substances are **amphetamines** (am-**FET**-ah-meens) and barbiturates (bar-**BIT**-yoo-rayts). Members of the amphetamine group, indicated by the suffix _____, are all "nitrogen-containing compounds." Members of the _____ group, in contrast, are all derivatives of **barbituric** (bar-bih-**TOO**-rik) **acid**.
amphetamines barbiturates	**250** The nitrogen-containing _____ (amphetamines/barbiturates) greatly stimulate the brain. The _____ (amphetamines/barbiturates), however, depress brain activity.
isotopes	**251** There are also many chemicals existing as simple **isotopes** (**IGH**-soh-tohps). These _____ are differing atoms of the same chemical element. They differ in the number of **neutrons** (**NOO**-trahns), or uncharged particles, within their nuclei.

isotopes	**252** Two _____ of the element **carbon (C)**, for example, are the **C-12** and **C-14** atoms.
radi/o/isotopes (**ray**-dee-oh-**IGH**-so-tohps)	**253** The isotopes of certain atoms have unstable nuclei that tend to break down and release "rays" (radi). These are technically called _____ / _____ / _____ , that is, "ray-isotopes."
radioisotope	**254** Since C-14 is radioactive and spontaneously decays, it is commonly classified as a _____.
ions	**255** When isotopes have too many or too few electrons (**ee-LEK**-trahns), negatively charged particles, they are called **ions** (**IGH**-ahns). Such _____ (charged particles) can be positively charged, such as **sodium (Na⁺),** or negatively charged, such as **chloride (Cl⁻).**
ions	**256** The negatively charged _____ (such as Cl⁻) have too many electrons, while those that are positively charged (such as Na⁺) have too few electrons.
ionto/phoresis (igh-**ahn**-toh-for-**EE**-sis)	**257** Ions can be expressed by the root **ionto** (igh-**AHN**-toh). The suffix **-phoresis** (for-**EE**-sis) means "carrying or transmission of (something)." Now we can build _____ / _____ , the "carrying or transmission of ions" into the body.
iontophoresis **aque/ous** (**AHK**-wee-us)	**258** **Aque** (**AHK**-wee) is a root for "water." The process of _____ (transmission of ions) is usually done using _____ / _____ ("watery") solutions. Here the "relating to" suffix for "watery" is **-ous.**
aqueous	**259** Most drugs are consumed in _____ ("watery") form, since the body fluids consist of about 60% water by volume.
stimulants **hypnotics** (hip-**NAHT**-iks) **narcotics** (nar-**KAHT**-iks) **tranquilizers** (**TRAN**-kwi-**ligh**-zers) **sedatives** (**SED**-ah-tivs)	**260** In addition to specific types of chemicals, chemotherapy includes the use of broad classes of drugs. Some of these include: _____ drugs that "arouse" **(stimul)** the nervous system _____ drugs that induce a trancelike "sleep" (**hypn/o**; **HIHP**-noh) _____ drugs that exert a powerful "sleepiness or numbness" (**narc/o**; **NAHR**-koh) _____ drugs that relieve tension and anxiety, creating a "calm" (**tranquil**; **TRAN**-kwil) state _____ drugs that "quiet" (**sedat**; seh-**DAYT**) the nerves
tranquilizers sedatives	**261** Mental patients in hospital wards are often "calmed" with _____ and "quieted" with _____.

stimulant	**262** The caffeine in your coffee is a _____, helping you stay awake and keep alert for studying.
hypnotic narcotics	**263** Other drugs do the opposite of caffeine. Taking a _____ makes you sleepy, as if in a trance. Extremely powerful sleep inducers that also relieve severe pain are called _____.
-algesia -esthesia	**264** Recall that *alges* denotes "feeling or sensitivity to pain," while *esthes* denotes "feelings or sensations" in general. Attach the suffix in hypochondria **(frame 114)** to the end of each to produce the large suffixes _____ and _____ **(frame 129)**, respectively.
an/algesia (**an**-al-**JEE**-zee-uh) an/esthesia (**an**-es-**THEE**-zee-uh)	**265** Remember that **an-**, like **a-**, is a prefix for "absence" or "without." Use this fact and those in the frame above to guide you in building: _____ /_____ "absence of feelings of pain" _____ /_____ "absence of feeling or sensation"
anesthesia analgesia	**266** Employment of _____ removes all sensations from the patient during surgery, while _____ removes the pain sensations only.
an/**esthesi**/o/**logist** (**an**-es-**thee**-zee-**AHL**-oh-jist)	**267** Just as a pharmacologist **(frame 246)** is "one who specializes in the study of drugs," an _____ /_____ /_____ /_____ is "one who specializes in the study of (conditions) lacking sensations."
anesthesiologist	**268** An _____ is usually a physician who oversees the anesthesia of a patient during surgery.
an/**esthet**/ic (**an**-es-**THEHT**-ik) an/**alges**/ic (**an**-al-**JEE**-zik)	**269** **Esthet** (es-**THEHT**) is a root with the same meaning as *esthes*. Consequently, _____ /_____ /_____, "pertains to a lack of feeling or sensation," with **-ic** being the suffix. Likewise, _____ /_____ /_____ "pertains to a lack of pain."
anesthetics analgesics	**270** Drugs that are _____ (analgesics/anesthetics) tend to block all types of sensations, while _____ (analgesics/anesthetics) remove pain sensations only.
an/**esthet**/ist (an-**ES**-theh-**tist**)	**271** "Lack of feeling" as found in anesthetic may be combined with the ending in pharmacist **(frame 242)** to produce _____ /_____ /_____, "one who specializes in lack of sensation."
anesthesiologist anesthetist	**272** Anesthetics and analgesics may be given by an _____ (a physician who specializes in knowledge about lack of sensation) or by an _____ (a nurse or other nonphysician who specializes in lack of sensation).

273 While anesthetics and analgesics remove sensations, other drugs act "against" (anti-) various things. There are, for instance, antibiotics (an-tih-bigh-**AH**-tiks) and antidotes (**AN**-tih-**dohts**).

anti/**bi**/o/tics

274 The root **bi (bigh)**, denotes "life." The combining form is bi/o. It appears within antibiotics, which is subdivided as _____ /____ /____ /_____. The prefix anti- means "against."

anti/**dot**/es

275 The root **dot (DOHT)** means "(something) given." Antidotes is dissected as _____ /_____ /____.

antibiotics

antidotes

276 Drugs called _____ literally act "against living" things, such as **bacteria** (bak-**TEE**-ree-ah), to inhibit their growth. Drugs that are "given against" the harmful effects of other drugs or poisons are called _____.

enter/al (**EN**-ter-al)

277 Drugs taken by mouth eventually reach the "intestine," or **enter** (**EN**-ter). This root takes the same "referring to" suffix as lethal (**frame 159**). The adjective _____ /____ thus "refers to the intestine."

par/**enter**/al (pahr-**EN**-ter-al)

278 The prefix par- **(PAHR)** means "other than." Build another adjective, _____ /_____ /____, that "refers to something other than the intestine."

enteral

parenteral

279 Drugs given by the _____ route pass through the mouth on their way to the intestine, while those given via the _____ route bypass the mouth and intestine.

280 There are many symbols and abbreviations used in pharmacology and chemotherapy. A few of them are listed below.

Abbreviation	Meaning
a	before (ante)
ac	before meals (antecibum)
bid	twice a day (bis in die)
c	cup
c, w/	with
cap(s)	capsules
hs	hour of sleep, bedtime (hora somni)
pc	after meals (postcibum)
prn	as needed or desired (pro re nata)
q	every (quaque)
qid	four times a day (quater in die)
s, w/o	without (sine)
stat	immediately (statim)
tab(s)	tablets
tid	three times a day (ter in die)

physi/o/therapy
(fih-zee-oh-**THEHR**-ah-pee)

281 Besides pharmacology or chemotherapy, there are many other non-chemical treatments available. **Physi** (**FIH**-zee), the root in physiology, means "nature." Using -**therapy**, build a term that literally means "treatment with nature": _____ /_____ /_____.

---

physiotherapy

282 The "natural treatments" of _____ are also known as **physiatrics** (**fih**-zee-**AT**-riks).

---

physiatrics
therm

283 The natural agents used in _____ (physiotherapy) include "heat," represented by the root _____ **(frame 216).**

---

dia/therm/y (DIGH-ah-ther-mee)

284 The prefix **dia-** **(frame 162)** means "through." Thus the "process of heating (something) through" is _____ /_____ /____; the -**y** serves as the suffix. Together therm and -**y** form a noun suffix.

---

diathermy

285 The technique of _____ entails a local heating of body tissues by means of a high-frequency current. This technique is often applied by a physiotherapist (**fih**-zee-oh-**THEHR**-ah-pist) to relieve muscular aches and pains.

---

physi/o/therap/**ist**

286 Physiotherapist is properly subdivided as _____ /_____ /_____ /_____. This word exactly translates as "one who specializes in natural treatments."

---

physiotherapist
aque

287 Still another natural tool of the _____ (physical therapist) is water. **Hydr/o** (**HIGH**-droh), like _____, the root in aqueous **(frame 258)**, means "water."

---

hydr/o/therapy
(**high**-droh-**THEHR**-ah-pee)

288 Using a similar word-synthesizing approach as for physiotherapy, build _____ /_____ /_____, the "process of treating with water."

---

hydrotherapy

289 A football player soaking his sore legs in a whirlpool bath would be receiving the benefits of _____ (water treatment).

---

prosthesis

290 Sometimes a prosthesis (**prahs-THEE**-sis), or artificial replacement, for a lost or damaged body part is required. The term _____ comes from Greek and means an "addition."

---

prosthesis

291 Fitting a _____ ("addition") to a body limb may require surgery.

292 A step beyond physiotherapy is surgery. The first step in surgery is usually making an incision into the skin. The suffix **-o/tomy** (**AHT**-oh-mee) means "making an incision into (something)."

oste
arthr

293 Remember from Chapter 1 **(frame 51)**, that _____ is a root for "bone," while _____ is one for "joint."

oste/o/tomy (**ah**-stee-**AHT**-oh-mee)
arthr/o/tomy
(**ahr-THRAHT**-oh-mee)

294 Take advantage of the roots mentioned in **frame 293** to construct _____ / _____ / _____ ("making an incision into bone") and _____ / _____ / _____ ("making an incision into a joint").

osteotomy
arthrotomy

295 The surgery called _____ is performed to open a bone, while _____ is done to reveal the interior of a joint.

296 An incision is temporary. The suffix **-o/stomy** (**AHS**-toh-mee) is the "forming of a permanent opening in (something)." Os comes from the Latin word meaning "hole or opening."

oste/o/stomy
(**ah**-stee-**AHS**-toh-mee)
arthr/o/stomy
(**ahr-THRAHS**-toh-mee)

297 Build a word that indicates "forming of a permanent opening in bone": _____ / _____ / _____. Do the same for "joint": _____ / _____ / _____.

osteotomy
arthrotomy

298 After cutting into a bone, an _____ is left permanently behind. After cutting into a joint, an _____ becomes a lasting hole.

oste/o/centesis
(**ahs**-tee-oh-sen-**TEE**-sis)
arthr/o/centesis
(**ahr**-throh-sen-**TEE**-sis)

299 The suffix **-centesis** (sen-**TEE**-sis) designates the "surgical puncture and tapping of (something)." For bones, this procedure is called _____ / _____ / _____. For a joint, the procedure is described as _____ / _____ / _____.

arthrocentesis
osteocentesis

300 A surgeon might carry out _____ to suction out excess fluid from a joint. The procedure called _____ may be indicated to suck out a sample of marrow from the interior of a bone.

301 Two related surgical suffixes are **-desis** (**DEE**-sis) and **-pexy** (**PEKS**-ee). The first root denotes a "binding together," the second a "surgical fixation."

---

oste/o/desis (**ahs**-tee-**AH**-dee-sis)
oste/o/pexy (**ahs**-tee-oh-**PEKS**-ee)
arthr/o/desis (**ahr**-throh-**DEE**-sis)
arthr/o/pexy (**ahr**-throh-**PEKS**-ee)

302 Following the pattern of the last few frames, create terms that mean the following:

_____ / ____ / _____   "binding together of bones"
_____ / ____ / _____   "surgical fixation of a bone"
_____ / ____ / _____   "binding together of joints"
_____ / ____ / _____   "surgical fixation of a joint"

---

osteodesis
osteopexy

303 The operation of _____ unites adjacent bones together. The procedure called _____ surgically fixes and stabilizes a loose bone.

---

arthrodesis
arthropexy

304 The technique of _____ links together neighboring joints, while _____ fixes a loose joint into its proper position.

---

oste/o/plasty
(**ahs**-tee-oh-**PLAS**-tee)
arthr/o/plasty
(**arth**-roh-**PLAS**-tee)

305 Sometimes a damaged structure must undergo a type of **-plasty** (**PLAS**-tee), or "surgical repair." A "surgical repair of bone" is called _____ / ____ / _____. The "surgical repair of a joint" is called _____ / ____ / _____.

---

osteoplasty
arthroplasty

306 A bone severely damaged in a fall from a bicycle may have to be repaired by _____. If an associated joint is torn apart, _____ may also be involved.

---

ost/ectomy (**ahs**-**TEK**-toh-mee)
arthr/ectomy
(**ahr**-**THREK**-toh-mee)

307 The suffix **-ectomy** (**EK**-toh-**mee**) indicates the "removal of (something)." Therefore, _____ / _____ is the "removal of bone," while _____ / _____ is the "removal of a joint."

---

ostectomy
arthrectomy

308 A skull bone crushed when a person slams through a car windshield may be removed by _____. If there is unrepairable damage to some joint, _____ may also be indicated.

---

oste/o/rrhaphy
(**ahs**-tee-**OR**-hah-fee)
arthr/o/rrhaphy
(ar-**THROR**-hah-fee)

309 Whenever surgery is through, the skin and involved structures must be sutured back together. The suffix **-o/rrhaphy** (**OR**-hah-fee) means a "suturing of (something)." Now build these words:

_____ / ____ / _____   "suturing of a bone"
_____ / ____ / _____   "suturing of a joint"

osteorrhaphy

arthrorrhaphy
-o/rrhexis (or-**EKS**-is)

enter/o/rrhexis (**en**-ter-oh-**REKS**-is)

Information Frame

310 The procedure of _____ closes a bone and its surrounding membrane after an operation. The procedure of
_____ closes a joint after an operation upon it.
Another suffix, ____ /_____ , (**frame 147**), refers to "rupture."
Build a term that means "rupture of the intestine":
_____ /____ /_____ .

311 Figure 4.1 illustrates the surgical procedures discussed in **frames 292 to
310,** using bone as an example. More specific applications of these procedures will be found in the chapters on the individual organ systems in
the body.

F I G U R E   4 . 1

General Types of Operative Procedures, Using Bone as an Example

Osteotomy
(cutting into a bone)

Osteostomy
(making a permanent
new opening in a bone)

Applied suction
for tapping

Catheter

Osteocentesis
(surgical puncture and
tapping of a bone)

Osteodesis
(binding together of bones)

Body
wall

Osteopexy
(surgical fixation of a bone)

Osteoplasty
(surgical repair of a
damaged bone)

Ostectomy
(removal of a bone)

Osteorrhaphy
(suturing of a bone)

Chapter 4 Surgery, Pharmacology, and Therapy in General

312 There are numerous abbreviations used in therapy and surgery. The following list presents a partial sampling of them.

Abbreviation	Meaning
AMB	ambulate (walk)
BRP	bathroom privileges
Bx	biopsy
CBR	complete bed rest
ER	emergency room
exc	excise
ICU	intensive care unit
I & D	incision and drainage
NPO	nothing by mouth
OR	operating room
PO	postoperative
RATx	radiation therapy
SOP	standard operating procedure
TC & DB	turn, cough, and deep breathe
Tx	treatment, traction, transplant
V, Y, W, Z, -plasty	several types of plastic surgery

Multiple Choice

1. The suffix for "bind together" is

    a. -o/rrhaphy   b. -desis   c. -phoresis   d. -amine

2. The suffix for "form a permanent opening" is

    a. -o/rrhexis   b. -o/stomy   c. -pexy   d. -desis

3. The combining form for "something given" is

    a. plast/o   b. ionto   c. dot/o   d. pharmac/o

4. Narc/o means

    a. "drug"   b. "dead"   c. "seizure"   d. "numb"

5. The prefix for "absence of" is

    a. pro-   b. par-   c. anti-   d. an-

6. The suffix for "removal" is

    a. -pexy   b. -ectomy   c. -o/rrhexis   d. -atrics

Meanings of Selected Roots

Add the correct combining vowel (cv) after each root. Then write the definition of each root in the space provided.

ROOT/CV   **DEFINITION**

1. aque/_____

2. hypn/_____

3. narc/_____

4. enter/_____

5. chem/_____

6. therapeut/_____

7. bi/_____

8. pharmac/_____

9. hydr/_____

10. pharmaceut/_____

Word Dissection and Translation

Analyze the following terms by dissecting them with slashmarks and identifying their word parts. To the right of each term, write its correct English translation.

Key: R (root), cv (combining vowel), P (prefix), S (suffix)

1. chemotherapy

_____ / _____ / _____   _____
     R   cv   S

2. arthrodesis

_____ / _____ / _____   _____
     R   cv   S

3. parenteral

_____ / _____ / _____   _____
     P   R   S

4. antidotes

_____ / _____ / _____   _____
     P   R   S

5. aqueous

_____ / _____   _____
     R   S

6. anesthesiologist

_____ / _____ / _____ / _____   _____
     P   R   cv   S

7. pharmacist

_____ / _____   _____
     R   S

8. therapeutic

_____ / _____   _____
     R   S

9. iontophoresis

_____ / _____   _____
     R   S

10. physiotherapist

_____ / _____ / _____ / _____   _____
     R   cv   R   S

Terms and Their Abbreviations

In the list below, when the term is given, write its abbreviation in the space provided. When the abbreviation is given, write its corresponding term.

TERM	ABBREVIATION
1. nothing by mouth	_____
2. _____	qid
3. _____	stat
4. _____	OR
5. _____	ICU
6. _____	pc
7. _____	prn
8. incision and drainage	_____

Word Spelling

Look at each of the terms listed below. Identify those that are misspelled by circling Y for "Yes." Write the correct spelling in the blank.

WORD	MISSPELLED?	CORRECT SPELLING
1. artherorraphy	Y/N	_____
2. osteotomy	Y/N	_____
3. barbiturate	Y/N	_____
4. hidrotherapy	Y/N	_____
5. enteral	Y/N	_____
6. narcotik	Y/N	_____
7. eyeontophoresis	Y/N	_____
8. amphetamines	Y/N	_____
9. farmasuitical	Y/N	_____
10. thairapewtik	Y/N	_____
11. pharmacology	Y/N	_____
12. fizzeatrics	Y/N	_____
13. sedative	Y/N	_____
14. prosthesis	Y/N	_____

New Word Synthesis

Using word parts that appear in this and previous chapters, build new terms with the following meanings:

1. _____ surgical puncture and tapping of the intestine

2. _____ relating to sleep and drugs

3. _____ treatment with ions

4. _____ pertaining to watery chemicals

5. _____ removal of a flat plate

6. _____ surgical repair of the intestine

7. _____ one who specializes in the study of water

8. _____ surgical fixation of the chest

9. _____ binding together of the intestine

10. _____ rupture of a wound

11. _____ calmness without feeling or sensation

12. _____ process of excessive nourishment

C ASE S TUDY

Read through the following operative report. Note the terms in bold print. A series of multiple choice questions probes your knowledge of these terms.

Operative Report

Pt: female, age 16

Dx: enterorrhexis of lower third of large intestine

Procedure: Enterectomy of lesioned area and **enterodesis** of the cut ends. **Enterotomy** was accomplished by an incision through the lower abdominal wall. The ruptured **enteral** segment was quite fragile and necrotic. Upon removal of the affected area, silk sutures were employed for **enterorrhaphy.**

Case Study Questions

1. The diagnosis of **enterorrhexis** (suffix in Chapter 3) implies that the intestine was

    (a) ruptured.

    (b) shriveled.

    (c) enlarged.

    (d) normal.

2. **Enterectomy** and **enterodesis** suggest that

    (a) surgical repair wasn't required.

    (b) suturing of the intestines was included.

    (c) removal and binding together of the intestines was performed.

    (d) the morbid zone and interior growths were removed.

3. Accomplishment of **enterotomy** means the damaged organ was

(a) removed.

(b) incised.

(c) repaired.

(d) punctured.

4. An **enteral** segment is one associated with the

(a) intestine.

(b) chest.

(c) stomach.

(d) joint.

5. **Enterorrhaphy** is a term for what general type of operative procedure?

(a) fixation

(b) suturing

(c) excision

(d) incision

CHAPTER 5 Structure and Function of the Human Body

INTRODUCTION

You have received the basics of medical terminology. Now it is appropriate to examine some of the terms involving the normal anatomy and physiology of the body as a whole.

As a start, let us view the body placed in the **anatomical position** (Figure 5.1). Note that the person is standing erect and looking forward, with the chin parallel to the floor, the feet slightly spread apart, the arms hanging loosely at the sides, and the palms facing forward. This is the common reference or standard road map used to name the relative positions of various body structures. We shall refer to this road map again and again as we discuss the terminology of locations on the body.

FIGURE 5.1   The Soma (Body) in the Anatomical Position

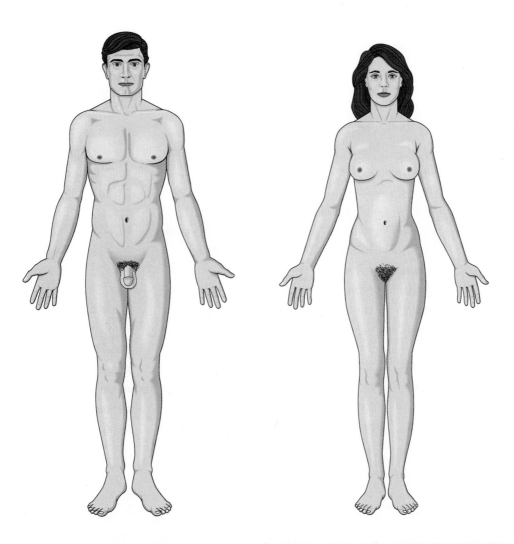

CHAPTER OBJECTIVES

By the end of this chapter, you should be able to:

1 Identify major prefixes, roots, suffixes, and abbreviations related to the structure and function of the entire body.

2 Dissect terms of general body structure and function into their component parts.

3 Translate terms of general body structure and function into their common English equivalents.

4 Build new terms associated with general body structure and function.

Normal A & P

Word Parts and Abbreviations Associated with Normal Anatomy and Physiology of the Whole Body

The following is a list of common word parts and an abbreviation associated with normal anatomy and physiology. Use this list to help you complete **frames 313 to 422.**

ab-	from; away from	epi-	upon	per-	through
abdomin/o	trunk midsection	ex-; exo-	outside	peri-	around
acr/o	body extremity	**extern/o**	outside	**physi/o**	nature
ad-	to; toward; near	extra-	outside	**poster/o**	behind
af-	toward	-form	resembling	pre-	before; in front of
ant	anterior	-gen	production	**proxim/o**	near
ante-	before; in front of	-genesis	production	retro-	behind; back
anter/o	in front of	**ili/o**	flank	**sagitt/o**	arrow
AP	anteroposterior	in-	in; into; not	**sinistr/o**	to the left of
caud/o	tail (end) of body	**infer/o**	below	**som/;**	
cephal/o	head	infra-	under, below	**somat/a**	body
circum-	around	inter-	between	sub-	under
constrict/o	narrow	**intern/o**	within	super-	above
coron/o	crown	intra-	within	supra-	above; upper
crani/o	skull	**later/o**	side	**thorac/o**	chest
cyst/o	bladder; sac of fluid	**lumb/o**	loins (lower back)	trans-	across; through
		medi/o	middle	**umbilic/o**	pit (the navel)
dextr/o	to the right of	-o/rrhea	flow	**ventr/o**	belly
dilat/o	widen	par-; para-	beside; near; beyond	**vers/o**	to turn
dist/o	distant			**vertebr/o**	backbone
dors/o	back	**pariet/o**	wall	**viscer/o**	guts (internal organs)
ecto-	outside	**pelv/i**	bowl		
en-	in; within				

---

anatomy and physiology	**313** The foundation of medical terminology is human _____ _____ _____ (A & P). The discipline is built around terms describing disorders of body structures and functions on a system-by-system basis.
som (SOHM) **somat (SOH**-mat) **som/a (SOH**-mah)	**314** A look back at Figure 5.1 reveals the entire "body," indicated by the roots _____ and _____ on the word list. Employing the shorter root and adding **-a**, we obtain _____ /____, "presence of the body."
soma	**315** The _____ is the major mass of the body. It primarily consists of the skin, bones, joints, and skeletal muscles.
somat/ic (soh-**MAT**-ik)	**316** Use the second root in **frame 314** and the suffix in analgesic **(frame 269)** to help you build _____ /____, "relating to the body."
somatic	**317** The _____ portion of the nervous system supplies nerves to the soma (skin, bones, joints, and skeletal muscles).
ana/tom/**y** ana- tom **-y**	**318** The soma is studied in anatomy. Recall **(frame 45)** that anatomy is sub-divided as: _____ /_____ /____. To help you, remember that _____ **(frame 46)** is a prefix for "up" or "apart," _____ **(frame 89)** is a root for "cut," and ____ **(frame 44)** is a suffix meaning "action, process, or condition of."
anatomy	**319** You may remember _____ defined previously **(frame 47)** as the "action of cutting (something) up or apart."
pertaining (relating, referring) to	**320** Anatomy becomes an adjective when the suffix **-ical (frame 91)**, which means "_____ ____," is added.
ana/tom/**ical**	**321** **Frame 92** mentioned the term _____ /_____ /_____, which "refers to cutting (something) apart."
cut (cutting)	**322** Both *anatomy* and *anatomical* contain a root for "_____" because they involve **dissection** (dih-**SEK**-shun), the cutting up of body parts. Formally speaking, then, anatomy is body structure and the study of body structures, primarily by means of dissection.
anatomical	**323** It is proper to speak of an _____ (anatomy/anatomical) position because this position provides a guideline for body dissection. Such dissections may be either real or imaginary. An **anatomical plane** is a flat imaginary dividing sheet that can be passed through the body at some particular angle. An **anatomical section** is an actual physical cut made through the body in the direction of a certain plane.

planes

sections

324 Imaginary anatomical _____ (planes/sections) are useful in separating body structures from one another for description. Actual anatomical _____ (planes/sections), however, are cuts that physically separate body parts.

Information Frame

325 Natural body landmarks are used to guide dissection whenever possible. Such landmarks include **sutures** (**SOO**-churs). These are narrow jagged cracks running like "seams" across the skull and facial bones. Figure 5.2 shows two such sutures present on the skull.

F I G U R E   5 . 2

Some Sutures ("Seams") on the Skull Used for Directional Terms

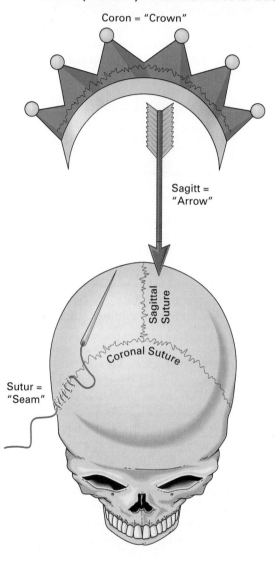

Coron = "Crown"

Sagitt = "Arrow"

Sagittal Suture

Coronal Suture

Sutur = "Seam"

---

sagitt/o (**SAJ**-it-oh)
coron/o (kor-**OHN**-oh)

326 Note from Figure 5.2 that_____ /____ means "arrow," while _____ /____ means "crown."

---

sagittal suture (**SAJ**-ih-tal)
coronal suture (kor-**OHN**-al)

327 Thus the _____ _____ is literally a "seam pertaining to an arrow," while the _____ _____ is a "seam pertaining to a crown."

Chapter 5 Structure and Function of the Human Body

sagittal

coronal

mid/sagitt/al (mid-**SAJ**-ih-tal)

midsagittal plane

para/sagitt/al (pair-uh-**SAJ**-ih-tal)

para/sagitt/al

midsagittal

328 The _____ suture appears to have been made by an arrow that flew too low and creased the top of the skull. The _____ suture appears to result from a heavy crown that cracked the skull.

329 Mid- means "middle." Thus one can create _____ /_____ /____, or "referring to the middle of the sagittal (suture)." A plane can be passed through this area.

330 A _____ _____ is a flat imaginary dividing sheet passed down through the middle of the sagittal suture. This plane is often called the **body midline,** because it subdivides the body into exactly equal right and left halves. (See Figure 5.3A.)

331 The two prefixes par- (**PAIR**) and para- (**PAIR**-uh) mean "beside, near, or beyond." Use the second prefix to help you synthesize _____ /_____ /____, "referring to (something) beside the sagittal (suture)."

332 A _____ /_____ /____ plane is any plane that runs parallel to the sagittal suture—that is, beside it. (See Figure 5.3B.) This is unlike the _____ plane, which passes directly through the middle of this suture.

F I G U R E   5 . 3   **Terms Associated with the Midsagittal Plane**

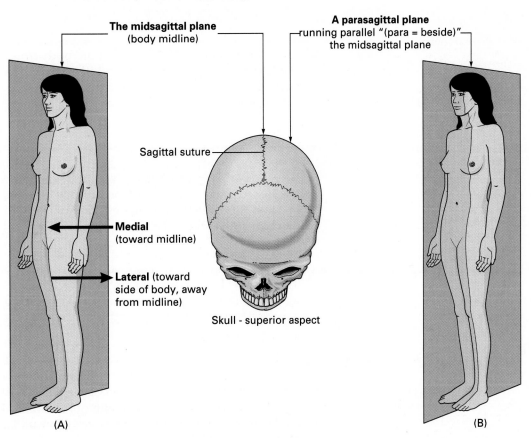

The midsagittal plane
(body midline)

A parasagittal plane
running parallel "(para = beside)"
the midsagittal plane

Sagittal suture

Medial
(toward midline)

Lateral (toward
side of body, away
from midline)

Skull - superior aspect

(A)

(B)

medi (**MEE**-dee)
later (**LAH**-ter)
medi/al (**MEE**-dee-al)
later/al (**LAH**-ter-al)

333 The chapter word list indicates that _____, like mid-, means "middle." A root for "side" is _____. So _____ / _____ "refers to the middle (body midline)," whereas _____ / _____ "refers to the side (of the body)."

medial

lateral

334 The ear is _____ to the shoulder, because it lies closer to the body midline (midsagittal plane). The shoulder, conversely, is _____ to the ear, because it lies farther from the body midline.

ad-
af-
ab-

335 Two prefixes in the word list, _____ and _____, mean "toward or near," while _____ means "from or away from." All of these prefixes, however, are not necessarily used in connection with the midsagittal plane only.

adductor
afferent
abductor

336 Pronounce the following three terms:
adductor (**a-DUKT**-or)
abductor (**ab-DUK**-tor)
afferent (**A**-fer-**ent**)
The two terms _____ and _____ contain prefixes that mean "toward or near." But _____ includes a prefix for "from or away from." (These terms will be explored further in later chapters.) Build a term using the prefixes ab-, ad-, af-, or look up a term for each using the medical dictionary.

dextr/al (**DEKS**-tral)
sinistr/al (**SIN**-ihs-tral)

337 The midline marks off one side of the body from the other. **Dextr** (**DEKS**-ter) is a root for "right," while **sinistr** (**SIN**-ihs-ter) is one for "left." Use the suffix in sagittal to build _____ / _____ ("pertaining to the right") and _____ / _____ ("pertaining to the left").

sinistral

dextral

338 A body part with a _____ location is positioned to the left side of the body midline. Two-thirds of the heart, for instance, usually lies to the left of the midline. A body part with a _____ location is positioned on the right side of the midline. Certain lobes of the liver, for example, lie mostly on the right.

339 The last few frames have chiefly involved body directions named according to the sagittal suture and midsagittal plane. Other directional terms refer to the _____ ("crown") suture.

coronal

coronal

340 A _____ ("crown"), or **frontal plane** is one passed down through the skull in the direction of the coronal suture. Since the coronal suture extends across the width of the skull, such a plane subdivides the body into front and back portions. (Consult Figure 5.4.)

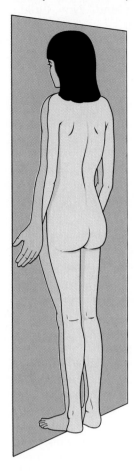

Information Frame	**341** A prefix, ante- (**AN**-tee), and a root, **anter** (**AN**-ter), both mean "in front of." So do the prefixes, pre- and pro-
post- **poster** (**PAHS**-ter)	**342** Glance back at the word list to find _____ and _____, two word parts that indicate "after" or "behind."
anter **poster**	**343** Let us work with the two opposite roots, _____ ("in front of") and _____ ("behind").
anter/i/or (an-**TEER**-ee-er) **poster/i/or** (pahs-**TEER**-ee-er)	**344** Each root can take **i** as a combining vowel and **-or** as a suffix. This combination results in _____ /____ /____ ("one that is in front") and _____ /____ /____ ("one that is behind").
posterior anterior	**345** The forehead, for instance, is _____ to the nose, being located behind it. Turning things around, the nose is _____ to the forehead, since it lies in front of it.
ant ante-	**346** Anterior is abbreviated with its first three letters as _____. Take care not to confuse this abbreviation with the somewhat similar four-letter prefix _____ ("in front of").

antero/poster/i/or (**AN**-ter-oh-**pohs-TEER**-ee-or)	**347** Antero- and postero- can also be considered prefixes. They still mean "in front of" and "behind." Now build a term that means, "one that passes from front to rear": _____ /_____ /_____ /_____. Note that in the word *anteroposterior,* antero- is the prefix while **poster/i** is the combining form.
anteroposterior	**348** Radiograms of fractured bones are sometimes taken in an _____ direction, from the front of the bone all the way toward its rear.
AP	**349** The two capital letters _____ _____ represent an abbreviation for antero-posterior, with each letter indicating a root in the word.
retro- (**REH**-troh)	**350** Another prefix on the word list, _____, like postero-, means "behind." Alternatively it means "back," like the root, **dors.**
dors	**351** The opposite of _____ ("back") is **ventr** (**VEN**-ter), or "belly."
dors/**al** (**DOR**-sal) ventr/**al** (**VEN**-tral)	**352** The roots for back and belly both take the suffix of dextral **(frame 337).** This yields _____ /_____ ("pertaining to the back") and _____ /_____ ("pertaining to the belly").
ventral dorsal	**353** For humans in the anatomical position, anterior and _____ indicate approximately the same direction, since the "belly" is always in "front." Posterior and _____ indicate a position toward the "back," which lies "behind." (See Figure 5.5.)

FIGURE 5.5 **Front and Behind = Belly and Back**

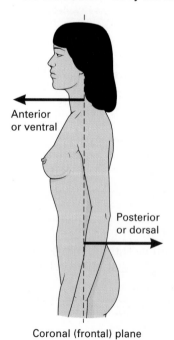

Anterior
or ventral

Posterior
or dorsal

Coronal (frontal) plane

Chapter 5 Structure and Function of the Human Body

dia- (**DIGH**-ah) per- trans- (**TRANZ**)	**354** Now it is time to identify some word parts that mean "across" or "through." Recall _____, the prefix in diagnosis **(frame 162)**. Two prefixes on the word list with this meaning are _____ and _____.
trans/**vers**/e (tranz-**VERS**)	**355** **Vers/e** is "a turning." Using trans- and -e, build _____ /_____ /_____, "a turning across." The prefix is trans- and the suffix is **-e**
transverse	**356** A _____, or **horizontal, plane** is one that is "turned" and passed "across" the body in a left-right "horizontal" direction.
horizontal	**357** A transverse (_____) plane subdivides the body into upper and lower portions.
transverse horizontal	**358** There are several directional terms related to _____ or _____ (left-right) planes.
crani/o (**KRAY**-nee-oh) **caud/o** (**KAW**-doh) **cephal/o** (**SEF**-al-oh) **infer/o** (**IN**-fer-oh) infra- (**IN**-frah) sub- super- (**SOO**-per) supra- (**SOO**-prah)	**359** Find these word parts related to transverse planes in the word list: _____ /_____ "skull" _____ /_____ "tail" _____ /_____ "head" _____ /_____ "below" _____ "under; below" _____ "under" _____ "above" _____ "above; upper"
super/i/or (soo-**PEER**-ee-or) infer/i/or (in-**FEER**-ee-or)	**360** Several of these word parts have been used to create whole terms related to transverse planes. Adopting the pattern of anterior and posterior, use super- to create _____ /_____ /_____ ("one that is above") and **infer** to make _____ /_____ /_____ ("one that is below").
superior inferior	**361** The eye is _____ to the cheek, but the cheek is _____ to the eye.
crani/al (**KRAY**-nee-al) **caud/al** (**KAW**-dal) **cephal/ic** (seh-**FAL**-ik)	**362** As with dorsal and ventral, use **crani** and **caud** to make _____ /_____ ("pertaining to the skull") and _____ /_____ ("pertaining to the tail"), respectively. Using **-ic**, we create _____ /_____ ("pertaining to the head").

cranial cephalic	**363** The eye is _____ (more toward the top of the skull) or _____ (more toward the top of the head) in relation to the cheek.
caudal	**364** The cheek is _____ (more toward the tail end of the body) in relation to the eye.
inferior cranial cephalic	**365** It should be obvious from **frames 360–364** that caudal indicates the same general direction as _____ , and that superior denotes the same general direction as _____ or _____ . All these terms relative to a transverse plane are shown in Figure 5.6.

FIGURE 5.6   **Terms Associated with Transverse (Horizontal) Planes**

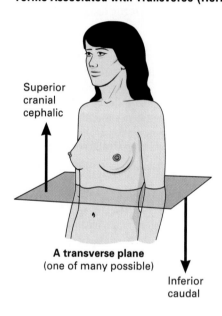

Superior
cranial
cephalic

A transverse plane
(one of many possible)

Inferior
caudal

366 Some word parts describing body locations are not associated with any
particular anatomical plane. Find these examples from your word list:

acr/o (**AK**-roh) circum- (**SIR**-kum) **dist/o** ecto- (**EK**-toh) ex- exo- **extern/o** (**EKS**-ter-noh) extra- (**EK**-strah) en- intra- (**IN**-trah) **intern/o** (**IN**-ter-noh) in- peri- (**PEHR**-ee) **proxim/o** (**PRAHKS**-ih-moh) epi- (**EP**-ee) inter- (**IN**-ter)	_____ / _____ "body extremity" _____ "around" _____ / _____ "distant" _____ "outside" _____ or _____ "outside" _____ / _____ "outside" _____ "outside" _____ "within" _____ "within" _____ / _____ "within" _____ "in; into; not" _____ "around" _____ / _____ "near" _____ "upon" _____ "between"

Chapter 5 Structure and Function of the Human Body

dist/al (DIS-tal)
proxim/al (PRAHKS-ih-mal)

367 Let us now practice our skills in terminology by working with several word parts of the preceding frame. To start, extract the suffix from dorsal and build: _____ /_____, "referring to (something) far or distant" from the origin of a body limb, and _____ /_____, "referring to (something) near or closer" to the origin of a body limb.

proximal

distal

368 The knee is considered _____ to the ankle, because it lies closer to the hip (the origin of the leg). Conversely, the ankle is _____ to the knee, because it lies farther from the hip.

distal

proximal

369 The wrist is considered _____ to the elbow, because it lies farther from the shoulder (the origin of the arm). The elbow is _____ to the wrist, because it lies closer to the shoulder.

intern/al

extern/al

370 Now let us switch focus to terms describing directions toward the body interior, or toward its surface. **Internal (in-TER-nal)** is an example. It is dissected as _____ /_____, using the ending in proximal. **External (eks-TER-nal)**, likewise, is subdivided as _____ /_____.

within
outside

371 Glancing back at **frame 366** allows you to translate internal as "pertaining to (something) _____" and external as "pertaining to (something) _____."

internal
external

372 Individual _____ structures are those lying deep within the body, whereas _____ structures are those lying outside the body or on the body surface.

external

373 One _____ structure readily visible to anyone looking at the ventral surface of the body is the umbilicus (um-**BIL**-ih-kus)—the "pit," or navel.

umbilic/**us**
umbilic (um-**BIL**-ik)

374 Umbilicus is analyzed as _____ /_____. Its suffix, **-us**, like **-e**, means "presence of." Its root, _____, means "pit."

umbilic/al (um-BIL-ih-kal)

375 Employ the suffix in external to help you build _____ /_____ ("referring to the navel").

umbilical

376 The _____ area is the region surrounding the pit, or navel.

377 The _____ region containing its pit is just one of nine different regions that can be marked off on the _____ (outer) aspect of the trunk midsection. (See Figure 5.7.)

FIGURE 5.7 The Nine Regions of the Abdomen

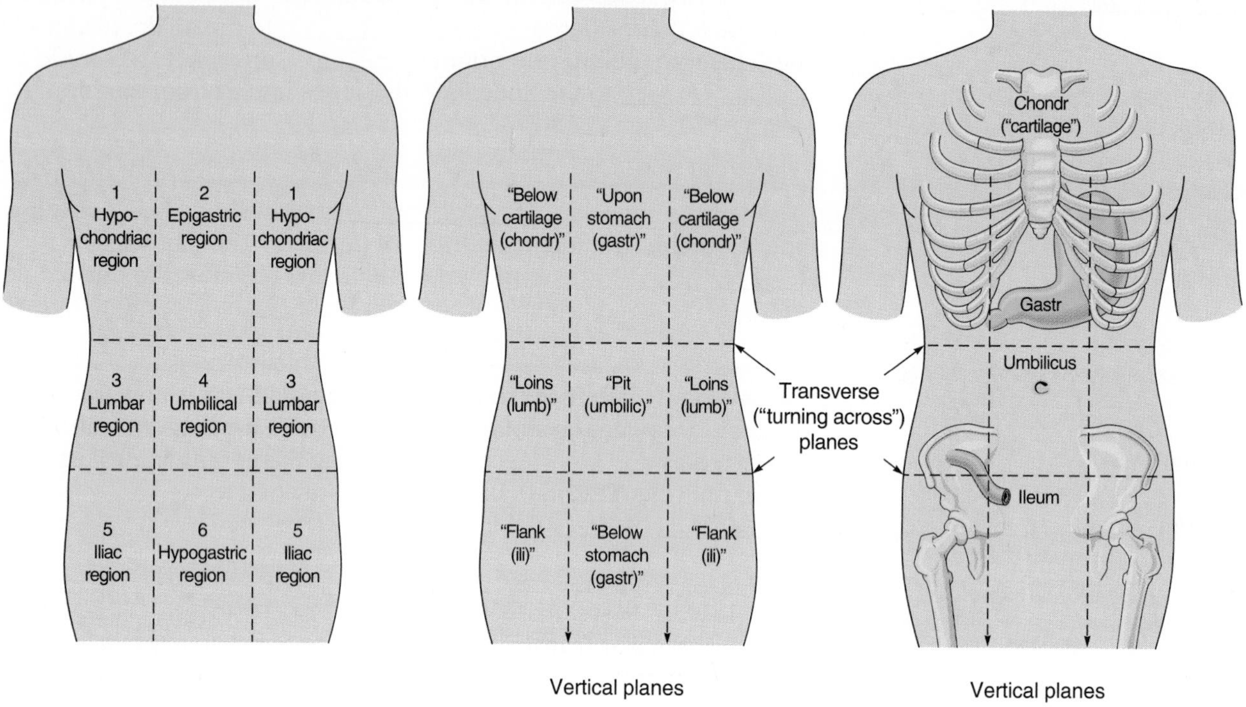

1 Hypo-chondriac region	2 Epigastric region	1 Hypo-chondriac region
3 Lumbar region	4 Umbilical region	3 Lumbar region
5 Iliac region	6 Hypogastric region	5 Iliac region

"Below cartilage (chondr)"	"Upon stomach (gastr)"	"Below cartilage (chondr)"
"Loins (lumb)"	"Pit (umbilic)"	"Loins (lumb)"
"Flank (ili)"	"Below stomach (gastr)"	"Flank (ili)"

Transverse ("turning across") planes

Chondr ("cartilage")
Gastr
Umbilicus
Ileum

Vertical planes   Vertical planes

Information Frame

378 The **abdomen** (**AB**-doh-**men**) is the "trunk midsection," but it is represented by the root **abdomin** (ab-**DAHM**-in) for most word-building purposes.

---

abdomin/al (ab-**DAHM**-ih-nal)

379 Extract the suffix from umbilical and construct _____ /____, "referring to the trunk midsection."

---

abdomen
abdominal
umbilical

380 The _____ (trunk midsection) is artificially demarcated into nine different _____ areas. Of these, the _____ (pit) area is the most centrally located.

---

lumbar (**LUM**-bar)

381 Figure 5.7 reveals that the central umbilical region of the abdomen is bordered on either side by a _____ region.

---

lumb/ar

382 Lumbar is correctly subdivided as _____ /____, keeping in mind that its suffix, -**ar**, is treated just like -**al** and means "pertaining to."

---

lumb

383 The root in lumbar is _____, which means "loins," the lower back area.

---

lumbar	**384** When a physician carries out a _____ puncture, a needle is inserted through the loins (lower back) and into the spine for withdrawing fluid.
ili (**IHL**-ee)	**385** Inferior and lateral to the umbilicus on either side is the **ilium** (**IL**-ee-um), or "flank." The suffix in this word is **-um**, which has the same meaning as **-us** in umbilicus **(frame 374)**. The root in ilium is _____.
ili/ac (**IHL**-ee-ak)	**386** *Ili* usually takes **-ac** as its "pertaining to" ending. Therefore, _____ /____ literally "pertains to the flank."
iliac	**387** The right and left _____ regions of the abdomen can be seen in Figure 5.7 as flanking either side of the **hypogastric** (**high**-poh-**GAS**-trik) region.
gastr/ic (**GAS**-trik)	**388** **Gastr/o** (**GAS**-troh) is a root/cv for "stomach." Just as cephalic **(frame 362)** "pertains to the head," _____ /____ "pertains to the stomach."
hypo/gastr/ic	**389** This knowledge helps you to understand hypogastric, dissected as _____ / _____ /____.
pertaining to (the region) below the stomach	**390** The prefix in hypogastric has the same meaning as it does in hypochondria **(frame 114)**. Hypogastric thus literally translates to mean "_____ _____ (the region) _____ _____ _____."
hypogastric	**391** Looking back at Figure 5.7 should allow you to see that the _____ region does lie considerably below the stomach, and also below the umbilical region.
epi/gastr/ic	**392** A term related to hypogastric is **epigastric** (**eh**-pih-**GAS**-trik). This term is analyzed with slashes as _____ / _____ /____.
epi-	**393** Reference back to **frame 366** shows that _____, the prefix in epigastric, means "upon."
pertaining to (the region) upon the stomach	**394** Epigastric literally means "_____ _____ (the region) _____ _____ _____."
epigastric	**395** A final glance at Figure 5.7 justifies the term _____, because of its abdominal location immediately upon the stomach.

abdomen

396 Figure 5.7 and the last few frames all focused on one major body area, the _____ (trunk midsection). Pronounce the following names for other major body areas:
thorax (THOR-aks)—"chest"
pelvis (PEL-vis)—bony "bowl" of the hips
vertebrae (VER-teh-bree)—the "backbones"

thorax
pelvis
vertebrae

397 The root for _____ ("chest") is **thorac (THOR**-ak). The one for _____ ("bony bowl") is **pelv (PELV)**. The root for _____ ("backbones") is **vertebr.**

thorac/ic (thor-AS-ik)
pelv/ic (PEL-vic)
vertebr/al (ver-**TEE**-bral)

398 Use the suffix in epigastric to form _____ / _____ "pertaining to the chest" and _____ / _____ for "referring to the bowl." The ending in abdominal allows us to build _____ / _____ for "pertaining to the backbones."

dorsal
cranial
vertebral

399 The terms in the preceding frame, as well as some of those in earlier frames, can be used to name various body cavities. Some of these cavities are displayed in Figure 5.8. Note that the large _____ cavity in the "back" consists of two smaller cavities: the _____ cavity within the "skull" and the _____ canal located within the "backbones."

FIGURE 5.8   **Some Major Body Cavities**

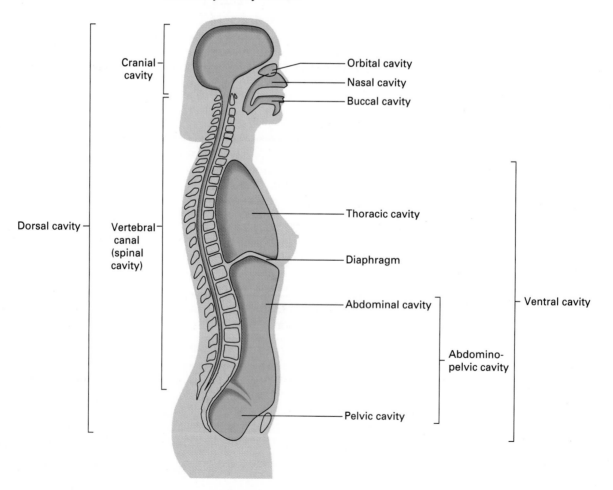

Cranial cavity

Orbital cavity
Nasal cavity
Buccal cavity

Dorsal cavity

Vertebral canal (spinal cavity)

Thoracic cavity

Diaphragm

Abdominal cavity

Ventral cavity

Abdomino-pelvic cavity

Pelvic cavity

ventral	**400** Another major cavity, the _____ cavity, is located on the "belly" side of the body and has several components. These are separated from one another by the **diaphragm** (**DIGH**-uh-**fram**)—a thin muscle that acts as a "barrier." The superior one is the _____ ("chest") cavity. Inferior ones are the _____ ("trunk midsection") and _____ ("bowl") cavities.
thoracic abdominal pelvic	

abdomin/o/pelv/ic (ab-**dahm**-ih-noh-**PEL**-vik)	**401** Observe from Figure 5.8 that there is no actual physical separation between the abdominal and pelvic cavities. Consequently the roots for the two names are often combined to create a compound word. The suffix of pelvic is added. This combination creates _____ /_____ /_____ /_____.

abdominopelvic	**402** The compound word _____ literally "pertains to the trunk midsection and the bowl."

abdominopelvic	**403** Injuries to the _____ area can very severely disrupt the function of various organs in the trunk midsection and bowl cavity between the hip bones.

pariet/al (pah-**RIGH**-eh-tal) **viscer/al** (**VIH**-ser-al)	**404** Whether we are considering the abdominopelvic or some other cavity, certain word parts are associated with cavities in general. Prominent among these are **pariet/o** (pah-**RIGH**-eh-toh), or "wall," and **viscer/o** (**VIH**-ser), for "guts" (internal organs). Extract the suffix of abdominal and build: "pertaining to wall" _____ /_____; "pertaining to guts" _____ /_____.

visceral	**405** The term _____ indicates a direction toward the "guts" or **viscer/a** (**VIH**-ser-ah), within a cavity. The noun viscera is a generic term referring to the internal organs.

viscera	**406** The internal organs, "guts," or _____ include **cysts (SISTS)**, "bladders" that are fluid-filled sacs. The **urinary bladder**, for instance, is a cyst.

parietal cysts	**407** The term _____ indicates a direction toward the wall of a body cavity. This term suggests movement away from any _____ (bladders) that may be present.

visceral parietal	**408** For example, one can say that a bullet passed in a _____ direction as it hit a cowboy in the stomach. However, the bullet penetrated all the way through the stomach and then traveled outward in a _____ direction, eventually exiting through the cowboy's back.

cyst/o/form (**SIST**-oh-**form**)

409   So far our discussion has primarily been centered on anatomy. In temporarily leaving this subject, we should be aware of the suffix **-form**. It means "resembling" or "in the shape of (something)." For instance, _____ /_____ /_____ , denotes something "in the shape of a bladder."

cystoform

410   A _____ structure will often look like a fluid-filled bladder on a roentgenogram.

physi/**o**/**logy**

411   Bladders are anatomical structures. Physiology, as you may remember **(frame 20)**, is body function and the study of body functions. It is subdivided as _____ /_____ /_____ **(frame 69).**

physi (**FIH**-zee)
study of
nature

412   The root in physiology is _____. It literally means "nature." Therefore physiology literally means the "_____ _____ _____."

physiology

413   The concept of "nature," however, is now far too broad to be accurate. Physiology involves body functions. We can then see _____ as the study of the "nature" of living things—the things that carry out functions.

bi-

414   The root **bi** indicates "life." (This is not to be confused with the prefix _____ in **frame 80**, which means "two.")

bi/o/logy (bigh-**AHL**-oh-jee)

415   Just as physiology is the "study of nature," _____ /_____ /_____ is the "study of life."

biology

416   The science of _____ commonly examines the physiology of living things.

physi/o/log/ical
(**fih**-zee-oh-**LAHJ**-ih-kal)
bi/o/log/**ical**
(**bigh**-oh-**LAHJ**-ih-kal)

417   Using the same suffix in anatomical **(frame 321)**, build _____ /_____ /_____ /_____ ("referring to the study of nature") and _____ /_____ /_____ /_____ ("referring to the study of life").

physiological
biological

418   Many _____ (functional) processes are expressed as word parts in the _____ (living) sciences.

constrict (kun-**STRIHKT**)
dilat (digh-**LAYT**)
-gen (**JEN**)
-genesis (**JEN**-eh-sis)
-o/rrhea (or-**EE**-uh)

419   Take a last look at the chapter word list and note these physiology-related entries:

_____   "narrow"
_____   "widen"
_____   "production; formation of"
_____   "production; formation of"
_____ /_____   "flow of; excessive flow of"

home/o
-stasis

home/o/**stasis**
(**hoh**-mee-oh-**STAY**-sis)

420 Related to the previous entries is the root _____ /_____ for "sameness or constancy" **(frame 88)** and the suffix _____ for "controlling or stopping" **(frame 99)**. Putting these word parts together yields _____ /_____ /_____.

homeostasis

421 Just as hemostasis **(frame 102)** denotes a "control of bleeding," _____ denotes a "control of sameness."

morbidity
mortality

422 Homeostasis represents a relative constancy or control of various aspects of the body's internal environment. We can usually look to disorders of homeostasis for most of the causes of _____ ("condition of illness," **frame 107**) and _____ ("condition of death," **frame 157**).

Multiple Choice

1. The brain is located in the _____ cavity.

   a. abdominal   b. cranial   c. thoracic   d. pelvic

2. The heart is located in the _____ cavity.

   a. abdominal   b. cranial   c. thoracic   d. pelvic

3. To describe an organ on the right side, use the term

   a. sinistral   b. lateral   c. medial   d. dextral

4. A sagittal plane divides the body into

   a. halves   b. front/back   c. left/right   d. top/bottom

5. The root exactly opposite in meaning to constrict is

   a. caud   b. crani   c. cephal   d. dilat

6. Abdominopelvic is a _____ word because it is composed of two roots.

   a. plural   b. noun   c. compound   d. singular

Meanings of Selected Roots

Add the correct combining vowel (cv) after each root. Then write the definition of each root in the space provided.

ROOT/CV   **DEFINITION**

1. vers/_____   _____

2. caud/_____   _____

3. dors/_____   _____

4. som/_____   _____

5. later/_____   _____

6. abdomin/_____ _____

7. intern/_____ _____

8. ventr/_____   _____

9. pelv/_____   _____

10. pariet/_____ _____

Word Dissection and Translation

Analyze the following terms by dissecting them with slashmarks and identifying their word parts. To the right of each term, write its correct English translation.

Key: R (root), cv (combining vowel), P (prefix), S (suffix)

1. anatomical

_____ / _____ / _____   _____
  P   R   S

2. anterior

_____ / ____ / _____   _____
    R   cv   S

3. transverse

_____ / _____ / _____   _____
  P   R   S

4. cranial

_____ / _____   _____
    R   S

5. inferior

_____ / ____ / _____   _____
    R   cv   S

6. cystoform

_____ / ____ / _____   _____
    R   cv   S

7. biology

_____ / ____ / _____   _____
    R   cv   S

8. physiological

_____ / ____ / _____ / _____   _____
    R   cv   R   S

9. visceral

_____ / _____   _____
    R   S

10. cephalic

_____ / _____   _____
    R   S

Terms and Their Abbreviations

In the list below, when the term is given, write its abbreviation in the space provided. When the abbreviation is given, write its corresponding term.

TERM	ABBREVIATION
1. anterior	_____
2. _____	A & P
3. anteroposterior	_____

Word Spelling

Look at each of the terms listed below. Identify those that are misspelled by circling Y for "Yes." Write the correct spelling in the blank.

WORD	MISSPELLED?	CORRECT SPELLING
1. meadeul	Y/N	_____
2. dorsal	Y/N	_____
3. sinistral	Y/N	_____
4. midsaggital	Y/N	_____
5. korohnal	Y/N	_____
6. thorassic	Y/N	_____
7. superior	Y/N	_____
8. umbilical	Y/N	_____
9. eeleac	Y/N	_____
10. inturnal	Y/N	_____
11. parasagittal	Y/N	_____
12. posteereor	Y/N	_____
13. abdominal	Y/N	_____
14. biolodgikal	Y/N	_____

New Word Synthesis

Using word parts that appear in this and previous chapters, build new terms with the following meanings:

1. _____ referring to (something) near a bladder
2. _____ the process of cutting a flank apart
3. _____ the study of internal organs
4. _____ pertaining to (something) around a bowl
5. _____ a barrier body
6. _____ the study of drugs and body functions
7. _____ pertaining to the stomach and intestines
8. _____ shaped like a navel
9. _____ in front of the intestine
10. _____ relating to a cutting across the chest

Read through the following partial autopsy report. Note the terms in bold print. A series of multiple choice questions probes your knowledge of these terms.

Autopsy Report

SUBJECT: Caucasian male, 5'11 ½", 115 lb

AGE: 84

CLINICAL DIAGNOSIS: After a **transverse** incision was made into the thoracic cavity, massive internal bleeding was noted due to rupture of a dissecting aneurysm (widening or dilation of a blood vessel). Clotted blood surrounds many viscera. A craniotomy was performed, and the **cephalic** region noted no abnormal pathology. Etiologic findings concluded a diagnosis of ruptured dissecting aortic aneurysm.

POSTMORTEM FINDINGS: **Thoracic** cavity—clotted blood surrounds many **viscera.**

Case Study Questions

1. A **transverse** incision means cutting

    (a) across.

    (b) in a curving direction.

    (c) vertically.

    (d) diagonally.

2. **Viscera** are the

    (a) abdominal organs.

    (b) internal organs.

    (c) cavity walls.

    (d) pelvic organs.

3. No abnormal pathology in the **cephalic** region means no disease

    (a) around the heart.

    (b) within the head.

    (c) at the base of the neck.

    (d) near the skull.

4. The **thoracic** cavity involves the

    (a) vertebrae.

    (b) cranium.

    (c) chest.

    (d) umbilicus.

CHAPTER 6 Cells and Oncology

INTRODUCTION

All body systems have something in common. Their basic individual units are cells. Cells represent the smallest living level of body organization. They are made up of even smaller **atoms** (such as hydrogen, **H,** and oxygen, **O**) and **molecules** (such as water, **H$_2$O**). Atoms and molecules are examples of **chemicals** (types of matter). Chemicals compose both cells and the fluid internal environment of the body that surrounds them. Therefore, this chapter includes some basic terms of **chemistry,** the study of matter and its reactions. Various atoms and molecules commonly found in the human body are depicted in Figure 6.1.

Although each cell is tinier than the head of a pin, it contains many important structures that keep it alive. Molecules are intricately arranged to create a number

---

FIGURE 6.1   **Some Common Atoms and Molecules in the Body**

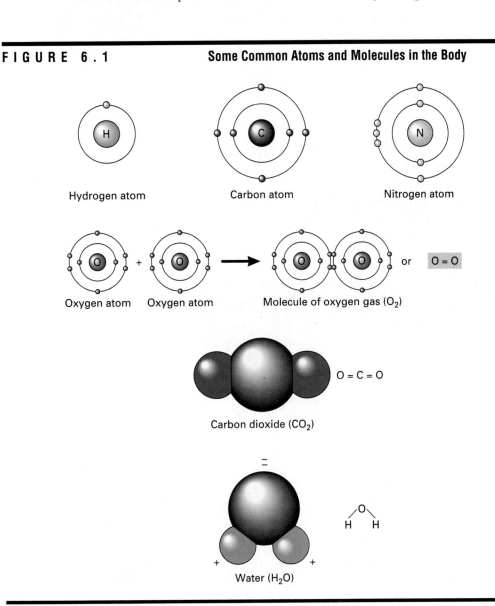

Hydrogen atom   Carbon atom   Nitrogen atom

Oxygen atom Oxygen atom   Molecule of oxygen gas (O$_2$)   or   O = O

O = C = O

Carbon dioxide (CO$_2$)

Water (H$_2$O)

of **organelles** (**or**-gan-**ELS**) within the cell. These organelles are miniature organlike structures that have their own specific functions. Figure 6.2 below provides a general view of cell anatomy and shows a number of organelles.

A basic understanding of normal anatomy and physiology of the cell is required before we can intelligently discuss various cell-based diseases. Two especially critical organelles are the **plasma membrane** (Figure 6.3) and the **centrioles** (**SEN**-tree-**ohlz**), shown enlarged in Figure 6.4.

F I G U R E   6 . 2   **A Basic Overview of Cell Anatomy**

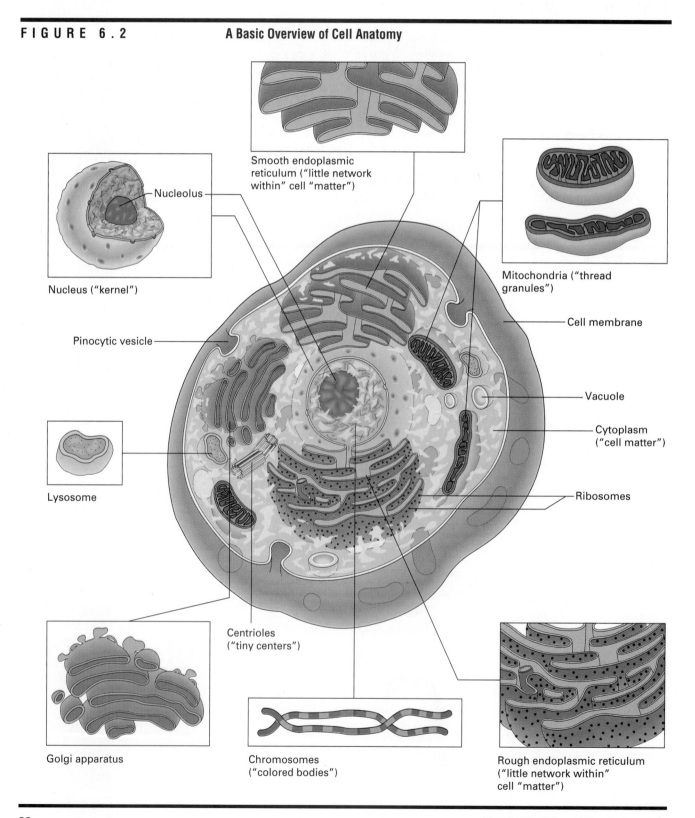

Smooth endoplasmic reticulum ("little network within" cell "matter")

Nucleolus

Nucleus ("kernel")

Pinocytic vesicle

Lysosome

Golgi apparatus

Centrioles ("tiny centers")

Chromosomes ("colored bodies")

Mitochondria ("thread granules")

Cell membrane

Vacuole

Cytoplasm ("cell matter")

Ribosomes

Rough endoplasmic reticulum ("little network within" cell "matter")

FIGURE 6.3

The Cell (Plasma) Membrane

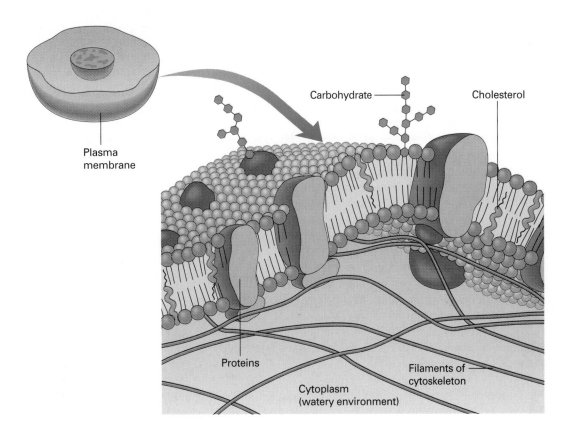

The plasma membrane, also called the **cell membrane,** is the thin envelope around each individual body cell. In Figure 6.3 you can see some of the types of molecules that make up the plasma membrane. The names of these molecules will become more understandable as you progress through the chapter. The plasma membrane (cell membrane) limits the size of the cell and determines what particles are able to enter or leave the cell. Any drugs or other therapies must be able to cross the plasma membrane, or at least interact with it, if they are going to have any direct effect on cellular (**SEL**-yoo-**lar**) **physiology.**

FIGURE 6.4

An Enlarged View of the Centrioles

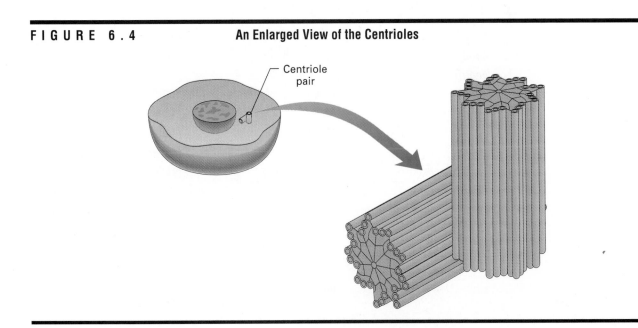

The centrioles are a pair of tiny bodies composed of bright central cores surrounded by nine rows of **microtubules** (**migh**-kroh-**TOO**-byools)—hollow "little tubes." The microtubules act like guidewires for the **chromosomes** (**KROH**-moh-**sohmz**)—dark "colored" wormlike "bodies" that contain most of the cell's hereditary material. The chromosomes migrate along the guiding microtubles of the centrioles as the cell undergoes division.

Cell division, when normal, serves to replace dead or damaged cells and to provide additional cells during body growth. When abnormal, cell division results in tumors. Abnormal cell growth involves the discipline of **oncology** (ahn-**KAHL**-oh-**jee**) and its related terms.

In summary, this chapter presents terms related to normal anatomy, physiology, and chemistry of the cell; terms related to cell disease; terms associated with lab tests and diagnoses involving cells; and terms describing surgery, pharmacology, and other therapies at the cellular level.

CHAPTER OBJECTIVES

By the end of this chapter, you should be able to:

1 Identify major prefixes, roots, suffixes, abbreviations, and symbols related to the cell.

2 Dissect cellular terms into their component parts.

3 Translate cellular terms into their common English equivalents.

4 Build new terms associated with the cell.

Word Parts Associated with Normal Anatomy, Physiology, and Chemistry of the Cell

The following is a list of common word parts and abbreviations associated with the normal structure, function, and chemistry of cells. Use this list to help you complete **frames 423 to 526.**

carb/o	carbon; charcoal	**ER**	endoplasmic reticulum	**molecul/o**	little mass
cellul/o	little cell			**organ/o**	carbon or organs
centr/i	central	extra-	outside		
chrom/o	colored; color	**gen/o**	gene; produce; form	**osm/o**	thrust
cyt/o	cell	**gluc/o**	sugar; sweet	**perme/o**	cross through
de-	down; away from	**glyc/o**	sugar; sweet	**phag/o**	eat
deoxy-	lacking an oxygen atom	**ICF**	intracellular fluid	**phosph/o**	phosphorus
		-icle	small	**plasm/o**	matter
diffus/o	scatter	**lip/o**	fat	**ribo**	ribose
DNA	deoxyribonucleic acid	**macr/o**	large	**RNA**	ribonucleic acid
		mei/o	lessening; reduction	**scop**	examine; appear
ECF	extracellular fluid			semi-	partial; half
electr/o	electric	**micr/o**	tiny; small	**solubl**	dissolved
endo-	inner; inside	**mit/o**	thread	**ton/o**	strength

cellul/**ar**	**423** A "cell" or "little cell" in general is indicated by the root **cellul** (**SEL**-yool). This root commonly takes the adjectival ending of lumbar (**frame 382**) to become _____ /_____ ("pertaining to little cells").
cellular soma	**424** Normal _____ ("little cell") anatomy and physiology is the basis for human survival. This is true because the _____ (**frame 315**) or major portion of the human "body" consists of trillions of living cells. To a very large extent, then, if these cells are healthy, the entire body is healthy.
scop/**e** scop	**425** One way of checking on the health of cells is to examine them. Recall (**frame 177**) that a _____ /_____ in general is "an instrument used to examine (something)." The root here, _____, also means "appear."
small	**426** Some things are "large" or **macr/o** (**MAH**-kroh); others are the exact opposite—"_____," or **micr/o** (**MIGH**-kroh).
micr/o/scop/e (**MIGH**-kroh-**skohp**)	**427** A special "instrument used to examine small (things)" is called a _____ /_____ /_____ /_____.
microscope	**428** Since human cells are too small to be examined with the naked eye, they must be studied under a _____.
scop/ic (**SKAHP**-ik)	**429** The root for "examine" or "appear" usually takes the "referring to" suffix of abdominopelvic (**frame 401**). This results in _____ /_____, "referring to appearance."
micr/o/scop/ic (**migh**-kroh-**SKAHP**-ik) **macr/o/scop/ic** (**MA**-kroh-**skahp**-ik)	**430** Now bring together the information of the last few frames to help you build _____ /_____ /_____ /_____, "referring to (things) that appear small," and _____ /_____ /_____ /_____, "referring to (things) that appear large."
microscopic macroscopic	**431** The cell organelles are all _____, since they are too small to be seen with the naked eye. The major body organs (such as the heart), however, are all _____, since they are large enough to be seen with the unaided eye.
a/tom tom **molecul/e**	**432** The atoms and molecules represent some of the smallest levels of organization within the cell. The term _____ /_____ means "not cuttable," where the prefix, **a-**, and the root for "cut," _____ (**frame 89**), are used. **Molecul/o** (mah-**LEK-yoo**-loh), in contrast, means "little mass." Consequently, _____ /_____ is literally "a little mass," where the suffix of microscope is adopted.

atoms

433 The _____ received their name because the early Greeks believed they were the most fundamental, "uncuttable" particles of matter. One such particle is **carbon,** denoted by the root **carb (KARB).**

molecule

434 One carbon atom may combine with another carbon (or some other type of atom) to create a _____ ("little mass").

atoms

435 A molecule, then, is a combination of two or more _____ held together by chemical bonds.

H
O

436 An example of a molecule is water, symbolized as H_2O. This symbolic formula indicates that a single water molecule consists of two ____ (hydrogen) atoms and one ____ (oxygen) atom, held together by chemical bonds.

437 Provided below are some additional symbols and names for several types of atoms and molecules found in the body.

Symbol/Formula	Name of Atom/Molecule
$C_6H_{12}O_6$	glucose (**GLOO**-kohs)
CO_2	carbon dioxide (digh-**AHK**-sighd)
O_2	oxygen (molecule)
N	nitrogen
P	phosphorus (**FAHS**-for-**us**)
S	sulfur

a/tom/ic (uh-**TAHM**-ik)
molecul/ar (mah-**LEK**- yoo-lar)

438 Atom takes the same "referring to" suffix as macroscopic, while molecul assumes the ending of cellular (**frame 423).** Thus we can build: ____ / _____ / ____ "referring to atoms or uncuttable particles" and _____ / ____ "referring to molecules or little masses."

atomic
molecular

439 The preceding table shows both _____ symbols for individual chemical particles and _____ formulas for groups of atoms held together by chemical bonds.

glucose
N

440 For instance, the molecular formula for _____ is $C_6H_{12}O_6$. The atomic symbol for nitrogen is _____ .

hydr

441 Glucose is a type of **carb/o/hydr/ate** (**kar**-boh-**HIGH-drayt**). Perhaps you can identify the root for "water" here as _____, as in hydrotherapy **(frame 288).**

carbohydrate

C (carbon)
H₂O (water)

442 Literally speaking, then, a _____ is "something that (contains) carbon and water." This chemical grouping can indeed be symbolized as **C(H_2O)**—as equal numbers of _____ atoms and _____ molecules.

carbohydrates	**443** The _____ are carbon-containing molecules that include glucose and other simple sugars. They play a major role as a source of body fuel.
pertaining to organs	**444** **Organ/ic** (or-**GAN**-ik) translates as "_____ ____ _____," but it also means "pertaining to carbon."
organ/ic in/**organ**/ic (**in**-or-**GAN**-ik)	**445** The **i**-beginning prefix in-, like a-, means "not or without." Since _____ /____ "pertains to (having) carbon," ____ /_____ /____ "pertains to not (having) carbon."
organic inorganic	**446** Carbohydrates are considered _____ molecules because they contain carbon atoms. Water is classified as _____ because its molecules contain no carbon atoms.
lip (**LIP**)	**447** Two other major categories of organic molecules are the **lipids** (**LIP**-ids) and **proteins** (**PROH**-teens). The root in lipid, _____, means "fat."
lipids	**448** The _____ are a group of organic molecules that include the "fats."
-ity	**449** Lipids are named for their **solubility** (**sahl**-yoo-**BIL**-ih-tee), that is, for their _____ ("condition or ability") to be "dissolved" (solubl).
in/**solubl**/e (in-**SAHL**-yoo-buhl)	**450** Lipids are **solubl/e** (**SAHL**-yoo-buhl), or "dissolvable," in electrically uncharged chemicals. These same substances are ____ /_____ /____, or "not dissolvable," in electrically charged chemicals, such as water.
lipids insoluble carbohydrates soluble	**451** The _____ ("fat" family) are organic molecules that are _____ ("not dissolvable") in water. Conversely, most of the _____, such as glucose, are readily _____ ("dissolvable") in water.
Information Frame	**452** Some lipids combine with phosphorus and oxygen. A combining form for phosphorus is **phosph/o** (**FAHS**-foh).
phosph/o/lip/ids (**FAHS**-foh-**lip**-ids)	**453** The _____ /____ /_____ /_____ are a group of "lipids" that contain "phosphorus" and oxygen.
phospholipids insoluble	**454** The plasma membrane surrounding the cell is largely composed of _____ ("phosphorus-containing lipids"). The lipid portions of these molecules are _____ ("not dissolvable") in water.

455 Besides carbohydrates and lipids, a third group of organic molecules are the _____ **(frame 477)**. Their name derives from the Greek **protos,** "first."

proteins

---

456 This name may reflect the fact that _____ were some of the first and most important molecules to appear on earth. These large nitrogen-containing organic molecules are readily _____ ("dissolvable") in water.

proteins

soluble

---

457 Some chemicals are not really proteins. They just resemble them. Such chemicals are described as _____ / _____ ("proteinlike" or "protein-resembling"), much as thyroid **(frame 93)** is described as "shieldlike."

protein/oid (PROH-ten-oyd)

---

458 Some scientists speculate that warm pools of _____ ("protein-resembling") substances may have preceded actual proteins on earth, far before life appeared.

proteinoid

---

459 Using the root in biology **(frame 415)** and the suffix in biological **(frame 417),** create a term that "refers to the chemicals of life": ____ / ____ / _____ / _____.

bi/o/chem/icals (bigh-oh-KEM-ih-kals)

---

460 Carbohydrates, lipids, and proteins are all considered _____, since these chemicals occur largely in living things.

biochemicals

---

461 Some _____ ("chemicals of life") are soluble in water; others are not. Both **solv (SAHLV)** and **solut (SAHL-yoot)** mean "dissolve," and they appear in such terms as:

biochemicals

solv/ent (SAHL-vent)	"one that dissolves"
solut/e	"thing that is being dissolved"
solut/ion	"the act or process of dissolving"

---

462 A _____ is a liquid "that dissolves" solid particles of _____ ("thing that is being dissolved"). A _____ is the mixture formed by the "dissolving process." In other words, the solution is created by the dissolving action of the liquid solvent on the particles of solute.

solvent
solute
solution

---

463 The sodium chloride **(NaCl)** crystal, for instance, is considered a _____ when it is being dissolved by water.

solute

electr	**464** NaCl solute is generally classified as an **electrolyte** (ee-**LEK**-troh-**light**). The suffix is the same as in solute. It will also be good to recall that _____ **(frame 216)** is a root for "electrical current." Analyze electrolyte by inserting slashmarks:
electr/o/lyt/**e**	_____ / _____ / _____ / _____ .

lyt	**465** The second root in electrolyte, _____, means "breakdown." An electrolyte is a substance that "breaks down" into ions in water solvent and is capable of conducting an "electrical current."

electrolyte Na$^+$ Cl$^-$ solution	**466** NaCl is a common _____. When dissolved by water solvent, it is broken down into individual _____ and _____ ions. The negatively charged electrons within an electrical current are attracted to all positively charged ions. This attraction allows the electrons to be conducted through the NaCl-H$_2$O _____. (Consult Figure 6.5.)

FIGURE 6.5   **Electrolytes and Solutions**

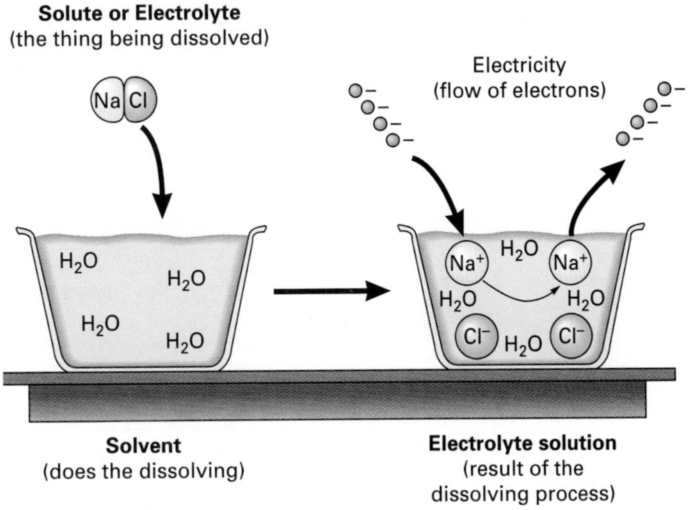

Solute or Electrolyte
(the thing being dissolved)

Electricity
(flow of electrons)

Solvent
(does the dissolving)

Electrolyte solution
(result of the
dissolving process)

	467 In addition to their ability to conduct an electrical current, solutions can also be classified according to their **tonicity** (**toh-NIH**-sih-tee). That is, they are classified according to the "strength (concentration)" of their solute. Looking back at the word list, note that a root for "strength" is
ton (**TOHN**)	_____ .

ton/**ic** (**TAHN**-ik)	**468** Adopt the suffix in atomic **(frame 438)** to build _____ / _____ , "pertaining to (solute) strength." Observe and pronounce each of the terms below involving solute "strength":
	isotonic (**igh**-so-**TAHN**-ik)
	hypotonic (**high**-poh-**TAHN**-ik)
	hypertonic (**high**-per-**TAHN**-ik)
	Each term can be analyzed on the basis of its prefix.

iso- (**IGH**-soh) iso/ton/ic	**469** The chapter word list tells you that _____ is a prefix for "same or equal." Therefore, _____ / _____ / ____ literally "pertains to equal strength (of solute)."
hypo- hyper-	**470** The prefix _____ (as in hypoalgesia, **frame 130**) means "below normal or deficient," while _____ (as in hyperalgesia, **frame 130**) means "above normal or excessive."
hyper/ton/ic hypo/ton/ic	**471** Following a pattern as for isotonic allows us to create: _____ / _____ / ____, "referring to an excessive strength or concentration (of solute)," and _____ / _____ / ____, "referring to a deficient strength or concentration (of solute)."
within extra- intra/cellul/ar (**in**-trah-**SEL**-yoo-lar) extra/cellul/ar (**eks**-trah-**SEL**-yoo-lar)	**472** You may remember that intra- **(frame 366)** is a prefix meaning "_____". Its opposite, _____, means "outside." Use this information to build: _____ / _____ / ____, "pertaining to (something) within little cells," and _____ / _____ / ____ "pertaining to (something) outside little cells."
intracellular fluid ECF	**473** The _____ _____, or ICF, is the "fluid within cells." Conversely, the extracellular fluid, or____ ____ ____, is the "fluid outside cells."
isotonic hypotonic hypertonic	**474** A solution is described as _____ if its concentration of solute is equal to that within the normal intracellular fluid. It is called _____ if its concentration of solute is less and _____ if its concentration of solute is greater than that of normal ICF.
extracellular	**475** The tonicity of _____("outside cells") solutions is depicted in Figure 6.6.

FIGURE 6.6

The Tonicity of Solutions

Hypertonic solution
(more particles outside cell)

Hypotonic solution
(fewer particles outside cell)

Isotonic solution
(equal particles inside
and outside cell)

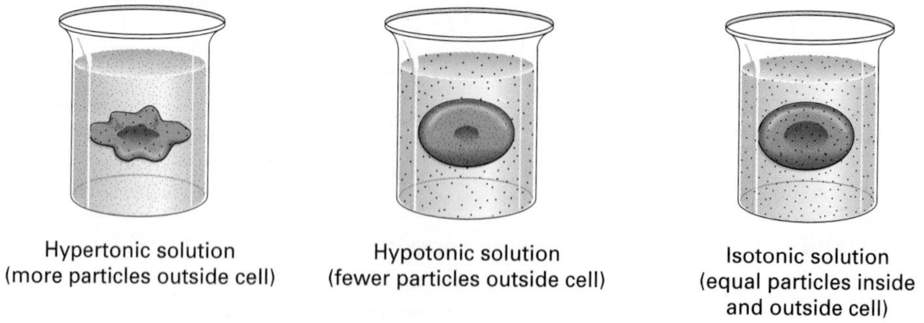

perme/ate -ate	**476** The tonicity of solutions is important because water and various solutes can **permeate** (**PER**-mee-**ate**), or "cross through," the cell membrane. You can subdivide permeate as _____ / _____, if you recall that _____ is the suffix (as in carbohydrate, **frame 441**).

permeate	**477** Water molecules can _____ ("cross through") the plasma membrane by moving through its small channels called pores.
perme/able (**PER**-mee-**ah**-buhl)	**478** If something is _____ /_____, it has the "ability to cross through," that is, permeate. The cell membrane often is said to be **selectively permeable.** It allows some substances to pass through it, others not to pass.
semi- **semi**/**perme**/able (**sem**-ee-**PER**-mee-ah-buhl)	**479** Chapter 2 **(frame 81)** spoke of four prefixes of proportion. Three of these, _____, **demi**-, and **hemi**-, indicate "partial or half." Use the **s**-beginning prefix to help you build _____ /_____ /_____, "partially able to cross through."
semipermeable	**480** The cell membrane, being _____, allows small particles, such as water molecules, ions, and small molecules to cross through it. Very large particles, such as proteins, however, usually cannot pass.
-ion	**481** **Osm/o** (**AHZ**-moh) is a root/cv for "thrusting," while **diffus** (dih-**FYOOZ**) is a root for "scattering." The first root takes the "condition of" suffix -o/sis. The second root adopts _____, the suffix in the word solution **(frame 461)**.
osm/o/sis (ahz-**MOH**-sis) **diffus**/ion (dih-**FYOO**-zhun)	**482** Use the above information to create _____ /____ /_____, a "condition of thrusting," and _____ /_____, a "process of scattering."
osmosis hypotonic permeate	**483** The term _____ reflects the occurrence of thrusting, pressure, or pushing when large numbers of water molecules are moving together in a particular direction. In a _____ ("low concentration of solute") solution, for instance, many water molecules _____ ("cross through") the plasma membrane, causing the cell to push out and swell.
diffusion	**484** The term _____ denotes the scattering of particles in general from an area where their concentration is high, to an area where their concentration is low.
phag/o/**cyt**/o/sis (**fay**-goh-sigh-**TOH**-sis)	**485** Some particles are simply too large to enter cells by diffusion or osmosis. The cell may just go ahead and eat them! The combining form **phag/o** (**FAY**-goh) means "eat," while **cyt/o** (**SIGH**-toh) denotes "cell." With the suffix -osis we obtain _____ /____ /_____ /____ /_____, a "condition of cell eating."

phagocytosis	**486** Certain cells in the human body actually engage in _____, engulfing **bacteria** (bak-**TEER**-ee-uh) and various other foreign invaders.
macr/o **macr/o/phag/e** (**MAH**-kroh-**fayj**)	**487** Using the combining form _____ /____ for "large," the root for "eat," and the "presence of" suffix in *solute,* we get _____ /____ /_____ /____ . This is literally a "large eating (cell)." Pronounce macrophage, noting the **"g" rule (frame 73).**
macrophages phagocytosis	**488** Special large cells called _____ can be on the prowl in human connective tissues. They carry out _____, engulfing any foreign invaders or cell debris that they encounter.
cyt/o/plasm cyt	**489** Once particles are taken into the cell, they enter the **cytoplasm** (**SIGH**-toh-**plaz**-im), or "cell matter." This term is subdivided as _____ /____ /_____ , with _____ being its root for "cell."
cytoplasm	**490** This _____ is actually a complex gel-like "matter" including both intracellular fluid and an intricate network of rods and tubes within the "cell."
cyt/o/plasm/ic (**sigh**-toh-**PLAZ**-mik)	**491** Cytoplasm is used as a noun. By adding the suffix in organic **(frame 444),** we can construct _____ /____ /_____ /____ , which literally "refers to cell matter."
cytoplasmic	**492** The _____ region within the boundaries of the cell surrounds and separates many of the organelles.
centr/i/oles (**SEN**-tree-ohlz)	**493** Organelles by definition are "little." Two suffixes indicating small size are **-icle** (**IHK**-el) and **-ole** (**OHL**). **Centr/i** (**SEN**-tree) is a combining form for "central." Here the combining vowel is **i.** Use this root plus **-oles** to create _____ /____ /_____ , literally "tiny centers."
centrioles	**494** You may recall from the Introduction that _____ are organelles that act as "tiny centers" for cell division, splitting apart to form a plate for the chromosomes.
chrom/o/som/e som **chrom (KROHM)**	**495** Chromosome is subdivided as _____ /____ /_____ /____ . Note the presence of _____ , a root for "body" **(frame 314).** The other root, _____ **(frame 87),** means "color" or "colored."
chromosomes	**496** The _____ are "colored bodies" that resemble worms within the nucleus of the cell. During cell division, when the nucleus disintegrates, these colored bodies line up along a network of microtubules involving the centrioles.

mit/o/sis (migh-**TOH**-sis)

mei/o/sis (migh-**OH**-sis)

497 The two basic kinds of cell division are indicated by the roots **mit (MIGHT)** for "thread" and **mei (MIGH)** for "lessening." So _____ /_____ /_____ is a "condition of threads," the "threads" being the chromosomes. A "condition of lessening" is _____ /_____ /_____ .

---

meiosis

498 In _____ (mitosis/meiosis) the number of chromosomes per cell is reduced by one-half after cell division takes place; hence the name.

---

mitosis

499 In _____ (mitosis/meiosis) the number of chromosomes ("threads" visible under a microscope) is not reduced in the cell after division. (Mitosis and meiosis are diagrammatically compared in Figure 6.7.)

FIGURE 6.7

Mitosis versus Meiosis

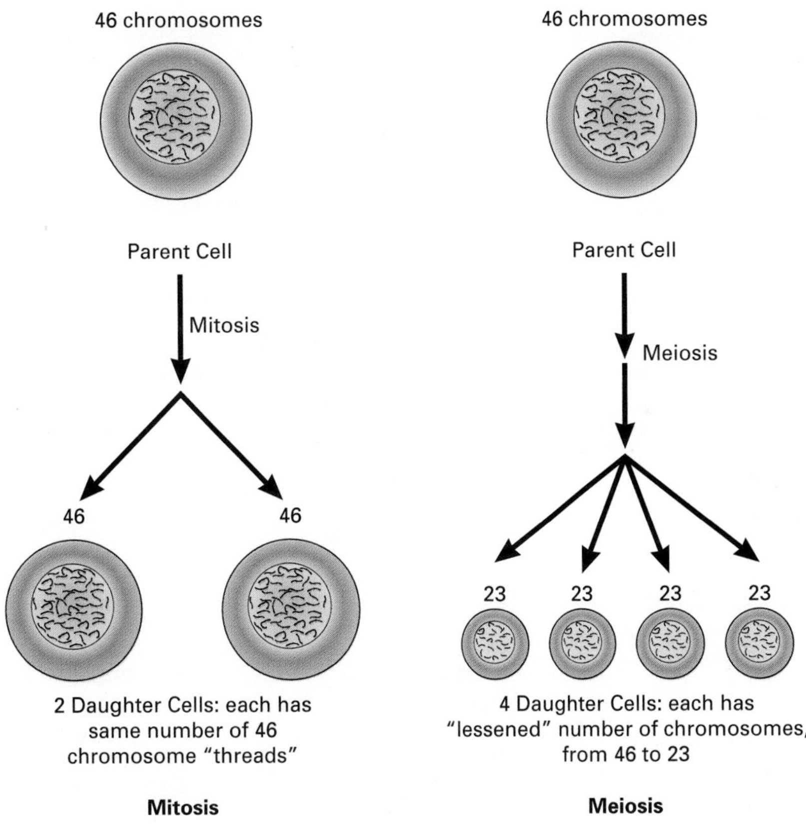

46 chromosomes

Parent Cell

Mitosis

46   46

2 Daughter Cells: each has same number of 46 chromosome "threads"

Mitosis

46 chromosomes

Parent Cell

Meiosis

23   23   23   23

4 Daughter Cells: each has "lessened" number of chromosomes, from 46 to 23

Meiosis

---

gen
genet (jeh-**NET**)

500 Each of the chromosomes affected by cell division contains a number of **genes (JEENS)**. The root in this case is _____ . Another root with the same meaning, "produce," is _____, extracted from **genetic (jeh-NET**-ik).

-gen

501 Both gen/o and genet/o mean "produce or production," as does the three-letter suffix _____ **(frame 419).**

| genes | 502 The _____ are the components of chromosomes largely responsible for "producing" proteins. |

| genet/ic | 503 Look at the term **genetic** (**jeh-NET**-ik). Subdivide this term with slashmarks:_____ /_____ . |

| genetic | 504 The genes serve as a _____ ("pertaining to producing") code for protein synthesis in the cell. |

| deoxyribonucleic acid
ribonucleic acid | 505 Genes are actually sections along a **deoxyribonucleic** (de-**ahk**-see-righ-boh-noo-**KLEE**-ik) **acid** molecule. Their code is interpreted by **ribonucleic** (**righ**-boh-noo-**KLEE**-ik) **acid** molecules during protein synthesis. **DNA** is an abbreviation for _____ _____ . RNA is an abbreviation for _____ _____ . |

| deoxyribo
ribo | 506 Observe that the **D** in DNA stands for _____ , while the **R** in RNA stands for _____ . |

| **oxy**
de/**oxy** | 507 The prefix de- means "away from." The root for the element **oxygen** (**O**) is _____ . Then _____ /_____ means "an oxygen atom is taken away from." Guess what deoxyribo means. (Examine Figure 6.8 carefully. How do the two molecules differ?) |

FIGURE 6.8

Ribose versus Deoxyribose

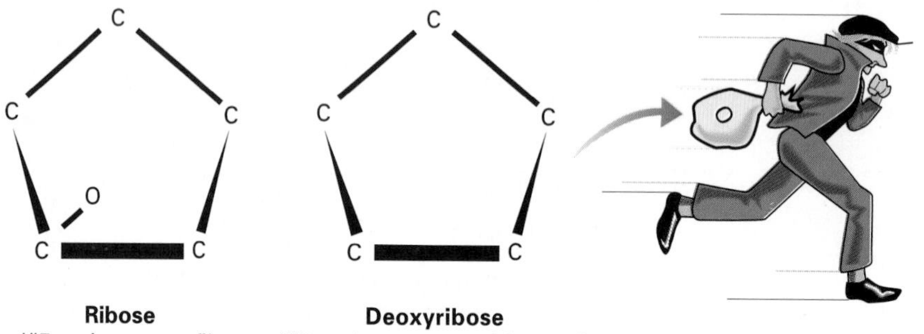

Ribose
("5-carbon sugar")
$C_5H_{10}O_5$

Deoxyribose
("5-carbon sugar with one O taken away")
$C_5H_{10}O_4$

| de/oxy/rib/o
oxygen
away from
ribose | 508 Analyze deoxyribo: _____ /_____ /_____ /_____ . Deoxyribo means "an _____ atom is taken _____ _____ the _____ ." |

| ribose | 509 Figure 6.8 tells you that ribo represents _____ , a particular 5-carbon organic sugar. |

RNA DNA	**510** Whereas the _____ (DNA/RNA) molecule contains the sugar ribose, the _____ (DNA/RNA) molecule contains the sugar deoxyribose.
nucle/**us** **-us**	**511** Both DNA and RNA are "acids" **(A)** found within the "nucleus" **(N).** Nucleus is dissected as _____ /_____ . Its "presence of" suffix, _____ , is the one also ending umbilicus **(frame 374).**
nuclei nuclei	**512** Chapter 3 **(frame 207)** spoke of atomic _____ ("kernels"). In this chapter we speak of cellular _____ ("kernels").
nucleus	**513** Each cellular _____ ("kernel present") contains the cell's chromosomes and most of its DNA.
nucle/**ar** nucle/**ic**	**514** **Frame 206** used _____ /_____ for "referring to a kernel." In the case of DNA and RNA, "referring to a kernel" takes the suffix of genetic. Hence, one speaks of the _____ /_____ acids DNA and RNA.
nucleic	**515** Proteins are produced under the direction of the _____ acids—in particular, segments of DNA comprising genes.
-um	**516** As new proteins are synthesized, they are circulated throughout a "little network" in the cell. **Reticul** (reh-**TIK**-yool) is a root for "little network." It usually takes _____ as its "presence of" suffix, as occurs in ilium **(frame 385).**
reticul/um (reh-TIK-yoo-lum)	**517** Use the information in the preceding frame to help you build _____ /_____ , "a little network." The **ul** in reticulum means "little."
plasm	**518** The prefix endo- **(EN**-doh) means "within." Further, note that _____ , a root in cytoplasm **(frame 489),** means "matter." This root follows the suffix pattern of nucleic.
endo/plasm/ic (en-doh-**PLAZ**-mik)	**519** The term _____ /_____ /_____ "pertains to (something) within matter."
endoplasmic reticulum	**520** Combining the facts of the three preceding frames results in _____ _____ , "a little network present within matter."
ER	**521** The endoplasmic reticulum, abbreviated as ____ ____ , is actually a network of tiny passageways that circulates proteins and other cell products throughout the cytoplasm.

glyc/o/gen (GLIGH-koh-jen)

522 Making proteins requires energy. Much of this energy comes from the breakdown of simple sugars, such as glucose. Glucose tastes sweet. **Glyc (GLIGHK)** means "sweet" or "sugar." Thus _____ /____ /_____ translates as "sweetness producer," where -gen is the suffix.

glycogen

523 A stored form of sugar, _____, is readily broken down into simple glucose, thereby "producing sweetness." This free glucose is then broken down.

thread

mit/o/chondr/i/on (migh-toh-KAHN-dree-uhn)

524 Much of the energy released from the breakdown of glucose is produced by the **mit/o/chondr/i/a (migh-toh-KAHN-dree-uh).** Remember that mit **(frame 497)** means "_____." Chondr **(KAHN-der),** introduced as "cartilage" **(frame 114),** also means "granule." So a _____ /____ /_____ /____ /____ is "a thread granule," where the "presence of" suffix is **-on**

mitochondrion

mitochondrion

525 A _____ is an energy-producing organelle. Mitochondria (the plural of mitochondrion) have different shapes. Some are thin like "threads"; others are rounded like "granules." (A glance back at Figure 6.2 will show this characteristic of the _____, or "thread granule.")

mitochondria

526 Energy produced by many _____ (mitochondrion/mitochondria) is constantly being used by cells, whether these cells are normal or diseased.

Diseases

Word Parts Associated with Disease at the Cellular Level

The following is a list of word parts associated with disease at the cellular level. Use this list to help you complete **frames 527 to 574.**

bacill/o	rod-shaped	**microbi/o**	tiny living creature	**sarc/o**	connective tissue
benign	nonspreading				
carcin/o	cancer	neo-	new	**staphyl/o**	bunch of grapes
cocc/o	berry-shaped	-oma	tumor of	**strept/o**	curved
dipl/o	double	**path/o**	disease	**theli**	nipples
lys/o	breakdown	**plas/o**	formation	**thel/o**	nipples
meta-	after; beyond	-plasm	growth; development	**vir/o**	poison

pathogen

527 A **path/o/gen (PATH-oh-jen)** is a "disease producer." Almost any disease-producing agent, whether it is chemical (like a poison), physical (like a burn), or biological (like an infecting organism), can be considered a _____ for body cells.

path/o/gen/ic (path-oh-JEN-ik)

528 Just as ton/ic **(frame 468)** "refers to (solute) strength," _____ /____ /_____ /____ "refers to production of disease."

pathogens pathogenic	**529** Cells can be "sick" because they are being attacked by foreign _____ or because they suffer some _____ abnormality of their own functions.
noun adjective	**530** In the preceding frame, pathogens acts as a(n) _____ (noun/verb/adjective), while pathogenic behaves as a(n) _____ (noun/verb/adjective).
microbi/al (migh-KROH-bee-uhl)	**531** Human cells are often attacked by **microbes** (**MIGH**-krohbs)—"tiny living" organisms. **Microbi** means "tiny life." Adding the suffix in visceral **(frame 404)** results in _____ /_____.
microbial	**532** Some _____ ("tiny living") agents are pathogenic and occur in a number of types. Probably the best known are the **bacteria** (**bak-TEER**-ee-uh) and the **viruses** (**VIGH**-rus-es).
vir/**us**	**533** Virus is subdivided as _____ /_____, with its ending being the same as in nucleus **(frame 511).**
vir (VIGHR)	**534** The root in virus, _____, actually means "poison." Viruses invade human cells and use them to grow and reproduce. When the cells are bulging with viruses, they break down and die, as if they had been "poisoned."
vir/al (VIGH-ral)	**535** We can build_____ /_____ for "pertaining to poison," much as we built microbial for "pertaining to tiny living" organisms.
viral	**536** Infections that are _____ (due to viruses) are difficult to treat. This is because viruses are not clearly alive. Rather, they exist on the foggy border between life and nonliving superchemicals.
viral virus	**537** The term _____ (viral/virus) is an adjective, modifying other words. The term _____ (viral/virus) is a noun, standing alone.
lyt/o	**538** **Lys/o** (**LIGH**-soh), like _____ /_____ within electrolyte **(frame 465),** means "breakdown."
lys/is (LIGH-sis)	**539** Using **-is** as the "presence of" suffix yields _____ /_____, "a breakdown."
lysis	**540** After cells undergo _____ ("breakdown"), any reproduced viruses are set loose to wreak more havoc.
bacter/i/a	**541** Indisputably alive are the bacteria. Bacteria is a plural term. This term is subdivided as _____ /_____ /_____, much like mitochondria **(frame 524).**

542 Way back in **frame 75,** Table 1.2, general rules for forming word plurals were stated. This table indicated that singular terms ending in either _____ , as in mitochondrion, or _____ , as in **bacterium** (**bak-TEER**-ee-um), form plurals with the letter -a.

543 Bacterium is properly analyzed as _____ /_____ /_____ . Especially note its suffix, _____ .

544 A _____ (bacteria/bacterium) is a single-celled plant-like microbe. The term _____ (bacteria/bacterium) denotes more than one of these microbes.

545 Bacteria can be found in several shapes, such as **bacill/i** (bah-**SIL**-igh), or "rods," and **cocc/i** (**KAHK**-sigh), or "berries."

546 Bacilli and cocci are both plural terms. Reference back to Table 1.2 reveals that singular terms ending in _____ form plurals using -i.

547 Use the information from the above frame to help you build: _____ /_____ , "a rod," and _____ /_____ , "a berry."

548 A _____ is one rod-shaped bacterium, while a _____ is one berry-shaped bacterium.

549 Although the _____ ("rods") are all pretty much the same, the _____ ("berries") can be grouped together in a variety of ways. Here are some word parts related to this bacterial type:

dipl/o (**DIHP**-loh)   "double"
staphyl/o (**STAF**-ih-loh)   "bunch of grapes"
strept/o (**STREHP**-toh)   "curved"

550 Use the information provided in the previous frame to help you build names for the following bacteria:
_____ /_____ /_____ /_____   "double berries"
_____ /_____ /_____ /_____   a "curved" chain of "berries"
_____ /_____ /_____ /_____   "berries" arranged like a "bunch of grapes"

551 The _____ occur in encapsulated pairs. The _____ are seen as long curvy chains when viewed under the microscope. And the _____ resemble bunches of grapes. Several types of bacteria are shown in Figure 6.9.

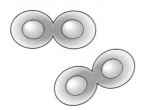

Diplococci

Streptococci

Staphylococci

Bacilli

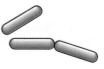

---

streptococci
staphylococci

552 Many of these bacteria are important pathogens. For instance, _____ ("curved berries") cause so-called **strep throat,** while _____ ("berries" arranged as "bunches of grapes") are often found in boils.

---

mitosis

553 Various other diseases arise not from pathogenic microbes, but from disorders of the body cells. Especially important are abnormalities of _____ ("condition of threads," **frame 497**).

---

plas/ia (PLAY-see-uh)

554 **Plas (PLAYS)** is a root for "formation." Attaching the suffix in hypochondria **(frame 114)** results in _____ /_____ ("an abnormal condition of formation").

---

hyper/**plas/**ia
(**HIGH**-per-**play**-see-uh)
hypo/**plas/**ia
(**HIGH**-poh-**play**-see-uh)

555 A very high rate of mitosis may result in _____ /_____ /_____, "an abnormal condition of excessive formation" of new tissue cells. A very low rate of mitosis may result in _____ /_____ /_____, "an abnormal condition of deficient formation" of new tissue cells. Here the prefixes for both hypertonic and hypotonic appear.

---

hyperplasia
hypoplasia

556 If a tissue exhibits _____, it probably will contain too many cells. Conversely, _____ often reveals itself as a definite decrease in the number of tissue cells observed.

---

hyperplasia

557 In addition to occurring too fast, mitosis during _____ ("excessive formation") may result in new cells with "bad" (abnormal) characteristics. The prefix dys- **(frame 132)** means "bad, difficult, or painful."

dys/plas/ia (dis-**PLAY**-see-uh)	**558** The term _____ / _____ / ____ can be built to denote "an abnormal condition of bad formation" of new tissue cells.
dysplasia	**559** When _____ happens, the resulting abnormal cells may have such problems as two or more nuclei.
hyperplasia dysplasia	**560** A _____ ("excessive formation") as well as _____ ("bad formation") can affect both connective and **epithelial** (**eh**-pih-**THEEL**-ee-uhl) tissue. Such rapid, abnormal mitosis results in growths or tumors. A suffix indicating "growth" is -**plasm** (**PLAZ**-im). A suffix for "tumor" is -**oma** (**OH**-mah).
neo/plasm (**NEE**-oh-**plaz**-im) neo-	**561** A _____ / _____ is a "new growth" of some kind, where _____ **(frame 82)** is the prefix for "new."
neoplasm	**562** A tumor is one kind of _____. If the tumor is **benign** (bee-**NIGHN**), or "kind," it is nonspreading and generally nonfatal. If it is **malignant** (**mah-LIG**-nant), or "wicked," it usually spreads and is often fatal.
malignant neoplasm	**563** The tumor-related adjective _____ actually means "to produce (something) bad." The "bad" thing usually resulting is a spreading _____ ("new growth").
-stasis	**564** The prefix meta- (**MET**-ah) means "after" or "beyond." Recall from **homeostasis (frame 420)** that _____ is a suffix for "controlling or stopping." It also means "standing or placing."
meta/stasis (meh-**TAH**-stah-sis)	**565** From the above, create a new term, _____ / _____, that means a "placing beyond." Note the accent change when meta- and -stasis are connected.
metastasis	**566** When a neoplasm moves "beyond" its original "place" in the body, _____ has occurred.
benign malignant metastasis	**567** If a neoplasm is _____ (malignant/benign), there is no spreading. If a neoplasm is _____ (malignant/benign), however, it will probably result in _____ of the tumor to other body sites.
malignant benign epi/theli/al	**568** Neoplasms, either _____ ("wicked") or _____ ("kind"), can occur in _____ / _____ / ____ tissue. This type of tissue literally lies "upon" (epi-) the "nipples," because theli (**THEE**-lee) or thel/o (**THEE**-loh) means "nipples."

epithelial	**569** Most _____ tissue covers the nipples or body surface. Another major type, connective tissue, either directly or indirectly connects body parts together.
Cancer **carcin/o**	**570** If you are a follower of astrology, you know that _____ is the sign of the "crab." A root for "crab" is **carcin** (**KAR**-sin). The combining form is _____ /_____ .
carcin/oma (**kar**-sin-**OH**-mah)	**571** Employing the suffix for "tumor" (**frame 560**) results in _____ /_____ , "crab tumor."
carcinoma cancer	**572** A _____ is a malignant neoplasm of epithelial tissue, as in _____ ("crab") of the skin. Perhaps the analogy to a crab is made because once cancer grabs hold, it is very hard to remove!
sarc/oma (sar-**KOH**-mah)	**573** Sarc (**SARK**) is a root for "flesh." A _____ /_____ , then, is literally a "fleshy tumor."
sarcoma	**574** In modern usage, _____ ("fleshy tumor") has come to mean a malignant neoplasm of connective tissue.

575 The following list presents some abbreviations related to neoplasms.

Abbreviation	Meaning
Ca	cancer
CIS	carcinoma in situ ("in place")
met, mets	metastasis

576 Whether malignant or benign, neoplasms must be diagnosed before they can be treated.

Lab Tests and Diagnoses

Word Parts Associated with Lab Tests and Diagnoses Involving Cells

The following is a list of word parts associated with lab tests and diagnoses involving cells. Use this list to help you complete **frames 577 to 604**.

aspir/o	to suck out	**-opsy**	vision of
onc/o	tumor	**-o/scopy**	process of examining

aspir (**AH**-spir)	**577** Before cells can be examined for morbid changes, they have to be extracted from the body. One way is simply to "suck them out," a process identified by the root, _____ .

aspir/a/tion (**as**-pih-**RAY**-shun)	**578** Use a pattern like that for auscultation **(frame 167)** to build _____ /_____ /_____, the "process of sucking (things) out."
aspiration	**579** An _____ ("sucking out") of cells is performed in order to view them under a microscope.
-**opsy** (**AHP**-see)	**580** Note that the suffix _____ in the word list means "vision of."
bi/**opsy**	**581** Dissect the term **biopsy** (**BIGH**-ahp-see): _____ /_____. This term contains the same root as biology **(frame 415).**
biopsy	**582** The literal meaning of _____ is a "vision of life." This is because the procedure withdraws samples of living tissue for examination.
aspiration biopsy	**583** Combining **frames 579 and 582** results in a new phrase, _____ _____. This is a "process of sucking out and viewing (things from the) living body."
aspiration biopsy	**584** Both living cells and fluid-borne body chemicals are obtained by _____ _____.
-o/scopy **micr**/o/scopy (**migh-KRAH**-skohp-ee)	**585** Most of the objects "sucked out" are microscopic. Use _____ /_____, a suffix for "the process of examining" **(frame 180),** and the root in microscopic to construct _____ /_____ /_____, "the process of examining tiny (things)."
microscopy	**586** Cells obtained from aspiration biopsy are often examined by _____.
micr/o/bi/o/logy (**migh**-kroh-bigh-**AHL**-oh-jee)	**587** The root and suffix in biology **(frame 415)** can be combined with the root of microscopy to yield _____ /_____ /_____ /_____ /_____.
microbiology	**588** The science of _____ involves both the formal study (as in reading) and direct examination (as by microscope viewing) of tiny living things.
radi/o/logist **micr**/o/bi/o/logist (**migh**-kroh-bigh-**AHL**-oh-jist)	**589** Recall that in radiology a specialist is called a _____ /_____ /_____ **(frame 211).** Similarly, in microbiology a specialist is called a _____ /_____ /_____ /_____ /_____.

microbiology microbiologist	**590** While _____ is the "study of tiny living (things)," a _____ is "one who specializes in the study of tiny living (things)."
cyt/o/**logy** (sigh-**TAHL**-oh-jee) **cyt**/o/**logist** (sigh-**TAHL**-oh-jist)	**591** Extract the root from cytoplasm **(frame 489)** and synthesize the following terms: _____ /_____ /_____, "the study of cells," and _____ /_____ /_____, "one who specializes in the study of cells."
Cytology cytologist	**592** Biopsy samples are often taken to a Department of _____ for careful examination by a _____, who specializes in the study of cells.
bacter/**i**/o/**logy** (bak-**teer**-ee-**AHL**-oh-jee) **bacter**/**i**/o/**logist** (bak-**teer**-ee-**AHL**-oh-jist)	**593** Extract the root from bacterium **(frame 543)** and synthesize these terms: _____ /_____ /_____ /_____, "the study of bacteria," and _____ /_____ /_____ /_____, "one who specializes in the study of bacteria."
bacteriology bacteriologist	**594** Advanced college students may sign up for a course in _____ if they really want to learn all about bacteria and perhaps become a _____.
vir/o/**logy** (veer-**AHL**-oh-**jee**)	**595** Extract the root from virus **(frame 533)** and build _____ /_____ /_____, or the "study of viruses."
bacteriology virology	**596** Bacteria are studied in _____, and viruses are studied in _____.
onc/o/**logy** (ahn-**KAHL**-oh-jee) **onc**/o/**logist** (ahn-**KAHL**-oh-jist)	**597** A root for "tumor" is **onc (AHNK).** As in the preceding few frames, we can build: _____ /_____ /_____, "the study of tumors," and _____ /_____ /_____, "one who specializes in the study of tumors."
oncology oncologist	**598** The science of _____ studies the causes of various neoplasms or tumors. A professional _____ may be called in to help diagnose and treat difficult cases of cancer.
carcinomas	**599** The causes of many cancers, or _____ ("crab tumors"), are environmental. For instance, most cancer of the lung is probably caused by long-term exposure to the **carcinogens** (kar-**SIN**-oh-**jens**) in cigarette smoke.
carcin/o/**gen** -gen	**600** Carcinogen is subdivided as _____ /_____ /_____, with the suffix _____, as in glycogen **(frame 522).**

cancer (crab) producer	**601** Much as glycogen translates as "sweetness producer," carcinogen translates as "_____ _____."
carcin/o/gen/ic (**kar**-sin-oh-**JEN**-ik)	**602** If we attach the "pertaining to" ending of endoplasmic **(frame 519)** to "cancer producer" we can build _____ / ____ / _____ / ____. In this case **gen** appears as a root rather than a suffix.
carcinogenic	**603** The term _____ means "cancer-producing" or "pertaining to the production of cancer."
carcinogenic	**604** Various _____ substances are heavily concentrated within cigarette smoke.
	605 When cancer strikes, the only remaining alternative is treatment.

Surgery and Therapies

Word Parts Associated with Surgery, Pharmacology, and Other Therapies Effective at the Cellular Level

The following is a list of word parts and an abbreviation associated with surgery, pharmacology, and other therapies effective at the cellular level. Use this list to help you complete **frames 607 to 619.**

anti-	against	**cyt/o**	cells
cry/o	cold	**DPT**	diphtheria-pertussis-tetanus (vaccine)

606 Recent advances in pharmacology and surgery permit medical interventions to be effective even down at the minute level of the cell.

anti-

607 Various drugs act "against" some pathogenic condition of the cell. Below is a list of such drugs. Note that all their names begin with _____, a prefix for "against" **(frame 83).**

antibacterial (**an**-tigh-bak-**TEER**-ee-al)
antibiotic (**an**-tigh-bigh-**AH**-tik)
antimicrobial (**an**-tigh-migh-**KROH**-bee-al)
antineoplastic (**an**-tigh-nee-oh-**PLAH**-stik)
antiviral (**an**-tigh-**VIGH**-ral)

antineoplastic
antibacterial
antibiotic
antimicrobial
antiviral

608 To reduce the size of a tumor, you would take an _____ drug. An _____ drug kills foreign bacteria, specifically. An _____ agent can be used against any living foreign invader. An _____ agent is given to destroy tiny living invaders. Finally, an _____ drug is effective in halting the growth of viruses.

antibacterial **DPT**	**609** A number of vaccines are commonly given because of their powerful _____ actions that make them so effective "against" harmful "bacteria." A good example is the combined **diphtheria (dif-THEER**-ee-ah)-**pertussis (per-TUHS**-is)-**tetanus (TET**-ah-nus) vaccine. This vaccine is abbreviated by the three letters ____ ____ ____ .
antibiotic	**610** **Penicillin** is an example of a broad-spectrum _____, in that it kills infecting bacteria and many other "living," invading cells.
radi pharmaceut	**611** Carcinomas and sarcomas are much more difficult to treat. Stubborn neoplasms may require treatment with **radiopharmaceutical (RAY**-dee-oh-**far**-muh-**SOO**-tih-kal) agents. Analyzing this term should allow you to find _____, a root in radiogram **(frame 191),** and _____, a root for "drug" **(frame 239).**
radiopharmaceutical	**612** Radioactive drugs called _____ agents tend to concentrate in particular body areas and destroy tumors.
micr/o/surgery (**migh**-kroh-**SURJ**-er-ee)	**613** Sometimes, however, microscopic surgery is necessary for cells. It is called _____ /____ /_____, "surgery" upon a very "minute" level of body organization.
microsurgery	**614** In _____, a microscope is used to guide ultrafine cuttings into cells for removing abnormal structures.
cry/o/surgery (**crigh**-oh-**SURJ**-er-ee)	**615** Sometimes the property of coldness is used for killing cancerous cells. A root for "cold" is **cry (KRIGH).** "Surgery using cold" is called _____ /____ /_____ .
cryosurgery	**616** One specific technique of _____ employs a supercooled probe to destroy cancers of the oral cavity, brain, and prostate gland.
cyt **cyt/o/therapy** (**sigh**-toh-**THEHR**-ah-pee)	**617** Various nonsurgical types of therapy can be used to treat cellular disorders. Remember that _____, as in cytology **(frame 591),** denotes "cells." Now build _____ /____ /_____, which literally means "cell therapy."
cytotherapy	**618** In _____, living foreign cells are administered to the patient. The idea is that dead or damaged cells in the patient will be replaced by new, healthy cells from a donor.
cytotherapy	**619** Bone marrow transplant may be considered a type of _____ .

E X E R C I S E S   F O R   C H A P T E R   **6**

Multiple Choice

1. The root for "examine" is

    a. log   b. scop   c som   d. plasm

2. The combining form mit/o means

    a. mass   b. thread   c. ribose   d. reduction

3. A term that means "colored body" is

    a. reticulum   b. ribosome   c. centriole   d. chromosome

4. The combining form for "thrust" is

    a. reticul/o   b. diffus/o   c. osm/o   d. ton/o

5. Phag/o is a

    a. word root   b. noun suffix   c. combining form   d. proportion suffix

6. Which of these prefixes means "outside"?

    a. endo-   b. intra-   c. inter-   d. extra-

Meanings of Selected Roots

Add the correct combining vowel (cv) after each root. Then write the definition of each root in the space provided.

ROOT/CV   **DEFINITION**

1. carcin/_____

2. vir/_____

3. plas/_____

4. mit/_____

5. molecul/_____

6. phag/_____

7. glyc/_____

8. macr/_____

9. perme/_____

10. ton/_____

Word Dissection and Translation

Analyze the following terms by dissecting them with slashmarks and identifying their word parts. To the right of each term, write its correct English translation.

Key: R (root), cv (combining vowel), P (prefix), S (suffix)

1. phagocytosis

   _____ / _____ / _____ / _____ / _____   _____
          R   cv   R   cv   S

2. macroscopic

   _____ / _____ / _____ / _____   _____
          R   cv   R   S

3. inorganic

   _____ / _____ / _____   _____
      P   R   S

4. electrolyte

   _____ / _____ / _____ / _____   _____
          R   cv   R   S

5. dysplasia

   _____ / _____ / _____   _____
      P   R   S

6. carcinoma

   _____ / _____   _____
          R   S

7. bacteriology

   _____ / _____ / _____ / _____   _____
          R   cv   cv   S

8. radiopharmaceutical

   _____ / _____ / _____ / _____   _____
          R   cv   R   S

9. antineoplastic

   _____ / _____ / _____ / _____   _____
      P   P   R   S

10. hypertonic

    _____ / _____ / _____   _____
       P   R   S

Terms and Their Abbreviations

In the list below, when the term is given, write its abbreviation in the space provided. When the abbreviation is given, write its corresponding term.

TERM	ABBREVIATION
1. endoplasmic reticulum	_____
2. _____	DPT
3. cancer	_____
4. _____	ICF
5. _____	DNA
6. extracellular fluid	_____
7. ribonucleic acid	_____

Word Spelling

Look at each of the terms listed below. Identify those that are misspelled by circling Y for "Yes." Write the correct spelling in the blank.

WORD	MISSPELLED?	CORRECT SPELLING
1. asperation	Y/N	_____
2. antibiotic	Y/N	_____
3. staphylocoxy	Y/N	_____
4. hypoplasia	Y/N	_____
5. microbiology	Y/N	_____
6. carsinogenic	Y/N	_____
7. antibacterial	Y/N	_____
8. biopsy	Y/N	_____
9. metastasis	Y/N	_____
10. pathojen	Y/N	_____
11. oncology	Y/N	_____
12. kneeohplahsim	Y/N	_____
13. molecolar	Y/N	_____
14. solvent	Y/N	_____

New Word Synthesis

Using word parts that appear in this and previous chapters, build new terms with the following meanings:

1. _____ pertaining to a curved stomach

2. _____ a deficiency of sweetness

3. _____ process of sucking (something) out (under) cold conditions

4. _____ the breakdown of cancer

5. _____ little eaters

6. _____ an instrument used to examine large (structures)

7. _____ relating to the strength of a body

8. _____ a new growth of large eaters

9. _____ one who specializes in the study of cell interiors

10. _____ a little network of threads

11. _____ breakdown by heat

12. _____ a vision of flesh

C A S E   S T U D Y

Read through the following partial cytology report. Note the terms in bold print. A series of multiple choice questions probes your knowledge of these terms.

CYTOLOGY REPORT

A 6-ml sample obtained by **aspiration biopsy** of an abdominal cyst revealed a murky **solution** of **bacterial** bodies. Most of these bodies were pathogenic **bacilli.** Further **cytological** studies are planned.

Case Study Questions

1. The **sample** was obtained by **aspiration biopsy,** or
   (a) removing an entire sac.
   (b) sucking out fluid from a sac.
   (c) heating and testing a bone.
   (d) stretching the viscera taut.

2. The **solution** consisted of
   (a) a mixture of dissolved particles and dissolving solution.
   (b) intracellular fluid only.
   (c) ECF alone.
   (d) heavy solutes.

3. **Bacterial** bodies means bodies that
   (a) always occur in pairs.
   (b) serve as pathways of intracellular transport.
   (c) are unicellular, living, and plantlike.
   (d) probably reflect the presence of viruses.

4. Pathogenic **bacilli** had what appearance under the microscope?
   (a) rodlike
   (b) slightly squared
   (c) oval
   (d) triangular

5. **Cytological** studies will probably involve
   (a) dissection of major viscera.
   (b) measurement of gross calorie consumption.
   (c) counting of different cell types present.
   (d) analysis of muscle mass.

CHAPTER 7 Tissues and the Integumentary System

INTRODUCTION

A **tissue** is a collection of similar cells plus the **intercellular** (in-ter-SEL-yoo-lar) **material** located between them. Figure 7.1 provides a diagrammatic view of a tissue as it might appear microscopically. There are four types of **basic tissues: epithelial tissue, connective tissue, muscle tissue,** and **nervous tissue.** Chapter 6 briefly mentioned epithelial and connective tissues.

FIGURE 7.1 **Diagrammatic View of Tissue**

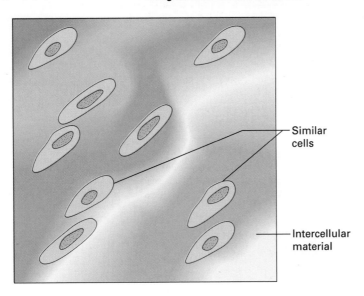

Similar cells

Intercellular material

Epithelial tissue is the body's major covering and lining tissue. This tissue typically consists of many cells tightly packed together, with little or no intercellular material. These cells lie upon a thin dark **basement membrane** of support. Epithelial cells can occur either as a single layer on the basement membrane or as multiple layers. A few common types of epithelial tissue are illustrated in Figure 7.2 on page 118.

Connective tissue either directly or indirectly connects body parts together. Connective tissue is generally characterized by a large amount of intercellular material between its widely spaced cells. The intercellular material sometimes contains **connective tissue fibers.** These fibers directly support and attach body structures to one another. Figure 7.3 (page 119) provides microscopic views of several specific types of connective tissue, some with, some without, connective tissue fibers.

Muscle tissue is involved in body movements, while nervous tissue is mainly responsible for coordinating and controlling the internal environment. Muscle and nervous tissues will be discussed in Chapters 9 and 10, respectively.

Some Common Epithelial Tissues

Simple Squamous Epithelium

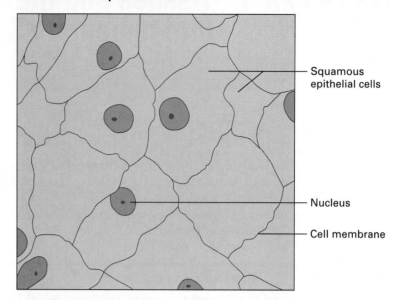

Squamous epithelial cells

Nucleus

Cell membrane

Simple Cuboidal Epithelium

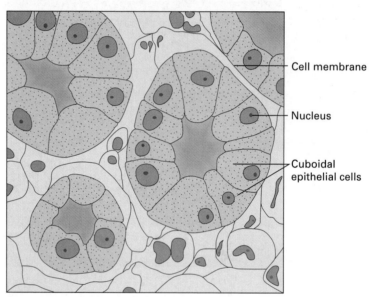

Cell membrane

Nucleus

Cuboidal epithelial cells

Simple Columnar Epithelium

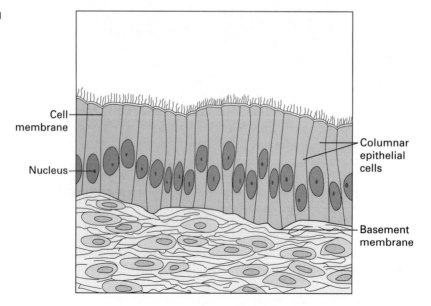

Cell membrane

Nucleus

Columnar epithelial cells

Basement membrane

FIGURE 7.3

Some Common Connective Tissues

Areolar (Loose) Connective Tissue

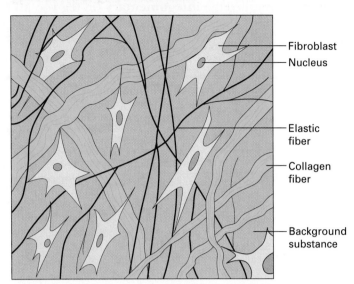

Fibroblast
Nucleus

Elastic fiber

Collagen fiber

Background substance

Dense Fibrous (Collagenous)
Connective Tissue

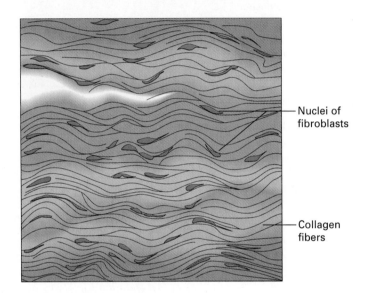

Nuclei of fibroblasts

Collagen fibers

Adipose Tissue

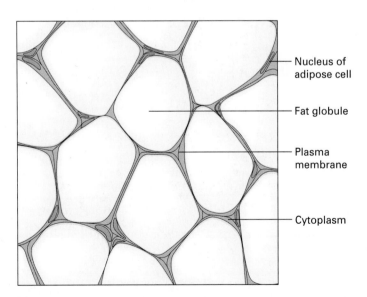

Nucleus of adipose cell

Fat globule

Plasma membrane

Cytoplasm

Some tissues form an **integument** (in-**TEG**-yoo-**ment**), that is, a body covering. The collection of all such covering tissues is called the **integumentary** (in-**teg**-yoo-**MEN**-tah-ree) system. The skin makes up most of the body's integumentary system. The layered structure of the skin is quite apparent in Figure 7.4.

FIGURE 7.4   **An Overview of Skin Anatomy**

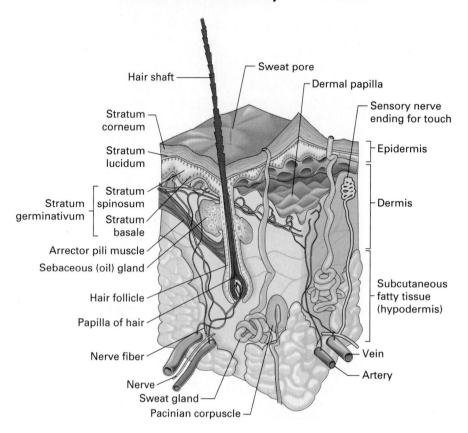

Hair shaft
Sweat pore
Dermal papilla
Sensory nerve ending for touch
Stratum corneum
Stratum lucidum
Epidermis
Stratum germinativum — Stratum spinosum / Stratum basale
Dermis
Arrector pili muscle
Sebaceous (oil) gland
Hair follicle
Papilla of hair
Subcutaneous fatty tissue (hypodermis)
Nerve fiber
Vein
Nerve
Artery
Sweat gland
Pacinian corpuscle

This chapter presents terms related to the normal anatomy and physiology of the skin and tissues; terms related to skin and tissue disease; terms associated with lab tests and diagnoses involving skin and tissues; and terms describing surgery, pharmacology, and other therapies applied to the skin and tissues.

CHAPTER OBJECTIVES

By the end of this chapter, you should be able to:

1 Identify major prefixes, roots, suffixes, and abbreviations related to the skin and tissues.

2 Dissect skin and tissue terms into their component parts.

3 Translate skin and tissue terms into their common English equivalents.

4 Build new terms associated with the tissues and skin.

Word Parts Associated with Normal Anatomy and Physiology of the Tissues and Skin

The following is a list of word parts associated with the normal structure and function of the skin and body tissues. Use this list to help you complete **frames 620 to 668.**

adipos/o	fatty	**derm/o**	skin	**seb/o**	grease
areol/o	little area	**dermat/o**	skin	**sebace/o**	grease
coll/a	glue	**fasci/o**	sheet	**ser/o**	watery
column/o	tall and column-shaped	**fibr/o**	fibers	**squam/o**	scale
		muc/o	slime	**strat/o**	layer
cutane/o	skin	**papill/o**	pimple; nipple		

cutane/o (kyoo-**TAY**-nee-oh)
derm/o (**DERM**-oh)
dermat/o (**DER**-mah-toh)

620 The terms of this chapter focus primarily on the skin and its associated tissues. Quickly examine the word list and note that _____ /____, _____ /____, and _____ /____ are all roots/cv for "skin."

cutane/ous (kyoo-**TAY**-nee-us)
derm/al (**DER**-mal)

621 Cutane usually takes **-ous** as its "pertaining to" suffix, while derm takes the ending in antimicrobial **(frame 531)**. This combination leads to _____ /_____ and _____ /____, respectively, for "pertaining to the skin."

cutaneous
dermal

622 A _____ or _____ structure is one associated with the skin.

derm/is (**DER**-mis)

623 Using the shorter **d**-beginning root for "skin" and the "presence of" ending **-is**, results in _____ /____, "presence of the skin."

dermis

624 A look back at Figure 7.4, however, reveals that the _____ is not the whole skin. Rather, it represents just the major connective tissue portion of the skin.

papill (**PAH**-pil)
papill/a (pah-**PIL**-ah)

625 Note from the chapter word list that _____ is a root for "pimple" or "nipple." A _____ /____, then, is "a pimple or nipple," where the noun-forming suffix is that found in soma **(frame 314)**.

papill/ae (pah-**PIL**-ee)
P

626 Words ending in **-a** can form plurals using either **-as** or **-ae**, for example, vertebra (singular, S), vertebras or vertebrae (plural, P). Papill, for instance, employs the second plural ending, resulting in _____ /____. Papillae is the ____ (S/P) form for pimple.

dermal **papillae**	**627** Use the adjective form of derm from **frame 621**, and the preceding frame, to help you build a new phrase: _____ _____ (more than one "pimple" from the "dermis").
dermal papillae	**628** The _____ _____ are small "pimple"-like projections from the surface of the "dermis." These structures, like the rest of the dermis, are rich in connective tissue fibers.
fibr/ous (FIGH-brus)	**629** **Fibr/o** (**FIGH**-broh) is a root/cv meaning "fiber." It can be said that the dermis and the dermal papillae have a _____ /_____ ("relating to fibers") nature. In this case the suffix of cutaneous is seen.
fibrous	**630** Tissue that is _____ can better resist pulling, because of its connective tissue fibers.
colla/gen **-gen**	**631** One of the main types of connective tissue fibers in the dermis is **collagen** (KAH-lah-jen). Subdivide this term as _____ /_____. For help, recall that _____, the same suffix, is also found in glycogen **(frame 522)** and means "formation" or "production."
collagen	**632** **Colla** (**KAH**-lah) is a root for "glue." Thus _____ means "glue producer" just as glycogen means "sweetness producer." These thick ropelike fibers in a sense glue body parts together.
fasci/a (FASH-ee-ah) fasci/ae (**FASH**-ee-igh)	**633** Collagen fibers can occur in large "sheets." A root for "sheet" is **fasci** (**FAH**-shee). Just as papilla denotes "a pimple," _____ /____ denotes "a sheet." Like papill**ae**, the plural of fascia is _____ /____.
fasciae	**634** There are _____, or "sheets," of fibrous connective tissue that envelope various organs and attach them to the undersurface of the skin.
adipos/e (AH-dih-pohs)	**635** Also under the skin is fatty tissue. **Adipos/o** (**AH**-dih-**poh**-soh) is a combining form for "fat." The root takes the ending in electrolyte **(frame 464)** to become either a noun or an adjective. Therefore _____ /_____ translates as either "presence of fat" or "pertaining to fat."
adipose	**636** Strip the skin off a piece of fried chicken. Note that a yellowish strip of _____ (fatty) tissue underlies the skin.
hypo/derm/is (high-poh-DER-mis)	**637** Using dermis as the naming reference, we can build _____ /_____ /_____, literally "presence of (something) below the skin." Here the prefix is identical to that in hypoplasia **(frame 555)**.

hypodermis	**638** What you see is _____ just internal to the skin of a raw or fried chicken.
hypodermis	**639** Another name for the _____ is the **subdermis** (sub-**DER**-mis), since it lies "under" (sub-) the dermis.
sub/derm/is **hypo-** **sub-**	**640** Subdermis is properly dissected as _____ / _____ / ____. Note that its word parts are identical to those in hypodermis, except for the prefix. The two prefixes meaning "under" are _____ and _____.
hypodermis subdermis	**641** The _____ or _____ is the thick layer of adipose tissue and fascia underlying the dermis of the skin.
areol/ar (ah-**REE**-uh-**lar**)	**642** **Areol/o** (**ah-REE**-oh-loh) means "little areas." Using the suffix appearing in extracellular **(frame 472)**, create _____ / ____, "referring to little areas."
areolar	**643** A microscopic view of _____ tissue shows many "little areas" or spaces existing among a loose arrangement of connective tissue fibers and cells.
Information Frame	**644** Remember the last time you saw raw chicken. Internal to the hypodermis or subdermis (yellow strip) is a clear, sticky webbing that connects the skin to the raw meat. This clear webbing is actually areolar connective tissue. It is an important part of the body fascia.
epi/derm/is (**ep**-ih-**DER**-mis)	**645** While the hypodermis literally lies "below the dermis," the _____ / _____ / ____ literally lies "upon the dermis." Here the prefix for "upon" is that in epithelial **(frame 568)**.
epidermis	**646** The _____ is the outermost epithelial portion of the skin.
epidermis epidermis dermal hypodermis subdermis	**647** Isn't it interesting that the only part of your skin that is visible to others is the _____, the outer layer? There are several layers to the skin: the outermost layer, or _____, the large _____ layer, and the adipose tissue and fascia under the skin existing as the _____ or _____.
strat/um (**STRAHT**-um)	**648** **Strat** (**STRAHT**) is a root for "layer." A _____ / ____ is "a layer," where the suffix is the one found in reticulum **(frame 517)**.

stratum	**649** Words that end in **-um** take plurals with **-a**. For instance, recall bacterium **(frame 543)**, which, like _____ ("a layer"), ends in **-um**
strat/a (STRAT-ah)	**650** Just as the plural of bacterium is bacteria, the plural of stratum is _____ /_____.
strata	**651** The _____ ("layers") of the skin include the epidermis.
epi/derm/al (**ep**-ih-**DER**-mal)	**652** **Epi/derm/is** takes the same adjectival ending as dermis. Therefore, just as derm/**al** "refers to the dermis or skin," _____ /_____ /_____ "refers to the epidermis or (something) upon the skin."
epidermal strata	**653** There are a number of _____ _____ ("layers of epidermis").
stratum	**654** Within each _____ ("layer") of the epidermis are epithelial cells of particular shapes. Figure 7.5 illustrates the three major shapes of individual epithelial cells. These are **columnar** (kuh-**LUM**-nar), **cuboidal** (kyoo-**BOYD**-al), and **squamous** (**SKWAH**-mus).

FIGURE 7.5   **Major Shapes of Individual Epithelial Cells**

Squamous cell   Cuboidal cell   Columnar cell

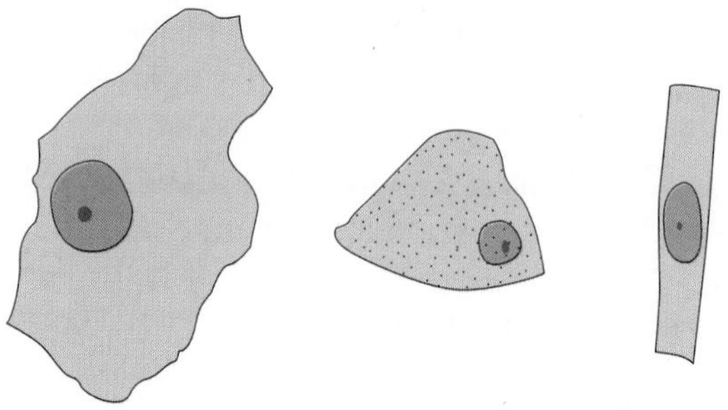

column/**ar** cuboid/**al** squam/**ous**	**655** Try your hand at word dissection and translation. Columnar is subdivided as _____ /_____, similar to areolar. Cuboidal is subdivided as _____ /_____, with its suffix being the same as in epidermal. Squamous is analyzed as _____ /_____, with an ending also found in cutaneous **(frame 621)**.
cuboidal columnar	**656** It is probably easy for you to guess that _____ "refers to (something) resembling cubes" and that _____ "refers to (something) resembling columns."

squamous	**657** **Squam/o** (**SKWAH**-moh) means "scale." Consequently _____ "refers to scales."
squamous	**658** The outermost stratum of the epidermis consists of several layers of dead _____ ("scale") cells.
cuboidal columnar	**659** **Glands** are secreting structures composed mainly of _____ ("cube-resembling") and _____ ("columnlike") epithelial cells specialized for the function of **secretion** (release of some useful product).
seb/um	**660** One useful secretion of cutaneous glands is **sebum** (**SEE**-bum), "grease." Sebum is subdivided as _____ /_____, with the same suffix as stratum.
sebum	**661** The skin is lubricated by the _____ ("grease") it contains.
sebace/ous (see-**BAY**-shus)	**662** Another root/cv for "grease" is **sebace/o** (see-**BAY**-see-oh). Thus _____ /_____ "refers to grease," just as cutaneous "refers to skin."
sebaceous	**663** Sebum is secreted by the _____ glands in the skin surface.
muc/ous **ser/ous**	**664** Pronounce **mucous** (**MYOO**-kus) and **serous** (**SEER**-us). Both these terms have the same suffix as sebaceous. Therefore, mucous is subdivided as _____ /_____ and serous as _____ /_____.
muc ser muc/o ser/o	**665** The root in mucous is _____, and it means "slime." The root in serous is _____, and it means "watery." The combining form for muc is _____ /_____ and for ser is _____ /_____.
serous mucous	**666** The term _____ "pertains to (something) watery," while the term _____ "pertains to slime."
mucous	**667** Because of their thick covering of "slime," the _____ membranes prevent the dehydration (drying out) of underlying cell layers. An example is the membrane lining our nostrils.

serous

668 Because of their release of "watery" fluid, the _____ membranes help reduce friction between moving body organs. Examples are the membranes immediately lining the wall of the thoracic cavity, serving to moisten the surface of the lungs.

669 Whatever the type of tissue or membrane (cutaneous, mucous, or serous), they are all subject to pathological changes under certain circumstances.

Diseases

Word Parts Associated with Diseases of the Tissues and Skin

The following is a list of word parts and abbreviations associated with diseases of the skin and body tissues. Use this list to help you complete **frames 670 to 725.**

alopec/o	bald	**herpes zoster**	girdle or zone spreading	**jaundic/o**	yellow
cicatric/i	connective tissue scar	**hidr/o**	sweat	**macul/o**	spot
decubit/o	bedsore	**HS**	herpes simplex; simple spreading	**papul/o**	small pimple
diaphor/o	sweat			**prurit/o**	itch
erythem/a	redness			**psorias/o**	itch
furuncl/o	boil	**HSV**	herpes simplex virus	**rubell/o**	little reddish
herpes	spreading			**rubeol/o**	little reddish
		icter/o	yellow	**seb/o**	sebum; grease
				terat/o	monster

dermat/o/sis (der-mah-**TOH**-sis)

670 Diseases of the skin are perhaps the most visible and bothersome. Utilizing **dermat** for "skin," we can build _____ / _____ / _____, "an (abnormal) condition of the skin." The ending here is that in phagocytosis **(frame 485)**.

dermat/o/ses (der-mah-**TOH**-seez)

671 Terms that end in -**o/sis** form plurals with -**o/ses** (**OH**-seez). Abnormal "conditions of the skin" are described as _____ / _____ / _____.

cyan/o
xanth/o
hidr/o (**HIGH**-droh)

672 A review way back to **frame 87** brings to mind that _____ / _____ is a combining form for "blue," while _____ / _____ is one for "yellow." Observe from this section's word list that _____ / _____ is a root for "sweat."

cyan/o/sis
hidr/o/sis
xanth/o/sis

673 Use your knowledge of word dissection to analyze cyanosis as _____ / _____ / _____, hidrosis as _____ / _____ / _____, and xanthosis as _____ / _____ / _____.

cyanosis
xanthosis

674 A blueness of the skin due to lack of oxygen in the blood is called _____. A yellowish discoloration of skin or other tissue that is degenerating is called _____.

hidrosis	**675** The term _____ indicates a condition of excessive sweating.
cyan/o/ses (sigh-ah-**NOH**-seez) **hidr/o/ses** (high-**DROH**-seez) **xanth/o/ses** (zanth-**OH**-seez)	**676** Now form three new terms using the plural suffix for "condition": "blue conditions" _____ /_____ /_____ "sweat conditions" _____ /_____ /_____ "yellow conditions" _____ /_____ /_____
diaphor/o (**DIGH**-ah-**for**-oh)	**677** Scan this section's word list and find another combining form for "sweat," _____ /_____.
diaphor/esis (digh-ah-for-**EE**-sis)	**678** **Frame 98** told you that -esis, like -o/sis, is a suffix for "condition of." Use this information and that in the preceding frame to build _____ /_____, "a condition of (excessive) sweating."
diaphoresis hidrosis	**679** A patient who is sweating profusely has a case of _____ or _____, both terms meaning essentially the same thing.
icter (IHK-ter) **jaundic (JAWN-dis)**	**680** Focusing on color, note that, in addition to xanth, two other roots on the word list indicate yellowing. These are _____ and _____.
icter/us (**IHK**-ter-us) **jaundic/e** (**JAWN**-dis)	**681** Icter takes the suffix in nucleus (**frame 511**), becoming _____ /_____. Jaundic assumes the ending of molecule (**frame 432**), becoming _____ /_____.
icterus jaundice	**682** The symptom of _____ or _____ is a yellowing of the skin, usually due to a back-up of yellow-brown bile in the bloodstream.
icter/ic (**IHK**-ter-ik)	**683** Use the root in icterus and the suffix in microscopic (**frame 430**) to help you build _____ /_____, "pertaining to yellowing."
icteric	**684** A patient with _____ skin is suffering from jaundice.
Information Frame	**685** Other color-related terms are: **albinism** (**AL**-bin-izm) **erythema** (**ee**-rih-**THEE**-mah) **melanism** (**MEH**-lah-**niz**-im) **melanoma** (mel-uh-**NOH**-mah) **melanocarcinoma** (**mel**-ah-noh-kar-sin-**OH**-mah) **rubella** (roo-**BELL**-uh) **rubeola** (**roo**-bee-**OH**-lah)

albin/ism
-ism

686 Return again to the color roots introduced in Chapter 2 **(frame 87)**, to help you dissect the terms in the preceding frame. We have, for instance, _____ /_____, an "abnormal condition of whiteness" of the skin. Here the suffix, _____ **(frame 113)**, denotes an "abnormal condition of."

---

melan/**ism**

687 A similar word-dissecting pattern holds for _____ /_____, an "abnormal condition of blackness" of the skin.

---

melanism
albinism

688 When a person suffers from _____, black areas appear on normally light skin. A person afflicted with _____ gets white areas appearing on normally dark skin.

---

melan/oma

689 The skin, like other body organs, can be stricken with tumors. A _____ /_____ is literally a "tumor of blackness" in the same way that sarcoma **(frame 573)** is a "tumor of flesh."

---

melanoma
melan/o/carcin/oma
carcinoma

690 A term closely related to _____ ("black tumor") is _____ /_____ /_____ /_____, a "tumor of black crabs." Remember that a _____ **(frame 571)** is a "crab tumor" in general.

---

melanoma
melanocarcinoma

691 Either _____ or _____ can be used to describe a blackish cancer of the skin. The chief etiology or cause of such cancers is probably chronic exposure to excessive sunlight.

---

erythem/a

692 Too much exposure to sunlight can also result in sunburn. **Frame 685** includes _____ /_____, "a redness," where the root is close to **erythr/o** and the suffix is that appearing in papilla **(frame 625)**.

---

erythema

693 The redness, or _____, of the skin during sunburn is actually a type of inflammation.

---

rubell/a
rubeol/a

694 Both rubella and rubeola in **frame 685** are subdivided the same as erythema. This provides us with _____/_____ and _____ /_____, respectively.

---

rubella
rubeola

695 Both _____ and _____ denote "little reddish" (things). In reality, these are little reddish spots, as found in German measles.

---

rubella
rubeola
erythema

696 Whereas _____ and _____ denote local inflammations of the skin, reflected as reddish spots, _____ involves redness due to a large-scale skin inflammation.

---

dermat/itis (der-mah-**TIGH**-tis)

697 "Inflammation of the skin" can be denoted by the root in dermatosis **(frame 670)** plus the ending in carditis **(frame 152)**. This combination allows us to build _____ /_____.

dermatitis

698 Erythema, rubella, and rubeola are all examples of _____ ("skin inflammation").

macul/e (**MAK**-yool)
papul/e (**PAP**-yool)

699 Dermatitis may involve the appearance of spots or pimplelike elevations. **Macul** (**MAK**-yool) is a root for "spot," while **papul** (**PAP**-yool) is one for "pimple." To create nouns describing a spot and a pimple, use the noun suffix in adipose **(frame 635)** with the roots macul and papul. Remember that **e** is a vowel, so the combining vowel is not necessary.
_____ /_____ "a spot"
_____ /_____ "a pimple"

macules

papules

700 The reddish spots of German measles are examples of _____ (macules/papules). The pimples of **common acne** (**AHK**-nee), or **acne vulgaris** (vul-**GAHR**-is), are examples of _____ (macules/papules).

acne vulgaris

701 Common acne, or _____ _____, is especially frequent during puberty and the teenage years.

furuncl/e (**FUR**-un-kil)

702 Closely related to pimples are boils. **Furuncl** (**FUR**-un-kil) is a root for "boil." Just as papule indicates "presence of a pimple," _____ /_____ indicates "presence of a boil."

furuncles
papules

703 "Boils," or _____, are generally larger than "pimples," or _____, and they contain pus rather than being solid.

papules
furuncles

704 Certain bacteria feed on excessive sebum, producing irritating acids than can result in _____ ("pimples") and _____ ("boils").

seb/o
seb/o/rrhea (seb-or-**EE**-uh)

705 Too much sebum is a common teenage problem. The root/cv in sebum **(frame 660)**, _____ /_____, can be combined with the suffix o/rrhea **(frame 419)**. The resulting term is _____ /_____ /_____, an "excessive flow of sebum."

seborrhea

706 Overactivity of sebaceous glands results in _____. Irritating bacteria feed on the excess sebum, resulting in a skin inflammation.

alopec/ia

707 Furuncles and seborrhea usually occur around hairs. **Alopecia** (al-loh-**PEE**-see-ah), or "presence of baldness," involves loss or thinning of hair. This term is subdivided as _____ /_____, where the suffix is identical to that in plasia **(frame 554)**.

alopec (ah-loh-**PEES**) **alopec/o** o	**708** The root in alopecia is _____. It indicates "baldness." The combining form is _____ /_____, where _____ is the combining vowel.
prurit (proo-**RIGHT**) **psorias** (sor-**IGH**-as)	**709** Other skin problems, the opposite of seborrhea, involve dry skin with itching and burning. One good example is **eczema** (**EHG**-zeh-muh). Note from the section word list that _____ and _____ indicate "itching."
prurit/us (proo-**RIGH**-tus) **psorias/is** (sor-**IGH**-ah-**sis**)	**710** Prurit takes the ending in icterus **(frame 681)** to become _____ /_____. Psorias assumes the suffix of hypodermis **(frame 637)** to become _____ /_____.
pruritus psoriasis	**711** An itching in general is called _____. In contrast, _____ involves itchy, reddish skin eruptions that are covered by silvery scales (Figure 7.6).

FIGURE 7.6

Skin Affected by Psoriasis
(Photograph courtesy of Armed Forces Institute of Pathology, negative 74-16637)

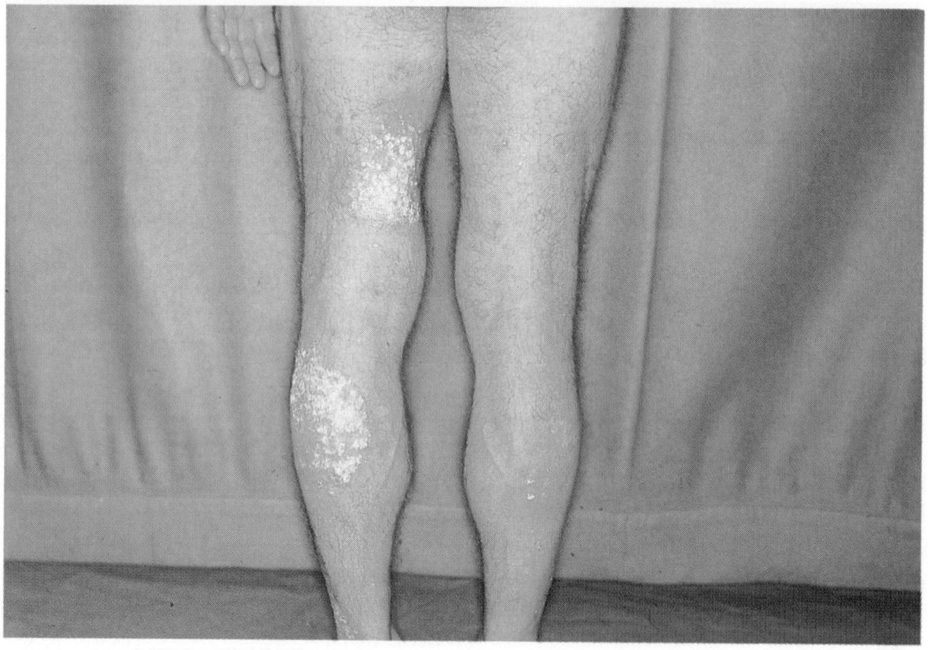

herpes (**HER**-peez) **herpes simplex** (**SIHM**-plex) **herpes zoster** (**ZAHS**-ter)	**712** A whole set of skin inflammations can be described as _____, or "spreading," on the word list. Two specific types are "simple spreading," or _____ _____, and "girdle or zone spreading," called _____ _____.
herpes herpes simplex	**713** Both types of _____ ("spreading") in the preceding frame are due to infection with viruses. **HS** (the abbreviation for _____ _____) is a simple type of viral infection wherein eruptions form near various mucous membranes, as on the corners of the lips. These eruptions are commonly known as cold sores.

herpes **simplex virus**	**714** The causative organism in herpes simplex is the _____ _____ _____, abbreviated as **HSV**.
HSV	**715** Cold sores on your lips are due to ____ ____ ____ ("herpes simplex virus").
herpes zoster	**716** The other type of herpes is _____ _____. This "spreading" disease occurs as a thin "zone" of eruptions on the skin along the course of a nerve. The disease is commonly called **shingles** (Figure 7.7).

FIGURE 7.7

Skin Affected by Shingles (Herpes Zoster)
(Photograph courtesy of Centers for Disease Control and Prevention)

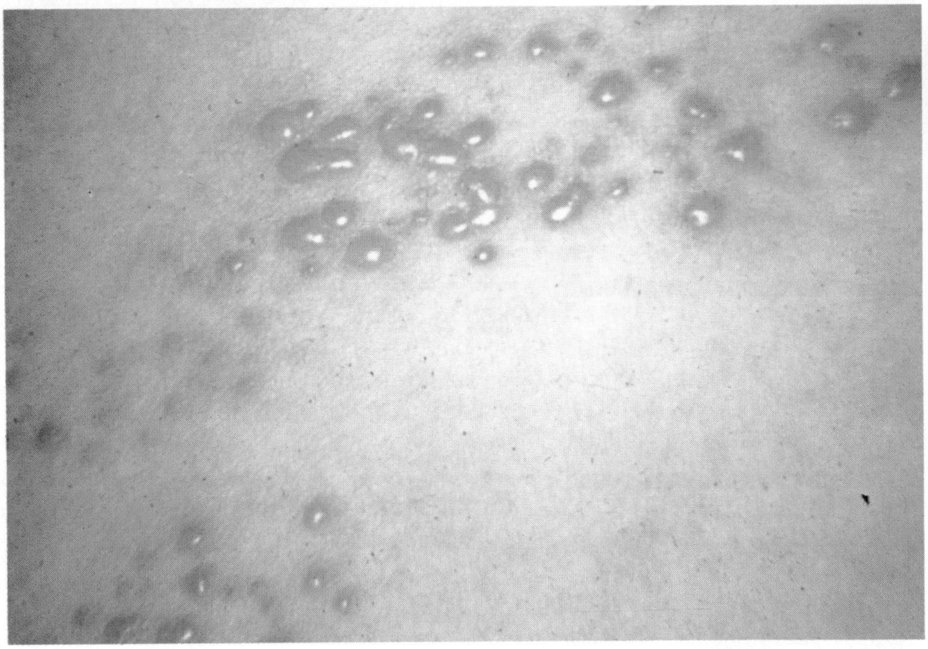

cicatric (**SIK**-ah-trik) **decubit** (dee-**KOO**-bit) **terat** (**TAHR**-at)	**717** Three separate roots on the section word list involve pathology of con- nective tissue, rather than just the skin. These roots are: _____ "connective tissue scar" _____ "bedsore" _____ "monster"
terat/oma (**tahr**-ah-**TOH**-mah)	**718** Employing the suffix in melanoma, build a term that means "monster tumor": _____ / _____.
teratoma -oma	**719** A _____ ("monster tumor") is a weird object consisting of a conglomeration of unrelated tissues or structures. Such a tumor may, like a carcin/_____, occur on the skin, but it might contain teeth and hair!

cicatric	**720** **Cicatrix** (**SIK**-ah-**triks**) means "a connective tissue scar." From **frame 717** you know that _____ is a root for such a scar. This root can help create a "pertaining to" word with the help of **i** as combining vowel and the ending in dermal:
cicatric/i/al (sik-ah-**TRISH**-al)	_____ /____ /____.

cicatricial	**721** The term _____ literally "pertains to a connective tissue scar."

cicatricial	**722** A cicatrix ("scar") consists of _____ tissue containing collagen and other connective tissue fibers. It serves to replace dead cells in the skin, brain, heart, and elsewhere.

decubit/us (dee-**KOO**-bih-**tus**)	**723** A possible source of severe scarring is a _____ /____, or "bedsore present," on the skin surface. Here the root is mentioned in **frame 717**, the suffix in **frame 681**.

decubitus **decubit/i** (dee-**KOO**-bih-**tigh**)	**724** Since _____ ("a bedsore"), like bacillus (**frame 547**), is a singular term ending in **-us**, it forms a plural as _____ /____ (**frame 546**).

decubiti	**725** One of the most frustrating problems in the long-term care of bedridden patients is the frequent occurrence of _____ ("bedsores") in skin of the buttocks, hips, back, and heels. Such sores are probably due to chronic interference of blood flow to these areas.

	726 A decubitus or other skin or tissue pathology should be promptly diagnosed.

Lab Tests and Diagnoses

Word Parts Associated with Lab Tests and Diagnoses Involving Tissues and the Skin

The following is a list of word parts describing lab tests and diagnostic procedures revolving around the tissues and skin. Use this list to help you complete **frames 727 to 747**.

acid/o acid	**chromat/o** color	**phil/o** love
bas/o alkali; base	**hist/o** tissue or web	**-tome** instrument used to cut

skin **hist (HIST)**	**727** Two terms especially signify the study and diagnosis of skin and tissue characteristics. One of them involves dermat, a root for "_____." The other involves _____, a root for "tissue" or "web" found on the section word list.

dermat/o/logy (**der**-mah-**TAHL**-oh-jee) **hist/o/logy** (his-**TAHL**-oh-jee)	**728** Use the "study of" suffix in cytology (**frame 591**) to help you synthesize two new terms: _____ /____ /_____, "study of skin," and _____ /____ /_____, "study of tissues."

histology	**729** The term _____ involves the study of tissues, some of which (like areolar connective tissue) do resemble webs.
histology	**730** A department of _____ often prepares slides of tissues for study.
dermatology	**731** The term _____ involves the study of skin, especially diseases of the skin.
cytologist **hist/o/logist** (**his-TAHL**-oh-jist) **dermat/o/logist** (**der**-mah-**TAHL**-oh-jist)	**732** Recall that a _____ **(frame 591)** is "one who specializes in the study of cells." In similar fashion, a _____ / _____ / _____ is "one who studies tissues," and a _____ / _____ / _____ is "one who studies the skin."
histologist dermatologist	**733** A _____ studies both normal and diseased tissues in general. A _____, however, concentrates on the skin.
tom	**734** Histologists have to cut body tissues into very thin slices for study. Remember that _____, a root for "cut," exists in both anatomy **(frame 44)** and tomogram **(frame 197).**
micr/o/tom/e (**MIGH**-kroh-**tohm**)	**735** Take the above information, a root in microbiologist **(frame 589)**, and the suffix in macule **(frame 699)** to build _____ / _____ / _____ / _____, an instrument used to make "tiny cuts."
microtome	**736** A _____ cuts extremely thin slices of tissues for study under the microscope.
color	**737** After being cut, tissues are treated with various biological dyes or stains. **Chromat** (**KROH**-mat), like chrom **(frame 87)**, is a root meaning "_____."
chromat/ic	**738** Applying the suffix of icteric **(frame 683)** helps us build _____ / _____, "pertaining to color."
chromatic	**739** The _____ properties of various biological dyes makes them extremely useful in coloring human and animal tissues for inspection.
hyper- **hyper/chromat/ic** (**high**-per-kroh-**MAT**-ik)	**740** Some coloring, however, can be "excessive," denoted by _____, the prefix in hypertonic **(frame 471)**. The term for "pertains to excessive color" then, is _____ / _____ / _____.

hyperchromatic	**741** Certain tissues are _____, meaning they stain excessively and thereby become intensely colored.
phil (FIHL) **phil/ic (FIHL-ik)**	**742** It is almost as if certain tissues "love" certain dyes. The word list cites _____ as a root for "love." Just as chromatic "pertains to color," _____ /____ "pertains to love."
bas/o (BAY-soh) **acid/o**	**743** Certain tissues seem to "love," that is, are heavily stained by, biological dyes having particular characteristics. These include either basic characteristics (with the combining form _____ /____) or acidic characteristics (with the combining form _____ /____).
bas/o/phil/ic (BAY-soh-fihl-ik) **acid/o/phil/ic (ah-SID-oh-fihl-ik)**	**744** For example, _____ /____ /_____ /____ "refers to the love for basic" dyes. Conversely, _____ /____ /_____ /____ "refers to a love for acid" dyes.
acidophilic basophilic	**745** Tissues that are _____ readily stain with acid dyes. Tissues that are _____ readily stain with basic dyes.
Gram	**746** A special kind of dye is **Gram's stain**. Hans _____, a Danish bacteriologist, noticed that certain types of bacteria react with iodine solution and stain a deep violet color. Other types are decolorized, not taking in the stain.
Gram-positive **Gram-negative**	**747** If something reacts, it is generally referred to as being "positive." If it doesn't react it is called "negative." Common sense thus tells you that _____ -_____ bacteria become deep violet with "Gram" stain. But _____ -_____ bacteria do not react with "Gram" stain.

Surgery and Therapies

Word Parts Associated with Surgery, Pharmacology, and Other Therapies Involving the Tissues and Skin

The following is a list of word parts and abbreviations associated with surgery, pharmacology, and other therapies involving the tissues and skin. Use this list to help you complete **frames 749 to 768.**

abras/o	rub	**subcu**	subcutaneous	**sq**	subcutaneous
lip/o	fat	**Subq**	subcutaneous	**top**	place; area
sc	subcutaneous				

748 The skin, especially, is convenient to treat. Its location at the body surface makes it highly accessible to instruments, medications, and physical agents of various kinds.

Information Frame

749 Two antibiotics, for instance, readily work against acne bacteria on the skin. These are **erythromycin** (eh-**rith**-roh-**MIGH**-sin) and **tetracycline** (**tet**-rah-**SIGH**-kleen).

erythromycin tetracycline	**750** Both _____ and _____ are often taken by mouth in conjunction with various **topical** (**TAH**-pih-**kal**) scrubs, soaps, and creams to treat a specific "place" (top)—the surface of the skin.
top/**ical** **derm/a/tom/e** (**DER**-mah-**tohm**)	**751** In cases of severe acne scarring, _____ /_____ applications to the skin surface "area" may be inadequate. The skin must be cut. Just as a microtome **(frame 735)** is an instrument used to make "tiny cuts," a _____ /____ /_____ /____ is a device employed for "skin cuts." In this case the root for "skin" is the one appearing in subdermis **(frame 640)**.
dermatome	**752** A _____ may be used to cut skin from a donor site (as on the anterior surface of the thigh) for transplantation to a severely burned site on the body.
dermatome **derm/abrasion** (**DERM**-ah-**bray**-zhun)	**753** Although a _____ cuts the skin, rubbing, or **abrasion** (ah-**BRAY**-zhun), of the skin may also be useful. The technical term for "process of skin rubbing" is _____ /_____. Here the "skin" root is identical to that for dermatome.
dermabrasion	**754** The technique of _____ is sometimes employed to literally rub off the upper layers of the skin, thereby removing acne scars.
collagen collagen	**755** Certain wrinkles, however, that are too deep to be simply rubbed away are treated by _____ ("glue producer," **frame 632**) **implantation**. This treatment is a controversial technique involving the insertion of thick, ropelike _____ fibers into the dermal area.
collagen implantation	**756** Theoretically, _____ _____ fills in the gaps formerly occupied by wrinkles.
sub/**cutane**/**ous** (**sub**-kyoo-**TAY**-nee-us)	**757** Sometimes it is necessary to inject or remove materials from the subdermal area, "below the skin," to obtain improvement in a person's looks. Recall that cutaneous **(frame 621)** "pertains to the skin." Therefore, _____ /_____ /_____ "refers to (something) below the skin," where the prefix for subdermis is used.
subcutaneous	**758** Abbreviations for _____ are **sc, subcu, Subq,** and **sq**.
sc/subcu/Subq/sq	**759** Injections are often made _____ (use any abbreviation for subcutaneously).
subcutaneous	**760** The adipose or fatty tissue has a _____ location within the hypodermis (subdermis).

hypo/derm/ic (high-poh-**DERM**-ik)

761 Hypodermis can have its "presence of" suffix switched for the ending in chromatic **(frame 738)**. Using that suffix results in the new term _____ / _____ /_____.

hypodermic

762 Subcutaneous injections are made in a _____ position "below the skin."

hypodermic injection

763 A _____ _____, like a Subq injection, is delivered into the fascia and adipose tissue below the dermis.

hypodermic

764 **Hypo** is an abbreviation for _____ injection.

hypo

765 The prefix **hypo-** means "under." But when used as an abbreviation, _____ means hypodermic injection.

lip

766 The fatty tissue below the skin is rich in blood vessels, into which the injected drug can readily enter. Recall that _____, as in lipid **(frame 447)**, is a root for "fat."

lip/o/suction (**LIP**-oh-**suhk**-shun)

767 If a person wants to spot-reduce, without dieting, it is possible to insert a device subcu and "suck out fat." The technical term is _____ / ____ / _____, "the process of sucking fat."

liposuction

768 The _____ ("fat-sucking") procedure is widely performed, but it may have some surgical complications.

Multiple Choice

1. In the term cuboidal, -oid means

a. "condition"   b. "presence"   c. "resemblance"   d. "state"

2. -gen means

a. "formation"   b. "presence"   c. "condition"   d. "state"

3. Areolar pertains to

a. ropelike   b. little areas   c. fatty   d. layered

4. Which of these does *not* mean "red"?

a. icter/o   b. erythr/o   c. rube/o   d. rubell/o

5. Which of these does *not* mean "yellow"?

a. xanth/o   b. jaund/o   c. icter/o   d. cyan/o

6. Strata refers to

a. skins   b. layers   c. sheets   d. tissues

Meanings of Selected Roots

Add the correct combining vowel (cv) after each root. Then write the definition of each root in the space provided.

ROOT/CV	DEFINITION
1. dermat/_____	_____
2. fasci/_____	_____
3. rubell/_____	_____
4. decubit/_____	_____
5. phil/_____	_____
6. cutane/_____	_____
7. muc/_____	_____
8. strat/_____	_____
9. areol/_____	_____
10. adipos/_____	_____

Word Dissection and Translation

Analyze the following terms by dissecting them with slashmarks and identifying their word parts. To the right of each term, write its correct English translation.

Key: R (root), cv (combining vowel), P (prefix), S (suffix)

1. papillae

‗‗‗‗‗‗‗‗‗‗/‗‗‗‗‗‗
     R   S   ‗‗‗‗‗‗‗‗‗‗‗‗‗‗‗‗‗‗‗‗

2. epidermis

‗‗‗‗‗/‗‗‗‗‗‗‗‗‗/‗‗‗‗
  P   R   S   ‗‗‗‗‗‗‗‗‗‗‗‗‗‗‗‗‗‗‗‗

3. cicatricial

‗‗‗‗‗‗‗‗/‗‗‗/‗‗‗‗
     R   cv   S   ‗‗‗‗‗‗‗‗‗‗‗‗‗‗‗‗‗‗‗‗

4. fibrous

‗‗‗‗‗‗‗‗‗/‗‗‗‗‗
     R   S   ‗‗‗‗‗‗‗‗‗‗‗‗‗‗‗‗‗‗‗‗

5. teratoma

‗‗‗‗‗‗‗‗‗/‗‗‗‗‗
     R   S   ‗‗‗‗‗‗‗‗‗‗‗‗‗‗‗‗‗‗‗‗

6. decubitus

‗‗‗‗‗‗‗‗‗/‗‗‗‗‗
     R   S   ‗‗‗‗‗‗‗‗‗‗‗‗‗‗‗‗‗‗‗‗

7. hyperchromatic

‗‗‗‗/‗‗‗‗‗‗‗‗‗/‗‗‗‗
  P   R   S   ‗‗‗‗‗‗‗‗‗‗‗‗‗‗‗‗‗‗‗‗

8. histologist

‗‗‗‗‗‗‗‗/‗‗‗/‗‗‗‗
     R   cv   S   ‗‗‗‗‗‗‗‗‗‗‗‗‗‗‗‗‗‗‗‗

9. acidophilic

‗‗‗‗‗‗‗‗/‗‗‗/‗‗‗‗‗‗‗‗/‗‗‗‗
     R   cv   R   S   ‗‗‗‗‗‗‗‗‗‗‗‗‗‗‗‗‗‗‗‗

10. subcutaneous

‗‗‗‗/‗‗‗‗‗‗‗‗‗/‗‗‗‗
  P   R   S   ‗‗‗‗‗‗‗‗‗‗‗‗‗‗‗‗‗‗‗‗

Terms and Their Abbreviations

In the list below, when the term is given, write its abbreviation in the space provided. When the abbreviation is given, write its corresponding term.

TERM	ABBREVIATION
1. herpes simplex virus	_____
2. _____	hypo
3. _____	sc

Word Spelling

Look at each of the terms listed below. Identify those that are misspelled by circling Y for "Yes." Write the correct spelling in the blank.

WORD	MISSPELLED?	CORRECT SPELLING
1. mykrotome	Y/N	_____
2. pruritus	Y/N	_____
3. herpeez simplex	Y/N	_____
4. dermutalogy	Y/N	_____
5. basophilic	Y/N	_____
6. erythromycin	Y/N	_____
7. addipose	Y/N	_____
8. sebaceeus	Y/N	_____
9. diaphoresis	Y/N	_____
10. zanthosis	Y/N	_____
11. areolar	Y/N	_____
12. subdurmas	Y/N	_____
13. dermahtoesas	Y/N	_____
14. sickatktrishal	Y/N	_____

New Word Synthesis

Using word parts that appear in this and previous chapters, build new terms with the following meanings:

1. _____	referring to love of skin
2. _____	inflammation of tissues
3. _____	excessive flow of scales
4. _____	a white tumor
5. _____	a condition under slime
6. _____	a fat cell
7. _____	referring to grease
8. _____	pertaining to color of a monster
9. _____	inflammation of a little area
10. _____	a columnlike (pattern) of baldness

CASE STUDY

Read through the following partial dermatology case referral. Note the terms in bold print. A series of multiple choice questions probes your knowledge of these terms.

Dermatology Case Referral

A 15-year-old male patient was referred for severe complications of **acne vulgaris** with **seborrhea.** Patient repeatedly picked at large **papules** with his fingernails, leading to formation of extensive furuncles on the right and left cheeks. Patient squeezed furuncles to release pus. This squeezing resulted in occurrence of widespread facial pitting and **cicatricial** lesions.

Case Study Questions

1. The patient's prior prognosis for successful recovery from **acne vulgaris** was

    (a) excellent.

    (b) poor.

    (c) permanent.

    (d) temporary.

2. A synonym for **papules** is

    (a) macules.

    (b) furuncles.

    (c) pimples.

    (d) spots.

3. **Seborrhea** means

    (a) "discharge of slime."

    (b) "flow of grease."

    (c) "bursting forth of pus."

    (d) "rupture of sebum."

4. **Cicatricial** lesions are

    (a) tumors.

    (b) pimples.

    (c) boils.

    (d) scars.

CHAPTER 8 The Skeletal System

INTRODUCTION

The skeleton is our collection of bones and their places of union, the joints. The entire skeleton can be conveniently subdivided into two major parts: the **axial** (**AK**-see-**ahl**) **skeleton** and the **appendicular** (**ap**-en-**DIHK**-yoo-lar) **skeleton** (Figure 8.1). The axial skeleton forms the main lengthwise axis, or central turning rod of the body. It includes the bones of the skull; face; **sternum** (**STER**-num), or "breastplate"; the ribs; and the **vertebral column**, or backbones. The appendicular skeleton is the one in our **appendages** (a-**PEN**-dih-**jez**), or "attachments" to the axial skeleton. These attachments are the arms and legs. Included here are all the bones of the shoulder, arm, wrist, hand, hip, leg, knee, ankle, and foot. We will be learning some terms dealing with specific bones and joints in the axial and appendicular skeletons.

FIGURE 8.1   **The Skeleton and Its Two Major Divisions**

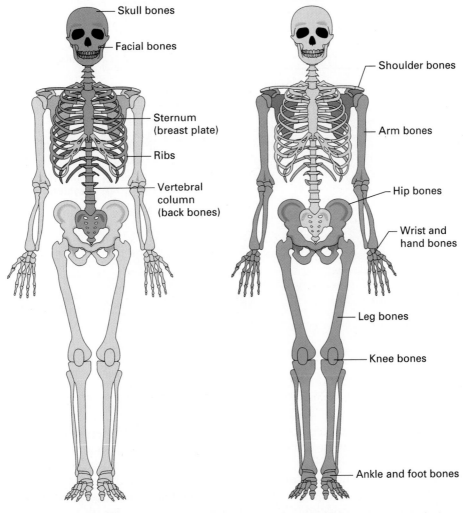

- Skull bones
- Facial bones
- Sternum (breast plate)
- Ribs
- Vertebral column (back bones)

- Shoulder bones
- Arm bones
- Hip bones
- Wrist and hand bones
- Leg bones
- Knee bones
- Ankle and foot bones

The Axial Skeleton (in blue)   The Appendicular Skeleton (in blue)

Two types of **special connective tissue**, cartilage and bone, make up most of the skeleton. The special connective tissues have something very special or unique about the intercellular material between their cells. The intercellular substance in cartilage tissue is a tough, rubbery gel (Figure 8.2A). The intercellular substance in bone tissue is a white, rock-hard, highly calcified material (Figure 8.2B). In both tissues, however, the pattern of cell occurrence is fairly similar. Both cartilage cells, called **chondrocytes** (**KAHN**-droh-**sights**), and bone cells, called **osteocytes** (**AH**-stee-oh-**sights**), occur singly or in small groups within saltwater-filled pools. These pools, called **lacunae** (lah-**KOO**-nee), are scattered here and there in the intercellular substance. Other terms describing the microscopic anatomy of bone and cartilage tissues will be analyzed and synthesized.

FIGURE 8.2

Osseous Tissue Versus Cartilage

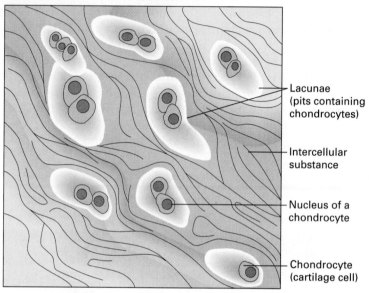

(A) Microscopic View of Cartilage

Lacunae (pits containing chondrocytes)

Intercellular substance

Nucleus of a chondrocyte

Chondrocyte (cartilage cell)

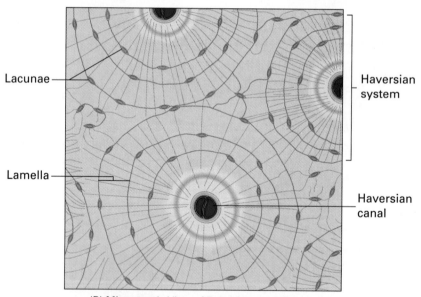

(B) Microscopic View of Dead Osseous Tissue

Lacunae

Lamella

Haversian system

Haversian canal

The bones largely serve as rigid protectors of the soft body viscera. The sternum and ribs, for instance, protect the heart and lungs, while the skull bones create a rock-hard casing for the delicate brain. Other bones (especially in the legs) act as rigid pillars for supporting the weight of the body against gravity. Movable bones act as **levers**—rigid bars that are pulled upon by contracting skeletal muscles. Such pulling results in body movement. The intercellular substance of bone serves as an essential storage bank for body calcium (Ca^{++}) and various other ions. Finally, many bones contain

marrow, a soft pulpy material (either red or yellow) that can store adipose tissue for reserve fuel or produce new blood cells.

Cartilage, being tough and rubbery, has some protective function. The mainly **cartilaginous** (**kar**-tigh-**LAJ**-ih-nus) skeleton of the unborn child, especially, has a protective function (Figure 8.3A). In the adult, cartilage tissue has largely been replaced by bone, but it is still present at particular locations. These include the ends of many bones, where the cartilage softens the contact between bones forming freely movable joints (Figure 8.3B).

FIGURE 8.3   **Body Locations of Cartilage Tissue**

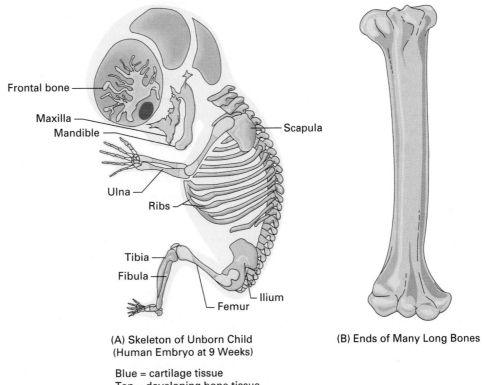
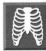

Frontal bone

Maxilla

Mandible

Scapula

Ulna

Ribs

Tibia

Fibula

Ilium

Femur

(A) Skeleton of Unborn Child
(Human Embryo at 9 Weeks)

(B) Ends of Many Long Bones

Blue = cartilage tissue
Tan = developing bone tissue

This chapter presents terms related to the normal anatomy and physiology of bone and cartilage tissues, as well as terms for a number of individual bones and types of joints. Terms related to bone, cartilage, and joint diseases and injuries are examined. Terms associated with lab tests and diagnoses for those conditions are also presented. Finally, terms describing surgery, pharmacology, and other therapies for such problems are discussed.

CHAPTER OBJECTIVES

By the end of this chapter, you should be able to:

1 Identify major prefixes, roots, suffixes, and abbreviations related to the skeleton.

2 Dissect skeletal terms into their component parts.

3 Translate skeletal terms into their common English equivalents.

4 Build new terms associated with the skeleton.

Word Parts Associated with Normal Anatomy and Physiology of the Skeleton

The following is a list of word parts associated with the normal structure and function of the skeleton. Use this list to help you complete **frames 769 to 879.**

articul/o	little joint	**fic/a**	make	**ossi/o**	bone
-blast	sprouter; former	**foramen**	hole	**ov/i**	egg
burs/o	small purselike sac	**foramin/o**	hole	**patell/o**	kneecap
		foss/o	ditch; bony depression	**ped/o**	foot
carp/o	wrist			**pod/o**	foot
cartilagin/o	cartilage (gristle)	**humer/o**	arm	**pub/o**	adult or grown-up
cervic/o	collar; neck	**ischi/o**	hip	**radi/o**	radius
clavic/o	key	**ligament/o**	band of fibers	**sacr/o**	something sacred
clavicul/o	little key	**mandibul/o**	lower jaw bone	**scapul/o**	shoulder blade
coccyg/e	cuckoo	**medull/o**	marrow	**tars/o**	ankle
condyl/o	knuckle	**myel/o**	marrow; spinal cord	**tempor/o**	temple
cost/o	rib			**tibi/o**	shin
femor/o	thigh	**nomin/o**	name	**uln/o**	elbow
fibul/o	little buckle	**osse/o**	bone		

---

osse/o (AHS-ee-oh)
ossi/o (AHS-ee-oh)

769 The skeleton is largely composed of "bone" or oste/o **(frame 51)**. Skim the word list and observe that two other combining forms starting with os mean "bone": _____ /_____ and _____ /_____.

---

osse/ous (AHS-ee-us)

770 When "referring to bone," use the term _____ /_____. To form this adjective we use **-ous**, much like cutaneous **(frame 621)** and osse.

---

osseous

771 The "bony," or _____, tissue in humans derives from either cartilage or primitive connective tissue. A root for "make" is **fic (FIHK)**.

---

ossi/fic/a/tion
(ah-sih-fih-**KAY**-shun)
osse/**ous**
ossification

772 Employ ossi and the suffix **-tion** to help you build _____ /_____ /_____ /_____, the "process of making bone" tissue. To describe "bony" use the term _____ /_____. To describe the "process of making bone" use the term _____.

---

ossification

773 During _____ ("bone formation"), certain bone-forming cells are active.

-blast (BLAST)

oste/o/blast (AHS-tee-oh-blast)

774 Note that _____ on the word list is a suffix for "sprouter" or "former." Combine this suffix with oste. The resulting term is _____ /_____ /_____, with **o**, as usual, being the combining vowel.

---

oste/o/blast

775 An _____ /____ /_____ is literally a "bone former." These immature bone cells are mainly responsible for laying down the rock-hard, calcium-rich background substance found in mature bone tissue.

oste/o/cyt/e (AHS-tee-oh-sight)

776 When immature, or **blast**, cells do become mature, they are called **cyt/es (SIGHTS)**, or "adult cells." So an _____ /____ /_____ /____ is a "mature bone cell present" after ossification has occurred.

osteocytes

777 The "mature bone cells," or _____, exist within lacunae (fluid-filled microscopic pits).

chondr

chondr/o/blasts
(KAHN-droh-blasts)
chondr/o/cyt/es
(KAHN-droh-sights)

778 Recall that _____, the root in hypochondriac **(frame 114)**, means "cartilage." Use this fact to help you synthesize: "cartilage-forming" cells, _____ /____ /_____, and "mature cartilage cells," _____ /____ /_____ /____.

chondroblasts
chondrocytes

779 Like osteoblasts, the _____ are immature cells. The _____, like the osteocytes, are mature connective tissue cells.

cartilagin/o (kar-tih-LAJ-in-oh)

780 Another combining form on the word list, _____ /____, like chondr/o, denotes "cartilage."

cartilagin/ous (kar-tih-LAJ-ihn-us)

781 Just as osseous **(frame 770)** "refers to bone" and cutaneous **(frame 621)** "refers to skin," _____ /_____ "refers to cartilage."

chondr/al (KAHN-dral)
cartilaginous

782 Chondr/o, unlike cartilagin/o, takes the "pertaining to" ending in dermal **(frame 621)**. Therefore, _____ /____ "pertains to cartilage," just as does _____, its counterpart ending in **-ous**

intra-
endo-
intra/cartilagin/ous
(in-trah-kar-tih-LAJ-ihn-us)
endo/chondr/al
(en-doh-KAHN-drul)

783 Recall different prefixes that mean "within." These include _____ (as in intracellular, **frame 472**) and _____ (as in endoplasmic, **frame 519**). Use the first prefix and cartilagin to synthesize _____ /_____ /_____, "pertaining to (something) within cartilage." Similarly, use the second prefix and chondr to synthesize _____ /_____ /____.

intracartilaginous
endochondral

784 Ossification that occurs within preexisting cartilage is called _____ or _____ ossification.

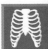

intracartilaginous
endochondral

785 Many **long bones** in the body (bones longer than they are wide) form largely from preexisting cartilage models in the unborn child. The bone is formed by an _____ or _____ process occurring within each cartilage model.

peri/oste/um
end/oste/um
oste

786 An individual bone in the body has both cartilaginous and osseous components. It also has membranes and cavities. Figure 8.4 shows a long bone with a **periosteum** (**pehr**-ee-**AHS**-tee-um), **endosteum** (**en-DAHS**-tee-um), and a **medullary** (**MED**-yoo-**layr**-ee) **cavity.** Subdivide the first two terms with slashmarks as: _____ /_____ /____ and _____ /_____ /____. The root in both is _____ ("bone").

FIGURE 8.4   **Anatomical Features of a Typical Long Bone**

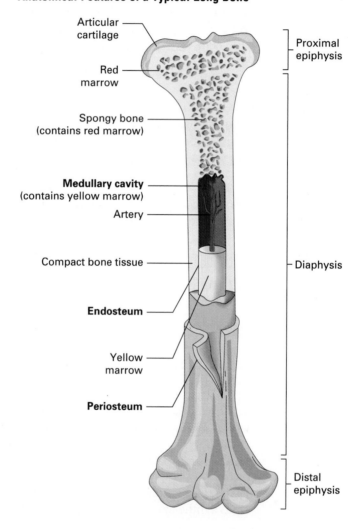

Articular cartilage
Red marrow
Spongy bone (contains red marrow)
Medullary cavity (contains yellow marrow)
Artery
Compact bone tissue
Endosteum
Yellow marrow
Periosteum
Proximal epiphysis
Diaphysis
Distal epiphysis

periosteum
endosteum

787 The _____ is a membrane "present around a bone." The _____ is a membrane "present within a bone."

endosteum
medullary

788 From Figure 8.4 you can see that the _____ (periosteum/endosteum) is the lining of the _____ cavity.

medull/ary **-ary** **medull** (**MED**-yool)	**789** Medullary is subdivided as _____ /_____. The suffix, _____, was first introduced back in **frame 91**. The root, _____, means "marrow."
myel/o (**MIGH**-eh-loh)	**790** Another root on the word list, _____ /____, means either "marrow" or "spinal cord."
pertaining to **myel/ic** (migh-**EL**-ik)	**791** The suffix **-ary** means "_____ ____." The suffix in philic **(frame 742)** has the same meaning. Use the root in **frame 790** and the suffix in philic to construct _____ /____, "pertaining to marrow or the spinal chord."
medullary myelic	**792** We have now discussed two terms that "pertain to marrow." These are _____ and _____. Marrow (specifically **yellow marrow**) is the soft, pulpy, blood-vessel-rich material contained within the deep interior cavity of a long bone.
medullary myelic	**793** One _____ or _____ function that "pertains to marrow" is acting as a storage place for osseous adipose tissue. 
arthr/o (**ARTH**-roh) articul/o (ar-**TIK**-yoo-loh) cellul	**794** At the ends of many bones are joints. Recall that _____ /____ **(frame 51)** is a combining form for "joint." A closely related combining form on the chapter word list, _____ /____, means "little joint." The **ul** portion of the second combining form means "little," and it generally indicates "smallness" of a body part. Recall, for instance, _____, or "little cell" **(frame 423)**.
arthr articul	**795** In common usage, however, _____ ("joint") and _____ ("little joint") are the same.
arthr/al (**ARTH**-ral) **articul/ar** (ar-**TIK**-yoo-lar)	**796** The "joint" root commonly takes the "referring to" ending in epithelial **(frame 568)**. But the "little joint" root usually takes the same ending as columnar **(frame 655)**. Now use this information to build: "referring to a joint," _____ /____, and "referring to a little joint," _____ /____.
arthral articular	**797** The _____ or _____ cartilage at either end of a long bone helps it make a joint with each of its neighbors.
-osis dermatosis	**798** A joint is simply the place of union between two or more bones. Joints come in different types or conditions. You may recall **(frame 670)** that a suffix ending for "condition of" is _____, as in "a condition of the skin," or _____.

arthr/o/sis (arth-ROH-sis)

799 Use the root in arthral plus the suffix in dermatosis to help you build
_____ /_____ /_____, "a condition (or type) of joint."

---

dermatoses
arthr/o/ses (arth-ROH-seez)

800 Just as the plural of dermatosis is _____ **(frame 671)**,
the plural of arthrosis is _____ /_____ /_____.

---

arthrosis
arthroses

801 An _____ is a general type of joint. Two or more of
these general types of joints are called _____.

---

arthroses

802 Two major joint types, or _____, are listed below:
diarthroses (**digh**-arth-**ROH**-seez)
synarthroses (**sin**-arth-**ROH**-seez)

---

di/arthr/o/sis
syn/arthr/o/sis

803 Subdivide diarthrosis with slashmarks:
_____ /_____ /_____ /_____. Do the same for synarthrosis:
_____ /_____ /_____ /_____.

---

diarthrosis
synarthrosis

804 Observe the important differences in meaning that can result from different prefixes only. Review of **frames 80** and **83** should enable you to translate "a type of double joint" as _____, and "a condition of together joint" as _____.

---

diarthrosis (**digh**-arth-**ROH**-sis)
synarthrosis (**sin**-arth-**ROH**-sis)

805 The singular form of diarthroses is _____. The singular form of synarthroses is _____.

---

two (double)

806 When you say someone is double-jointed, you really mean that the person has an unusually high degree of mobility at certain joints (such as those between the finger bones). These freely movable joints are called diarthroses. Examples include the knee, hip, and shoulder joints. In the term diarthroses, the prefix **di-** means "_____."

---

synarthroses

with
together

807 Other joints are immovable. In this group, the adjacent bones are strapped together by collagen fibers, such that no movement is possible. Chief examples of the suture joints, or _____, are the jagged seams between adjacent skull and facial bones. In the term synarthroses, **syn-** means "_____" or "_____."

---

ligament

808 Diarthroses (freely movable joints) exist as closed sacs (Figure 8.5). The bones forming the joints are held together by ligaments (**LIG**-ah-**ments**), or "bands." Each band, or _____, consists of stretchy elastic and tough collagen fibers.

Chapter 8 The Skeletal System

ligament/ous (**lig**-ah-**MEN**-tus)	**809** Just as the term cartilaginous "refers to cartilage" **(frame 781)**, the term _____ /_____ "refers to bands."
ligamentous	**810** Straps of _____ tissue create tough bands that make a joint capsule around the ends of freely movable bones.

FIGURE 8.5   **Anatomy of a Freely Movable Joint**

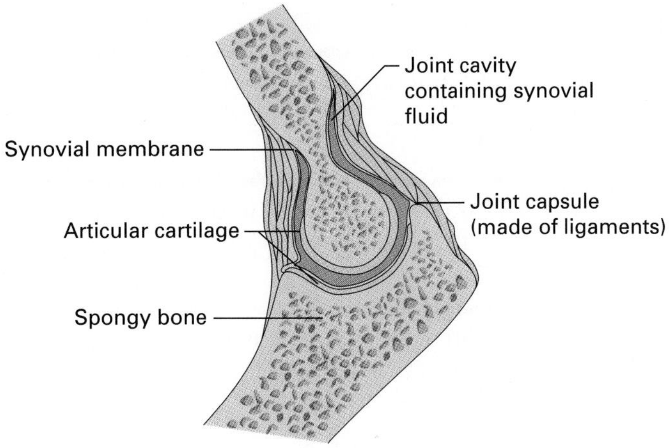

- Joint cavity containing synovial fluid
- Synovial membrane
- Articular cartilage
- Joint capsule (made of ligaments)
- Spongy bone

syn/ov/i/al	**811** Within the joint capsule is a **synovial** (**sin-OH**-vee-al) **membrane.** Using the prefix of synarthrosis and the "pertaining to" ending of endo-chondral **(frame 783)**, dissect synovial with slashes: _____ /_____ /_____ /_____. Note **i** rather than **o** is the combining vowel in this case.
ov (OHV)	**812** The root in synovial, _____, means "egg." This term therefore indicates that synovial fluid is a clear syrupy fluid that resembles the whites of many "eggs" poured "together"!
synovial	**813** The function of _____ fluid is lubrication. It serves as a type of joint oil, lubricating the ends of adjoining bones and reducing their friction and wear.
burs/a (**BUR**-sah) papilla	**814** Near many freely movable joints are bursae (**BUR**-see), or "purses." The singular form of bursae is _____ /_____ , just as _____ **(frame 625)** is the singular form of papillae.
bursa bursae	**815** A _____ near a joint is typically a small fluid-filled "purse" or sac. Cushioning by _____ prevents overlying parts of muscles and bones from rubbing too hard against one another during body movements.

condyl (**KAHN**-dighl)
foramen (for-**A**-men)
foss (**FAHS**)

816 Look up in the word list these roots describing anatomical features that are parts of many bones:

_____ bony "knuckle"

_____ "hole" in a bone

_____ "ditch or depression" in a bone

---

condyl/e (**KAHN**-dighl)

foss/a (**FAH**-sah)

817 The "knuckle" root assumes the "presence of" ending in osteocyte **(frame 776)** to become _____ /_____. The "ditch or depression" root assumes the "presence of" suffix in bursa to yield _____ /_____.

---

fossa
condyles

818 Sometimes a "depression," or _____, will occur between two _____ ("knuckles").

---

foss/ae (**FAH**-see)

819 Just as bursae is the plural of bursa, _____ /_____ is the plural of fossa.

---

fossae
condyles

820 In your mind, visualize _____ (fossae/condyles) as dents on a bone, whereas _____ (fossae/condyles) are bony bumps.

---

epi-
epi/condyl/es
(**eh**-pih-**KAHN**-dighls)
epicondyles

821 The prefix in epidermal **(frame 652)**, _____, can be used to fashion a new term, _____ /_____ /_____, which denotes literally "(something) present upon bony knuckles." If we visualize condyles as bumps or knuckles, then _____ are bumps lying on those bumps.

---

foramen

822 Looking back at **frame 816** shows that a _____ is a hole rather than a bump.

---

foramen

foramin/a (for-**AH**-mih-nah)

823 When _____ ("hole") is used as a root in combination with other word parts, it is spelled **foramin** (for-**A**-min). The plural form takes **-a**. Consequently, _____ /_____ are "holes" in the bones.

---

foramina

824 There are _____ ("holes") in most bones for the passage of nerves and blood vessels.

---

fossa
fossae
condyle
condyles
epicondyle
epicondyles
foramen
foramina

825 Figure 8.6 depicts a bone with certain characteristics or markings. Identify the single and plural names for each:

_____ (a single depression)

_____ (a group of depressions)

_____ (a single knuckle-like bump)

_____ (a group of knuckle-like bumps)

_____ (a single bump on a bump)

_____ (a group of bumps on other bumps)

_____ (a single hole)

_____ (a group of holes)

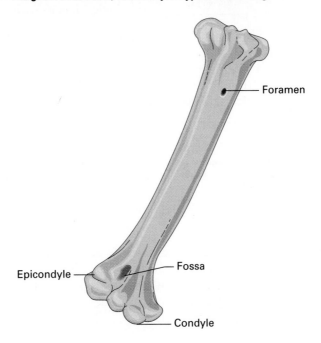

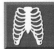

826 In addition to having prominent structural features, bones also occur in groups within certain body areas. Some of these body areas are denoted by the following roots (found on the word list):

carp (KARP)
cervic (SER-vik)
ped (PEED)
pod (POHD)
tars (TARS)

_____ "wrist"
_____ "collar; neck"
_____ or _____ "foot"
_____ "ankle"

827 Adopt the ending of synovial **(frame 811)** to help you build _____ /_____ ("pertaining to the wrist"); _____ /_____ ("referring to the neck"); _____ /_____ or _____ /_____ ("relating to the foot"); and _____ /_____ ("pertaining to the ankle").

carp/al (KARP-al)
cervic/al (SER-vik-al)
ped/al (PEE-dal)
pod/al (POH-dal)
tars/al (TAR-sal)

828 The wrist, or _____; ankle, or _____; and foot, or _____ (_____) bones are all classified as part of the appendicular skeleton. The collar or _____ bones, being vertebrae, are considered part of the axial skeleton.

carpal
tarsal
pedal (podal)
cervical

829 The roots for "wrist" and "ankle" take the "presence of" suffix found in pruritus **(frame 710)**. This combination yields _____ /_____, "the wrist," and _____ /_____, "the ankle."

carp/us (KAR-pus)
tars/us (TAR-sus)

carpus tarsus	**830** The _____, or "wrist," contains smaller bones. Likewise, the _____, or "ankle," has its own complement of bones.
cervical thoracic lumbar	**831** The "neck," or _____, area in adults contains 7 vertebrae. Inferior to these are 12 _____ ("pertaining to the chest," **frame 398**) vertebrae. Even more caudally located are 5 _____ ("referring to loins," **frame 383**) vertebrae.
Information Frame	**832** Two additional combining forms that represent regions of the vertebral column are **sacr/o** (**SAY**-kroh) and **coccyg/o** (**KAHK**-sih-goh). The first indicates something "sacred," the second, a "cuckoo" bird!
coccyg sacr **sacr/um** (**SAY**-krum)	**833** The root for "cuckoo" is _____. Used alone, however, the term **coccyx** (**KAHK**-siks) is employed. The root for "sacred," _____, usually takes the "presence of" ending found in endosteum **(frame 786)**. The result is _____ /____, the "presence of (something) sacred."
sacrum	**834** The strange word origins in the preceding frame suggest that the early anatomists had quite vivid imaginations! The _____, or "sacred" bone, is large, pointed, and spade-shaped (Figure 8.7A). This unusual shape, legend has it, caused a belief that the bone was somehow sacred. It was thought to be a bone from which an entire human body could be reincarnated after death.
coccyx	**835** The _____, or "cuckoo," somewhat resembles the thick stubby beak of a cuckoo bird (Figure 8.7A). Hence its name. In nonclinical usage, however, the bone is called the "tailbone."
sacr/al (**SAY**-kral) **coccyg/e/al** (**kahk-SIJ**-ee-al)	**836** The roots for both "cuckoo" and "sacred" assume the "referring to" suffix of cervical. The "cuckoo" root, however, takes **e** as a combining vowel. Use this information to help you build _____ /____, "referring to the sacrum," and _____ /____ /____, "referring to the coccyx."
sacrum sacral coccyx coccygeal	**837** In most adults, the single large _____ ("sacred" bone) actually consists of five smaller _____ vertebrae that have fused together inferior to the last lumbar vertebra. The single _____ ("cuckoo") likewise consists of four smaller _____ vertebrae fused together to form the caudal tip of the vertebral column. The entire vertebral column and its regions are shown in Figure 8.7B.

Detailed Anatomy of the Vertebral Column

(A) The Sacrum and Coccyx

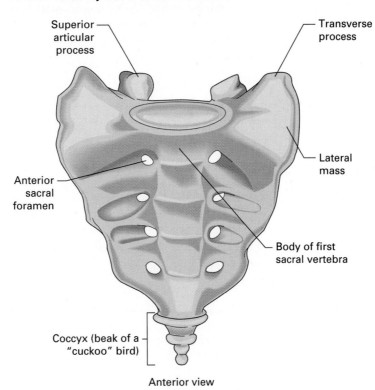

Superior articular process

Transverse process

Lateral mass

Anterior sacral foramen

Body of first sacral vertebra

Coccyx (beak of a "cuckoo" bird)

Anterior view

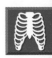

(B) The Vertebral Column and Its Regions

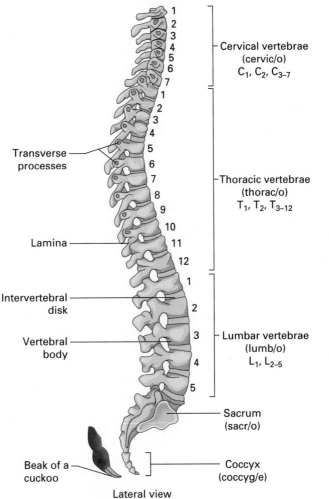

Cervical vertebrae (cervic/o)
C_1, C_2, C_{3-7}

Transverse processes

Thoracic vertebrae (thorac/o)
T_1, T_2, T_{3-12}

Lamina

Intervertebral disk

Vertebral body

Lumbar vertebrae (lumb/o)
L_1, L_{2-5}

Sacrum (sacr/o)

Beak of a cuckoo

Coccyx (coccyg/e)

Lateral view

838 Another intriguing bone consisting of smaller fused members is the hip, or **innominate** (ih-**NAH**-mih-**nut**) bone. **Nomin** (**NAH**-min) is a root for "name." Innominate has the same prefix as inorganic **(frame 445)** and the suffix **-ate**, which means "_____ _____" **(frame 92)**.

something that

839 Use the above facts to help you dissect innominate as
_____ / _____ / _____.

in/**nomin**/ate

840 Innominate literally translates as "something that (has) no name." This _____ bone has no single name because it is actually the result of three smaller bones that fuse together in early childhood. These bones are called the **ilium, ischium** (**ISH**-ee-**um**), and **pubis** (**PYOO**-bis).

innominate

841 You may remember the _____ **(frame 385)** as the "flank present" on either side of the umbilicus. This bone forms the broad, flared flank of each innominate bone (Figure 8.8).

ilium

842 Containing the same suffix as ilium is its bony neighbor, the _____ /_____. The root in this case is **ischi** (**ISH**-ee), the "hip" or "socket of the hip joint." This bone is the stirrup-shaped inferior portion of the innominate and is named for the deep fossa in its lateral aspect. This depression is the socket for the hip joint.

ischi/um

843 The third bony member of the innominate mentioned in **frame 840**, the _____, takes **-is** as its "presence of" ending.

pubis

844 Pubis is therefore analyzed with slashmarks as _____ /_____. Its root, _____, means "adult" or "grown-up."

pub/is
pub (**PYOOB**)

845 The root in the preceding frame takes the suffix of hyperchromatic **(frame 740)** for its "pertaining to" usage. Therefore, _____ /_____ means "presence of an adult or grown-up," while _____ /_____ "pertains to an adult or grown-up."

pub/is
pub/ic (**PYOOB**-ik)

846 The _____ is the solid, narrow, barlike anterior portion of the innominate. Originally the name referred only to the hair-covered _____ area containing the sex organs of "grown-ups." (The innominate and its three subparts are depicted in Figure 8.8.)

pubis

pubic

FIGURE 8.8

The Innominate Bone and Its Subparts

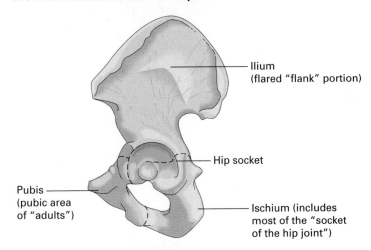

- Ilium (flared "flank" portion)
- Hip socket
- Pubis (pubic area of "adults")
- Ischium (includes most of the "socket of the hip joint")

Information Frame

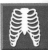

847 There are approximately 206 bones in the adult human skeleton. The names of these individual bones and their characteristics or markings are often derived from highly imaginative and entertaining analogies and concepts. We can touch upon only a few here. It is helpful to group bones according to body region. Pronounce the terms and roots listed in Table 8.1. These are all related to the upper body (skull, shoulder, ribs, and arms).

TABLE 8.1

Some Names and Roots for Bones in the Upper Body

Bone Name	Root	Meaning
clavicle (**KLA**-vih-kl)	clavic (**KLA**-vik)	key: the collar bone
	clavicul	little key
scapula (**SKAP**-yoo-lah)	scapul (**SKAP**-yool)	shoulder blade
costa	cost (**KAHST**)	coast: a rib
mandible	mandib (man-**DIB**)	a chewer: jaw
	mandibul (man-**DIB**-yool)	a little chewer
temporal (**TEM**-por-al)	tempor (**TEM**-por)	a temple
humerus (**HYOO**-mer-us)	humer (**HYOO**-mer)	the shoulder: upper arm bone
radius (**RAY**-dee-us)	radi	a ray, rod, or spoke of a wheel: a forearm bone
ulna (**UL**-nah)	uln (**ULN**)	the elbow

---

mandible
temporal

mandib/le
tempor/al

848 Let us now work with two terms from Table 8.1 that are related to the skull. These bones are the _____, or lower jaw bone, literally called "a chewer," and the _____ bones, which form part of the sides of the skull, "a temple" for the brain. The first term is subdivided as _____ /____, the second as _____ /____.

mandib	**849** The **-le** suffix after _____, the root in mandible, indicates something "little." The other root indicating mandible is _____, which itself means "little chewer."
mandibul	

temporal	**850** The adjective _____ "refers to a temple." Build a term that "refers to a little chewer," where the "referring to" ending is that in areolar **(frame 642)**: _____ /____.
mandibul/ar (man-**DIB**-yoo-**lar**)	

mandibular	**851** A knuckle-like bump on the mandible, called the_____ condyle, fits into a socket on the _____ (temple) bone.
temporal	

scapul/ar	**852** Pronounce **scapular** (**SKAP**-yoo-**lar**) and **ulnar** (**UL**-nar). Dissecting each of them as you did mandibular yields _____ /____ and _____ /____.
uln/ar	

scapular	**853** Table 8.1 suggests that _____ "refers to the shoulder blade," while _____ "refers to the elbow."
ulnar	

scapul/a	**854** Figure 8.9 reveals that the _____ /____ is "the shoulder blade" and the _____ /____ is "the elbow" bone. Both these terms contain the "presence of" ending in fossa **(frame 817).**
uln/a	

FIGURE 8.9   **Some Bones of the Upper Body**

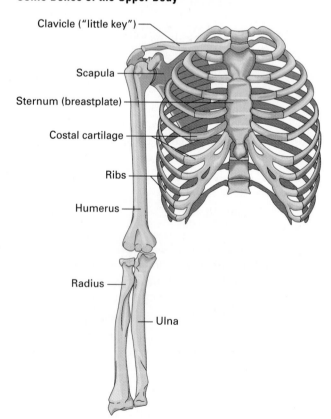

Chapter 8 The Skeletal System

scapula cost	**855** The _____, or shoulder blade, is the spadelike bone lying just posterior to the upper ribs. Table 8.1 cites _____ as the root for costa, meaning "rib."
cost/al (KAHS-tal)	**856** The adjective _____ /_____ "pertains to ribs," just as temporal "pertains to temples."
costal	**857** The _____ **cartilages** are those that attach the anterior ends of the ribs to the breastplate.
clavicle	**858** The ribs do not form a joint with the scapula. The _____, or collar bone, however, does.
clavic/**le**	**859** Clavicle is subdivided as _____ /_____, just as mandible is.
clavicle	**860** Table 8.1 defines the _____ as a "little key." The bone was named for its somewhat curved S shape, like an ancient door key.
clavic clavicul	**861** The root of clavicle is _____. Another root with the same meaning in Table 8.1 is _____.
clavicul	**862** Just as mandibul has a **ul** to indicate smallness, _____ (root for "little key") has one as well.
clavicul/ar (klah-**VIK**-yoo-**lar**)	**863** Mandibul/**ar** means "referring to a little chewer," and we can create _____ /_____ for "referring to a little key."
clavicular	**864** The lateral end of the clavicle makes a _____ ("little key") joint with the scapula.
humer	**865** The clavicle and scapula together create most of the shoulder. Note in Table 8.1 that _____, however, is a root for "shoulder."
radi	**866** Recall that _____ **(frame 211)** is a root for "ray" or "radiation." It can also denote a "rod" or "spoke," as of a wooden wagon wheel.

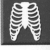

humer/us (**HYOO**-mer-**us**)
radi/us (**RAY**-dee-**us**)

867 Both of the roots in the preceding two frames assume the suffix of tarsus (**frame 829**) for "presence of." This combination yields _____ /_____ ("presence of the shoulder") and _____ /_____ ("presence of a rod"), respectively.

---

humerus
radius

868 The _____ is the long bone of the upper arm, named for its jointing with the scapula at the "shoulder." The _____ is the long bone forming a "rod" on the thumb side of the forearm. (Look back at Figure 8.9.)

---

humer/al (**HYOO**-mer-**al**)
radi/al (**RAY**-dee-**al**)

869 Cost/al provides an adjective-forming pattern for the roots in both humerus and radius. This pattern is reflected as _____ /_____ ("relating to the shoulder") and _____ /_____ ("relating to a rod").

---

radial
humeral

870 The _____ (humeral/radial) pulse is the heartbeat felt in the wrist. The _____ (humeral/radial) pulse is detectable in the upper arm.

Information Frame

871 Another grouping of bones can be associated with the lower body. Pronounce the names and roots of some of these bones, which are listed in Table 8.2 below.

T A B L E   8 . 2

Some Names and Roots for Bones in the Lower Body

Bone Name	Root	Meaning
femur (**FEE**-mer)	**femor** (**FEH**-mor)	thigh
patella (**pah-TEH**-lah)	**patell** (**pah-TEL**)	little pan; knee pan; kneecap
tibia (**TIH**-bee-**ah**)	**tibi** (**TIH**-bee)	pipe; flute; shin bone
fibula (**FIH**-byoo-lah)	**fibul** (**FIH**-byool)	little buckle or clasp; a bone of the lower leg

---

patell/a
tibi/a
fibul/a

872 All of the bones mentioned in Table 8.2 are illustrated in Figure 8.10. Note that the names of three of these bones—the _____ /_____ ("little pan"), _____ /_____ ("pipe"), and _____ /_____ ("little buckle")—end in the same way as scapula and ulna.

---

patella
tibia

fibula

873 The _____, or kneecap, is named for its rough resemblance to a small shallow pan. The _____, or shin bone, is the larger, more medial bone of the lower leg. In ancient times this bone was taken from birds and used as a pipe or flute. Finally, the _____ is the smaller, more lateral bone of the lower leg. It resembles the pointed clasp of an ancient buckle.

---

femur
femor

874 The _____ is simply named for its body location—the upper leg or "thigh." It is denoted by the root _____.

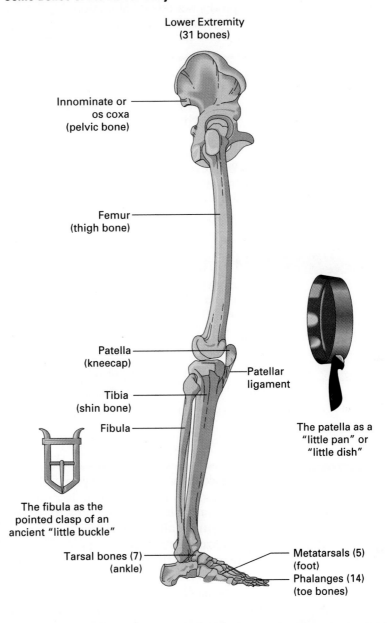

Lower Extremity
(31 bones)

Innominate or
os coxa
(pelvic bone)

Femur
(thigh bone)

Patella
(kneecap)

Patellar
ligament

Tibia
(shin bone)

Fibula

The patella as a
"little pan" or
"little dish"

The fibula as the
pointed clasp of an
ancient "little buckle"

Tarsal bones (7)
(ankle)

Metatarsals (5)
(foot)

Phalanges (14)
(toe bones)

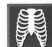

---

patell/ar (pah-**TEH**-ler)
femor/al (**FEM**-or-al)

875 The roots for both the kneecap and the thigh bone generally take the "relating to" suffix in clavicular. Using that suffix results in _____ /____ ("relating to a little pan or kneecap") and _____ /____ ("relating to the thigh").

---

femoral
patellar

876 The athlete had _____ pain in the thigh area when she landed too hard and overpulled her _____ ("kneecap") tendon.

---

fibul
fibul/ar (**FIH**-byoo-ler)

877 Like femor and patell, _____, the root for "little buckle," takes -**ar** as its "pertaining to" suffix. The result is _____ /____—"pertaining to a little buckle."

tibi/al (**TIH**-bee-al)

878 The root in tibia, however, usually assumes -**al** for "pertaining to." The product of this combination is _____ /____, which "pertains to the shin bone or pipe."

tibial

fibular

879 Tiny hairline fractures may result in _____, or shin bone, pain when a person runs too far or too frequently. Because the "little buckle" bone plays no major role in weight bearing, _____ pain is less likely.

880 Whatever the names of the individual bones and joints, they are susceptible to several types of diseases and injuries.

Diseases

Word Parts Associated with Diseases of the Skeletal System

The following is a list of word parts and abbreviations describing diseases and injuries of the skeletal system. Use this list to help you complete **frames 882 to 921.**

Fx	fracture	**OA**	osteoarthritis	**scoli/o**	crookedness
FxBB	fracture of both bones	**rachi/o**	spine	**spicul/o**	little point
kyph/o	hump	**rheum/o**	painful change	**spondyl/o**	backbone
lord/o	bending backward	**rheumat/o**	painful change		

881 Disorders of the skeletal system may involve problems with the bones themselves. Recall that oste is a root for "bone." Pronounce these terms:
osteoarthritis (**ahs**-tee-oh-arth-**RIGH**-tus)
osteoma (**ahs**-tee-**OH**-mah)
osteomalacia (**ahs**-tee-oh-mah-**LAY**-shuh)
osteomyelitis (**ahs**-tee-oh-my-eh-**LIGH**-tus)
osteoporosis (**ahs**-tee-oh-por-**OH**-sis)
osteosarcoma (**ahs**-tee-oh-sar-**KOH**-mah)

-oma
sarcoma

oste/oma
oste/o/sarc/oma

882 Perhaps you remember from Chapter 6 that _____ (**frame 560**) is a suffix for "tumor," while a _____ (**frame 573**) is a "fleshy tumor." Use this information to identify and subdivide
_____ /_____ ("bone tumor") and
_____ /____ /_____ /_____ (a "fleshy bone tumor").

osteoma

osteosarcoma

883 An _____, or bone tumor, in general is not necessarily malignant. From what we have learned about sarcomas, however, an _____ is by definition a malignant bone tumor.

-malacia

oste/o/malacia

884 You learned earlier (**frame 147**) that _____ is a suffix for "destructive softening." Thus "destructive softening of bone" is given by the term _____ /____ /_____ (first introduced in **frame 148**).

osteomalacia	**885** An _____ of bone makes it soft and weak with a tendency to buckle and deform under the body's weight.
chondr/oma (kahn-**DROH**-mah) **chondr/o/malacia** (**kahn**-droh-mah-**LAY**-shuh)	**886** Cartilage, like bone, can also have tumors or a destructive softening. Use a root from chondrocytes **(frame 778)** to help you build _____ /_____ , "tumor of cartilage," and _____ /_____ /_____ , "destructive softening of cartilage."
chondroma chondromalacia	**887** Like an osteoma, a _____ , or neoplasm of cartilage, is not necessarily malignant. Like osteomalacia, _____ is a destructive softening of bone-related connective tissue that may promote limb deformity.
oste/o/porosis	**888** Osteoporosis, subdivided as _____ /_____ /_____ , is an "abnormal condition of holes or pores" in a "bone." Its suffix was introduced in **frame 147**.
osteoporosis	**889** A chronic deficiency in dietary calcium, which is stored in bone tissue, is a main cause of _____ ("condition of pores in bones").
osteoporosis	**890** A person with _____ has fragile bones with holes or pores that are much larger than normal. This increased fragility makes bones more susceptible to fracture. Figure 8.11 shows a severe deformity of the tibia and fibula from a fracture and this condition of excessive holes.

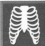

FIGURE 8.11

A Severe Skeletal Deformity Associated with Osteoporosis
(From R. Carlton and A. Adler, *Principles of Radiographic Imaging: An Art and a Science,* Albany, NY: Delmar Publishers Inc., 1992)

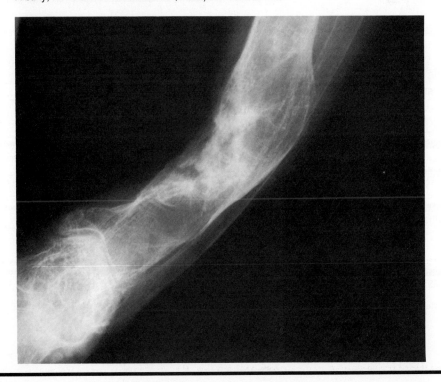

Fx
FxBB

891 A fracture is a break in the structural continuity of a bone. The word list cites _____ as a two-letter abbreviation for fracture. Fracture of both bones is abbreviated as _____.

Fx

FxBB

892 The great force of a man falling forward onto his hand from a moving bicycle may result in a fracture or _____, of his clavicle. Such a single fracture of the clavicle is shown in Figure 8.12. A fracture of both bones in the lower arm would be abbreviated as _____.

F I G U R E   8 . 1 2   **Complete Fracture and Severe Displacement of the Clavicle**

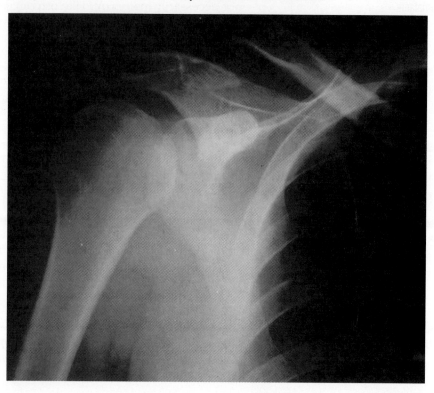

myel/itis (migh-eh-**LIGH**-tis)
oste/o/myel/itis

893 Bone and joints, like skin tissue, can suffer from inflammation. Extract the suffix from dermatitis **(frame 697)** and the root in myelic **(frame 791)** to help you build _____ /_____, "marrow inflammation," and _____ /_____ /_____ /_____, "inflammation of bone marrow."

myelitis
osteomyelitis

894 Technically, _____ is a form of _____, because any marrow that is "inflamed" is located in a "bone."

myel/oma (migh-eh-**LOH**-mah)

895 Another disease involving marrow is _____ /_____, or a "tumor of marrow."

myelomas
myelitis

896 Any _____ ("marrow tumors") present may be associated with _____ ("marrow inflammation"). Symptoms can include fever and pain.

arthr/itis (arth-**RIGH**-tis) **oste/o/arthr/itis**	**897** Diseases of joints are also common. Use the root in arthral **(frame 796)** to help you build _____ /_____, an "inflammation of joints." Technically, this condition is referred to as _____ /_____ /_____ /_____ ("inflammation of bony joints").
arthritis osteoarthritis	**898** A case of _____ is technically a case of _____, because "bone" tissue adjacent to the "inflamed joints" is almost always involved.
OA	**899** The two roots in osteoarthritis lead to its abbreviation as _____ _____.
OA	**900** Osteoarthritis, or _____ _____, is generally accompanied by joint pain.
arthr/algia (arth-**RAL**-juh)	**901** Use a root in osteoarthritis and the suffix **-algia (frame 127)** to build _____ /_____, or "joint pain."
arthralgia	**902** Often _____, or "joint pain," accompanies various harmful changes in the joints. **Rheum (ROOM)** and **rheumat (ROO-mat)** are roots for "painful change."
-oid **rheumat/oid** (**ROO**-mah-toyd)	**903** Incorporating the second root in the preceding frame with the _____ suffix for "resembling" **(frame 93)** results in _____ /_____. This term translates as "resembling painful changes."
rheumatoid	**904** More severe than osteoarthritis is _____ **arthritis.** This is an "inflammation" involving "painful changes" and gross deformity in "joint" structure.
rheumat/ic (roo-**MAT**-ik)	**905** Rheumat usually takes the ending in pubic **(frame 845)** for its "pertaining to" suffix. Consequently, _____ /_____ "refers to painful changes."
rheumatic	**906** A condition called _____ **fever** involves an elevation of body temperature accompanied by painful changes in the muscles and joints.
bunion bursa	**907** Also painful are **bunions** (**BUN**-yuns), or "mounds." In reality, a _____ is an inflammatory swelling of the _____ (fluid-filled "purse," **frame 815**) overlying the joint of the big toe. This inflammation forms a "mound" on the big toe, but it is not a form of arthritis.

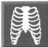

bunion	**908** Besides _____ (inflamed bursa over the big toe), other bumps or mounds may occur on the bony tissue itself. Look at **exostosis (eks-ahs-TOH-sis)** and **spicule (SPIK-yool)**. The first term contains the suffix in dermatosis **(frame 670)**, the second term the suffix in macule **(frame 699)**. Dissect exostosis with slashmarks as ____ /_____ /____ /_____. Dissect spicule as _____ /____.
ex/**ost**/o/**sis** spicul/e	

spicul (SPIK-yool) a little point	**909** The root in spicule, _____, means "little point." Therefore, **spicul/e** translates as "presence of ____ _____ _____."

ex- outside bone	**910** The prefix in exostosis, _____, means "outside" **(frame 366)**. Consequently, exostosis literally indicates an "abnormal condition of (something sticking) _____ _____."

exostosis spicule	**911** In general, an "abnormal bony projection" is called a/an _____, especially if it is blunt or rounded. The term _____ is usually reserved for abnormal bony projections that are slender and "pointed."

spicules	**912** Figure 8.13 contrasts a normal big toe joint on the left foot with a big toe joint bearing two _____ ("little points") on the right. One of these abnormal projections is just anterior to the joint, while the other is immediately posterior to it.

FIGURE 8.13

Normal versus Abnormal Big Toe Joint
(A) Big Toe Joint on the Right Foot (Showing Spicules)
(B) Normal Big Toe Joint on the Left Foot

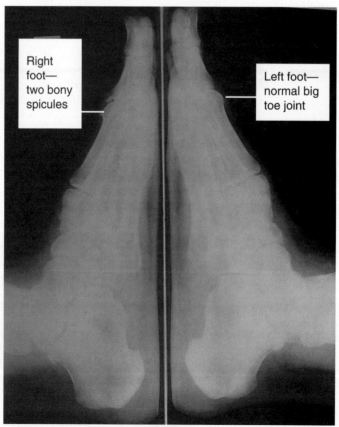

Right foot— two bony spicules

Left foot— normal big toe joint

(A) **(B)**

spondyl/o/sis (**spahn**-dil-**OH**-sis)

913 Finally, the backbone (spine or vertebral column) may suffer various abnormalities. A root for "spine" is **rachi** (**RAH**-kee). A root for "backbone" is **spondyl** (**SPAHN**-dil). Use the second root and the suffix in exostosis to build _____ / _____ / _____. This term translates as "an abnormal condition of the backbone."

---

spondylosis

914 A deterioration and stiffening of the spine is referred to as

_____.

Information Frame

915 Another major problem of the vertebral column is a great exaggeration of its normal curves. Here are some roots describing such exaggerations:
kyph (**KIGHF**) "hump-backed"
lord (**LORD**) "bending backward"
scoli (**SKOH**-lee) "crookedness"

---

kyph/o/sis (kigh-**FOH**-sis)
lord/o/sis (lor-**DOH**-sis)
scoli/o/sis (**skoh**-lee-**OH**-sis)

916 Add the suffix of spondylosis to each of the roots described in the preceding frame. The three new terms produced are
_____ / _____ / _____   "condition of being hump-backed"
_____ / _____ / _____   "condition of bending backward"
_____ / _____ / _____   "condition of crookedness"

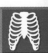

---

kyphosis

917 The problem of _____, or "humping of the back," is due to an exaggeration of the normal thoracic curve (Figure 8.14A).

---

lordosis

918 The problem of _____, also called sway-back, is a "bending backward" and straining due to an exaggeration of the normal lumbar curve (Figure 8.14B). This condition temporarily occurs in pregnant women with protruding abdomens; it usually subsides after delivery.

---

scoliosis

919 The problem of _____ is a right or left lateral curvature ("crookedness") of the spine from its normal position along the body midline. (See Figure 8.14C.)

---

kyph/o/scoli/o/sis
(**kigh**-foh-**skoh**-lee-**OH**-sis)

920 The roots for "hump-backed" and "crookedness" can be combined to create another abnormal condition called
_____ / _____ / _____ / _____ / _____.

---

kyphoscoliosis

921 In persons suffering from _____, a painful dorsal humping is accompanied by a marked shift of the vertebral column to either the right or left of the body midline. (See Figure 8.14D.)

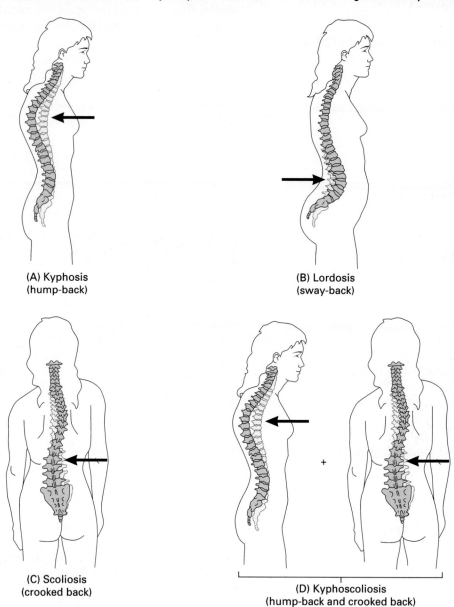

(A) Kyphosis
(hump-back)

(B) Lordosis
(sway-back)

(C) Scoliosis
(crooked back)

(D) Kyphoscoliosis
(hump-back and crooked back)

922 There are a number of terms describing diagnostic procedures for the skeletal system.

Lab Tests and Diagnoses

Word Parts Associated with Lab Tests and Diagnoses for the Skeletal System

The following is a list of word parts associated with diagnostic tests for the skeletal system. Use this list to help you complete **frames 923 to 933.**

-centesis	puncture and tapping of fluid	**-o/scopy**	process of examining
-gram	x-ray image	**scan**	use of radioactive isotopes

arthr/o/scop/e (ARTH-roh-**skohp**)

923 Some diagnostic procedures focus on examining joints, others on bone itself. Take, for example, the root in arthritis **(frame 897)**. Combine it with a root and suffix in microscope **(frame 427)**. The result, _____ /____ /_____ /____, translates as "an instrument used to examine joints."

arthroscope

924 An _____ is an endoscope **(frame 180)** that is inserted directly into joints to examine their interior.

micr/o/scopy

arthr/o/scopy (arth-**RAH**-skoh-**pee**)

925 Recall that _____ /____ /_____ **(frame 585)** is "the process of examining tiny (things)." A similar term is _____ /____ /_____, "the process of examining joints."

stern/al (**STER**-nul)

926 Examination can also be done by aspirating marrow from bones. The **sternum**, or "breastplate," is a large surface bone convenient for such sampling. The procedure is formally called _____ /____ ("pertaining to the breastplate") **puncture**, where the "pertaining to" ending of synovial **(frame 811)** is adopted.

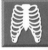

sternal puncture

927 The _____ _____ is actually a type of needle biopsy performed on the breastplate. Marrow cells are sucked out and examined later under the microscope.

rachi

rachi/o/centesis
(**ray**-kee-oh-sen-**TEE**-sis)

928 Sometimes the spinal column, like an individual bone, is punctured for diagnosis. Remember that _____ **(frame 913)** is a root for "spine." Combine this root with the suffix in arthrocentesis **(frame 299)**. The product is _____ /____ /_____, "puncture and tapping of the spine."

rachiocentesis

929 A formal term indicating a surgical "puncture and tapping of fluid from the spine" is called _____.

rachiocentesis

930 Fluid withdrawn from the interior of the vertebral column by _____ can be analyzed in the lab for its chemical and microscopic content.

arthr/o/gram (ARTH-roh-**gram**)

931 At times, bones and joints must be examined indirectly. Techniques include radiograms and the injection of radioactive isotopes. An _____ /____ /_____, for instance, is an x-ray "record of joints," much as a tomogram **(frame 197)** is an x-ray "record of a (thin) slice."

arthrogram

932 An _____ can reveal details of joint structure that cannot be observed directly using the arthroscope.

bone scan

933 Another technique is the **bone scan**. In the _____ _____, radioactive isotopes are injected into the blood leading into "bones." The bone locations where these isotopes become concentrated are then "scanned." Such concentrated bone activity may suggest the presence of bone tumors or other problems.

934 When bone or joint disorders are detected, it is only natural to try to do something to correct them.

Word Parts Associated with Surgery, Pharmacology, and Other Therapies for the Skeletal System

The following is a list of word parts and an abbreviation associated with surgery, pharmacology, and other therapies for the skeletal system. Use this list to help you complete **frames 935 to 953.**

amput/a	pruning	**ortho-**	straight; normal
ASA	acetylsalicylic acid	**paed**	child
-desis	binding together		

closed

open

935 Some common injuries, such as bone fractures (partial or total bone breakage), must have prompt treatment. Several phrases have been coined to describe these treatments. Two such terms are **closed reduction** and **open reduction.** One treatment, _____ (open/closed) reduction, requires the manipulation of the broken bone back into proper position. This position is then fixed from the outside (closed to the body interior), by means of a cast, splint, or traction. The other treatment, _____ (open/closed) reduction, conversely, involves an opening into the body interior to fix the bones back into proper position for healing. Plates, screws, or even nails may have to be inserted into the bones.

ped

936 Open or closed reductions of fractures are performed to straighten broken bones and place them into normal alignment. The prefix ortho- (**OR**-thoh) means "straight" or "normal." The root _____ **(frame 826)**, like pod, means "foot." An alternate meaning is "child." In fact, **paed (PAID)**, another root meaning the same thing, derives from the Greek for "child."

ortho/ped/ics
ortho/paed/ics

937 Dissect **orthopedics** (or-thoh-**PEE**-diks) as _____ / _____ / _____ and **orthopaedics** (or-thoh-**PAY**-diks) as _____ / _____ / _____. Note that both terms include the suffix appearing in myelic **(frame 791)**, with a terminal **s** added.

orthopedics
orthopaedics

938 The literal meaning of _____ or _____ is "pertaining to straightening children." This meaning reflects the history of the medical specialty. It originally focused on correcting deformities in the spine, bones, and joints of children.

-ist	**939** Remember that _____, the suffix in anesthetist **(frame 271)**, means "one who specializes in (something)." Use this fact to help you build two terms that indicate "one who specializes in straightening children": _____ / _____ / _____ or _____ / _____ / _____.
ortho/ped/ist (**or**-thoh-**PEE**-dist) **ortho/paed/ist** (**or**-thoh-**PAY**-dist)	
orthopedist orthopaedist	**940** An _____ or _____ may have to perform various operations on the bones and joints. Observe and pronounce the list of operations below: **amputation** (**am**-pyoo-**TAY**-shun) **arthrotomy** (review **frame 294**) **arthrodesis** (review **frame 302**) **arthroplasty** (review **frame 305**) **bunionectomy** (**bun**-yun-**EK**-toh-mee) **bursectomy** (burs-**EK**-toh-mee) **ostectomy** (review **frame 307**) **synovectomy** (**sin**-oh-**VEK**-toh-mee)
arthrotomy -o/tomy	**941** One of the first steps in joint surgery is _____, or "incision into a joint" **(frame 294)**. This term contains the suffix _____ / _____. 
arthrodesis arthroplasty	**942** Other surgical terms involving joints include _____, or "binding together of joints" **(frame 302)**, and _____, or "surgical repair of joints" **(frame 305)**.
arthrodesis arthroplasty	**943** The technique of _____ involves the "binding together" of nearby structures to surgically fix and stabilize a "joint." This procedure is thus a specific type of _____ in which "joints" are "surgically repaired."
ostectomy	**944** Various bone and joint structures may also be surgically removed. **Frame 307** mentioned that _____ is the "removal of bone."
bunion burs **bunion/ectomy** **burs/ectomy**	**945** Recollect _____, a root for "mound" **(frame 907)**, and _____, a root for "purse" **(frame 814)**. Use them to help you create two new surgical terms: _____ / _____, "removal of a mound," and _____ / _____, "removal of a purse."
bunionectomy bursectomy	**946** Both _____ ("bunion removal") and _____ ("removal of an overlying 'purse'-like sac") may have to be done for correction of severe swelling and deformities of joints in the big toe.
syn/ov/ectomy	**947** A _____ / _____ / _____ is a procedure that "removes the synovial" membrane **(frame 811)** lining the freely movable joints.

synovectomy	**948** A _____ may have to be performed if the lining of the knee joint is so inflamed that it interferes with normal movement.
bone grafting	**949** If the broken ends of a fractured bone fail to unite, then **bone grafting** may be carried out. This _____ _____ procedure involves the transplantation of bony tissue from one part of the body to another.
amput/a/tion	**950** **Amput (am-PYOOT)** is a root for "pruning." Therefore _____ / ____ / _____ is a "process of pruning." The "process of" ending in this term **(frame 169)** is also seen in aspiration **(frame 578)**.
amputation	**951** The pruning or removal of diseased or damaged body limbs is called _____.
Information Frame	**952** Amputation or other surgical procedures may result in chronic pain. One of the oldest and most effective pain killers is aspirin. Its active ingredient is **acetylsalicylic** (ah-**see**-til-**sal**-ih-**SIL**-ik) **acid**, abbreviated as **ASA**.
acetylsalicylic acid	**953** **Aspirin** is the so-called **trade name** for its chemical component, _____ _____ (ASA). This substance is useful in relieving pain in damaged structures of nearly all body systems.

Multiple Choice

1. The root for "make" is

   a. foss   b. fic   c. fibul   d. femor

2. To build "freely movable joints," use the prefix

   a. un-   b. di-   c. bi-   d. syn-

3. The root for "arm" is

   a. radi   b. uln   c. humer   d. femor

4. Spondylosis is "a condition of the"

   a. scapula   b. sacrum   c. vertebra   d. cranium

5. Which term indicates malignancy?

   a. osteoma   b. osteosarcoma   c. myeloma   d. chondroma

6. Mandibular refers to

   a. lower jaw   b. upper jaw   c. cheek   d. collar bone

Meanings of Selected Roots

Add the correct combining vowel (cv) after each root. Then write the definition of each root in the space provided.

ROOT/CV	DEFINITION
1. cartilagin/_____	_____
2. carp/_____	_____
3. arthr/_____	_____
4. kyph/_____	_____
5. rheumat/_____	_____
6. tars/_____	_____
7. ossi/_____	_____
8. myel/_____	_____
9. condyl/_____	_____
10. ped/_____	_____

Word Dissection and Translation

Analyze the following terms by dissecting them with slashmarks and identifying their word parts. To the right of each term, write its correct English translation.

Key: R (root), cv (combining vowel), P (prefix), S (suffix)

1. patella

_____/_____
R   S

_____

2. claviculotomy

_____/_____/_____
R   cv   S

_____

3. arthralgia

_____/_____
R   S

_____

4. kyphoscoliosis

_____/_____/_____/_____/_____
R   cv   R   cv   S

_____

5. sternal

_____/_____
R   S

_____

6. arthroplasty

_____/_____/_____
R   cv   S

_____

7. bunionectomy

_____/_____
R   S

_____

8. orthopaedics

_____/_____/_____
P   R   S

_____

9. chondrocyte

_____/_____/_____/_____
R   cv   R   S

_____

10. intracartilaginous

_____/_____/_____
P   R   S

_____

11. rheumatospicular

_____/_____/_____/_____
R   cv   R   S

_____

12. sacroiliac

_____/_____/_____/_____
R   cv   R   S

_____

Terms and Their Abbreviations

In the list below, when the term is given, write its abbreviation in the space provided. When the abbreviation is given, write its corresponding term.

TERM	ABBREVIATION
1. fracture	_____
2. _____	FxBB
3. osteoarthritis	_____

Word Spelling

Look at each of the terms listed below. Identify those that are misspelled by circling Y for "Yes." Write the correct spelling in the blank.

WORD	MISSPELLED?	CORRECT SPELLING
1. fibyula	Y/N	_____
2. osseous	Y/N	_____
3. sinoveal	Y/N	_____
4. articular	Y/N	_____
5. endokondrul	Y/N	_____
6. myeleyetus	Y/N	_____
7. scoliosis	Y/N	_____
8. ahstektohmee	Y/N	_____
9. osteoporosis	Y/N	_____
10. arthraalguh	Y/N	_____
11. tibial	Y/N	_____
12. arthrowgram	Y/N	_____
13. ampewtayshun	Y/N	_____
14. arthroses	Y/N	_____

New Word Synthesis

Using word parts that appear in this and previous chapters, build new terms with the following meanings:

1. _____	resembling a little point
2. _____	pertaining to bands
3. _____	presence of (something) within cartilage cells
4. _____	removal of cartilage or gristle
5. _____	tumor of the collar bone
6. _____	inflammation of joints and skin
7. _____	relating to the thigh and kneecap
8. _____	surgical incision into the shin bone
9. _____	one who studies tissues and bones
10. _____	an abnormal condition of pores and crookedness

CASE STUDY

Read through the following diagnostic summary. Note the terms in bold print. A series of multiple choice questions probes your knowledge of these terms.

Diagnostic Summary

A 68-year-old female Caucasian fell off a tall kitchen stool and landed on her left side. She reported severe **arthralgia** in the left **innominate area. Arthrography** revealed a compound fracture of the **left ischial spine.**

Case Study Questions

1. One of the patient's symptoms, **arthralgia,** was

   (a) bone pain.

   (b) joint pain.

   (c) head rupture.

   (d) muscle paralysis.

2. You would look for the **innominate area** in the

   (a) hip.

   (b) shoulder.

   (c) knee.

   (d) ankle.

3. Compound fracture was revealed by the technique of **arthrography,** which is

   (a) surgical puncture and tapping.

   (b) x-raying.

   (c) applying ultrasound waves.

   (d) measuring body temperature.

4. The **left ischial spine** would be roughly located in the

   (a) buttocks.

   (b) neck.

   (c) lumbar area.

   (d) thoracic curve.

CHAPTER 9 The Muscular System

INTRODUCTION

The muscular system is a large grouping of over 600 individual muscle organs. There are three basic types of muscle tissue: **smooth muscle** (located in the walls of many viscera), **cardiac** (**KAR**-dee-**ak**) **muscle** (located in the wall of the heart), and **skeletal muscle** (attached to the bones of the skeleton). Microscopic views of these muscle tissue types are provided in Figure 9.1.

FIGURE 9.1   **The Three Types of Muscle Tissue**

(A) Smooth Muscle Fibers (Nonstriated)

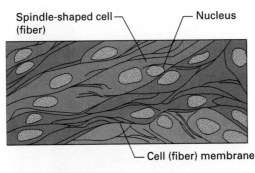

(B) Skeletal Muscle Fibers (Striated)

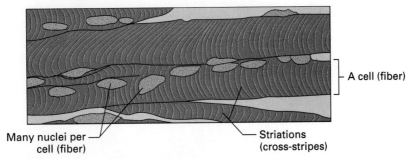

(C) Cardiac Muscle Fibers (Striated)

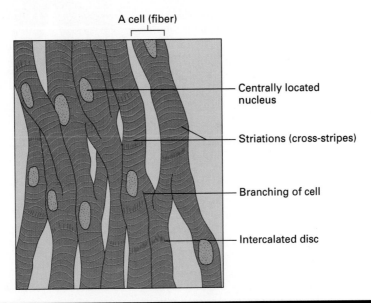

Observe from Figure 9.1 that all three types of muscle tissue consist primarily of **muscle fibers.** These are simply long, thin muscle tissue cells. Smooth and cardiac muscle fibers bear a single nucleus. Skeletal muscle fibers, in contrast, are **multinucleate** (**mul**-tee-**NOO**-klee-ayt), containing "many nuclei." You can see in Figure 9.1B that each skeletal muscle fiber has many small dark nuclei scattered along its periphery. (Picture a breadstick dotted with sesame seeds.)

Muscle fibers can also differ in the presence or absence of **striations** (strigh-**AY**-shuns)—that is, cross-stripes. Muscle cells are either **striated** (**STRIGH-ay**-ted) ("striped") or **nonstriated** (**NAHN-strigh**-ay-ted) (lack cross-stripes). Both skeletal and cardiac muscle fibers are striated. The skeletal muscle fibers, especially, bear a distinct zebralike cross-striping pattern. As their name indicates, however, smooth muscle fibers are without any such banding or striping pattern.

The chief function of all three types of muscle tissue is **contraction**—a shortening. Muscle cells appear thin and fiberlike because they are being pulled upon at either end. When the muscle fibers contract and pull back, body movement occurs. For smooth muscle, this contraction may create a narrowing of the major blood vessels. For cardiac muscle, fiber contraction may cause blood to spurt out of a chamber of the heart. For skeletal muscle, the contraction may produce movement of a body limb.

FIGURE 9.2   **Major Muscles Near the Body Surface**

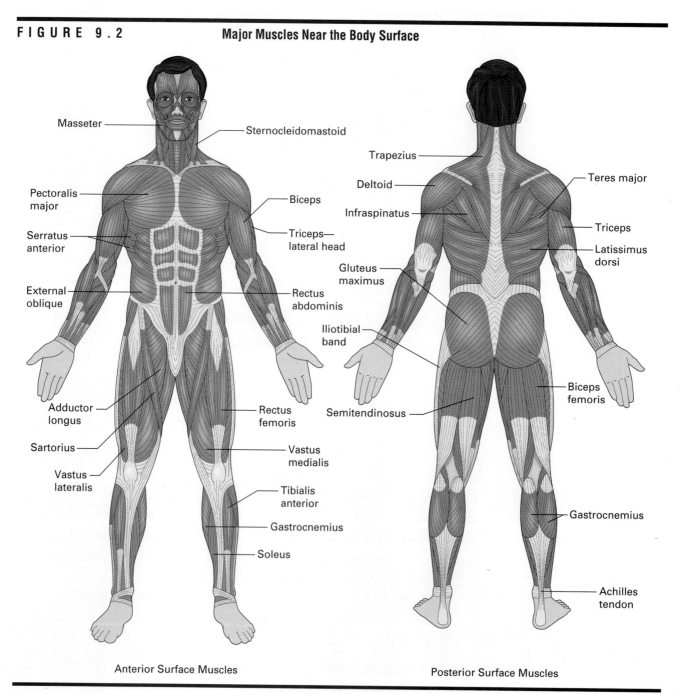

Anterior Surface Muscles

Posterior Surface Muscles

Our primary focus in this chapter is the skeletal muscles. Figure 9.2 provides an overall view of the skeletal muscles near the body surface.

Figure 9.3 shows how contraction, or shortening, of a skeletal muscle pulls on its **tendon.** (A tendon is a strap of fibrous connective tissue that anchors a skeletal muscle to a bone.) The tendon in turn pulls upon a bone. Finally, this bone moves relative to some other bone at the joint between them. Movement of a body part then results.

FIGURE 9.3   **Action of a Skeletal Muscle through Its Tendons**

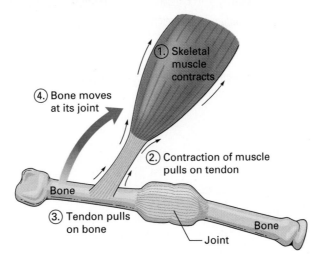

Movement is an example of physiology, while tendons and skeletal muscles exemplify anatomy. The first group of terms to be studied in this chapter reflect the normal anatomy and physiology of the muscular system. The sections that follow introduce terms associated with diseases of the muscular system, terms linked to lab tests and diagnoses of muscular diseases, and terms describing surgery, chemotherapy, and other therapies for muscular problems.

CHAPTER OBJECTIVES

By the end of this chapter, you should be able to:

1 Identify major prefixes, roots, suffixes, and abbreviations related to the muscular system.

2 Dissect muscular terms into their component parts.

3 Translate muscular terms into their common English equivalents.

4 Build new terms associated with the muscular system.

Word Parts Associated with the Normal Anatomy and Physiology of the Muscular System

The following is a list of word parts associated with the normal structure and function of the muscular system. Use this list to help you complete **frames 954 to 1003**.

brachi/o	arm	**glute/o**	rump	**pron/a**	place face down
delt/o	triangle	**kinesi/o**	movement	**rect/o**	vertical; straight
duct/o	move	**lemm/o**	husk (membrane)	**sartori/o**	tailor
extens/o	stretch; straighten	**muscul/o**	muscle (little mouse)	**supin/a**	place on back
		my/o	muscle	**ten/o**	tendon
flex/o	bend	**myos/o**	muscle	**tenon/o**	tendon
gastrocnemi/o	belly of the leg	**neur/o**	nerve	**tendin/o**	tendon
		pector/o	nipples; chest	**trapezi/o**	table

---

muscul/o (**MUS**-kyoo-loh)
my/o (**MIGH**-oh)
myos/o (**MIGH**-oh-soh)
sarc

954 The word list gives three combining forms for "muscle": _____ /_____, _____ /_____, and _____ /_____. You may recall another root, _____, that appears in sarcoma **(frame 573)**. This root denotes "flesh." The idea of "flesh" is essentially identical to that of "muscle." You will thus find all four of these roots appearing often in the terminology of skeletal muscle.

Information Frame

955 Let us consider muscul/o in particular. It is thought to have arisen from **musculus** (**MUS**-kyoo-**lus**)—Latin for "a little mouse." This name may have been given because of the way muscles ripple like "little mice" when they move under the skin.

---

muscul/ar (**MUS**-kyoo-**lar**)

956 You can use the "little mouse" root plus the ending in articular **(frame 796)** to help you build _____ /_____. This term "pertains to" either "muscles" or "little mice."

---

neur/o/muscul/ar
(**noo**-roh-**MUS**-kyoo-lar)

957 **Neur/o** (**NOO**-roh) means "nerve." Consequently, _____ /_____ /_____ /_____ "pertains to nerve and muscle."

---

neuromuscular

958 The _____ junction is a "nerve-muscle" joining place—the place where a nerve fiber nearly contacts a muscle fiber and excites it to contract.

---

sarc/o/lemm/a (**sar**-koh-**LEH**-mah)

959 Lemm (**LEM**) is a root for "husk." Adopt the root for "flesh" **(frame 573)** and the suffix in patella **(frame 872)** to construct _____ /_____ /_____ /_____, "a flesh husk."

---

sarcolemma	**960** The _____ is a "flesh husk" in the sense that it is actually the plasma membrane surrounding each individual muscle fiber.
-plasm	**961** The "flesh" root tends to be used with various other word parts to create terms describing muscle fiber organelles. Consider, for instance, _____, in cytoplasm **(frame 489)**, which means "matter."
sarc/o/plasm (**SAR**-koh-**plaz**-im)	**962** Use the information in the preceding frame to synthesize _____ /_____ /_____, "flesh matter."
sarcoplasm	**963** The _____ is just a special name for the cytoplasm muscle cells.
sarcoplasm **duct (DUKT)** **kinesi** (kih-**NEE**-zee)	**964** The _____ (muscle cell cytoplasm) contains glucose that provides energy for muscle contraction and body movement. Two roots on the word list, _____ (starting with **d**) and _____, indicate "movement."
-or a**d**/**duct**/**or** a**b**/**duct**/**or**	**965** The **o**-beginning suffix _____ **(frame 99)**, means "one that" or "one who." You pronounced both adductor and abductor earlier **(frame 336)**. Use the information in this and the preceding frame to help you dissect adductor as _____ /_____ /_____ and abductor as _____ /_____ /_____.
abductor adductor **ab-** **ad-**	**966** The prefix in _____ is **ab-**, and that in _____ is **ad-**. You may remember **(frame 335)** that _____ means "away from," and _____ means "toward."
a**b**/**duct**/**or** (ab-**DUHK**-tor) a**d**/**duct**/**or** (ad-**DUHK**-tor)	**967** An _____ /_____ /_____ is a muscle "that moves (a body part) away from" the midline. Conversely, an _____ /_____ /_____ is a muscle "that moves (a body part) toward" the midline.
adductor abductor	**968** A muscle acts as a **horizontal** _____ of the arm if it swings the arm horizontally toward the body midline. A muscle acts as a **horizontal** _____ if it swings the arm horizontally away from the midline.
Information Frame	**969** Now observe and pronounce the following terms describing specific types of body movements: **extension** (eks-**TEN**-shun) **flexion** (**FLEK**-shun) **pronation** (proh-**NAY**-shun) **supination** (soo-pih-**NAY**-shun)

-ion
-tion

extens/ion
flex/ion
pron/a/tion
supin/a/tion

---

970 The first two terms in the preceding frame contain the same "process of" suffix, _____ (as in **frame 98**). The second two terms have the "condition of" suffix, _____ (also in **frame 98**). This information (and consultation with the word list) should allow you to deduce the following meanings:

_____ /_____ "process of straightening"
_____ /_____ "process of bending"
_____ /____ /_____ "process of placing face down"
_____ /____ /_____ "process of placing on the back"

---

extension

flexion

971 The process of _____ occurs as a person unbends the lower arm and offers someone a candy bar. The process of _____ occurs as a person accepts the candy bar and bends the forearm, placing the candy into her mouth.

---

pronation

supination

972 The act of _____ occurs when a person turns her hands "face" down—such that the palms face backward in the anatomic position. The act of _____ occurs when a person turns her hands onto their "backs"—such that the palms face forward in the anatomical position. The various movements discussed in the last few frames are diagrammed in Figure 9.4.

---

ten (TEN)
tenon (TEN-ahn)
tendin (TEN-din)
tendin/ous (TEN-dih-nus)

973 Body movements occur when contracting muscles pull on their tendons. Note that the word list cites three roots for "tendon." These are _____, _____, and _____. Take the longest of these roots and use the suffix in osseous **(frame 770)** to build _____ /_____, "referring to tendons."

---

tendinous

974 Skeletal muscles pull on the bones by means of their _____ ("relating to tendon") attachments.

---

bi-
tri-
quadri-

975 Some muscles have more than one tendon attached at each end. There is a tendon for each **cep (SEP)**, or "head" (that is, each major division), of a skeletal muscle. You may recall from Chapter 2 **(frame 80)** some prefixes indicating number. There are _____ and **di-** for "two"; _____ for "three"; and _____ for "four."

---

bi/ceps (**BIGH**-seps)
tri/ceps (**TRIGH**-ceps)
quadri/ceps (**QUAD**-rih-ceps)

976 Extract appropriate information from the preceding frame to help you construct these terms:
____ /_____ "two heads"
_____ /_____ "three heads"
_____ /_____ "four heads"

---

femor
brachi

977 Terms for number of muscle heads can be combined with those for muscle location. For example,
brachi/i (BRAY-kee-igh)
femor/is (FEM-or-is)
Note that femoris contains _____, the root for "thigh" **(frame 874)**. The root in brachii, _____, denotes "arm."

Some Basic Types of Body Movements

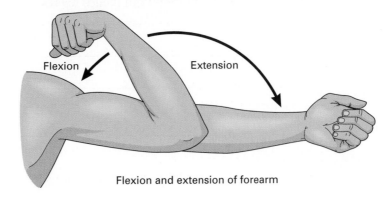

Flexion and extension of forearm

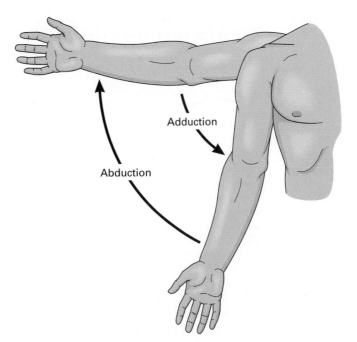

Vertical adduction and abduction of arm

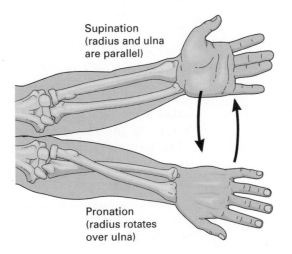

Pronation and supination of the hand

biceps brachii

triceps brachii

biceps femoris

quadriceps femoris

978 Combining terms for number of heads with those for body location results in two-word names for several individual skeletal muscles:

_____ _____ a "two-headed" muscle in the upper "arm"

_____ _____ a "three-headed" muscle in the upper "arm"

_____ _____ a "two-headed" muscle on the posterior aspect of the "thigh"

_____ _____ a "four-headed" muscle group on the anterior aspect of the "thigh"

These multiheaded muscles are shown in detail in Figure 9.5.

gastrocnemi/us
(**gas**-trahk-**NEE**-mee-us)
glute/us (**GLOO**-tee-**us**)

979 A few other roots for body location are **gastrocnemi** (**gas**-trahk-**NEE**-mee) for "calf" or "belly of the leg" and **glute** (**GLOO**-tee) for "rump." Both of these roots assume the "presence of" ending in radius (**frame 867**). Adding **-us** gives us _____ /_____ ("the calf") and _____ /_____ ("the rump").

gastrocnemius

980 The _____ muscle bulges out the posterior aspect of the calf. Hence it is named for the "belly of the leg."

gluteus

981 The _____ , or "rump," is "present" as the buttocks.

noun

glute/al (**GLOO**-tee-uhl)

982 We know that gluteus is a(n) _____ (adjective/verb/noun) because of the meaning of its suffix. If we change the suffix to that in synovial (**frame 811**), the result is _____ /_____, an adjective that "pertains to the rump."

gluteal

983 The _____ region is the buttocks, or "rump." This region actually includes several different muscles.

gluteal
macr
maxim/us (**MAKS**-ih-**mus**)

984 One _____ (buttock) muscle is especially large. **Maxim** (**MAKS**-im), like _____, the root in macroscopic (**frame 430**), means "large." Therefore, _____ /_____ indicates the "presence of (something) large" just as gluteus indicates the "presence of the rump."

gluteus maximus

985 The _____ _____ is literally the "large rump" muscle "present" in the buttocks.

gluteus maximus

986 When you sit around all day, you spend a lot of time on your _____ _____ , or "big rump" muscle!

Some Multiheaded Limb Muscles

Biceps Brachii and
Triceps Brachii
(Upper Arm)

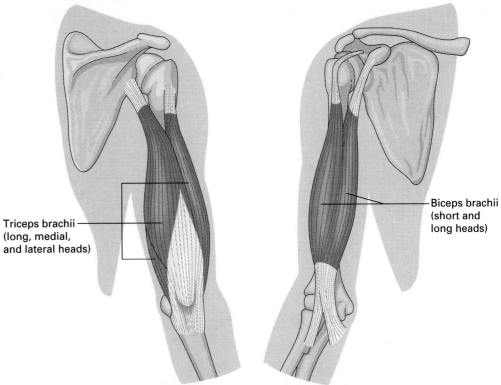

Triceps brachii
(long, medial,
and lateral heads)

Biceps brachii
(short and
long heads)

Biceps Femoris and
Quadriceps Femoris
(Upper Leg)

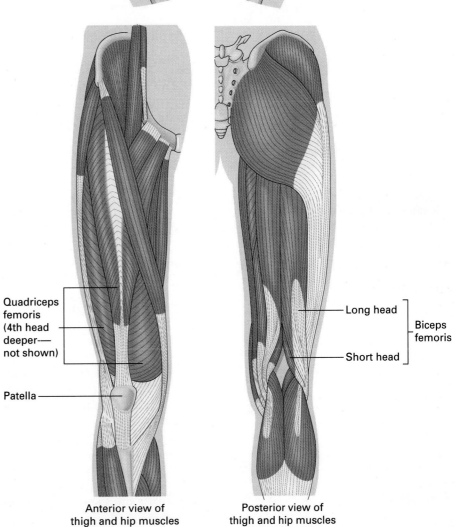

Quadriceps
femoris
(4th head
deeper—
not shown)

Patella

Long head

Short head

Biceps
femoris

Anterior view of
thigh and hip muscles

Posterior view of
thigh and hip muscles

thorac **pectoral/is (pek**-tor-**AL**-is)	**987** **Pector** (**PEK**-tor) or **pectoral** (**PEK**-tor-**al**), like _____ **(frame 397)**, means "chest." Employing the second root with the ending in femoris yields _____ /____ ("presence of the chest").
pectoralis major	**988** **Major**, like **maximus**, means "large." We can thus name the _____ _____ as the "large" muscle of the "chest."
pectoralis	**989** Following the same pattern as in **frame 988**, we can say that the _____ **minor** is the "small" muscle of the "chest."
inter/cost/al	**990** The name of another muscle group focuses exclusively on its body location. This is the **intercostal** (**in**-ter-**KAHS**-tal) group of muscles. You can subdivide this term as _____ /_____ /____. It will help you to recognize the root in costal **(frame 856)** and the suffix in gluteal.
costal	**991** Remember that _____ "pertains to the ribs." It can be combined with the prefix inter- for "between."
intercostal	**992** The _____ muscles lie "between the ribs" and assist their up-and-down movements during breathing.
rect/us (REKT-us)	**993** **Rect (REKT)** means "straight," "vertical," or "upright." Much as gluteus indicates "presence of the rump," _____ /____ denotes "presence of (something) straight or upright."
-is abdomin **abdomin/is (ab-DAHM**-ih-nus)	**994** Besides -**us**, another "presence of" suffix often used to name muscles is _____, the ending of pectoralis. Combine this ending with _____, the root for abdomen **(frame 378)**. The result is _____ /____, "presence of the abdomen or trunk midsection."
rectus abdominis	**995** Putting the names in the previous frames together allows you to generate _____ _____, a muscle in the "abdomen" having "upright" fibers.
rectus abdominis flexion	**996** The _____ _____ muscle, having vertical fibers that pull in a "straight," up-and-down direction, is the main muscle involved in doing sit-ups. It produces a_____ ("bending") of the trunk. Figure 9.6 displays some of the chest and abdominal muscles.
sartori/us **sartori (sar-TOR**-ee)	**997** A muscle with a most unusual name is the **sartorius** (**sar-TOR**-ee-us). Subdivide it with slashmarks: _____ /____. You will see that its suffix is the same as that in rectus. Its root, _____, means "tailor."

FIGURE 9.6

Some Chest and Abdominal Muscles

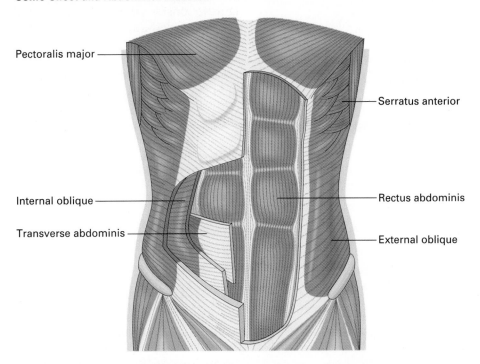

Pectoralis major

Serratus anterior

Internal oblique

Rectus abdominis

Transverse abdominis

External oblique

sartorius

998 The _____ is literally the "tailor's" muscle. The odd name derives from the fact that this thigh muscle flexes and rotates the lower extremity to permit sitting in a cross-legged manner. (Tailors in bygone days would sit cross-legged while they stitched, shown in Figure 9.7.)

FIGURE 9.7

The Sartorius: A Cross-Legged Tailor Uses This Muscle in Each Thigh

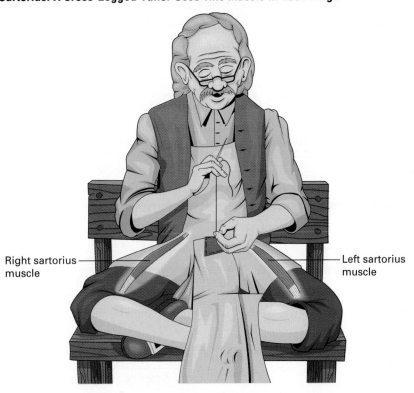

Right sartorius muscle

Left sartorius muscle

999 Some muscles are named for their resemblance to simple geometric figures. Consider **delt (DELT)** for "triangle" and **trapezi** (trah-**PEE**-zee) for a four-sided top of a "table."

delt/oid (**DEL**-toid)

1000 Use the above facts plus the suffix from rheumatoid **(frame 903)** to build _____ /_____, "resembling a triangle."

deltoid

1001 As you can see from review of Figure 9.2, the _____ muscle does have a somewhat triangular appearance as it forms the fleshy pad of the shoulder.

trapezi/us (trah-**PEE**-zee-**us**)

1002 Affixing the suffix of sartorius to the root for "table" in **frame 999** results in _____ /_____, "a table."

trapezius

1003 The _____ is a large "table"-shaped muscle forming much of the flesh of the upper back.

1004 There are many individual skeletal muscles with a great variety of names. Nevertheless, most of their pathology is the same.

Diseases

Word Parts Associated with Diseases of the Muscular System

The following is a list of word parts and an abbreviation for diseases associated with the muscular system. Use this list to help you complete **frames 1005 to 1029**.

-asthenia	weakness	**mort**	death
MD	muscular dystrophy	**rigor**	stiffness

-pathy

1005 Remember that path is a root for "disease" in general. You may recall that _____ **(frame 111)** is a larger suffix including this root, and it means a "disease of (something)."

my/o/pathy (**migh-AH**-pah-thee)

1006 Using **my** as the root for "muscle," build _____ /_____ /_____, a "disease of muscle."

myopathy

1007 A _____ may lead to disturbed or weakened muscle movements.

my/o/path/ies (**migh-AH**-pah-thees)

1008 Words whose singular ends in **-y** generally form plurals with **-ies** Therefore, _____ /_____ /_____ /_____ are "muscle diseases" in general.

myopathies

1009 The _____ ("muscle diseases") share several of the same types of problems as do bones and other tissues.

osteoma osteosarcoma **my/oma** (**migh-OH**-mah) **my/o/sarc/oma** (**migh**-oh-sar-**KOH**-mah)	**1010** Recall that an _____ (**frame 882**) is a "bone tumor" and that an _____ (**frame 882**) is a "fleshy bone tumor." Use a similar approach and a root in myopathies to help you build: ____ /_____ "muscle tumor" ____ /____ /_____ /_____ "fleshy tumor of muscle"
myoma myosarcoma	**1011** A _____, or "muscle tumor," usually involves an excessive and abnormal mitosis of connective tissue cells in a muscle. A _____ is a "muscle tumor" that has become "malignant."
myelitis **my/itis** (**migh-IGH**-tis) **myos/itis** (**migh**-oh-**SIGH**-tis)	**1012** Again returning to bone, remember that _____ (**frame 893**) denotes an "inflammation of marrow." Similarly, ____ /_____ indicates an "inflammation of muscle." An alternate term having the same meaning uses **myos** as the root: _____ /_____.
myitis myositis	**1013** Overuse of a muscle may lead to its inflammation, resulting in _____ or _____.
tendin/itis (**ten**-din-**IGH**-tis)	**1014** A similar problem can afflict tendons. Extract the root from tendinous (**frame 973**). Now synthesize _____ /_____, an "inflammation of tendons."
tendinitis	**1015** Enthusiastic tennis players may suffer _____ of the elbow when they overdo it and inflame their lower arm tendons.
my/asthenia -asthenia	**1016** People cannot overdo muscle use, or even do much moving at all, if they suffer from severe **myasthenia** (**migh**-as-**THEE**-nee-ah). This term may be dissected as ____ /_____. Word dissection is easier if you remember that _____ (**frame 144**) is a suffix meaning "weakness of (something)."
weakness of muscle	**1017** Myasthenia literally means "_____ ____ _____."
myasthenia	**1018** "Muscle weakness," or _____, may be associated with muscular atrophy due to severing of the nerves to a muscle.
myasthenia gravis	**1019** **Gravis** (**GRAH**-vis) is Latin for "heavy." A disease called _____ _____ translates as a "heavy muscular weakness."

myasthenia gravis	**1020** In _____ _____ there is a great "weakness" and perception of "heaviness" of the "muscles" of the face and neck. This form of muscle weakness is not accompanied by muscular atrophy.
dys- dys/troph/y (DIS-truh-fee)	**1021** Remember that the prefix _____, as in dysplasia **(frame 558)**, means "bad, difficult, or painful." Much as a/troph/y **(frame 141)** indicates "a condition without nourishment," _____ /_____/_____ denotes "a condition of bad nourishment."
dystrophy	**1022** In a case of atrophy, body parts that were once fully developed undergo a shrinking and wasting. In a case of _____, developing tissue never forms properly.
muscular dystrophy	**1023** Applied to muscles, we can create the phrase _____ _____, "a condition of bad nourishment of muscles."
muscular dystrophy atrophy	**1024** What is meant by _____ _____, of course, is a "bad" and "painful" situation for muscle tissue. The inherited presence of certain genes for this disease causes severe muscle _____, or wasting, and its replacement by adipose tissue.
MD	**1025** Muscular dystrophy, abbreviated as ____ ____, often occurs in childhood. Therefore, growing muscle tissue never fully develops, and what muscle is present begins to deteriorate.
muscular dystrophy mortality	**1026** The disease of MD, or _____ _____, can lead to _____, a "condition of death" **(frame 157)**.
mort/is (MOR-tis)	**1027** **Mort**, like mortal, is a root for "death." The term _____ /____ suggests "presence of death" in the same way that abdominis **(frame 994)** suggests "presence of the abdomen."
rigor mortis	**1028** **Rigor** (**RIH**-gor) means "stiffness." Using this fact and your learning from the previous frame, you can create the phrase _____ _____, when "death stiffness" is "present."
rigor mortis	**1029** The phenomenon of _____ _____ is a "stiffening" of partially contracted muscles a few hours after "death."
	1030 With proper diagnostic and lab tests, morbid conditions may be detected before they lead to mortal consequences.

Word Parts Associated with Lab Tests and Diagnoses for the Muscular System

The following is a list of some word parts and an abbreviation associated with lab tests and diagnoses of problems affecting the muscular system. Use this list to help you complete **frames 1031 to 1046**.

chir/o	hand	-iatrist	physician who specializes in
EMG	electromyogram	-iatry	process of being a physician

kinesi

1031 One way of detecting potential abnormalities in the muscular system is by studying body movements. You have already learned **(frame 964)** that _____, like duct, is a root for "movement."

kinesi/o/logy
(**kih**-nee-zee-**AHL**-oh-jee)

1032 Extract the suffix from dermatology **(frame 728)** and construct _____ /_____ /_____, "study of movement."

kinesiology

1033 Some movements studied in the science of _____ are normal, in the sense that they are associated with little or no bone-joint-muscle morbidity. Others have been shown to be related to injury or disease.

-graphy

1034 Various aspects of body motion can be observed and recorded. Remember that _____, as appearing in thermography **(frame 220)**, is a suffix meaning "process of recording."

my/o/graphy (migh-AH-grah-fee)

1035 Isolate the appropriate root from myopathy **(frame 1006)** and write out a new term, ____ /____ /_____, the "process of recording muscle (activity)."

myography

electr/o/my/o/graphy
(ee-**lek**-troh-migh-**AH**-grah-fee)

1036 One specific technique in _____ ("recording of muscle") involves electrical activity (electr). Add an appropriate root to help you build _____ /____ /____ /____ /_____. This is a technical term for the "process of recording the electrical activity (within) a muscle."

electromyography

1037 The technique of _____ "records" the "electrical" activity taking place within "muscles" as the body goes through various movements.

my/o/gram (MIGH-oh-**gram)**

1038 Much as a thermogram **(frame 223)** provides a "heat record," a ____ /____ /_____ provides a "muscle record."

myogram **electr/o/my/o/gram** (ee-**lek**-troh-**MIGH**-oh-gram)	**1039** Let us treat _____ ("muscle record") as we did myography. Add a root to create a term for a "record of muscle electrical activity": _____ /_____ /_____ /_____ /_____.
electromyogram	**1040** An _____ (abbreviated as **EMG**) might show excessive electrical activity in a muscle that is normally relaxed during a particular body movement. This activity could suggest an abnormal muscle strain that calls for further investigation.
EMG	**1041** An _____ _____ _____ (abbreviation for electromyogram) may show abnormal activity in muscles involving the feet.
pod/iatrist (poh-**DIGH**-uh-**trist**)	**1042** **Pod (POHD)**, like ped, means "feet." The suffix **-iatrist** denotes "a physician who specializes in (something)." Use this information to build _____ /_____, "a physician who specializes in the feet."
pod/iatry (poh-**DIGH**-uh-tree)	**1043** The closely related suffix **-iatry** (**IGH**-uh-tree) indicates "the process of being a physician," that is, the process of diagnosing and healing. Now use this information to create a new term, _____ /_____, diagnosing and healing problems of the "feet."
podiatrist podiatry	**1044** A _____ (foot specialist) usually holds a degree in the specialty of _____.
chir/o/pod/y (**chur-AH**-poh-dee)	**1045** **Chir (CHUR)** is a root for "hand." Add the root in podiatry to the one for "hand," then attach a terminal **-y**. Did you get _____ /_____ /_____ /_____? Did you remember to insert the combining vowel between roots?
chiropody	**1046** The discipline of _____ is really the same thing as podiatry. Rather oddly, the term includes a root for "hand." It has been speculated that this term originally indicated that the hands were used to treat and manipulate the feet.
	1047 Podiatry (chiropody) deals with treatments of muscles in the feet, if they are damaged.

Word Parts Associated with Surgery, Pharmacology, and Other Therapies for the Muscular System

The following is a list of word parts and abbreviations associated with surgery, pharmacology, and other types of therapy for the skeletal muscles. Use this list to help you complete **frames 1048 to 1069**.

ACh   acetylcholine: common type of natural muscle stimulant

-ant   things which; one which

IM   intramuscular: pertaining to (something) within muscle

-tasis   surgical stretching

---

relaxants

1048 The pharmacology of muscles includes the use of -**ant** for "things which" or "one which." There are various types of **muscle stimulants**, "things which" stimulate muscles and cause them to contract. There are also **muscle _____**, things which inhibit muscles and cause them to "relax." Muscular therapy can find both approaches useful.

---

acetylcholine

1049 Some muscle stimulants work at the neuromuscular junction. One of these is called acetylcholine (**ah**-SEE-til-**KOH**-leen). The drug _____, usually abbreviated as **ACh**, is essentially the same as the natural product released from the ending of a nerve fiber as it impinges on a muscle fiber.

ACh
neuromuscular junction

1050 Acetylcholine (abbreviated as ____ ____ ____) diffuses across the _____ _____ ("nerve-muscle joining place," **frame 958**) and excites the sarcolemma of a muscle fiber, causing the fiber to contract.

Valium

1051 There are many types of muscle relaxants. The drug **diazepam** (**digh-AZ**-eh-pam), commonly known as **Valium** (**VAL**-ee-um), is a type of muscle relaxant that operates across the neuromuscular junction. Diazepam, or _____, inhibits the nerves acting upon muscle fibers.

---

diazepam

1052 Valium (_____), by operating chiefly upon the nerve ending, can be considered an indirect relaxant of muscles.

---

neuromuscular

neuromuscular blocker
succinylcholine

1053 Certain drugs, the _____ ("nerve-muscle") **blockers**, actually deactivate the nerve-muscle joining area. An example of a _____ _____ is **succinylcholine** (**suhk**-sin-il-**KOH**-leen). This drug _____ is also called **Anectine** (**ah-NEK**-teen).

neuromuscular blockers	**1054** By temporarily inactivating the neuromuscular junction, the _____ _____ strongly relax muscles and prevent their reflex contractions during surgery.
Anectine	**1055** Succinylcholine (_____) is the most frequently used type of neuromuscular blocking agent for surgery.
dantrolene	**1056** Other types of relaxants act directly on the skeletal muscle itself, bypassing the neuromuscular junction. One of these is **dantrolene** (**DAN**-troh-leen), also called **Dantrium** (**DAN**-tree-um). This _____, or Dantrium, thus differs from Anectine in its mode of action.
intra/muscul/ar (**in**-trah-**MUS**-kyoo-lar)	**1057** Drugs that act directly on muscles may be injected right into them. Remember that muscular "pertains to muscle." You can extract the prefix from intracellular **(frame 472)** and build a new term, _____ / _____ / ____, "pertaining to (something) within muscle."
intramuscular	**1058** The _____ ("within muscle") route of injection gets a drug directly into contact with muscle tissue.
IM	**1059** Intramuscular (abbreviated as ____ ____) injection is also carried out for other drugs that are to be slowly absorbed into the bloodstream.
intramuscular dermatome **my/o/tom/e** (**MIGH**-oh-tohm)	**1060** Sometimes IM, or _____, surgery is required. There are a number of terms related to muscle surgery. You may remember that a _____ **(frame 751)** is an instrument used to make "skin cuts." Following similar thinking, use the root in myogram **(frame 1038)** to help you build ____ / ____ / _____ / ____, a knife used to "cut muscle."
myotome	**1061** A _____ may be used to slice through muscle in the process of entering the body cavities for surgery.
my/o/tomy (**migh-AH**-toh-mee) osteotomy arthrotomy	**1062** "Making an incision into muscle," or ____ / ____ / _____, follows the word-building pattern in both _____ ("making an incision into a bone") and _____ ("making an incision into a joint"), which were discussed in **frame 294**.
myotomy	**1063** A myotome is used for _____, "cutting" through layers of skeletal "muscles" to reach the interior of the abdominopelvic cavity.

ten/o/tomy (ten-**AH**-toh-mee)

my/o/ten/o/tomy
(**migh**-oh-ten-**AH**-toh-mee)

1064 Recall that ten, like tendin **(frame 973)**, is a root for "tendon." Just as myotomy is "incision into a muscle," _____ /_____ /_____ is "incision into a tendon." Combining the two roots produces _____ /_____ /_____ /_____ /_____, "cutting into a muscle and its tendon."

---

tenotomy
myotenotomy

1065 If one surgically interrupts a tendon only, the procedure is called a _____. If one surgically interrupts both a muscle and its tendon, the procedure is properly called a _____.

---

my/o/tasis (migh-**AHT**-ah-sis)

1066 The suffix **-tasis** (**TAY**-sis) means "a stretching." Now build _____ /_____ /_____, "a stretching of muscle."

---

myotasis

1067 The procedure of _____ ("muscle stretching") may be performed to hook a loosened muscle back onto its proper site of bony attachment.

---

osteorrhaphy

my/o/rrhaphy (**migh-OR**-hah-fee)

1068 Muscle, like bone, can be sutured. Just as _____ **(frame 309)** denotes a "suturing of bone," _____ /_____ /_____ indicates a "suturing of muscle."

---

myorrhaphy

1069 The procedure of _____ is performed to safely close up a muscle after myotomy.

Multiple Choice

1. Which type of muscle is nonstriated?

    a. branching   b. cardiac   c. skeletal   d. visceral

2. The combining form for "straight" is

    a. rect/o   b. abdomin/o   c. glute/o   d. femor/o

3. Which of the following move away from the midline?

    a. abductors   b. adductors   c. pronators   d. supinators

4. The suffix for "process of recording" is

    a. -graph   b. -gram   c. -graphy   d. -grapher

5. Which is a root for "husk"?

    a. sarc   b. rect   c. delt   d. lemm

6. Which of these indicates "difficult nourishment"?

    a. myasthenia   b. dystrophy   c. myositis   d. sartorius

Meanings of Selected Roots

Add the correct combining vowel (cv) after each root. Then write the definition of each root in the space provided.

ROOT/CV	DEFINITION
1. pod/_____	_____
2. muscul/_____	_____
3. lemm/_____	_____
4. kinesi/_____	_____
5. chir/_____	_____
6. neur/_____	_____
7. rect/_____	_____
8. pector/_____	_____
9. duct/_____	_____
10. ten/_____	_____

Word Dissection and Translation

Analyze the following terms by dissecting them with slashmarks and identifying their word parts. To the right of each term, write its correct English translation.

Key: R (root), cv (combining vowel), P (prefix), S (suffix)

1. intercostal

_____/_____/_____   _____
  P   R   S

2. rectus

_____/_____   _____
    R   S

3. neuromuscular

_____/____/_____/_____   _____
   R   cv   R   S

4. podiatry

_____/_____   _____
    R   S

5. gastrocnemius

_____/_____   _____
    R   S

6. myasthenia

_____/_____   _____
    R   S

7. quadriceps

_____/_____   _____
  P   R

8. electromyography

_____/____/_____/____/_____   _____
   R   cv   R   cv   S

9. myotenotomy

_____/____/_____/____/_____   _____
   R   cv   R   cv   S

10. abductor

_____/_____/_____   _____
  P   R   S

11. myosarcosis

_____/____/_____/____/_____   _____
   R   cv   R   cv   S

12. tendinoplasty

_____/____/_____   _____
   R   cv   S

Terms and Their Abbreviations

In the list below, when the term is given, write its abbreviation in the space provided. When the abbreviation is given, write its corresponding term.

TERM	ABBREVIATION
1. acetylcholine	_____
2. _____	EMG
3. intramuscular	_____

Word Spelling

Look at each of the terms listed below. Identify those that are misspelled by circling Y for "Yes." Write the correct spelling in the blank.

WORD	MISSPELLED?	CORRECT SPELLING
1. cheerohpody	Y/N	_____
2. Valium	Y/N	_____
3. myotome	Y/N	_____
4. abdominis	Y/N	_____
5. sartorius	Y/N	_____
6. myomas	Y/N	_____
7. podietrast	Y/N	_____
8. succinylcoline	Y/N	_____
9. tenotomy	Y/N	_____
10. diassepahm	Y/N	_____
11. tendinous	Y/N	_____
12. myopathys	Y/N	_____
13. distrophy	Y/N	_____
14. kinesiology	Y/N	_____

New Word Synthesis

Using word parts that appear in this and previous chapters, build new terms with the following meanings:

1. _____ referring to flesh and bone
2. _____ incision into a triangle
3. _____ process of straightening muscles
4. _____ process of turning a nerve onto its back
5. _____ recording of joint movements
6. _____ suturing of a tendon
7. _____ disease of muscle and cartilage
8. _____ inflammation of muscle and bone and marrow
9. _____ a physician who specializes in joints
10. _____ the process of bending the spine
11. _____ embryonic muscle cell
12. _____ herniation of muscle tissue

C A S E S T U D Y

Read through the following partial surgical report. Note the terms in bold print. A series of multiple choice questions probes your knowledge of these terms.

Surgical Report

A 38-year-old Oriental female suffered a severe right **gastrocnemial** tear during training for the summer Olympics. **Dystrophic** changes were observed in the main muscle bundle. Upper tendon rupture was also noted. Surgical correction proceeded after **IM** injection of 10 mg Valium. **Myotomy** was employed to isolate and excise the damaged muscle.

Case Study Questions

1. The **gastrocnemial** tear was located in the patient's

    (a) knee.

    (b) calf.

    (c) neck.

    (d) chest.

2. **Dystrophic** changes indicated that the main muscle bundle had

    (a) torn in half.

    (b) fused with another muscle.

    (c) suffered degenerative changes.

    (d) relaxed prematurely.

3. Valium was injected **IM**, or

    (a) directly into the muscle.

    (b) around the affected joint.

    (c) into a vein.

    (d) beneath the skin.

4. The surgical procedure of **myotomy** included

    (a) fixation of the nearby joint.

    (b) excision of the overlying skin.

    (c) repair of extensive bone.

    (d) division of the affected muscle.

CHAPTER 10 The Nervous System

INTRODUCTION

The **nervous system** is the body's major communication and control system. As Figure 10.1 illustrates, it has two main components. The **central nervous system,** or **CNS,** consists of the brain and spinal cord. The **peripheral nervous system,** or **PNS,** consists of the **nerves** and **sensory receptors** (specialized nerve endings that respond to particular changes in the environment).

FIGURE 10.1   **The Structural Organization of the Nervous System**

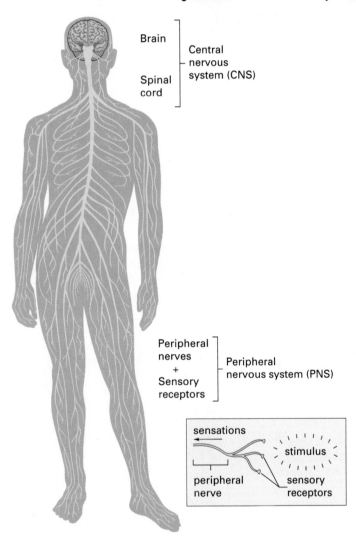

The central nervous system is named for its central location, straddling either side of the body midline. The brain is the portion of the CNS located within the skull. The brain consists of a complex combination of smaller parts, shown in Figure 10.2: the **cerebrum** (seh-**REE**-brum), the **cerebellum** (**sahr**-uh-**BEL**-um),

and the **brainstem**. Both the cerebrum and the cerebellum consist of right and left **hemispheres**, or "half" spheres. They are somewhat like the cap on a mushroom. Plugging into this cap from below is the brainstem. The brainstem is the narrow, stemlike, inferior portion of the brain. It merges caudally with the superior end of the spinal cord. The spinal cord is the portion of the central nervous system located within the **vertebral canal**, a cavity coursing through the vertebral column.

F I G U R E   1 0 . 2   **Major Components of the CNS (Central Nervous System)**

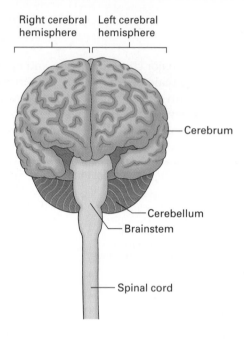

The cerebrum is where most conscious thought occurs. The cerebellum, brainstem, and spinal cord are primarily involved in regulating various **reflexes**, or automatic responses.

The peripheral nervous system derives its name from the fact that it largely consists of nerves that enter or leave the CNS from the body **periphery** (**per-IF**-er-ee), or edge. Some of these nerves carry **sensory information** about the environment, informing the CNS of both external and internal body conditions. Other nerves carry motor (movement) information from the CNS, directing the **body effectors** (muscles and glands) to move or secrete.

As shown in Figure 10.3, the PNS is subdivided into two major parts: the **autonomic** (**aw**-toh-**NAH**-mik) **nervous system**, or **ANS**, and the **somatic nervous system**, or **SNS**. The autonomic nervous system automatically controls the viscera (internal organs). The somatic nervous system primarily acts upon the gross body soma, such as the skeletal muscles, bones, joints, and skin.

Finally, the autonomic nervous system splits into the **sympathetic** (**sim**-pah-**THET**-ik) **nerves** and the **parasympathetic** (**pahr**-ah-sim-pah-**THET**-ik) **nerves**, which literally run "beside" them.

This chapter considers terms describing normal structure and function of the human nervous system, followed by terms of nervous disease, terms of lab tests and diagnoses, and terms of surgery and therapy for nervous system problems.

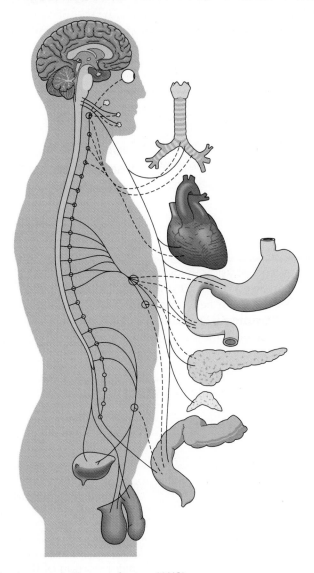

The Autonomic Nervous System (ANS)

Sympathetic and parasympathetic
nerves to the viscera

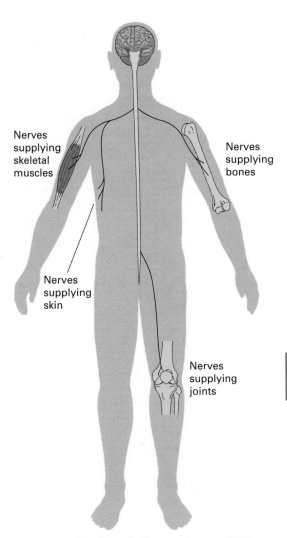

Nerves
supplying
skeletal
muscles

Nerves
supplying
bones

Nerves
supplying
skin

Nerves
supplying
joints

The Somatic Nervous System (SNS)

CHAPTER OBJECTIVES

By the end of this chapter, you should be able to:

1 Identify major prefixes, roots, suffixes, and abbreviations related to the nervous system.

2 Dissect nervous system terms into their component parts.

3 Translate nervous system terms into their common English equivalents.

4 Build new terms associated with the nervous system.

Word Parts Associated with Normal Anatomy and Physiology of the Nervous System

The following is a list of word parts and abbreviations associated with the normal structure and function of the nervous system. Use this list to help you complete **frames 1070 to 1138**.

ambul/a	walk	**CSF**	cerebrospinal fluid	**mes-**	middle
ax/i	axle			**tel-**	end
cerebell/o	little brain	**encephal/o**	brain	**thalam/o**	bedroom
cerebr/o	main brain mass	**gli/o**	glue	**vag/o**	wander
		hypophys/o	undergrowth	**vascul/o**	little vessel
cortic/o (cortex)	thin bark or covering	**mening/o**	membrane	**ventricul/o**	little belly

---

1070 The normal anatomy and physiology of the nervous system is a broad area, but it can be narrowed down to several key topics. First, of course, we know that the brain lies "within the head." Remember that _____ **(frame 362)** means "pertaining to the head." The prefix en-, like intra-, endo-, and end-, means "_____."

cephalic
within

1071 From the preceding frame, it should be evident that the root **encephal** (en-**SEF**-al) means "_____ _____ _____," that is, the "brain," because _____ means "within."

within the head
en-

1072 Extract the "presence of" suffix from mitochondrion **(frame 524)** and use it to build _____ /_____, "presence within head" or "the brain."

encephal/on (en-**SEF**-ah-**lahn**)

1073 The brain, or _____, is the major portion of the _____ _____ _____, or CNS, located within the head. Specifically, the brain lies "within the skull."

encephalon
central nervous system

1074 Tel- **(TEL)** is a prefix for "end," while mes- **(MES)**, like _____, the root in medial **(frame 333)**, means "middle." Use this information to help you synthesize two new terms:
_____ /_____ /_____ "the (front) end brain"
_____ /_____ /_____ "the midbrain"

medi

tel/**encephal**/on
(**tel**-en-**SEF**-ah-lahn)
mes/**encephal**/on
(**mes**-en-**SEF**-ah-lahn)

1075 The _____, or "(front) end brain," consists of most of the cerebrum involved in thinking activity. The _____, or "midbrain," in contrast, is the "middle" portion of the brainstem. It is mainly involved in unconscious reflex activity.

telencephalon

mesencephalon

---

neur/on
ax/on

1076 In addition to encephalon, two other terms on the word list that use the **-on** ending are **neuron** (**NOO**-rahn) and **axon** (**AKS**-ahn). These are subdivided as _____ / ____ and ____ / ____, respectively.

nerve
axon

1077 You may recall that the neur root, as appearing in neuromuscular **(frame 957)**, means "_____." The root in _____ means "axle." Its combining form is **ax/i** (**AKS**-ee).

neuron

axon

1078 The _____ is the main type of "nerve" cell "present" within the nervous system. Each of these nerve cells has its own individual _____, a long, "axle"-like, terminal cable. (Consult Figure 10.4.)

FIGURE 10.4   **Basic Microanatomy of the Neuron**

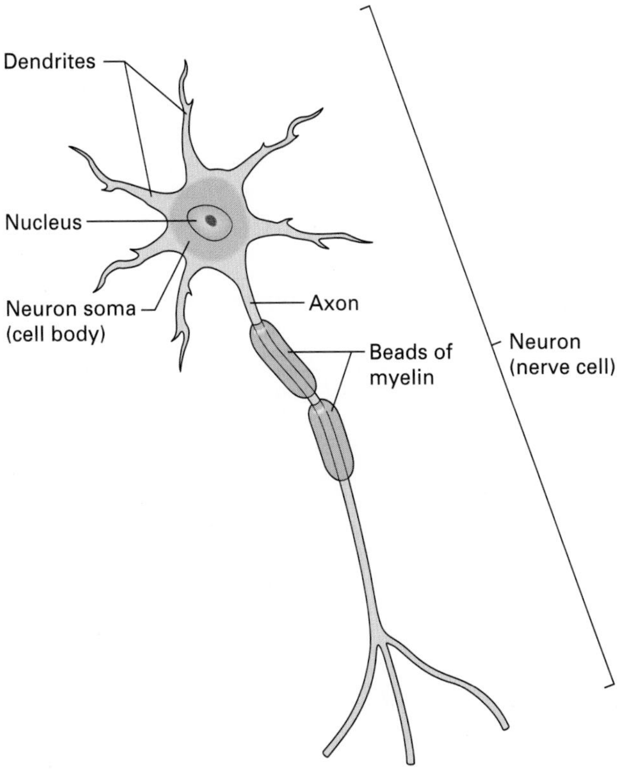

axons
myel

1079 The _____ ("axles") of many neurons are covered by beads of **myelin** (**MIGH**-eh-**lin**). This term contains _____, the root in myelic **(frame 791)**, which means either "marrow" or "spinal cord."

myel/in
-in

1080 Analyze myelin by inserting slashmarks: _____ / ____. The suffix in myelin, _____, denotes "a substance."

myelin	**1081** The term _____ denotes "a substance that (resembles) marrow."
myelin	**1082** Technically speaking, _____ is a fatty, white, "marrow"-like insulating material that speeds up the conduction of nerve impulses.
spinal cord **myel/encephal/on** (**migh**-el-en-**SEF**-ah-lahn)	**1083** The other meaning of myel, "_____ _____," becomes evident when we combine this root with the term for "presence of brain": _____ / _____ / _____.
myelencephalon	**1084** The _____ is literally "the spinal cord brain." This name indicates the part of the brainstem just superior to the spinal cord.
medull	**1085** The root in medullary (**frame 789**), _____, also means "marrow." This root, too, can be translated as "spinal cord."
medull/a (meh-DOO-lah)	**1086** Combine the root in medullary with the "presence of" suffix of bursa (**frame 814**). The result is _____ / _____.
medulla myel/o medull/o	**1087** Just as myelencephalon means "a spinal cord brain," _____ means "a spinal cord." The two combining forms for "spinal cord" are _____ / _____ and _____ / _____.
medulla **oblongata**	**1088** **Oblongata** (**ahb**-long-**GAH**-tah) denotes something "oblong," that is, something that is longer than it is wide. The name, _____ _____, therefore indicates "an oblong (brain region leading into) the spinal cord."
medulla oblongata myelencephalon	**1089** The _____ _____ is really the _____, or "spinal cord brain." Either name for this region can be used. Figure 10.5 depicts this most inferior portion of the brainstem, as well as several other structures.
mesencephalon myelencephalon **pons (PAHNS)**	**1090** Observe in Figure 10.5 that between the _____, or "midbrain present," above, and the _____, or "spinal cord brain," below, the brainstem includes the _____, which comes from the Latin for "bridge."
pons	**1091** The _____, or "bridge," includes transverse fibers that interconnect the right and left halves of the brainstem across the body midline.

cerebr/o/spin/al (**seh-REE**-broh-**SPIGH**-nal)	**1106** Combining word elements from the last few frames allows you to build _____ /____ / _____ /____, "pertaining to the main brain mass and the spinal cord."
cerebrospinal	**1107** Activity described as _____ involves both the cerebrum and the spinal cord.
cerebrospinal **CSF**	**1108** There is also a _____ ("main brain mass and spinal cord") **fluid**. This phrase is abbreviated by the initial letters of its three roots as ____ ____ ____.
cerebrospinal fluid	**1109** The _____ _____ (CSF) is a clear watery fluid that circulates both within and around the brain and spinal cord. It carries nutrients to, and harmful waste products from, the nervous tissue.
ventr **ventr/icle**	**1110** The CSF circulates within certain bellylike cavities, the **ventricles** (**VEN**-trih-**kuhls**). Using the root for "belly," _____ **(frame 351)**, dissect ventricle as _____ /_____.
-icle	**1111** The suffix in ventricle, _____, means "little."
little belly	**1112** Ventricle literally means a "_____ _____."
ventricles	**1113** The _____ are "little belly"-like chambers that contain the cerebrospinal fluid.
cerebellar	**1114** **Ventricul** (ven-**TRIK**-yool) and **vascul** (**VAS**-kyool) are roots indicating "little belly" and "little vessel or vessel," respectively. Both roots take the adjective-forming ending seen in _____ ("referring to the minor brain mass," **frame 1101**).
ventricul/ar (ven-**TRIK**-yoo-lar) **vascul/ar** (**VAS**-kyoo-lar)	**1115** "Referring to little bellies" can be written as _____ /____. "Referring to little vessels" can be written as _____ /____.
ventricular vascular	**1116** The _____ cavities are "little bellies" filled with cerebrospinal fluid. The CSF in turn has a _____ origin, since it is formed from the blood within certain "vessels."
cerebr/o/vascul/ar (seh-**ree**-broh-**VAS**-kyoo-lar)	**1117** The vessels in which cerebrospinal fluid is formed are located within the cerebrum. We can use the same pattern as in cerebrospinal to build _____ /____ /_____ /____, "pertaining to vessels" in "the main brain mass."

cerebrovascular

1118 Normal _____ function maintains brain health and proper brain blood circulation.

mening/e (meh-**NIN-jee**)

1119 The actual brain tissue is mostly isolated from direct physical contact with the blood by means of various membranes. **Mening** (meh-**NINJ**) means "membrane." Add to this root the suffix in myotome **(frame 1060)**. The word yielded is _____ / _____, that is, "a membrane."

meninges

1120 The _____ are a set of "membranes" that enclose and protect the central nervous system. Figure 10.6 shows these coverings and the ventricular system containing the CSF.

FIGURE 10.6   **The Meninges and Ventricles (Note: Ventricular System Is Denoted by Pink Color)**

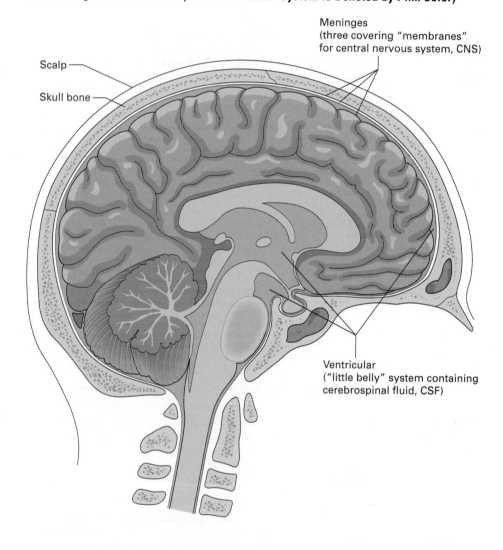

Meninges
(three covering "membranes"
for central nervous system, CNS)

Scalp

Skull bone

Ventricular
("little belly" system containing
cerebrospinal fluid, CSF)

in/voluntary (IN-vahl-en-**tahr**-ee)

1121 When the CNS is protected, it is able to properly carry out its important functions. Some of these are **voluntary** (under our conscious control). Others are classified as _____ / _____ ("not" under our conscious control), where the prefix for "not" is the same as that in insoluble **(frame 450)**.

voluntary involuntary	**1122** One body function usually considered _____ ("consciously controlled") is walking. The jerking of the lower leg when the knee tendon is tapped is generally considered _____ ("not consciously controlled").
Information Frame	**1123** A root for "walk" is **ambul (AM-byool)**. The suffix -ism **(frame 113)**, means "abnormal condition" or just "condition."
ambul/ism (**AM**-byoo-**lizm**)	**1124** Build a new term, _____ /_____, for a "condition of walking," especially an odd or abnormal walking.
ambulism	**1125** While _____ ("walking") is considered voluntary, the reflexes helping to maintain the body in an upright state are largely involuntary. These reflexes are regulated by the cerebellum.
Information Frame	**1126** When a dangerous or irritating stimulus (such as stepping on a nail) is encountered, other brain areas create a sense of pain. One of these areas is the **thalamus** (**THAL**-ah-**mus**)—a large "bedroom"-like structure at the top of the brainstem.
thalam/us **thalam** (**THAL**-ahm) **-us**	**1127** Thalamus contains the suffix in rectus **(frame 993)**. Consequently, this term is subdivided as _____ /____. The root in thalamus, _____, means "bedroom," and _____, its suffix, denotes "presence of."
thalamus	**1128** When the cerebrum is cut in midsagittal section (see Figure 10.5), the _____ does indeed appear like a "bedroom" or inner chamber "present." The large ventricle in this brain area resembles a "room" or "bedroom."
hypo- **hypo/thalam/us** (**high**-poh-**THAL**-ah-mus)	**1129** Recall that _____, the prefix in hypodermis **(frame 637)**, means "below." Thus, if thalamus denotes "presence of a bedroom," then _____ /_____ /____ indicates something "present below a bedroom."
hypothalamus	**1130** The _____ is the portion of the brainstem located immediately "below the thalamus" (see Figure 10.5). It is a broad funnel-shaped region containing a number of vital **reflex centers**—organizing areas for such automatic states as hunger and thirst.
hypophys/is **hypophys** (hih-**PAHF**-is)	**1131** Related in word structure to hypothalamus is **hypophysis** (hih-**PAHF**-ih-sis). The suffix in this term is the same as that in mortis **(frame 1027)**. The term is properly dissected with only one slashmark as _____ /____; hypo- is incorporated as part of the entire root, _____, an "undergrowth." Note how the accent and pronunciation change when hypo- and physis are combined. Say the word several times before continuing.

hypophysis	**1132** The _____ is a gland literally existing as an "undergrowth present" below the hypothalamus. It has secretions important for normal physiology.
hypophysis autonomic nervous system	**1133** The thalamus, hypothalamus, and _____ (the "undergrowth") influence much of the subconscious, involuntary activity of the nervous system. They all have a close connection to the _____ _____ _____, or ANS (see the Introduction).
vag/us	**1134** Various sympathetic and parasympathetic nerves arise from the thalamus and hypothalamus. A major parasympathetic nerve is the **vagus** (**VAY**-gus), which "wanders" to most of the viscera. Dissect vagus the way you dissected thalamus: _____ / ____.
vag (VAYG)	**1135** You can discover from the above frame that _____ is a root for "wander." **Vag/o** is the combining form.
vagus	**1136** The _____ nerve is "a wanderer" in that it supplies branches to most of the body viscera, rather than just one or a few.
-al **vag/**al (**VAY**-gal)	**1137** Vag assumes _____, the ending in cerebral, as its "referring to" suffix. Build a new term that "refers to a wanderer": _____ / ____.
vagal	**1138** Stimulation of _____ ("wandering") activity results in an automatic slowing of the heart rate.
	1139 The vagus nerve carries certain impulses that are interpreted by the brain as painful. Normal anatomy and physiology of the nervous system must be studied before its problems can be understood.

Diseases

Word Parts Associated with Diseases of the Nervous System

The following is a list of word parts and abbreviations associated with diseases and injuries of the nervous system. Use this list to help you complete **frames 1140 to 1181.**

concuss/o	violent shaking	**MS**	multiple sclerosis	**-plegia**	paralysis of
CVA	cerebrovascular accident	**noct/o**	night	**psych/o**	mind
		phas/o	speech	**schiz/o**	split
delus/o	play false; deceive	**phob/o**	unreasonable or insane fear	**syncop/o**	fainting
hallucin/o	to wander in mind	**phren/o**	mind	**tax/o**	order; arrangement; muscular coordination

-plegia (**PLEE**-jee-ah)

1140 Disorders of the nervous system may have either physical causes, mental/emotional causes, or some combination of those two types of causes. On the word list, for example, find a suffix that means "paralysis of": _____. Such paralysis may be due to a variety of causes.

quadri-
hemi-

1141 Remember that _____, as in quadriceps (**frame 976**), is a prefix indicating "four," while _____, like semi- and demi- (**frame 81**), means "partial" or "half."

hemi/plegia
(**heh**-mih-**PLEE**-jee-ah)
quadri/plegia
(**kwah**-drih-**PLEE**-jee-ah)

1142 Employy the information in the above two frames to help you build:
_____ /_____ "paralysis of half (the body)"
_____ /_____ "paralysis of four (body limbs)"

hemiplegia

quadriplegia

1143 The problem of _____ occurs when a stroke (blockage or rupture of cerebral blood vessels) causes muscles on either the right or left "half" of the body midline to be "paralyzed." When a stroke is so extensive that all "four" body limbs become "paralyzed," the condition is called _____.

cerebrovascular

1144 A more formal name for a stroke is a _____ ("pertaining to vessels" in "the main brain mass," **frame 1117**) **accident**.

cerebrovascular accident

1145 A stroke, or _____ _____ can indeed strike a person down. In fact, the ancient name for stroke is **apoplexy** (**A**-poh-**pleks**-ee), which is Greek for "a striking down."

CVA

1146 A stroke, apoplexy, or cerebrovascular accident (abbreviated by the three letters ____ ____ ____) often involves "a striking down" of the victim. There is a sudden loss of consciousness, which is frequently accompanied by a loss of feeling and body movement.

syncop/e

1147 Passing out or "fainting" in general is called **syncope** (**SIN**-koh-**pee**). This term contains the same suffix as meninge (**frame 1119**). It is therefore analyzed as _____ /____.

syncope
cerebrovascular accident

1148 Fainting, or _____, is not necessarily related to the occurrence of a _____ _____ (CVA). It can occur, for instance, in response to a sudden drop in blood pressure when one stands up too quickly.

concuss/ion (kun-**KUS**-shun)

1149 Trauma to the cerebrum can also cause syncope. A root for such a trauma, **concuss** (kun-**KUS**), means "violent shaking." This root can assume the "process of" ending in flexion (**frame 970**), becoming _____ /_____.

concussion	**1150** Violent head trauma, or _____, is usually associated with a severe headache, as well as temporary loss of consciousness.
-algia	**1151** You may recall that the **a**-beginning suffix _____ **(frame 127)**, like -**dynia**, means "condition of pain." Use the root in cephalic **(frame 362)** and the **a**-beginning suffix to create
cephal/algia (**sef**-al-**AL**-juh)	_____ /_____, "head pain" or "headache."
cephalalgia concussion	**1152** Symptoms of _____ ("headache") may reflect _____ ("process of violent shaking") or something as simple as nervous tension.
	1153 Brain damage due to trauma may also result in **tremors** (**TREH**-murs) and **vertigo** (**VER**-tih-**goh**), "uncontrollable shaking" and "dizziness," respectively. One common disease of the nervous system is **Parkinson's disease**. It involves slowness of movement and limb
tremors	_____ ("uncontrollable shaking").
vertigo tremors	**1154** A person affected by _____ ("dizziness") may or may not also experience limb _____ ("shaking").
tax/ia (**TAKS**-ee-ah)	**1155** Tax (**TAKS**) is a root for "order; arrangement; or muscular coordination." Combined with the "abnormal condition" ending in hypochondria **(frame 114)**, we get _____ /_____, "an abnormal condition of muscular coordination."
a /**tax/ia** (**a**-**TAKS**-ee-ah)	**1156** Remember that the prefix in atrophy **(frame 141)** means "without" or "lacking." Use this fact to help you construct _____ /_____ /_____, "an abnormal condition lacking muscular coordination."
CVA Parkinson's ataxia tremors vertigo	**1157** A ____ ____ ____ (stroke) as well as _____ disease **(frame 1153)**, may result in _____ ("lack of muscular coordination"). Such a lack of coordination may contribute directly to occurrence of limb _____ ("shaking") and indirectly to occurrence of _____ ("dizziness").
phas/ia (**FAYZ**-ee-ah)	**1158** **Phas (FAYZ)** is a root for "speech." Use the same format as for taxia to create _____ /_____, "an abnormal condition of speech."
a /**phas/ia** (ah-**FAY**-zhuh)	**1159** Extract the prefix from ataxia to assist you in making _____ /_____ /_____, "an abnormal condition lacking speech."
aphasia ataxia	**1160** A person with _____ would be mute, while one with _____ would tend to fall easily.

multiple
sclerosis (skleh-ROH-sis)
sclerosis

1161 Another disease state involving limb tremors is _____ _____, abbreviated as MS. You can see that the second part of this disease's name is _____, an "abnormal condition of hardening." (**Frame 147** treats this term as a suffix.)

MS

1162 The condition of multiple sclerosis (or ____ ____) is a progressive degenerative disease involving the "hardening" and loss of myelin at "multiple" sites on neuron axons.

multiple sclerosis

ataxia

1163 The problem of _____ _____ ("hardening" of "multiple" neuron axons) often manifests itself in severe limb tremors and _____ ("lack of muscular balance").

-itis

1164 Various kinds of inflammations can also occur that involve the brain or spinal cord. Recall that _____ is a suffix for "inflammation of," as in myositis **(frame 1012)**.

mening/itis (meh-nin-JIGH-tis)
encephal/itis (en-sef-ah-LIGH-tis)

1165 Adopt the root for "membrane" **(frame 1119)** and the one for "presence within head" or "brain" **(frame 1072)** to help you build:
_____ /_____ an "inflammation of the membranes"
_____ /_____ an "inflammation of the brain"

meningitis
encephalitis

1166 Both _____ ("inflamed meninges") and _____ ("brain inflammation") are often associated with high fever.

gli/oma (glee-OH-mah)

1167 Other brain problems may include various tumors. The glia (neuroglia), being connective tissue cells, are capable of excessive mitosis, thereby resulting in tumors. Follow a word-building pattern like that for myoma **(frame 1010)** and synthesize _____ /_____, "tumor of glue (glia cells)."

glioma
gli/o/sis
-o/sis

1168 A _____ ("tumor of glia") is a type of gliosis (**glee-OH-sis**). Dissect gliosis as _____ /____ /_____. Any ____ /_____ is by definition a "condition of" or an "abnormal condition of" something.

neur
neur/o/sis (noo-ROH-sis)
psych/o/sis (sigh-KOH-sis)

1169 Such "abnormal conditions" can occur for both the "nerves" (indicated by the root _____) and the "mind," indicated by the root **psych (SIGHK)**. Then a _____ /____ /_____ is literally "an abnormal condition of the nerves," while a _____ /____ /_____ is one involving the "mind."

neurosis

psychosis

1170 A _____ ("nerve condition") is formally considered a functional disorder of the nervous system, one with no clear physical cause. A _____ is a severe emotional disorder of the "mind," one involving loss of contact with reality.

noct/ambul/ism
(**nahkt-AM**-byoo-lizm)

1171 Some emotional problems are manifested in our sleep at "night." **Noct (NAHKT)** is a root for "night." Combining this with the term for "abnormal condition of walking" **(frame 1124)** results in _____ /_____ /_____.

---

noctambulism

1172 Sleepwalking, or "nightwalking," technically called _____, may reflect unresolved emotional problems—a neurosis of some kind.

Information Frame

1173 Potentially severe mental or emotional problems are represented by the following roots:
delus (deh-LOOZ) "false belief"
hallucin (hah-LOO-sin) "unreal sensation"
phob (FOHB) "unreasonable or insane fear"

---

delus/ion (deh-LOO-zhun)

1174 Extract the suffix in concussion **(frame 1149)** and consult **frame 1173** to build _____ /_____, "process of (having) a false belief."

---

delusion

1175 A man suffering from a _____ might think he was Napoleon. Such a "false belief" could never be changed by logical arguments.

---

hallucin/a/tion
(ha-**loo**-sih-**NAY**-shun)

1176 Follow the pattern in supination **(frame 970)** and consult **frame 1173** to build _____ /____ /_____, "a process of (having) unreal sensations."

---

hallucination

1177 A woman who sees "microbes" running up and down her living room curtains obviously is experiencing some sort of _____!

---

phob/ia (FOH-bee-ah)

1178 Extract the "abnormal condition" suffix in taxia **(frame 1155)** and consult **frame 1173** to help you build _____ /____, "an abnormal condition of unreasonable or insane fear."

---

phobia

1179 A person who avoids heights probably has a _____ about high places.

---

schiz/o/phren/ia
(**skiz**-oh-**FREN**-ee-uh)

1180 An emotional tug-of-war may result in a "split," or **schiz (SKIZ)**, of the "mind," which is **phren (FREN)**. Put these elements together and generate _____ /____ /_____ /____, much as you generated phobia.

---

schizophrenia

1181 An "abnormal condition of split mind" is technically called _____. It is a form of psychosis in which one "splits," or withdraws, from close relationships with others.

1182 Whether nervous system disease is mainly physical or mainly emotional, a major task for the health professional is proper diagnosis of the problem.

Lab Tests and Diagnoses

Word Parts Associated with Lab Tests and Diagnoses for the Nervous System

What follows is a list of some word parts and an abbreviation associated with lab tests and diagnoses concerning the nervous system. Use this list to help you complete **frames 1184 to 1200**.

EEG	electroencephalogram	**radi/o**	ray; x-ray
encephal/o	brain	**ventricul/o**	brain ventricles

Information Frame

1183 One of the simplest means of examining the nervous system for problems is to stimulate the body in certain areas and watch for the appearance of reflexes (automatic responses). Some early work by **Joseph Babinski (bah-BIN-**skee), a French physician, has contributed much to our understanding of the clinical value of reflexes.

---

flexion

Babinski

1184 When the sole of the foot is lightly stroked, the big toe should undergo _____, a "process of bending" **(frame 970)**. Babinski noticed that when certain nerve fibers from the cerebral cortex are damaged, the opposite reaction may occur. This reaction, named for its discoverer, is called a **positive** _____ **reflex**.

Babinski reflex

1185 The _____ _____ is an abnormal extension of the big toe (rather than flexion) after light stroking of the sole of the foot.

---

encephal

encephal/o/meter
(en-**sef**-ah-**LAH**-meh-ter)

1186 Some terms describe procedures for assessing the _____ (root for "brain") itself. Use the suffix in thermometer **(frame 226)** to help you build _____ /_____ /_____, an "instrument used to measure the brain."

---

encephalometer

1187 An _____ is a "device" used to mark the relative locations of various structures within the "brain."

---

neur/o/radi/o/logy
(**noo**-roh-**ray**-dee-**AHL**-oh-jee)

1188 Other means of assessing the brain involve radiology. Technically, the proper term is _____ /_____ /_____ /_____ /_____, "study of rays and nerves."

---

neuroradiology

1189 In _____, x-rays are used to study the CNS.

---

encephal/o/gram
(en-**SEF**-ah-loh-**gram**)

1190 For example, an _____ /_____ /_____ is a radiogram of the "brain."

---

encephalogram	**1191** An _____ can sometimes provide evidence suggestive of brain tumor.
ventricul	**1192** Recall that _____, the root in ventricular **(frame 1115)**, means "little belly." So just as radiography is the "process of recording x-ray (images)" in general, _____ / ____ / _____ is the "process of recording the little bellies" within the brain.
ventricul/o/graphy (ven-**trik**-yoo-**LAHG**-rah-fee)	
ventriculography	**1193** The technique of _____ involves an "x-raying" of the brain "ventricles."
ventricul/o/scopy (ven-**trik**-yoo-**LAH**-skoh-pee)	**1194** Ventriculography may provide suspicious-looking x-ray images suggesting a partially blocked flow of the cerebrospinal fluid. An endoscope may then be inserted into the brain. Adopt the suffix in arthroscopy **(frame 925)** to help you build _____ / ____ / _____, the "process of examining ventricles."
ventriculoscopy	**1195** By means of an inserted endoscope, _____ permits a direct visualization of the interior of the brain ventricles.
lumbar	**1196** For an examination of the cerebrospinal fluid itself, a _____ ("pertaining to the loins," **frame 382**) **puncture** is often made. The "low back" area within the vertebral canal has enough space to allow insertion of a needle, and it is generally below the body or main mass of the spinal cord. Therefore, the danger of stabbing into the spinal cord by accident is minimized.
lumbar puncture	**1197** A _____ _____ permits thorough examination of the contents of a small quantity of CSF withdrawn from the low back area.
electr/o/encephal/o/gram (ee-**lek**-troh-en-**SEF**-uh-loh-gram)	**1198** Another way of studying the brain is by looking at its electrical activity. Remember that an electromyogram **(frame 1039)** is a "record of muscle electrical (activity)." In similar fashion, an _____ / ____ / _____ / ____ / _____ is a "record of brain electrical (activity)."
electroencephalogram	**1199** An _____ can reveal whether neurons are producing electrical wave patterns of appropriate height and frequency.
EEG	**1200** An electroencephalogram, or ____ ____ ____, is a valuable tool for diagnosing potential abnormalities in neuron activity. If such abnormalities are detected, therapy is often required.

Word Parts Associated with Surgery, Pharmacology, and Other Therapies Involving the Nervous System

The following is a list of word parts associated with surgery, pharmacology, and other therapies for the nervous system. Use this list to help you complete **frames 1201 to 1229**.

mimet/o	mimic; imitate	**sympathet/o**	the sympathetic nerves
psych/o	mind	**trephin/a**	borer
sympath/o	the sympathetic nerves		

---

psych
neur

1201 The types of therapies administered for nervous system problems depend to some extent on the type of professional person from whom treatment is sought. Recall now that _____ is a root for "mind" (as found in psychosis, **frame 1169**) and that _____ is a root for "nerve" (as found in neurosis).

---

psych/o/logy (**sigh-KAHL**-oh-jee)
neur/o/logy (**noo-RAHL**-oh-jee)

psych/iatry (**sigh-KIGH**-ah-tree)

1202 Put the roots of the preceding frame together with suffixes for various medical specialities. With the suffix in dermatology **(frame 728)** we obtain:

_____ /_____ /_____ "study of the mind"
_____ /_____ /_____ "study of the nerves"
With the suffix in podiatry **(frame 1043)** we get
_____ /_____, "the process of being a physician for the mind."

---

psych/o/logists
(**sigh-KAHL**-oh-jists)
neur/o/logists
(**noo-RAHL**-oh-jists)

1203 Just as dermatologists are "studiers of the skin," other professionals are:

_____ /_____ /_____ "studiers of the mind"
_____ /_____ /_____ "studiers of the nerves"

---

podiatrists
psych/iatrists
(**sigh-KIGH**-ah-trists)

1204 And just as _____ **(frame 1042)** are "physicians who specialize in the feet," _____ /_____ are "physicians who specialize in the mind."

---

psychology
psychologists
neurology
neurologists

psychiatry
psychiatrists

1205 The discipline of _____, practiced by _____, primarily "studies" how thinking in the "mind" affects behavior. The discipline of _____, practiced by _____, mainly "studies" physical damage to the "nerves." The "process of being a physician for the mind" (_____) is practiced by _____, who focus on ways to diagnose and treat emotional disorders.

---

psych/o/therapy
(**sigh**-koh-**THEHR**-uh-pee)

1206 Another name for psychiatry is
_____ /_____ /_____, "therapy for the mind."

psychotherapy **neur/o/surgery** (**noo**-roh-**SURJ**-er-ee)	**1207** Sometimes psychiatry (_____) can't solve a nervous problem, such as that associated with a glioma or other brain tumor. At such times _____ /____ /_____, that is, "surgery of the nerves," is required.
neurosurgery	**1208** Actually, _____ is just as likely to involve cutting of the brain or spinal cord as cutting of the nerves themselves.
crani/o/**tomy** (**kray**-nee-**AH**-toh-mee)	**1209** Withdraw the suffix from myotenotomy **(frame 1064)** and the root in cranial **(frame 362)** and use them to help you build _____ /____ /_____, or "incision of the skull."
craniotomy neurosurgery	**1210** The procedure of _____ must be performed before _____ ("nerve surgery") on the brain can begin.
craniotomy	**1211** The operation of _____ often involves boring a hole in the skull bones. **Trephin/e** (**TREE**-fihn) means "a borer."
trephine	**1212** A _____ is actually a cylindrical saw used to "bore" out flat disks of bone.
trephin/a/**tion** (**treh**-fihn-**AY**-shun)	**1213** Use the word-building pattern of hallucination **(frame 1176)** to construct _____ /____ /_____, a term for the "process of boring."
trephination	**1214** The operation of _____ ("boring") into the skull was performed by ancient people to relieve severe cephalalgia.
trephination **thalam**/o/**tomy** (**thal**-am-**AH**-toh-mee)	**1215** Various techniques of neurosurgery require craniotomy by _____ ("boring") first. Among these techniques is _____ /____ /_____, "cutting into the bedroom, or thalamus."
thalamotomy	**1216** The operative procedure of _____ may be performed to help relieve pain sensations, whose perception usually involves the "thalamus."
neur/o/**surgeon** (**noo**-roh-**SUR**-jun)	**1217** Thalamotomy is only one of many possible procedures in neurosurgery. A person might be "suffering" (path) "with" (sym-) various nervous problems. A _____ /____ /_____ ("nerve surgeon") may perform both **-otomies** and **-ectomies** ("removals") of numerous types.

sympath/ectomy
(**sim**-path-**EK**-toh-mee)
neur/ectomy (**noo-REK**-toh-mee)

1218 A _____/_____, for instance, is literally a "process of removing sympathetic (suffering-with)" nerves. This procedure is a specific type of _____ /_____, "process of nerve removal."

neurectomy

sympathectomy

1219 The surgery of _____ is a general procedure whereby various "nerves" are "removed" or interrupted. The removal or interruption of particular sympathetic nerves, however, is _____. This operation may be performed when, say, particular sympathetic nerves are overstimulating the heart muscle to contract too fast.

vagus

vag/o/tomy (**vay-GAH**-toh-mee)

1220 Extremely large nerves, such as the _____, or "wanderer" (**frame 1134**), cannot be removed completely. They are simply incised (cut into). A _____ /____ /_____ is a "cutting into the wanderer."

vagotomy

1221 The _____ procedure (**frame 1220**) is sometimes performed to relieve severe pain arising from some cancerous organ, such as the stomach.

1222 Fortunately, pharmacological approaches are often adequate to treat many nervous and emotional disorders. Drugs are given "against" the abnormal states. The prefix here is the one appearing in antibiotics (**frame 274**). Use this prefix to complete the names of the drugs listed below:

anti/**depress**/ants
(**AN**-tih-**de-PRES**-ahnts)
anti/**psych/o/tic**
(**AN**-tih-**sigh-KAH**-tik)
anti/**parkinson**
(**AN**-tih-**PAR**-kin-sun)

_____ /depress/**ants**
_____ /psych/o/**tic** tranquilizers
_____ /parkinson drugs

antiparkinson
antidepressants
antipsychotic

1223 The _____ drugs are administered to combat the effects of Parkinson's disease. The _____ are given to relieve severe, chronic depression. The _____ tranquilizers are prescribed to calm down and relieve symptoms of patients who have lost contact with reality.

mimet/ic (mih-**MET**-ik)

1224 Still other drugs mimic the effects of natural body actions or secretions. **Mimet** (mih-**MET**) is a root for "mimic" or "imitate." Just as tonic (**frame 468**) "pertains to strength," _____ /____ "pertains to imitating."

mimetic

1225 Drugs that are _____ can "imitate" the effects of natural physiological substances.

sympath
sympath/o/mimet/ic
(**sim-PATH**-oh-mih-**MET**-ik)

1226 The root in sympathectomy, _____, for example, can be used to build _____ / _____ / _____ / _____, "pertaining to imitation of the sympathetic" nerves.

sympathomimetic

1227 The _____ drugs "mimic" the body-arousing effects caused by the natural activity of the "sympathetic" nerves. An example of such a drug is **adrenaline** (ah-**DREN**-ah-**lin**).

para/sympath/o/mimet/ic
(**pahr**-ah-sim-**PATH**-oh-mih-**MET**-ik)

1228 The _____ / _____ / _____ / _____ / _____ drugs likewise "imitate" the "parasympathetic" nerves in their actions.

parasympathomimetic

1229 A variety of _____ agents, such as **atropine** (**A**-troh-**peen**), produce body effects similar to what would happen if parasympathetic nerves were being stimulated. A specific instance is a marked decrease in the pulse (heart rate).

Multiple Choice

1. Mr. Jones has quadriplegia. He will require care to

  a. the lower limbs   b. one side of the body

  c. the whole body below the neck   d. the area below the waist

2. Which of the following means "fainting"?

  a. vertigo   b. tremor   c. syncope   d. ataxia

3. Which does *not* belong to the brainstem?

  a. pons   b. medulla   c. midbrain   d. cerebellum

4. The word root for "glue" is

  a. oglia   b. gli   c. myel   d. myelgia

5. Schizophrenia is a

  a. neurosis   b. phobia   c. psychosis   d. delusion

6. Hydrophobia is a _____ of water.

  a. falsehood   b. fallacy   c. fear   d. dislike

Meanings of Selected Roots

Add the correct combining vowel (cv) after each root. Then write the definition of each root in the space provided.

ROOT/CV   **DEFINITION**

1. cerebell/_____   _____

2. gli/_____   _____

3. thalam/_____   _____

4. mimet/_____   _____

5. encephal/_____   _____

6. ambul/_____   _____

7. delus/_____   _____

8. psych/_____   _____

9. vag/_____   _____

10. cerebr/_____   _____

Word Dissection and Translation

Analyze the following terms by dissecting them with slashmarks and identifying their word parts. To the right of each term, write its correct English translation.

Key: R (root), cv (combining vowel), P (prefix), S (suffix)

1. sympathomimetic

_____/____/_____/_____   _____
     R   cv   R   S

2. neuroglia

_____/____/_____/_____   _____
     R   cv   R   S

3. trephination

_____/____/_____   _____
     R   cv   S

4. encephalitis

_____/_____   _____
     R   S

5. schizophrenia

_____/____/_____/_____   _____
     R   cv   R   S

6. psychologist

_____/____/_____   _____
     R   cv   S

7. ventricular

_____/_____   _____
     R   S

8. thalamotomy

_____/____/_____   _____
     R   cv   S

9. ambulism

_____/_____   _____
     R   S

10. quadriplegia

_____/_____   _____
     P   R

11. psychotherapeutic

_____/____/_____/_____   _____
     R   cv   R   S

12. microcephalus

_____/____/_____/_____   _____
     R   cv   R   S

Terms and Their Abbreviations

In the list below, when the term is given, write its abbreviation in the space provided. When the abbreviation is given, write its corresponding term.

TERM	ABBREVIATION
1. somatic nervous system	_____
2. electroencephalogram	_____
3. _____	CNS
4. _____	PNS
5. cerebrospinal fluid	_____
6. _____	ANS
7. _____	CVA
8. multiple sclerosis	_____

Word Spelling

Look at each of the terms listed below. Identify those that are misspelled by circling Y for "Yes." Write the correct spelling in the blank.

WORD	MISSPELLED?	CORRECT SPELLING
1. auntiedepressants	Y/N	_____
2. neurologists	Y/N	_____
3. ensephulometer	Y/N	_____
4. cerebrovoskewlar	Y/N	_____
5. axon	Y/N	_____
6. myelin	Y/N	_____
7. hypophysis	Y/N	_____
8. ventrikyoular	Y/N	_____
9. encephalon	Y/N	_____
10. cerebellum	Y/N	_____
11. auntieparkinson	Y/N	_____
12. craniotomy	Y/N	_____
13. qwadripleejih	Y/N	_____
14. sefalalgia	Y/N	_____

New Word Synthesis

Using word parts that appear in this and previous chapters, build new terms with the following meanings:

1. _____ presence of imitation

2. _____ abnormal condition of the main brain mass

3. _____ relating to wandering little vessels

4. _____ a fainting speech

5. _____ lack of dizziness

6. _____ removal of a straight nerve

7. _____ inflammation of nerves and muscles

8. _____ pertaining to (a condition) without the cerebrum

9. _____ process of violently shaking the cerebellum

10. _____ abnormal condition of split nerves

11. _____ of mental origin

12. _____ herniation of meninges and spinal cord

C A S E   S T U D Y

Read through the following partial case history. Note the terms in bold print. A series of multiple choice questions probes your knowledge of these terms.

Case History

A 55-year-old black male was admitted to the hospital with complaints of **nocturnal hemiplegia**, which disappeared upon arising from bed in the morning. His wife, however, reported seeing him **noctambulating** frequently. **Psychiatric** evaluation uncovered various **hallucinations**.

Case Study Questions

1. **Nocturnal hemiplegia** means

   (a) anesthesia of all body limbs.

   (b) paralysis of half the body at night

   (c) pyrexia during the day.

   (d) paralysis of four limbs.

2. **Noctambulating** by the patient suggests

   (a) sleepwalking.

   (b) tremors.

   (c) pyrexia.

   (d) paralysis.

3. **Psychiatric** evaluation of the patient implies that he received

   (a) neurosurgery.

   (b) chemotherapy.

   (c) psychotherapy.

   (d) physical therapy.

4. The uncovering of various **hallucinations** implies that the patient suffered

   (a) organic nerve disease.

   (b) phobic attacks.

   (c) psychotic episodes.

   (d) false ideations.

CHAPTER 11 Special Senses: The Eye and Ear

INTRODUCTION

The **special senses** are those senses above and beyond such general feelings as touch, pain, pressure, cold, and warmth. Primary among these special senses are those of vision and hearing. The sense of vision is reflected in the anatomy and physiology of the eye, the sense of hearing in the anatomy and physiology of the ear. Figure 11.1 (A and B) presents an overall image of the structure of the eye, and Figure 11.2 does so for the ear. We will be referring to these images as we discuss the terms of normal structure and function for the eye and ear.

FIGURE 11.1A   **Structures of the Eye—External View**

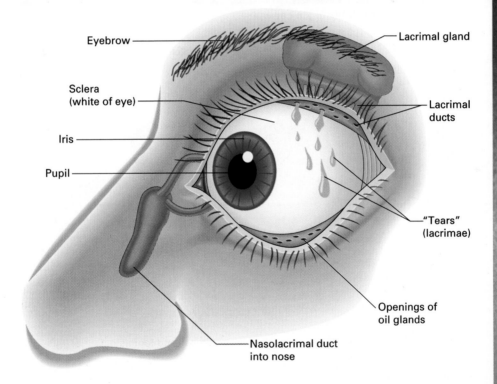

Eyebrow

Sclera (white of eye)

Iris

Pupil

Lacrimal gland

Lacrimal ducts

"Tears" (lacrimae)

Openings of oil glands

Nasolacrimal duct into nose

FIGURE 11.1B   Structures of the Eye—Lateral View of the Eyeball Interior

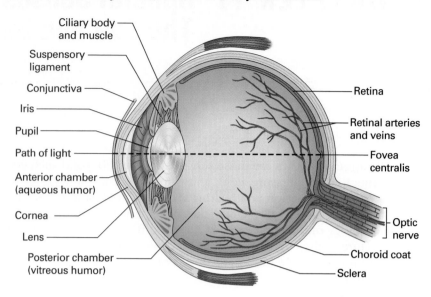

- Ciliary body and muscle
- Suspensory ligament
- Conjunctiva
- Iris
- Pupil
- Path of light
- Anterior chamber (aqueous humor)
- Cornea
- Lens
- Posterior chamber (vitreous humor)
- Retina
- Retinal arteries and veins
- Fovea centralis
- Optic nerve
- Choroid coat
- Sclera

FIGURE 11.2   Structures of the Ear

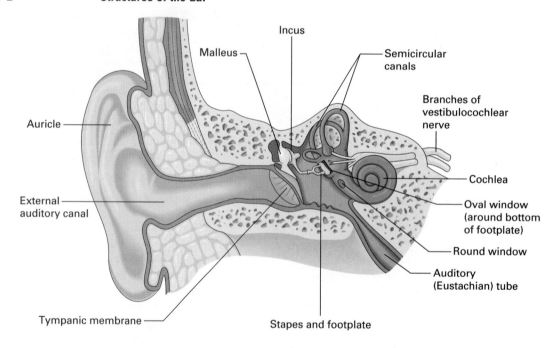

- Incus
- Malleus
- Semicircular canals
- Branches of vestibulocochlear nerve
- Auricle
- Cochlea
- External auditory canal
- Oval window (around bottom of footplate)
- Round window
- Auditory (Eustachian) tube
- Tympanic membrane
- Stapes and footplate

Although the physiology of human vision is quite complex, it is summarized simply in Figure 11.3. In brief, light rays enter the eye through its **pupil**. The rays are bent by the **lens** (somewhat like a camera lens). The rays continue through the **posterior chamber** of the eyeball (behind the lens). The rays come to focus on the **retina** (**RET**-ih-**nah**), the highly vascular interior lining at the extreme rear of the eyeball. The image is focused upside down on the retina! (Imagine trying to read this book with all the pages inverted!) The inverted image is changed into **electrochemical signals** by the **retinal** (**RET**-ih-**nal**) cells, or **visual receptors**. The **rods** are the light-dark visual receptors, and the cones are sensitive to color. The electrochemical signals from the rods and cones leave the eyeball via the **optic** (**AHP**-tik) **nerve**. This nerve carries the signals to the **primary visual area** at the dorsal tip of the cerebrum. Here the cerebrum somehow adjusts the inverted image, so that we perceive things upright.

FIGURE 11.3

Overview of Human Vision

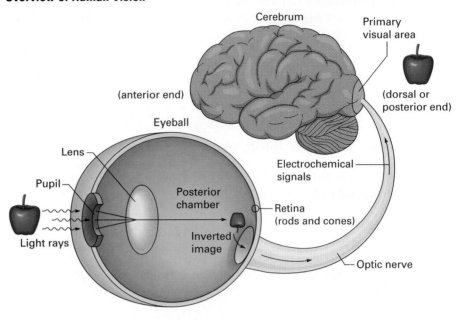

The complex physiology of human hearing is briefly summarized in Figure 11.4. Sound waves enter the **external ear** and travel into the **Eustachian (yoo-STAY-shun) tube (external auditory canal)**. The sound waves vibrate the membranous **eardrum**, or **tympanum** (tim-**PAN**-um). The active vibrating of the eardrum sets the three tiny bones of the **middle ear cavity** into motion. The **malleus (MAL-ee-us)** pushes on the **incus (IHNG-kus)**. The incus pushes against the **stapes (STAY**-peez). The stapes in turn pushes on a tiny oval window of the inner ear cavity. The oval window moves in and out, somewhat like a toilet plunger. The fluid within the snail shell-shaped **cochlea (KAHK**-lee-ah) is compressed by this plunging action. The microscopic **hair cells** lining the cochlea are the receptors for hearing. They are bent by the pressure and send electrochemical signals over the **auditory (AW**-dih-**tor**-ee) **nerve**. The signals finally reach the **primary auditory area** along the lateral aspect of the cerebrum. These signals are somehow perceived as meaningful language and sounds.

FIGURE 11.4

Overview of Human Hearing

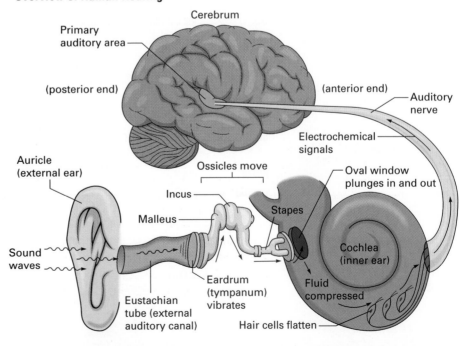

This chapter considers the terminology of the normal anatomy and physiology of the eye and ear, the terminology of their diseases, terms involving lab tests and diagnoses of eye-ear problems, and terms describing surgery, pharmacology, and other therapies for visual or hearing difficulties.

CHAPTER OBJECTIVES

By the end of this chapter, you should be able to:

1 Identify major prefixes, roots, suffixes, and abbreviations related to the eye and ear.

2 Dissect eye and ear terms into their component parts.

3 Translate eye and ear terms into their common English equivalents.

4 Build new terms associated with the eye and ear.

Normal A & P

Word Parts Associated with Normal Anatomy and Physiology of the Eye and Ear

The following is a list of word parts and abbreviations associated with the normal structure and function of the eye and ear. Use this list to help you complete **frames 1230 to 1280**.

acous/o	hear	**corne/o**	tough; hornlike	**ophthalm/o**	eye
acoust/o	hear	**dacry/o**	tear	**opt/o**	eye; vision
AD	right ear (auris dextra)	**inc/o**	anvil	**OS**	left eye (oculus sinister)
		ir/o	rainbow; iris		
AS	left ear (auris sinistra)	**irid/o**	rainbow; iris	**ossic/o**	bone
		kerat/o	tough; cornea	**ot/o**	ear
audit/o	hear	**lacrim/o**	tear	**palpebr/o**	eyelid
auric/o	ear	**malle/o**	mallet; hammer	**retin/o**	net
blephar/o	eyelid	**meat/o**	opening; passage	**scler/o**	hard
cochle/o	snail shell	**myring/o**	eardrum	**staped/o**	stirrup
conjunctiv/o	binding together (eyelid lining)	**ocul/o**	little eye	**tympan/o**	eardrum
		OD	right eye (oculus dexter)	**vestibul/o**	small entrance room
cor/o	pupil				
core/o	pupil				

---

auric/o (**OR**-ih-koh)
ot/o (**OH**-toh)

1230 Scan the word list and find two combining forms for "ear." These are _____ /_____ and _____ /_____.

Chapter 11 Special Senses: The Eye and Ear

ocul/o (**AHK**-yoo-loh)
ophthalm/o (**AHF-thal**-moh)
opt/o (**AHP**-toh)

1231 Scan the word list and find three combining forms for "eye" or "little eye": _____ /_____, _____ /_____, and _____ /_____.

auric/le (**OR**-ih-kul)

1232 Now let us build some terms related to the eye and ear. For building "a little ear," _____ /_____, use **auric** (**OR**-ik), following the same pattern used in ventricle (**frame 1111**). Note that here, however, the root already includes **ic**.

ocul/us (**AHK**-yoo-lus)

1233 For building "a little eye," _____ /_____, use **ocul** and the same suffix appearing in thalamus (**frame 1127**).

auricle
oculus

1234 For a student to learn, he or she must have an open _____ ("little ear"), open _____ ("little eye"), and an open **psych/e** (**SIGH**-kee, "mind")!

auris dextra
auris sinistra

1235 Closely related to auricle is **auris** (**OR**-is). **Dextra** (**DEKS**-trah) means "right," and **sinistra** (**SIN**-is-trah) means "left." Use these facts to create new phrases:
_____ _____ "ear" on the "right"
_____ _____ "ear" on the "left"

AD

AS

1236 Auris dextra, abbreviated as _____ _____, is often used in medical records to indicate the "right ear." Auris sinistra, abbreviated as _____ _____, is often used in medical records to indicate the "left ear."

oculus dexter
oculus sinister

1237 Using oculus, a similar strategy employs **dexter** (**DEKS**-ter) for "right" and **sinister** for "left," to yield:
_____ _____ "eye" on the "right"
_____ _____ "eye" on the "left"

OD

OS

1238 Oculus dexter, abbreviated as _____ _____, is often used in medical records to indicate the "right eye." Oculus sinister, abbreviated as _____ _____, is often used in medical records to indicate the "left eye."

ocul/ar (**AHK**-yoo-**ler**)

1239 The "little eye" root in oculus assumes the "pertaining to" suffix in vascular (**frame 1115**), thereby becoming _____ /_____.

ocular

ophthalm/**ic**
opt/**ic**
ot/ic (**OH**-tik)

1240 Structures that are _____ ("eye"-related) can also be described using **ophthalmic** (**ahf-THAL**-mik) and optic. The first term is subdivided as _____ /_____, the second as _____ /_____. For ot, this strategy produces _____ /_____, "relating to the ear."

ocular ophthalmic optic otic	**1241** Many terms describe detailed features of _____, _____, or _____, that is, "eye," anatomy. The terms for _____ ("ear") anatomy will be discussed later.
palpebr/a (pal-**PEE**-bruh)	**1242** The eye is protected by the "eyelid," indicated by the two roots/cv, **blephar/o** (**BLEF**-ah-roh) and **palpebr/o** (**pal-PEE**-broh). Using the second root, we can build _____ /____ ("an eyelid") as we did medulla **(frame 1086)**.
conjunctiv/a (kun-**JUNK**-tih-vuh) palpebra	**1243** **Conjunctiv** (**kun-JUNK**-tiv) means "binding together." Using the same suffix as in the preceding frame, build _____ /____. This is a membrane that "binds together" the interior of the _____ ("eyelid") with the frontal surface of the eyeball. It is in a sense, then, the "lining of the eyelid." (Review Figure 11.1 if desired.)
conjunctiva **corne** (**KOR**-nee) scler **scler/a** (**SKLAIR**-ah)	**1244** The _____ "binds" to the surface of the **corne/a** (**KOR**-nee-ah). The root in this term, _____, like **kerat** (**KEHR**-at), indicates something "tough" and "hornlike." Find in the word list a root, _____, that means "hard." A term that uses the same suffix as cornea and indicates that something "hard" is "present" is _____ /____.
cornea sclera	**1245** The _____ is the "tough, hornlike," transparent front of the eyeball. The _____ is the "hard," white portion of the eyeball surrounding this central hornlike area.
cor (**KOR**) **core** (**KOR**-ee)	**1246** At the middle zone of the cornea, one finds the **pupil**. This large dark opening is represented by two roots, _____ and _____, on the word list.
core/us (**KOR**-ee-us)	**1247** Add the suffix in hypothalamus **(frame 1129)** to the longer root for "pupil" and get _____ /____, "presence of the pupil."
coreus core	**1248** The term _____, and its root, _____, are usually used to indicate the "pupil" scientifically.
Information Frame	**1249** The name **pupil**, itself, means "little girl" or "doll." The colored ring around the pupil, called the **iris** (**IGH**-ris), denotes "a rainbow." These very imaginative terms show how early scholars used everyday analogies to help them name body structures. Apparently, **pupil** derives from the fact that a woman can see herself reflected back as a "little girl" or "doll" in the pupil of another person! Since the **iris** can occur in various colors, it was named as "a rainbow" around the "little girl"! (See Figure 11.5.)

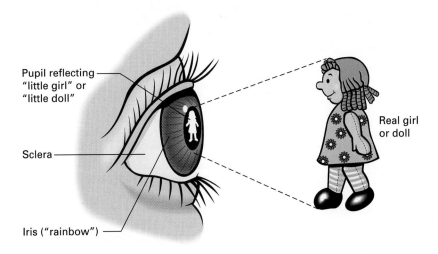

Pupil reflecting
"little girl" or
"little doll"

Sclera

Iris ("rainbow")

Real girl
or doll

---

ir/is

1250 Iris contains the same ending as abdominis **(frame 994)**.
Consequently, it is analyzed as _____ /_____, "presence of a rainbow."

---

iris

1251 The _____ ("rainbow") regulates the diameter of the pupil, hence
the amount of light entering the eye.

---

ir (IR)
irid (IR-id)

irid/ectomy

1252 The root in iris, _____, is not the only root for that eye part. Find
another root for iris, _____, on the word list. This second root is
often used with other word parts to indicate pathology or treatment of
the iris. With **-ectomy**, for instance, we have "removal of part of the
iris," or _____ /_____.

---

refract/ion (ree-**FRAK-shun**)

1253 Light rays are bent by the lens in the eye. **Refract** (ree-**FRAKT**) means
"bend." The "process of bending" light rays,
_____ /_____, takes the same "process of" suffix as concussion **(frame 1149)**.

---

refraction

1254 The "bending," or _____, of light rays by the lens
causes them to be projected onto the retina at the posterior wall of the
eyeball.

---

retin/a

1255 Retina contains the same suffix as sclera **(frame 1245)**. Therefore, retina is subdivided as _____ /_____.

---

retin
net

1256 Retina means "a net." Its root, therefore, is _____, which means
"_____."

---

retina

1257 The _____ is actually a "net" of visual receptor cells in the
posterior wall of the eyeball. From here, visual images are sent back
toward the brain via the optic nerve.

dacry/o (DAK-ree-oh)
lacrim/o (LAK-rih-moh)

1258 The eye must be kept moist and clean in order to see. This is one of the functions of tears. The word list shows two combining forms, _____ /____ and _____ /____ that mean "tears."

lacrim/al (LAK-rih-mal)

1259 The second root in the preceding frame can be used with the ending in cerebral **(frame 1099)** to result in _____ /____, which "pertains to tears."

lacrimal

1260 The _____ **glands** produce "tears," which serve to lubricate the eyes and help wash out foreign matter.

acous/o (ah-KOOS-oh)
acoust/o (ah-KOOS-toh)
audit/o (AW-dih-toh)

1261 Next in importance after vision and the eyes is hearing and the ears. Locate three roots on the word list that mean "hear." Cited alphabetically, with their combining vowels, these are _____ /____, _____ /____, and _____ /____.

acoust/ic (ah-KOOS-tik)

audit/ory (AW-dih-tor-ee)

1262 For "pertaining to," the second root in the above frame assumes the suffix in otic, becoming _____ /____. The third root in the sequence adopts the ending -ory, which, like -ary **(frame 91)**, means "pertaining to." The resulting term is _____ /_____.

acoustic
auditory

1263 Both _____ and _____ have essentially the same translation. They both "refer to hearing."

auricle

meat/us

1264 Hearing is caused by sound waves that enter the _____ ("little ear," **frame 1232**). They do so through a **meatus** (mee-AY-tus). This term is analyzed as _____ /____, similar to the method for oculus **(frame 1233)**.

meat (mee-AYT)

1265 The root in meatus is _____. It means "opening" or "passage."

meatus

1266 The **external auditory**, or **acoustic**, _____ is literally the "outside hearing passage" through which sound waves enter the head.

Information Frame

1267 At the end of this canal, also called the Eustachian tube, is the "eardrum." Two combining forms for "eardrum" are **myring/o** (MEER-in-goh) and **tympan/o** (TIM-pan-oh).

tympan/um (tim-PAN-um)

1268 Tympan associates with the "presence of" suffix in cerebellum **(frame 1098)**. The product of these two elements is _____ /____, "presence of the eardrum."

tympanum

1269 The _____ ("eardrum") vibrates when sound waves strike it. This vibration sets into motion a group of three **ossic/les** (AH-sih-kuls).

ossic (**AH**-sik)

presence of little
bones

1270 See if you can correctly translate ossicles. For help, realize that the root, _____, like ossi **(frame 769)**, means "bone." The suffix has the same meaning as the one in ventricle **(frame 1111)**. Ossicles therefore translates as "_____ ____ _____ _____."

---

ossicles

1271 The auditory _____ are the three "little bones present" in the middle ear cavity. These bones are named after some shapes of objects in a blacksmith's shop. Examine the following combining forms:
malle/o (**MAH**-lee-oh) "mallet" or "hammer"
inc/o (**INK**-oh) "anvil"
staped/o (**STAY**-peh-doh) "stirrup"

---

malle/us (**MAL**-ee-us)
inc/us (**IHNG**-kus)
stap/es

1272 The first two roots in the preceding frame take the "presence of" ending in meatus **(frame 1264)**. The third root assumes its "presence of" form as **stapes** (**STAY**-peez). We consequently have _____ /____ for "a hammer," _____ /____ for "an anvil," and _____ /____ for "a stirrup."

---

malleus
incus
stapes

1273 A quick look at Figure 11.6 will show you that the _____ does indeed resemble a wooden "mallet," the _____ a broad, flat "anvil" for shaping horseshoes, and the _____ a "stirrup" of a saddle.

F I G U R E   1 1 . 6   **The Three Ossicles**

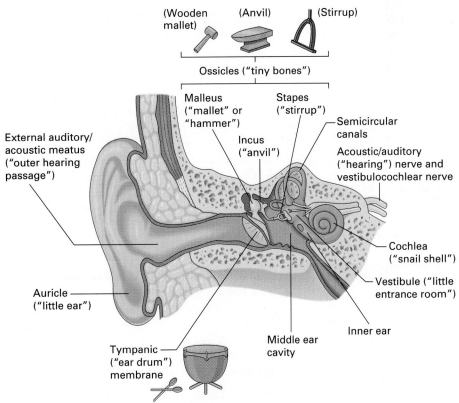

(Wooden mallet)   (Anvil)   (Stirrup)

Ossicles ("tiny bones")

Malleus ("mallet" or "hammer")   Stapes ("stirrup")

Incus ("anvil")

Semicircular canals

Acoustic/auditory ("hearing") nerve and vestibulocochlear nerve

External auditory/ acoustic meatus ("outer hearing passage")

Cochlea ("snail shell")

Vestibule ("little entrance room")

Auricle ("little ear")

Inner ear

Middle ear cavity

Tympanic ("ear drum") membrane

vestibul/e (**VES**-tih-**byool**)	**1274** When the tympanum vibrates, the three auditory ossicles move as a group. The stapes pushes on a tiny membrane, the oval window. This oval window is attached to a "little entrance room" for the inner ear. **Vestibul** (**VES**-tih-**byool**) means "little entrance room." It takes the ending in meninge **(frame 1119)**. The result is _____ /_____, "a little entrance room."
vestibule	**1275** When the oval window in the wall of the _____ ("little entrance room") plunges in and out with the movements of the stapes, it creates fluid pressure.
semi/**circul**/**ar** **semi-** **circul**/**ar**	**1276** This pressure is modified in the semicircular (**sem**-ee-**SER**-kyoo-lar) canals. Subdivide semicircular as _____ /_____ /_____. Note that the prefix is _____, as in semipermeable **(frame 479)**. Much as ventricular **(frame 1115)** "relates to little bellies," _____ /_____ "relates to a little circle."
semicircular	**1277** The _____ ("partially circular") canals are bony passageways containing fluid under pressure from the oval window.
cochle/**a** **cochle** (**KAHK**-lee)	**1278** Fluid from the vestibule and semicircular canals moves under pressure to the cochlea. Cochlea is divided as _____ /_____, like cornea **(frame 1244).** The root in cochlea, _____, means "snail shell" from its appearance.
cochlea	**1279** The _____ is a "snail shell"–like structure that contains the hair cells—minute auditory receptors. The pressure from sound waves, moving through the fluid chambers of the vestibule and semicircular canals, flattens these hair cells.
auditory acoustic	**1280** The flattening of the hair cells in the cochlea triggers impulses in the _____, or _____, ("pertaining to hearing") nerve. This cranial nerve finally relays the information to the hearing regions of the cerebral cortex.
	1281 Because of their great importance, defects and diseases of the eye and ear can be very disabling. You should therefore be well motivated to study their associated terminology.

Diseases

Word Parts Associated with Diseases of the Eye and Ear

The following is a list of word parts and an abbreviation associated with diseases of the eye and ear. Use this list to help you complete **frames 1282 to 1314**.

ambly/o	dull; dim	**my/o**	squinting	**strabism/o**	distorted squinting
cataract	waterfall	**OM**	otitis media	**tinnit/o**	ringing
glauc/o	bluish green	**ot/o**	ear		

ot	**1282** The two-letter root for "ear" is _____, as found in otic **(frame 1240)**. It is combined with many other roots and suffixes to create terms for diseases of the ear. For disorders of the "eye," the shortened root **op** (**OHP**) is often used.
-ia **op/ia** (**OHP**-ee-uh)	**1283** Recall that the suffix, _____, as found in phobia **(frame 1178)**, indicates a "condition of" something. Added to the shortened root for "eye," this gives _____ /_____, "a condition of the eye."
ambly/op/ia (**am**-blee-**OHP**-ee-uh)	**1284** The root **ambly** (**AM**-blee) means "dull" or "dim." So _____ /_____ /_____ means "a condition of dim eyes."
amblyopia	**1285** In _____, there is a "dimming of vision."
dipl/op/ia (dih-**PLOHP**-ee-ah)	**1286** Take the prefix in diplococci **(frame 550)** and use it to create _____ /_____ /_____, "a condition of double vision." Note that the **o** in the prefix is dropped.
diplopia	**1287** In _____, a person would "see two" images when looking at a single person.
hyper- **hyper/op/ia** (high-per-**OHP**-ee-ah)	**1288** Recall that _____, the prefix in hyperplasia **(frame 555)**, means "excessive." Therefore, _____ /_____ /_____ is literally "a condition of excessive vision."
hyperopia	**1289** More precisely, _____ is "excessively" far "vision"—that is, farsightedness.
my/op/ia (migh-**OHP**-ee-ah)	**1290** **Myo** (**MIGH**-oh), shortened to my, here means "squinting" rather than "muscle." Build a term that denotes "a condition of squinting vision": _____ /_____ /_____.
myopia	**1291** In _____, also called nearsightedness, the affected person tends to "squint" when attempting to view distant objects.
hyperopia myopia	**1292** In _____, the eyeball is too short, such that light rays come into focus at an "excessive" distance, beyond the retina. In _____, the eyeball is too long. The person tends to "squint" at far-off objects because light rays entering the eye come into focus in front of the retina.

ot/itis (oh-**TIGH**-tus) encephalitis	**1293** Considering the ear, we often suffer from _____ /_____, or "inflammation of the ear." The pattern here is like that seen in _____ ("inflammation of the brain," **frame 1165**).
media **externa**	**1294** An **otitis** _____ (**media/externa**) is an inflammation of the "middle" ear or tympanum, while an **otitis** _____ (**media/externa**) is an inflammation of the auditory/acoustic meatus.
OM	**1295** The disease of otitis media is abbreviated as _____ _____.
otitis media	**1296** In OM, or _____ _____, there may be both a sensation of pain and a discharge from the inflamed ear.
ot/algia (**oh-TAL**-juh)	**1297** Extract the suffix from cephalalgia (**frame 1151**) and create _____ /_____ ("condition of pain in the ear").
ot/o/rrhea (oht-**or-EE**-uh)	**1298** The suffix -o/rrhea means "flow" or "discharge." Use this fact to help you build _____ /_____ /_____, a "discharge" from the "ear."
otitis media otalgia otorrhea	**1299** The problem of _____ _____ (OM) may be accompanied by both _____ ("earache") and _____ ("ear discharge").
ot/o/sclerosis (**oh**-to-skleh-**ROH**-sis)	**1300** If otitis is severe enough, it may contribute to "an abnormal hardening of the (ossicles in) the ear." Adopt the ending in arteriosclerosis (**frame 148**) to help you make _____ /_____ /_____, which has this meaning.
otosclerosis	**1301** A "hardening" of the middle ear bones, or _____, is a serious problem that may lead to deafness.
tinnit/us (**TIN**-ih-tus)	**1302** **Tinnit** (**TIN**-iht) is a root for "ringing." Adapting from malleus (**frame 1272**) allows us to build _____ /_____, "a ringing" in the ears.
tinnitus	**1303** The symptom of _____ (ear "ringing") has many possible causes.
conjunctiv/itis (kun-**junk**-tih-**VIGH**-tis)	**1304** The eye, like the ear, can suffer from various symptoms. For example, there is _____ /_____, or "inflammation of the conjunctiva."

conjunctivitis	**1305** When sand blows into a person's eyes, _____ may occur if the "eyelid lining" becomes "inflamed" with dust specks.
dacry **dacry/o/rrhea** (**dak**-ree-oh-**REE**-uh)	**1306** When the eye is inflamed, it often tears. Recall that _____, as well as lacrim **(frame 1258)**, denotes "tears." Therefore _____ /_____ /_____ is literally a "flow of tears."
dacryorrhea	**1307** When dust is trapped under the eyelid, _____ often occurs in response to the inflammation, helping to wash ("flow") the dust out of the eye with "tears."
strabism/us (strah-**BIZ**-mus)	**1308** If debris gets trapped under the eyelids, there may be a "distorted squinting." **Strabism/o** (strah-**BIS**-moh) means "distorted squinting." Using the ending in tinnitus **(frame 1302)**, build _____ /_____, "presence of distorted squinting."
strabismus	**1309** The "distorted squinting" of _____ is due to a lack of coordination between the eyes. A so-called cross-eyed condition is a familiar example.
glauc/oma **glauc** (**GLAWK**)	**1310** Two related terms deal with internal conditions within the eyeball itself. These are **glaucoma** (glaw-**KOH**-mah) and **cataract** (**KAT**-ah-**rakt**). Remembering such earlier terms as glioma **(frame 1167)**, you can easily dissect glaucoma as _____ /_____. The root, _____, means "bluish green," and the suffix, **-oma**, means "tumor." Cataract comes from the Latin word meaning "waterfall."
glaucoma cataract	**1311** The term _____ literally translates as "bluish-green tumor." This condition really involves no tumor at all. A related word, _____, indicates a darkness of the lens.
glaucoma	**1312 Hippocrates**, the Father of Modern Medicine, used the term _____ to describe the "bluish-green," darkened appearance of many cataracts. It was not until hundreds of years later that cataracts were distinguished from glaucoma.
intra/ocul/ar (**in**-trah-**AHK**-yoo-ler)	**1313** Recall that ocular **(frame 1239)** "pertains to the eye." Look again at intracellular **(frame 472)**. Now synthesize a new term, _____ /_____ /_____, "pertaining to (something) within the eye."
intraocular	**1314** Glaucoma is primarily due to a great increase in the _____ pressure "within the eye." Such great pressure can damage the optic nerve, thereby resulting in permanent blindness.

1315 If glaucoma or other auditory or visual problems are detected early enough, effective treatment is often possible.

Lab Tests and Diagnoses

Word Parts Associated with Lab Tests and Diagnoses for the Eye and Ear

The following is a list of word parts and an abbreviation associated with lab tests and diagnoses of visual and hearing problems. Use this list to help you complete **frames 1316 to 1338**.

audi/o	hearing	**EENT**	eye, ear, nose, and throat specialist
dil/o	widening	**laryng/o**	larynx; voicebox
dilat/o	widening		

---

ophthalm/o/logy
(ahf-thal-**MAHL**-oh-**jee**)
ot/o/logy (oh-**TAL**-oh-jee)

1316 Several medical specialties are involved in diagnosing and testing for defects in the visual and hearing senses. Using ophthalm suggests _____ /_____ /_____ ("study of the eye"), and ot, _____ /_____ /_____ ("study of the ear"). In each case, the suffix of neurology **(frame 1202)** is adopted. Many of the terms we will consider come from one of those disciplines.

---

otology

1317 A sister of _____ ("study of the ear") is "study of the ear and voicebox." **Larynx** (**LAHR**-inks) is "the voicebox." When combined with other word parts, however, "voicebox" becomes **laryng/o** (**LAHR**-in-goh).

---

ot/o/laryng/o/logy
(**oh**-toh-**lahr**-in-**GAHL**-oh-jee)

1318 We can build the medical specialty _____ /_____ /_____ /_____ /_____, "study of the ear and voicebox."

---

otolaryngology

1319 The specialty of _____ technically involves the treatment and diagnosis of disorders of the "ear," nose, and throat, including those of the **laryngeal** (lah-**rin-JEE**-al), or "voicebox," area. Note the "**g**" rule for pronunciation as found in **frame 73**.

---

laryng/e/al
pertaining to the voicebox

1320 You can subdivide laryngeal as _____ /_____ /_____. It translates as "_____ ____ _____ _____."

---

ophthalm/o/logist
(**ahf**-thal-**MAHL**-oh-jist)
ot/o/logist (oh-**TAHL**-oh-jist)

ot/o/laryng/o/logist
(**oh**-toh-**lahr**-in-**GAHL**-oh-jist)

1321 Extract the suffix from neurologist **(frame 1203)** and use it to build the following terms:
_____ /_____ /_____
"one who specializes in studying the eyes" alone
_____ /_____ /_____
"one who specializes in studying the ears" alone
_____ /_____ /_____ /_____ /_____
"one who specializes in studying the ears and voicebox"

---

otolaryngologist laryngeal ophthalmologist otologist	**1322** Of the specialists listed in the preceding frame, you should choose an _____ for a problem of pain in your _____ ("voicebox") area. Eye problems would require an _____, and ear problems an _____.
otolaryngologist EENT	**1323** Related to the _____ ("ear-and-voicebox doctor") is the **eye, ear, nose, and throat** specialist, abbreviated by the four letters ____ ____ ____ ____.
eye, ear, nose, and throat	**1324** The EENT, or _____, _____, _____, and _____ specialist combines some of the duties of the ophthalmologist with those of the otolaryngologist.
ophthalm/o/scop/e (ahf-**THAL**-moh-**skohp**) **ot/o/scop/e** (**OH**-toh-**skohp**)	**1325** Remove the ending from fluoroscope **(frame 183)** and add it to the root in ophthalmology, producing _____ /____ /_____ /____, "an instrument used for examining the eyes." Doing the same for the root in otology yields ____ /____ /_____ /____, "an instrument used for examining the ears."
ophthalmoscope otoscope	**1326** An ophthalmologist uses an _____ for studying the eyes. An otologist uses an _____ for examining the ears.
audi (**AW**-dee)	**1327** Several alternative roots are heavily used in diagnostic terms relating to the eye and ear. The root from optic is extracted for use, for instance. Further, the root in auditory is shortened by one letter, yielding _____ for "hearing."
audi/o/logy (aw-dee-**AHL**-oh-jee) **audi/o/logist** (aw-dee-**AHL**-oh-jist)	**1328** The "study of hearing" is called _____ /____ /_____, and it is performed by an _____ /____ /_____, "one who specializes in the study of hearing."
audiologist otologist	**1329** An _____ who "specializes in hearing assessment" is usually a nonphysician, whereas an _____ is an "ear doctor" or "ear specialist."
-metry -meter	**1330** Measurement differs somewhat from studying and examining per se. Recall that _____, the suffix in thermometry **(frame 226)**, means the "process of measuring," while _____, the suffix in thermometer **(frame 226)**, denotes "an instrument used to measure (something)."
audi/o/metry (aw-dee-**AH**-meh-tree) **opt/o/metry** (ahp-**TAH**-meh-tree)	**1331** Now let us apply some suffixes for measuring to the cases of hearing and vision. The "process of measuring hearing" is _____ /____ /_____. Using the root of optic **(frame 1240)**, _____ /____ /_____ is the "process of measuring the (vision) of the eyes."

dilat/ion (digh-LAY-shun)

1332 **Dil** (**DIHL**) and **dilat** (**DIGH**-lat) are roots for "widening." The second root gives us _____ / _____ as the "process of widening," much as delusion **(frame 1174)** is the "process of (having) a false belief."

optometry
dilation

1333 Before _____ ("vision measurement"), drops are often placed into the eyes, causing _____ ("widening") of the pupils. The interior of the eyeballs can then be thoroughly examined, and certain measurements of vision can be more effectively carried out.

audiometry
audi/o/meter (aw-dee-**AH**-meh-ter)

1334 During _____, the "act of measuring hearing," a special instrument, the _____ / _____ / _____, is utilized.

audiometer

1335 The _____ is an electrical instrument that "measures" the threshold of "hearing" for pure tones.

audi/o/gram (**AW**-dee-oh-**gram**)

1336 It is also possible to create records with the audiometer. The appropriate suffix is found in electroencephalogram **(frame 1198)**. Use it to build _____ / _____ / _____, or a "record of hearing."

audi/o/metrist
(aw-dee-**AH**-meh-trist)
opt/o/metrist (ahp-**TAH**-meh-trist)

1337 A -metrist (**MEH**-trist) is "one who specializes in measuring (something)." Therefore an _____ / _____ / _____ is "one who specializes in measuring hearing," and an _____ / _____ / _____ is "one who specializes in measuring (vision) of the eyes."

audiogram
audiometrist
optometrist

1338 An _____ "record" would be of great interest to an _____ ("measurer of hearing"). Such a record would be of only minor interest to an _____ ("measurer of vision").

1339 Many of the specialists who detect or diagnose hearing or visual problems are also involved in their treatment.

Surgery and Therapies

Word Parts Associated with Surgery, Pharmacology, and Other Therapies for the Eye and Ear

The following is a list of word parts associated with surgery, pharmacology, and other therapies for visual and hearing problems. Use this list to help you complete **frames 1341 to 1358**.

blephar/o	eyelid	-ectasia	stretching or dilation
cor/o	pupil	**myring/o**	tympanic membrane (eardrum)

1340 You will recognize many of the roots for ear and eye structures in terms describing their surgery and therapy.

cor	**1341** You may recall, for instance, that _____ **(frame 1246)** is a three-let-ter root for "pupil." Find a suffix, _____, on the word list that means "stretching or dilation." Use this information to create _____ / _____, a "dilation of the pupil."
-ectasia (ek-**TAY**-zee-uh)	
cor/ectasia (**kor**-ek-**TAY**-zee-uh)	

corectasia	**1342** "Widening or dilation of the pupil," _____, occurs whenever a person is excited, such that the sympathetic nerves are active or the actions of the parasympathetic nerves are blocked.

lyt	**1343** Remember that _____, a root in electrolyte **(frame 465)**, means "breakdown." It can also be interpreted as "blockage." Thus _____ / _____ "refers to a blockage," where the ending is that in optic **(frame 1240)**.
lyt/ic (**LIT**-ik)	

para/sympath/o/lyt/ic (**pahr**-ah-sim-**path**-oh-**LIT**-ik)	**1344** Just as para/sympath/o/mimet/ic drugs **(frame 1228)** "mimic the parasympathetic nerves," _____ / _____ / _____ / _____ / _____ **drugs** serve to "block the parasympathetic nerves."

parasympatholytic	**1345** The _____ drugs, such as atropine, tend to "block" the effects of "parasympathetic nerve" activity. For instance, since parasympathetic nerves tend to constrict (narrow) the pupils, these drugs do the exact opposite; they relax the pupils and result in corectasia.

blephar/ectomy (**blef**-ar-**EK**-toh-mee)	**1346** Sometimes surgery must be performed on the eye. When the **b-**starting root for "eyelid" **(frame 1242)** is used, we can create several surgical terms. Just as neurectomy **(frame 1218)** is the "process of removing a nerve," _____ / _____ is the "process of remov-ing the eyelid." Just as myorrhaphy **(frame 1068)** is a "suturing of muscle," _____ / _____ / _____ is a "suturing of the eyelids."
blephar/o/rrhaphy (**blef**-ar-**OR**-hah-fee)	

blepharorrhaphy	**1347** The operation of _____ might be performed when the "eyelids" have been accidentally torn. If the eyelids developed large malignant tumors, a _____ might become nec-essary.
blepharectomy	

sclera	**1348** Recall that the _____ **(frame 1245)** is the "hard," white por-tion of the cornea. The appropriate term for removal of the sclera is _____ / _____.
scler/ectomy (**skleh-REK**-toh-mee)	

scler/o/stomy (**skleh-RAHS**-toh-mee)	**1349** Extract the surgical suffix from arthrostomy **(frame 297)**. Combine it with the root appearing in **frame 1348** above: _____ / _____ / _____.

sclerostomy sclera	**1350** The operation of _____ involves "making a perma-nent new opening" within the "sclera," just as scler/**ectomy** is "removal of" part of the "_____."
sclerostomy sclerectomy	**1351** A _____ could help drain off excessive fluid build-up within the eye. A _____ would simply extract all or part of the white of the eye.
    myring tympan	**1352** The suffixes in arthrotomy **(frame 941)** and arthroplasty **(frame 305)** can be effectively added to various eye-and-ear roots. For example, do you remember **(frame 1267)** that "eardrum" is represented by two roots, _____ and _____ ?
myring/o/tomy (**meer**-in-**GAHT**-oh-mee) **tympan/o/plasty** (tim-**PAN**-oh-**plas**-tee)	**1353** Use myring to help you build _____ /_____ /_____ ("making an incision into the eardrum"). Use tympan for constructing _____ /_____ /_____ ("surgical repair of the eardrum").
myringotomy tympanoplasty	**1354** The procedure of _____ is usually done first, to "cut open" the membrane of the "eardrum." It is then that _____ and "correction" of any "eardrum" defects can be carried out.
kerat **kerat/o/plasty** (kair-**AT**-oh-**plas**-tee) **ot/o/plasty** (**OH**-toh-**plas**-tee)	**1355** Let us create two other terms involving surgical repair. Using _____ **(frame 1244)**, a root for "tough" or "hornlike," build _____ /_____ /_____, "surgical repair of (something) tough or hornlike" (that is, the cornea). Using the root in otorrhea **(frame 1298)**, build _____ /_____ /_____ ("surgical repair of the ear").
keratoplasty otoplasty	**1356** The operation of _____ "fixes" damage to the outer "hornlike" layer of the eyeball (the cornea), while an _____ might be called an "ear job."
staped **staped/ectomy** (**stay**-pee-**DEK**-toh-mee)	**1357** Otoplasty usually involves plastic surgery of the auricles. Deep surgery may reach the middle ear ossicles. Remember that _____ **(frame 1271)**, not stapes, for instance, is actually the root for "stirrup." Therefore, _____ /_____, means "removal of the stirrup."
stapedectomy	**1358** The procedure of _____ may be indicated if the "stapes" has completely degenerated because of a severe case of otitis media.

Multiple Choice

1. A combining form for "ear" is
   a. acoust/o   b. auric/o   c. phon/o   d. opt/o

2. Cataract is an opaqueness of the
   a. retina   b. iris   c. lens   d. pupil

3. To repair a blepharoptosis the surgeon may perform a(n)
   a. -al   b. -plasty   c. -ectomy   d. -itis

4. Which of these means "opening"?
   a. ot/o   b. auric/o   c. malle/o   d. meat/o

5. A combining form for "net" is
   a. palpebr/o   b. retin/o   c. vestibul/o   d. meat/o

6. If a client suffers from otosclerosis, the surgeon may perform a(n)
   a. otopexy   b. otoplasty   c. myringotomy   d. dacryocystectomy

Meanings of Selected Roots

Add the correct combining vowel (cv) after each root. Then write the definition of each root in the space provided.

ROOT/CV	DEFINITION
1. inc/_____	_____
2. ossic/_____	_____
3. dacry/_____	_____
4. ambly/_____	_____
5. audi/_____	_____
6. scler/_____	_____
7. kerat/_____	_____
8. dilat/_____	_____
9. opt/_____	_____
10. ophthalm/_____	_____

Word Dissection and Translation

Analyze the following terms by dissecting them with slashmarks and identifying their word parts. To the right of each term, write its correct English translation.

Key: R (root), cv (combining vowel), P (prefix), S (suffix)

1. audiogram

_____/_____/_____   _____
         R   cv   S

2. conjunctivitis

_____/_____   _____
         R   S

3. meatus

_____/_____   _____
         R   S

4. amblyopia

_____/_____/_____   _____
         R   R   S

5. ocular

_____/_____   _____
         R   S

6. semicircular

_____/_____/_____   _____
      P   R   S

7. otitis

_____/_____   _____
         R   S

8. tinnitus

_____/_____   _____
         R   S

9. otolaryngology

_____/_____/_____/_____/_____   _____
         R   cv   R   cv   S

10. optometrist

_____/_____/_____   _____
         R   cv   S

11. corneoblepharon

_____/_____/_____/_____   _____
         R   cv   R   S

12. iridorrhaphy

_____/_____/_____   _____
         R   cv   S

Terms and Their Abbreviations

In the list below, when the term is given, write its abbreviation in the space provided. When the abbreviation is given, write its corresponding term.

TERM	ABBREVIATION
1. otitis media	_____
2. _____	AD
3. auris sinistra	_____
4. _____	EENT

Word Spelling

Look at each of the terms listed below. Identify those that are misspelled by circling Y for "Yes." Write the correct spelling in the blank.

WORD	MISSPELLED?	CORRECT SPELLING
1. vestigabool	Y/N	_____
2. diplopia	Y/N	_____
3. strabismus	Y/N	_____
4. audiometer	Y/N	_____
5. miringotomy	Y/N	_____
6. palpeebra	Y/N	_____
7. auditory	Y/N	_____
8. otosclerosis	Y/N	_____
9. intraoculer	Y/N	_____
10. opthalmoscope	Y/N	_____
11. cochlea	Y/N	_____
12. semeesircular	Y/N	_____
13. oculus	Y/N	_____
14. conjunktivah	Y/N	_____

New Word Synthesis

Using word parts that appear in this and previous chapters, build new terms with the following meanings:

1. _____ removal of nets

2. _____ instrument that measures bones

3. _____ one who specializes in the study of tears

4. _____ the process of examining bending (actions)

5. _____ a condition of squinting of the voicebox

6. _____ inflammation of the eardrum and nerves

7. _____ presence of a little doll and bedroom

8. _____ abnormal hardening of the sclera

9. _____ measurement of the spinal cord and iris

10. _____ suturing of the eardrum

11. _____ discharge from the ear

12. _____ instrument to measure eye muscles

C A S E   S T U D Y

Read through the following partial diagnostic workup. Note the terms in bold print. A series of multiple choice questions probes your knowledge of these terms.

Diagnostic Workup

A 43-year-old Caucasian female complained of severe **tinnitus**, **AS**. **Otoscopic** exam revealed advanced **otitis externa**. Antibacterial therapy is strongly suggested.

Case Study Questions

1. The patient's chief symptom, **tinnitus**, appeared to involve

   (a) wandering vision.

   (b) discharge from both ears.

   (c) ringing in the ears.

   (d) chronic earache.

2. The symptom was primarily localized in the **AS**, or

   (a) left ear.

   (b) left eye.

   (c) right ear.

   (d) right eye.

3. The **otoscopic** exam was carried out by

   (a) visual inspection of the cornea.

   (b) an instrument placed into the external acoustic meatus.

   (c) an instrument that pierced the eardrums.

   (d) vision exam with Snellen chart.

4. The major cause of the patient's symptom appears to be **otitis externa**, or

   (a) inflammation of the middle ear cavity.

   (b) lack of ability to see distant objects.

   (c) infection of the conjunctiva.

   (d) inflammation of the outer ear canal.

CHAPTER 12 The Glands

INTRODUCTION

Chapter 7 considered the tissues and skin. You may remember that the epidermis of the skin is primarily cellular in nature. It consists mainly of strata, or layers, of epithelial cells. Although epithelium is important for covering and lining, it can be modified to form **glands**. Glands are collections of epithelial cells specialized for the function of **secretion**—the release of some useful product.

Glands can be subdivided into two broad types (Figure 12.1): **exocrine (EKS-oh-krin) glands** and **endocrine (EN-doh-krin) glands**. The exocrine glands are glands of external secretion of some useful product into a duct. This duct then carries the secretion to some body surface. A good example of an exocrine gland is the sweat gland, which releases sweat into its sweat duct. When carried to the skin surface, the sweat helps to cool the body as it evaporates.

Endocrine glands internally secrete **hormones** (chemical messengers) directly into the bloodstream within the gland itself. The endocrine glands are often nicknamed the "ductless glands." After entering the blood within the gland itself, the hormone circulates throughout the bloodstream. Therefore, no duct or other passage for secretion is required.

FIGURE 12.1   **Endocrine versus Exocrine Glands**

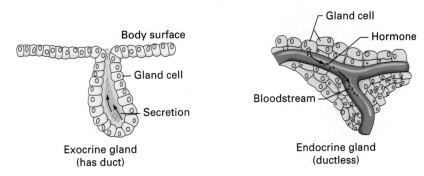

A good example of an endocrine gland is the **thyroid (THIGH-royd) gland** in the neck. The thyroid secretes several hormones. Among these is **thyroxine (thigh-RAHKS-in)**. The thyroid gland cells release thyroxine into the vascular network within the thyroid, which then carries the thyroxine out to the body at large.

Not all parts of the body react to thyroxine or any particular hormone. Each hormone acts upon certain sensitive **target cells**. The target cells for thyroxine include the adipose cells. Target cells respond to a hormone by altering some aspect of their function. The adipose cell targets for thyroxine, for instance, speed up the metabolism of their stored fat content.

Sweat glands are but one example of many exocrine glands, and the thyroid is a member of a large family of endocrine glands. Figure 12.2A shows some of the major exocrine glands of the human body, and Figure 12.2B illustrates some major endocrine glands.

FIGURE 12.2   **Some Major Glands in Males and Females**

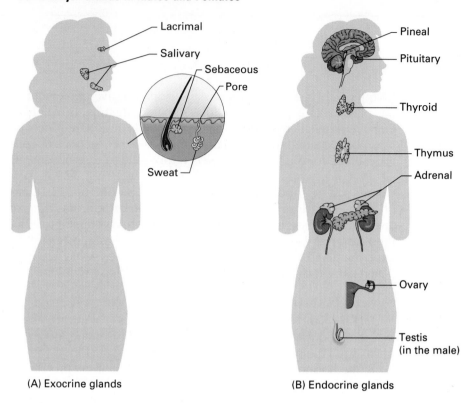

Lacrimal
Salivary
Sebaceous
Pore
Sweat

Pineal
Pituitary
Thyroid
Thymus
Adrenal
Ovary
Testis (in the male)

(A) Exocrine glands   (B) Endocrine glands

This chapter introduces terms related to the normal structure and function of the glands, terms describing the diseases of glands, terms of lab tests and therapy for **glandular** (**GLAN-dyoo**-lar) problems, and terms describing surgery and other treatment approaches for glands.

CHAPTER OBJECTIVES

By the end of this chapter, you should be able to:

1 Identify major prefixes, roots, suffixes, and abbreviations related to the glands.

2 Dissect glandular terms into their component parts.

3 Translate glandular terms into their common English equivalents.

4 Build new terms associated with the glands.

Word Parts Associated with Normal Anatomy and Physiology of the Glands

The following is a list of word parts and abbreviations associated with the normal structure and function of the glands. Use this list to help you complete **frames 1360 to 1421**.

ACTH	adrenocorticotrophic hormone	**-ine**	a substance	**-sterone**	a steroid
adren/o	toward the kidney; adrenal gland	**insul/o**	little island	**test/o**	eggshell
		nephr/o	kidney	**thyr/o**	shield; thyroid gland
cortic/o	cortex; covering; bark	**ovari/a**	egg	**thyrox/o**	shield; thyroid gland
		pancreat/o	the pancreas	**troph/o**	stimulation; nourishment
creat/o	flesh	**pituit/o**	mucus; phlegm		
-erone	a steroid	**ren/o**	kidney	**trop/o**	turn; change
estr/o	mad desire (sex drive)	**ster/o**	solid oil substance	**TSH**	thyroid-stimulating hormone
gest/o	bearing				

1359 There are many endocrine and exocrine glands. Examine and pronounce the partial list of endocrine glands provided in Table 12.1 below.

TABLE 12.1　　**Some Endocrine Glands in Humans**

adrenal (ad-**REE**-nal) **cortex**

adrenal medulla

ovary (**OH**-var-**ee**), singular; **ovaries** (**OH**-var-**eez**), plural

pancreas (**PAN**-kree-**ahs**)

pituitary (pih-**TOO**-ih-**tahr**-ee)

testis (**TES**-tis), singular; **testes** (**TES**-teez), plural

thyroid (**THIGH**-royd)

---

pituitary
pituit/**ary**

1360 Observe on this list the _____ gland, whose name begins with **pi**. It is subdivided as _____ /_____, with the "pertaining to" suffix used in medullary **(frame 789)**.

---

pituit (pih-**TOO**-it)
pertaining to
mucus
phlegm

1361 The root in pituitary, _____ , means "mucus" or "phlegm." Pituitary therefore translates as "_____ ____ _____ or _____." The reasoning behind this odd name becomes apparent when you realize that the pituitary gland is also known as the hypophysis or "undergrowth" **(frame 1131)** on the brain. Being located inferior to the hypothalamus and posterior to the nose, the pituitary gland (hypophysis) was thought in ancient times to release mucus or phlegm and to channel it into the nose!

---

pituitary

1362 The _____ ("referring to mucus") gland is actually a combination of several endocrine glands. It secretes a number of **trophic** (**TROHF**-ik) or **tropic** (**TROHP**-ik) hormones.

troph/**ic**	**1363** The "pertaining to" suffix in acoustic **(frame 1262)** is extracted, so that trophic is subdivided as _____ /_____ and tropic as _____ /_____.
trop/**ic**	

troph	**1364** You may recall that _____, the root in both trophic and hypertrophy **(frame 139)**, means "nourishment." It can also be considered as "stimulation." The root in tropic, _____, means "turn" or "change."
trop (TROHP)	

trophic	**1365** The term _____, then, literally "pertains to nourishment or stimulation;" _____, on the other hand, "pertains to turning or changing." In practice, the two terms are interchangeable. These types of hormones from the pituitary gland in a sense "nourish, stimulate, and turn on" the activity of other endocrine glands.
tropic	

Information Frame	**1366** Let's take a glance at the names of the **adrenocorticotrophic** (ad-**ree**-noh-**kor**-tih-koh-**TROHF**-ik) and **adrenocorticotropic** (ad-**ree**-noh-**kor**-tih-koh-**TROHP**-ik) hormones. Do not shrink from the task of subdividing these giants! Just relax and start whittling them down to size! Dealing with troph/**ic** and trop/**ic** at the end of each should be no problem. In each you see **cortic** (**KOR**-tik), a root for "cortex" or "bark." **Ren** (**REEN**) is a root for "kidney." The prefix **ad-** is familiar from terms such as adductor **(frame 966)**.

ad/ren/o/cortic/o/troph/**ic**	**1367** Use the information of the preceding frame to dissect adrenocorticotrophic as _____ /_____ /_____ /_____ /_____ /_____ /_____ and adrenocorticotropic as _____ /_____ /_____ /_____ /_____ /_____ /_____ . In both these terms, the word fragment _____ /_____ /_____ /_____ means the "cortex toward the kidney."
ad/ren/o/cortic/o/trop/**ic**	
ad/ren/o/cortic	

ad/ren/**al** (ad-**REE**-nal)	**1368** Use information from **frame 1366** plus the suffix in lacrimal **(frame 1259)** to help you build a new term, _____ /_____ /_____, "pertaining to (something) toward the kidney."

adrenal	**1369** Figure 12.2B showed the _____ as a single large gland located "toward the kidney," more or less lying upon it. Look back at Table 12.1 and identify the two portions of this gland. There is an outer _____ _____ which, like the cerebral cortex **(frame 1100)**, forms a thin external "bark." Further, there is an inner _____ _____, which, like bone "marrow" **(frame 1086)**, is "present" more toward the middle of the gland body. (Examine Figure 12.3.)
adrenal cortex	
adrenal medulla	

FIGURE 12.3   **The Two Portions of the Adrenal Gland**

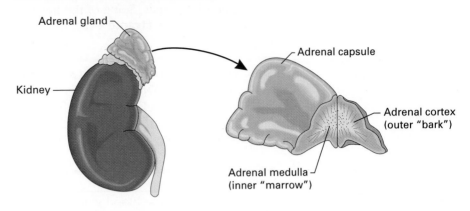

adrenal cortex	**1370** You can probably guess that **adrenocortic** refers to the _____ _____ (adrenal cortex/adrenal medulla).
ad/ren/o/cortic/o/troph/ic ad/ren/o/cortic/o/trop/ic	**1371** Retrieve the information from **frame 1368** to rebuild ____ / _____ / ____ / _____ / ____ / _____ / ____, "pertaining to stimulating the adrenal cortex," and ____ / _____ / ____ / _____ / ____ / _____ / ____, "pertaining to turning (on) the adrenal cortex."
adrenocorticotrophic	**1372** Of the two very long terms, _____ ("pertaining to stimulating the adrenal cortex") is more commonly used.
adrenocorticotrophic hormone	**1373** Putting **hormone** after the term in the above frame results in a new phrase, _____ _____.
A C T H	**1374** Adrenocorticotrophic hormone is abbreviated by the four letters— ____ (for **adreno**), ____ (for **cortico**), ____ (for **trophic**), and ____ (for **hormone**).
ACTH	**1375** As its name implies, ____ ____ ____ ____ (adrenocorticotrophic hormone) is a trophic hormone from the pituitary that stimulates the adrenal cortex to increase its output of hormones.
ster/oid	**1376** The hormones of the adrenal cortex are mainly **steroids** (STEHR-oyds). You can probably subdivide steroid fairly easily as _____ / _____.
-oid	**1377** The suffix _____ is one you have seen again and again for "like" or "resembling" something.
solid oil-like	**1378** If **ster (STEHR)** means "solid oil," then steroid literally means "_____ _____–_____," just as proteinoid **(frame 457)** is "proteinlike."

steroids	**1379** The _____ are "solid oil-like" substances incorporated into many hormones. Some of the hormones from the adrenal cortex affect blood glucose **(frame 440)**, represented by **gluc/o** (GLOO-koh).
cortic **gluc/o/cortic/oid** (**gloo**-koh-**KORT**-ih-koyd)	**1380** The suffix **-oid**, when used for hormone names, usually denotes "steroid." Combine this information with that of the above frame, plus _____, the root for "cortex." The result is _____ / ____ / _____ / _____, a "steroid (from) the (adrenal) cortex (that affects blood) glucose."
glucocorticoids	**1381** The _____, once released from the adrenal cortex, tend to raise the blood glucose level. The major hormone in this group is called **cortisol** (**KOR**-tih-**sahl**).
cortisol	**1382** Secretion of _____ (the main glucocorticoid) is raised whenever ACTH is released from the pituitary gland.
thyr/oid	**1383** **Thyr/o (THIGH-roh)** means "shield." Referring to **frame 1377**, create _____ / _____, denoting a "shield-resembler."
thyroid	**1384** A glance at Figure 12.4 should reveal that the _____ gland does indeed "resemble" the twin "shields" of warriors!

FIGURE 12.4   **The Thyroid Gland "Shields"**

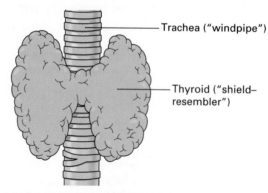

Trachea ("windpipe")

Thyroid ("shield–resembler")

Anterior view

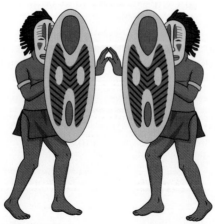

Oblong shields of African warriors

thyroid-stimulating hormone

1385 The thyroid gland, like the adrenal cortex, is strongly influenced by certain trophic (tropic) hormones. Note on the word list that there is a trophic hormone, _____-_____ _____ (TSH), that literally is "thyroid-stimulating."

TSH

1386 Thyroid-stimulating hormone, abbreviated as ____ ____ ____, stimulates the thyroid gland to increase the output of its own individual hormones.

thyr

1387 **Thyrox (THIGH-rahks)**, like _____, means "shield." The suffix **-ine (IN)**, like the **-in** in myelin **(frame 1080)**, denotes "a substance."

thyrox/ine (thigh-RAHKS-in)

1388 Apply the facts in the above frame to help you build _____ /_____, "a substance" from the "shield."

thyroxine
thyroid-stimulating
hormone

1389 The secretion of _____ by the thyroid gland is greatly increased when TSH (_____-_____ _____) is activating the thyroid. This hormone generally serves to raise the metabolic rate of adipose cells, such that they burn their stored fat faster.

testes

1390 Various steroid hormones affected by trophic hormones are also secreted by the ovaries in females and the _____ (a **t**-beginning gland; plural) in males.

ovary
testis

1391 Table 12.1 indicated that the singular of ovaries is _____ and the singular of testes is _____.

ov/ary

1392 Ovary contains the same root as synovial **(frame 812)** and is dissected the same way as pituitary **(frame 1360)**: ____ /_____.

ov

1393 Recall that _____, the root in both ovary and synovial, means "egg."

pertains to an egg

1394 Ovary therefore "_____ ____ ____ _____" in the same manner that pituitary "pertains to mucus."

ovaries

1395 The right and left _____ in adult females do look somewhat like hard-boiled "eggs" attached to either side of the womb!

ovari/es

1396 The _____ /____ are literally "eggs present" in the female.

ovari (OH-var-ee)

1397 In **frame 1396** you can see that _____, like ov, is a root for "egg."

test/is	**1398** Surprisingly similar in meaning is testis, which is subdivided like iris **(frame 1250)**: _____ /____.
test (TEST) an eggshell	**1399** The root in testis is _____ , and it means "eggshell." Testis therefore denotes "____ _____" in the same manner that iris denotes "a rainbow."
test/es	**1400** We can consequently describe the right and left _____ /____ in the male, which are named for their resemblance to intact "eggshells"!
test/o/sterone (tes-**TAHS**-ter-ohn)	**1401** Combine the root of testes with **-sterone** (stir-**OHN**), which indicates "steroid": _____ /____ /_____.
testosterone	**1402** As its name suggests, _____ is a "steroid" hormone secreted by the "testes." It is responsible for many of the physical characteristics (such as a beard) usually associated with the male sex.
-gen	**1403** The ovaries, like the testes, secrete steroid hormones. One of these is **estrogen** (**ES**-troh-jen). The other is **progesterone** (proh-**JES**-terohn). **Estr** (**ES**-ter) is a root for "mad desire." Recall that _____, the suffix in collagen **(frame 631)**, means "producer."
estr/o/gen	**1404** We can analyze estrogen as _____ /____ /_____, which translates as "producer of mad desire."
estrogen	**1405** The literal meaning of _____ reflects the fact that **estrus** (**ES**-trus), or heat (a time of maximum sex drive in nonhuman females), is largely due to increased estrogen secretion.
Information Frame	**1406** **Gest** (**JEST**) is a root for "bearing" (a child). The suffix **-erone** (ehr-**OHN**), means the same as **-sterone**, that is, "a steroid."
pro/**gest/erone** pro-	**1407** Applying the knowledge gained from the preceding frame allows us to analyze progesterone as _____ /_____ /_____. Remember that the prefix _____, like **pre-** **(frame 341)**, means "before" (or "in front of").
progesterone	**1408** The term _____ translates as "before-bearing steroid."
progesterone	**1409** Since _____ is present in especially high levels in the blood of pregnant females, its name indicates an association with "bearing" children.

pan- sarc	**1410** Certain glands are found in both sexes. Two examples are the adrenal medulla and the pancreas. A **p**-beginning prefix for "all" is _____ **(frame 81)**. Both **creas** (**KREE**-ahs) and **creat** (**KREE**-at), like _____, a root in sarcolemma **(frame 959)**, mean "flesh."
pancreas **pancreat** (**pan**-kree-**AT**)	**1411** The _____, or "all flesh," gland contains both endocrine and exocrine parts. Note that pan- and creas are put together as a single word element, rather than as a separate prefix and root. Using **creat** rather than **creas** results in a single large root, _____.
pancreat/ic (**pan**-kree-**AT**-ik)	**1412** Extract the ending from tropic **(frame 1363)** and build _____ /____, "pertaining to all flesh (the pancreas)."
pancreas pancreatic	**1413** The endocrine portion of the _____ ("all flesh") secretes a number of _____ ("referring to all flesh") hormones.
pancreatic	**1414** Among the most important of the _____ ("pancreas-occurring") hormones is **insulin** (**IN**-suh-**lin**).
insul/**in** **insul** (**IN**-sul)	**1415** Containing the same suffix as myelin **(frame 1080)**, insulin is subdivided as _____ /____. Its root, _____, denotes "little island."
insulin	**1416** Its name suggests that _____ is literally "a substance" secreted from "little islands" within the pancreas. This hormone acts to lower blood glucose levels when they are high (as after eating a carbohydrate-rich meal).
adrenal/in (ah-**DREN**-ah-lin) **adrenal/ine**	**1417** The whole term adrenal can take the suffix found in insulin. The result is _____ /____. Alternatively, it can assume the ending in thyroxine **(frame 1388)** to become _____ /_____.
adrenalin adrenaline	**1418** Both _____ and _____ translate as "a substance (from) the adrenal." Specifically, the hormone is released from the adrenal medulla gland.
epi- epi/**nephr**/**ine** (**ep**-ih-**NEF**-rin)	**1419** Recall that _____, the prefix in epigastric **(frame 392)**, means "upon." **Nephr** (**NEF**-er), like **ren**, is a root for "kidney." Construct a new term using nephr and the suffix of adrenaline. The term is _____ /_____ /_____, "a substance" (secreted from a gland) "upon the kidney."

epinephrine cortex medulla	**1420** Adrenalin, adrenaline, and _____ are simply alterna- tive names for the same hormone. The adrenal _____ ("bark") plus adrenal _____ (inner "marrow") make up one **adrenal body**, which is located "upon" the cranial pole of each "kidney." Hence, the three equivalent hormone names.
epinephrine	**1421** The same chemical (adrenaline, adrenalin, or _____) is a major hormone secreted by the adrenal medulla under stressful conditions. It is closely associated with the functioning of the sympa- thetic nervous system (Chapter 10).
	1422 Whether the body is under stress or not, disorders of its glands and hormones are of tremendous clinical importance. This is because the functioning of almost all body cells is dramatically affected by particu- lar hormones.

Diseases

Word Parts Associated with Diseases of the Glands

The following is a list of word parts and an abbreviation associated with diseases of the glands. Use this list to help you complete **frames 1423 to 1463**.

acr/o	body extremity	**diuret**	excessive urination	**MODM**	maturity onset
aden/o	gland	**-emia**	blood condition of		diabetes mellitus
diabet/o	siphon	**goitr/o**	goiter; throat	**pancreat/o**	all flesh; pancreas
diures	excessive urination	**mellit/o**	honey	**thyroid/o**	thyroid gland
				secret/o	secretion

secret/**ion**	**1423** **Secret (see-KREET)** is a root for "secretion," the release of some man- ufactured product. Hence _____ /_____ is the "process of secreting," just as refraction **(frame 1253)** is the "process of bending."
hyper- hypo- hyper/**secret**/**ion** (**high**-per-see-**KREE**-shun) hypo/**secret**/**ion** (**high**-poh-see-**KREE**-shun)	**1424** Too much or too little secretion of various hormones can have severe effects on body metabolism. Recall that _____, the prefix in hyperopia **(frame 1288)** means "excessive," while its opposite **(frame 114)**, _____, means "deficient." We can therefore coin two terms: _____ /_____ /_____ "a process of secreting excessively" _____ /_____ /_____ "a process of secreting deficiently"
hyposecretion hypersecretion	**1425** A process of _____ usually results in a "deficient" state of some aspect of body metabolism affected by a hormone. A process of _____ generally produces an "excessive" state of some aspect of metabolism within hormone target cells.

hyposecretion	**1426** **Addison's** (**A**-dih-**suns**) **disease**, for instance, is due to a chronic _____ ("deficient secretion") of hormones from the adrenal cortex. **Cushing's** (**KOOSH**-ings) **syndrome** reflects the opposite, _____ ("excessive secretion") of glucocorticoids from the adrenal cortex.
hypersecretion	

Cushing's syndrome	**1427** The disease called _____ _____ (hypersecretion of glucocorticoids) results in an excessively high glucose level in the blood.

glyc	**1428** Remember that _____, the root in glycogen **(frame 522)**, means "sweet" or "sugar." The suffix -emia (**EE**-mee-ah) denotes "a blood condition of (something)." Putting all this together results in _____ /_____, "a condition of blood sugar."
glyc/emia (**gligh-SEE**-mee-ah)	

glycemia	**1429** Use the prefix from hypersecretion **(frame 1424)** along with _____ ("blood sugar condition") and build _____ /_____ /_____. This new term translates as "a condition of excessive blood sugar."
hyper/glyc/emia (**high**-per-gligh-**SEE**-mee-ah)	

hyperglycemia	**1430** The condition of _____ is one of the major signs associated with Cushing's syndrome.

hypo/glyc/emia (**high**-poh-gligh-**SEE**-mee-ah)	**1431** The exact opposite of hyperglycemia is _____ /_____ /_____, "a condition of deficient blood sugar." (Refer to **frame 1424**.)

hypoglycemia Addison's disease	**1432** The "low-sugar blood condition" called _____ is sometimes associated with _____ _____ (hyposecretion of adrenocortical hormones, **frame 1426**), because not enough hormone molecules are released to boost the blood sugar level.

diabet/es	**1433** Hyperglycemia is sometimes a symptom of **diabetes** (**digh**-ah-**BEE**-teez). **Diabet** (**digh**-ah-**BEET**) is a root for "siphon." A siphon is a bent tube for drawing off water. Therefore _____ /_____ adds -es to denote "a siphon for drawing off water."

diabetes	**1434** The term _____ itself indicates excessive urination: water is, in a sense, being "siphoned off" from the body in large amounts.

diabet/ic (digh-ah-**BET**-ik)	**1435** Use the root in diabetes plus the suffix in adrenocorticotrophic **(frame 1371)** to build _____ /____, "pertaining to (being) siphoned off."
diabetic **diures** (digh-yoo-**REES**) **diuret** (digh-yoo-**RET**)	**1436** A person suffering from an untreated _____ condition will probably experience excessive urination. Note from the word list that _____ and _____ are a pair of roots that indicate "excessive urination."
diures/is (digh-yoo-**REE**-sis) **diuret/ic** (digh-yoo-**RET**-ik)	**1437** Diures takes the suffix of testis **(frame 1398)**. Diuret assumes the ending of diabetic **(frame 1435)**. The results are _____ /____ for the first root and _____ /____ for the second.
diuretic diuresis	**1438** From your remembrance of their endings, you know that _____ "pertains to excessive urination," while _____ denotes "presence of an excessive urination."
diuresis	**1439** Excessive urination, or _____, is a chief complaint in diabetes, resulting in a siphoning off of too much body water.
mellit/us (meh-**LIGH**-tus)	**1440** In the most common form of diabetes, the urine contains glucose and is sweet, like honey. **Mellit** (meh-**LIGHT**) means "honey." So _____ /____ denotes "presence of honey," where the "presence of" ending is that in incus **(frame 1272)**.
diabetes mellitus	**1441** The most common type of diabetes, _____ _____, literally means "honeyed siphon"!
diabetes mellitus diuresis	**1442** The disease name of _____ _____ indicates that there are both _____ ("excessive urination") and an abnormal excretion of glucose in the urine, making it like "honey." This problem ultimately derives from a hyposecretion of insulin and the presence of hyperglycemia.
MODM	**1443** Diabetes mellitus most often strikes during later life, in the years of "maturity." This condition is technically called **maturity onset diabetes mellitus**. It is abbreviated by the four letters ____ ____ ____ ____.
maturity onset diabetes mellitus	**1444** Diabetes mellitus acquired in later life, called _____ _____ _____ _____ (MODM), is a disease of the pancreas. The thyroid gland is also quite susceptible to various problems. Both glands, for instance, can suffer from inflammation.

otitis **pancreat/itis** (**pan**-kree-ah-**TIGH**-tis) **thyroid/itis** (**thigh**-royd-**IGH**-tis)	**1445** Just as _____ **(frame 1293)** denotes an "inflammation of the ear," _____ / _____ indicates an "inflammation of the pancreas" and _____ / _____ an "inflammation of the thyroid."
pancreatitis thyroiditis	**1446** The disease of _____ ("pancreatic inflammation") may cause abdominal pain, while _____ ("thyroid inflammation") often generates pain in the anterior neck region.
-ism **hyper/thyroid/ism** (**high**-per-**THIGH**-royd-izm) **hypo/thyroid/ism** (**high**-poh-**THIGH**-royd-izm)	**1447** There are other disease conditions besides inflammation. You might recall that _____ (as in albinism, **frame 686**) indicates "an (abnormal) condition of (something)." Using thyroid and the prefixes in hyperglycemia **(frame 1429)** and hypoglycemia **(frame 1431)** gives us _____ / _____ / _____, "an (abnormal) condition of excessive thyroid (activity)," and _____ / _____ / _____, "an (abnormal) condition of deficient thyroid (activity)."
hypothyroidism hyperthyroidism	**1448** "Deficient" activity of the "thyroid" gland is technically called _____. Conversely, _____ is an "excessive" activity of the "thyroid" gland.
hyperthyroidism	**1449** The disease of _____ (hypothyroidism/hyperthyroidism) can result in blood thyroxine levels that are far "above normal." One function of thyroxine is to stimulate body growth.
Information Frame	**1450** Probably the chief hormone that stimulates the body to add muscle and bone tissue is the **pituitary growth hormone**. After maturity, when the bones cannot get any longer, this hormone, if present in an excessive amount, causes the bones to become thicker. The bones of the jaw and the extremities are especially likely to thicken.
-megaly	**1451** The root **acr** (**A**-ker) means "body extremity." Search your memory for _____ **(frame 138)**, an **m**-beginning suffix that means "enlargement of (something)."
acr/o/megaly (a-kroh-**MEG**-ah-lee)	**1452** Putting those facts together allows you to build _____ / _____ / _____, an "enlargement of the body extremities."
acromegaly	**1453** Persons afflicted with _____ have a distinct thickening and coarsening of their features, especially those of their jaw, feet, and hands. (Consult Figure 12.5.)

Acromegaly: Note the Markedly Enlarged Jaw, Nose, and Hands (From E. E. Chaffee and I. M. Lytle, *Basic Physiology and Anatomy*, 4th ed. Philadelphia: J. B. Lippincott, 1980)

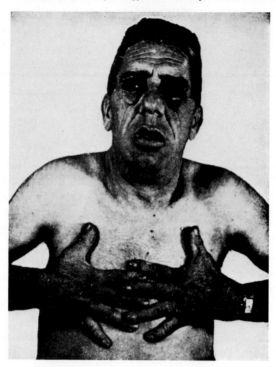

Information Frame	**1454** Another kind of body enlargement is **goiter** (**GOY**-ter), which technically means "throat." A root/cv for "goiter" or "throat" is **goitr/o** (**GOY**-troh).
goiter	**1455** An enlargement in the region of the "throat" is called _____. It represents an abnormally large thyroid gland, usually due to a chronic deficiency of iodine in the diet.
goitr/o/gen (**GOY**-troh-jen)	**1456** Use the suffix in estrogen **(frame 1403)** to help you build a new term, _____ /____ /_____, "producer of goiter."
goiter goitrogens	**1457** The principal cause of _____ ("enlarged thyroid") is dietary iodine deficiency. Certain types of foods, including plants in the cabbage family, also appear to act as _____ ("goiter-producers").
Information Frame	**1458** Practically any "gland," or **aden** (**A**-den), can have a diseased state. Remember that "muscle" can suffer from myopathy **(frame 1006)**, a diseased state.
aden/o/pathy (**a**-den-**AH**-pah-thee)	**1459** While myopathy is a diseased state of muscles, _____ /____ /_____, is "a condition of gland disease."

adenopathies
(**a**-den-**AH**-pah-theez)

1460 There are any number of _____ ("conditions of diseased glands").

---

aden/o/sclerosis
(a-den-oh-skleh-**ROH**-sis)
aden/itis (a-den-**IGH**-tis)

aden/oma (a-den-**OH**-mah)

aden/o/carcin/oma
(a-den-oh-**kar**-sin-**OH**-mah)

1461 Using knowledge of previously introduced suffixes, see how many types of adenopathies you can name below:
_____ / ____ / _____ "abnormal condition of hardening of the glands" (see otosclerosis, **frame 1300**)
_____ / _____ "inflammation of the glands"
(see thyroiditis, **frame 1446**)
_____ / _____ "tumor of a gland"
(see glaucoma, **frame 1310**)
_____ / ____ / _____ / _____ "crab tumor of a gland"
(see melanocarcinoma, **frame 690**)

---

adenitis

adenosclerosis

1462 If a set of "glands" are "inflamed," suffering _____, they may become abnormally hardened, technically called a condition of _____.

---

adenoma

adenocarcinoma

1463 A "tumor" in a "gland," technically termed an _____, may turn out to be benign. If malignant **(frame 572)**, however, it is properly called an _____, or "cancer" of the "gland."

1464 All types of adenopathies mentioned must be identified by testing and characterized by diagnosis.

Word Parts Associated with Lab Tests and Diagnoses of Glandular Disorders

The following is a list of word parts and abbreviations associated with lab tests and diagnoses of glandular disorders. Use this list to help you complete **frames 1466 to 1489**.

crin/o	secrete	**immun/o**	not serving (disease)	**nodul/o**	small knot or node
GTT	glucose tolerance test	**nod/o**	a knot; a knot-like body	**RIA**	radioimmunoassay

---

Information Frame

1465 There are various ways to detect abnormalities in endocrine glands. One of the simplest is palpation with the fingertips through the skin. The clinician may feel an abnormal **node (NOHD)**, or "knot," on a gland or perhaps a **nodule (NAHD**-yool), or "little knot," on, say, the thyroid.

---

nod/e
nodul/e

1466 If a _____ / ____ is a "knot present" on a gland, then a _____ / ____ is a "little knot present." The **ul** designation for something "little" mirrors its previous occurrence in the cellul root **(frame 423)** for "little cell."

---

nodules
node

1467 Many _____ ("little knots") or one large _____ ("knot") on the thyroid might suggest it was cancerous.

---

nodul/ar (**NAHD**-yoo-lar)

1468 Extract the ending from ocular **(frame 1239)** and construct
_____ /_____, "referring to little knots."

nodular

1469 The palpation of _____ ("little knot") tissue on the thyroid
would likely be followed up by a **thyroid scan**.

thyroid scan

1470 The _____ _____ is a technique wherein the "thyroid"
gland is "scanned" to detect the location of radioactively labeled
tumors or nodules.

scan

1471 In addition to the thyroid _____, the thyroid can be monitored by
means of its **radioactive iodine uptake**.

radioactive
iodine uptake

1472 Because the thyroid takes up iodine from the bloodstream and then
incorporates that element into thyroxine, a _____
_____ _____ test can be performed to measure this
ability.

radi/o

1473 The combining form in radioactive ("rays," **frame 188**),
_____ /_____, can be combined with **immun/o** (ih-**MYOO**-noh),
which denotes "not serving (disease)." An **assay** (**AS**-say) is a measure
of the quantity of something.

radi/o/immun/o/assay
(**ray**-dee-oh-**im**-yoo-noh-**AS**-say)

1474 Use the facts in the preceding frame to build a single long term,
_____ /_____ /_____ /_____ /_____, "an assay of
rays not serving (disease)."

radioimmunoassay

1475 The term _____ actually indicates a measuring, or
assay, of hormones attached to radioactively labeled **antibodies** (**AN**-
tih-**bah**-dees) in the blood.

RIA

1476 Radioimmunoassay, abbreviated as ____ ____ ____, can provide a
useful measure of hormone concentration within the bloodstream,
since many hormones attach to antibodies.

antibodies

immun/e (ih-**MYOON**)

1477 We can describe _____ literally as chemical "bodies"
that fight "against" (anti-) disease. They are therefore part of the
body's _____ /_____, or "not serving (disease)" system. This lat-
ter term takes the ending in ophthalmoscope **(frame 1325)**.

immune

1478 The _____ system includes antibodies to which hormones
can be attached. In general, the higher the concentration of such antibodies, the greater the person's resistance to disease.

Information Frame	**1479** Besides hormones themselves, substances affected by hormones can be measured and evaluated. An example is blood glucose concentration and urine glucose concentration. These factors are assessed by the **glucose tolerance test**.
glucose tolerance test	**1480** The _____ _____ _____ measures the amount of glucose that a person can ingest before the blood concentration rises to the point where glucose spills over into the urine.
GTT	**1481** The glucose tolerance test, abbreviated as ____ ____ ____, is a common screening device for diabetes mellitus.
Information Frame	**1482** Such tests for endocrine diseases are highly valuable. **Crin**, the root in endocrine, means "secretion."
endo/crin/e	**1483** Endocrine is subdivided as _____ / _____ / ____, with the same prefix found in endoplasmic **(frame 519)** and the same suffix as in immune **(frame 1477)**.
secretion within	**1484** Use the messages provided in the preceding frame to help you translate endocrine to mean "presence of a _____ _____."
endocrine	**1485** The literal meaning of _____ ("a secretion within") should help you understand why such glands are called glands of "internal secretion."
endo/crin/o/logy (**en**-doh-krih-**NAHL**-uh-jee)	**1486** These glands are so vital that their own special science has evolved. Just as otology **(frame 1316)**, for instance, indicates "study of the ear," _____ / _____ / ____ / _____ denotes a "study of secretion within."
endocrinology	**1487** The medical specialty of _____ focuses on diseases of the "internally secreting" glands.
endo/crin/o/logist (**en**-doh-krih-**NAHL**-oh-jist)	**1488** The specialty of endocrinology, like that of otology, has its own specialists. Just as an otologist **(frame 1321)** is "one who specializes in the study of the ear," an _____ / _____ / ____ / _____ is "one who specializes in the study of internal secretions."
endocrinologist	**1489** A person suffering from diabetes mellitus might well consider consulting an _____, because the affected gland, the pancreas, includes many internally secreting cells.

1490 An endocrinologist can also be of great value in carrying out treatment for various glandular problems.

Surgery and Therapies

Word Parts Associated with Surgery, Pharmacology, and Other Therapies for the Glands

The following is a list of word parts and an abbreviation associated with surgery, pharmacology, and other therapies related to the glands. Use this list to help you complete **frames 1491 to 1504**.

aden/o	a gland	**cry/o**	cold
andr/o	man; male	**DES**	diethylstilbestrol; synthetic estrogen

aden/ectomy (a-den-**EK**-toh-mee)

1491 If a "gland" is giving you trouble, the simplest thing to do is "remove" it! The formal term for "removal of a gland" is
_____ /_____, which follows the general word-building pattern of stapedectomy **(frame 1357)**.

adenectomy

thyroid
hypophysis
pancreas

1492 There are many specific types of _____ ("gland removal"). A partial list of glands that can be removed includes the _____ ("shield-resembler," **frame 1383**), the _____ ("an undergrowth," **frame 1131**), and the _____ ("all flesh," **frame 1411**).

thyroid/ectomy
(**thigh**-royd-**EK**-toh-mee)
hypophys/ectomy
(hih-**pah**-fih-**SEK**-toh-mee)
pancreat/ectomy
(**pan**-kree-at-**EK**-toh-mee)

1493 From the above information we can build:
_____ /_____ "removal of the shield-resembler"
_____ /_____ "removal of the undergrowth"
_____ /_____ "removal of the pancreas"

hypophysectomy
thyroidectomy

pancreatectomy

1494 Hypersecretion of growth hormone from tumors on the pituitary gland **(frame 1361)** might call for _____. Hypersecretion of thyroxine might make the operation of _____ necessary. Malignant neoplasms on the pancreas may make _____ a necessity.

Information Frame

1495 **Cry (KRIGH)** is a root for "cold." Delicate surgical procedures sometimes require the use of extremely cold baths or instruments.

cry/o/hypophys/ectomy
(**krigh**-oh-**high**-poh-fiz-**SEK**-toh-mee)

1496 An operation with a very long name is
_____ /____ /_____ /_____, "a removal of the undergrowth (involving) coldness."

cryohypophysectomy

1497 The procedure of _____ actually entails the destruction of the pituitary gland by the application of a freezing-"cold" probe.

Information Frame	**1498** Any type of adenectomy usually requires **hormone replacement therapy** afterward. Replacement is especially important after cryohypophysectomy.
hormone replacement therapy	**1499** The procedure called _____ _____ _____ involves the systematic use of certain "hormones" to "replace" those lost because of disease or injury of their secreting gland.
Information Frame	**1500** Here are the names of some synthetic hormones often employed in hormone replacement therapy: **levothyroxine** (**lee**-voh-thigh-**RAHKS**-in) **Calcimar** (**KAL**-sih-mar) **diethylstilbestrol** (digh-**eth**-il-**stil**-**BES**-trahl) **Cortef** (**KOR**-tef)
diethylstilbestrol Calcimar Cortef levothyroxine	**1501** See how well you can match the synthetic hormone names in the preceding frame with the natural hormones cited below: _____ synthetic estrogen **(DES)** _____ trade name for **calcitonin** (**kal**-sih-**TOHN**-in); a thyroid hormone that increases uptake of calcium into bones _____ trade name for cortisol; helps reduce inflammation _____ synthetic thyroxine
andr/o/gen (**AN**-droh-jen) estrogen	**1502** Some synthetic hormones produce characteristics like that of a "male" or a "man," denoted by the root **andr** (**AN**-der). A hormone that "produces a man" is called an _____ /____ /_____, much as a hormone that "produces mad desire" is called an _____ **(frame 1404)**.
synthetic androgens	**1503** Something that is synthetic was manufactured artificially. Thus _____ _____ are "artificially manufactured male-producers."
synthetic androgens	**1504** The _____ _____ are actually testosterone-like drugs that produce such "manly" body characteristics as a deep voice, large skeletal muscles, and extensive facial hair.

EXERCISES FOR CHAPTER 12

Multiple Choice

1. An adjectival form for "causing masculinization" is

   a. endogen   b. estrogenic   c. androgenic   d. progesterone

2. Which of the following means "secrete"?

   a. troph/o   b. diabet/o   c. cry/o   d. crin/o

3. The prefix in exocrine means

   a. "in"   b. "not"   c. "out"   d. "from"

4. A root for "siphon" is

   a. ren   b. test   c. diabet   d. crin

5. A combining form for "shield" is

   a. gluc/o   b. test/o   c. thyrox/o   d. gli/o

6. Another term for adrenalin is

   a. androgen   b. epinephrine   c. goitrogen   d. testerosterone

Meanings of Selected Roots

Add the correct combining vowel (cv) after each root. Then write the definition of each root in the space provided.

ROOT/CV	DEFINITION
1. crin/_____	_____
2. pituit/_____	_____
3. test/_____	_____
4. diabet/_____	_____
5. acr/_____	_____
6. aden/_____	_____
7. nodul/_____	_____
8. mellit/_____	_____
9. andr/_____	_____
10. cry/_____	_____

Word Dissection and Translation

Analyze the following terms by dissecting them with slashmarks and identifying their word parts. To the right of each term, write its correct English translation.

Key: R (root), cv (combining vowel), P (prefix), S (suffix)

1. diabetes mellitus

   _____ / _____ _____ / _____   _____
       R   S   R   S

2. thyroxine

   _____ / _____   _____
       R   S

3. hyposecretion

   _____ / _____ / _____   _____
     P   R   S

4. adenocarcinoma

   _____ / ___ / _____ / _____   _____
       R   cv   R   S

5. endocrinology

   _____ / _____ / ___ / ___   _____
     P   R   cv   S

6. hypophysectomy

   _____ / _____   _____
       R   S

7. androgen

   _____ / ___ / ___   _____
       R   cv   S

8. adrenocorticotrophic

   _____ / _____ / ___ / _____ / ___ / _____ / _____   _____
     P   R   cv   R   cv   R   S

                                                 _____

9. pancreas

   _____ / _____   _____
     P   R

10. acromegaly

    _____ / ___ / _____   _____
        R   cv   S

Terms and Their Abbreviations

In the list below, when the term is given, write its abbreviation in the space provided. When the abbreviation is given, write its corresponding term.

TERM	ABBREVIATION
1. glucose tolerance test	_____
2. _____	TSH
3. _____	RIA
4. adrenocorticotrophic hormone	_____

Word Spelling

Look at each of the terms listed below. Identify those that are misspelled by circling Y for "Yes." Write the correct spelling in the blank.

WORD	MISSPELLED?	CORRECT SPELLING
1. hypoglycemia	Y/N	_____
2. dyuresis	Y/N	_____
3. pituitary	Y/N	_____
4. glucocortycoyd	Y/N	_____
5. cortisol	Y/N	_____
6. insulin	Y/N	_____
7. epenefrine	Y/N	_____
8. diarrheasis	Y/N	_____
9. goiter	Y/N	_____
10. nodule	Y/N	_____
11. stearoid	Y/N	_____
12. hyperglycemia	Y/N	_____
13. endocrynology	Y/N	_____
14. cryohipofysectomy	Y/N	_____

New Word Synthesis

Using word parts that appear in this and previous chapters, build new terms with the following meanings:

1. _____	a honeyed body extremity
2. _____	a substance upon a shield-resembler
3. _____	removal of a cold gland
4. _____	condition of an undergrowth (in) the blood
5. _____	inflammation of the kidneys
6. _____	pertaining to changed mucus
7. _____	producer of rainbows
8. _____	the process of secreting all or everything
9. _____	one who specializes in the study of the eyes and glands
10. _____	inflammation of bark or cortex

CASE **S**TUDY

Read through the following partial autopsy report. Note the terms in bold print. A series of multiple choice questions probes your knowledge of these terms.

Autopsy Report

Examination of post-mortem remains of a 23-year-old white female killed in an auto accident. A multilobed **adenocarcinoma** of the **adrenal cortex** was discovered, measuring approximately 15 cm in diameter, which extended into the **renal capsule**. "Buffalo-hump" obesity suggests complications of **Cushing's disease**.

Case Study Questions

1. The finding of **adenocarcinoma** means that

   (a) a benign neoplasm was present.

   (b) overstretching of a muscle had occurred.

   (c) a malignant neoplasm of connective tissue was observed.

   (d) a malignant neoplasm of glandular tissue was present.

2. The **adrenal cortex** would be located

   (a) on the person's heart.

   (b) as a thin bark or rind around the glands located upon each kidney.

   (c) as the deep inner core or marrow within the adrenals.

   (d) around the pancreas.

3. The **renal capsule** is the capsule that

   (a) hugs the surface of the kidney.

   (b) envelopes the lungs and heart.

   (c) protects the thyroid.

   (d) surrounds the eyeball.

4. Complications of **Cushing's disease** suggests that the person may have suffered

   (a) hyposecretion of the adrenocortical hormones.

   (b) hyposecretion of certain sex hormones.

   (c) hypersecretion of the adrenocortical hormones.

   (d) hypersecretion of thyroxine.

CHAPTER 13 The Cardiovascular System

INTRODUCTION

The **cardiovascular** (**kar**-dee-oh-**VAS**-kyoo-lar), or **circulatory** (**SER**-kyoo-lah-**tor**-ee), **system** is one of the most important in both clinical medicine and natural science. Its general functional diagram (Figure 13.1) illustrates the reasons for such prominence. The four major functions of this system are (1) blood storage, (2) blood pumping, (3) blood filtration, and (4) blood circulation. This involvement of blood is crucial because blood carries life-giving nutrients such as oxygen and glucose to the trillions of body cells and transports poisonous waste products such as carbon dioxide away from the cells.

FIGURE 13.1   **General Functional Diagram of the Cardiovascular System**

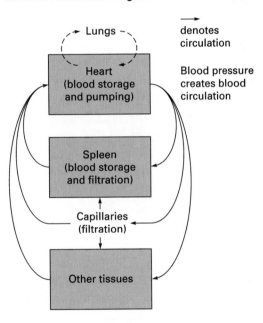

Note from Figure 13.2 that the cardiovascular (circulatory) system includes two major circulations. There is the **pulmonary** (**PUL**-muh-**nayr**-ee) **circulation**, which carries blood to, through, and from the lungs. The lungs receive low-oxygen blood from the heart and send blood back toward the heart after enriching it with oxygen. The **systemic** (**sis**-**TEM**-ik) **circulation**, as its name suggests, supplies blood to all major body "systems" except for the lungs. The major pump for the pulmonary circulation is the right side of the heart. The major pump for the systemic circulation is the left side of the heart.

FIGURE 13.2   **General Structural Diagram of the Cardiovascular Sysytem**

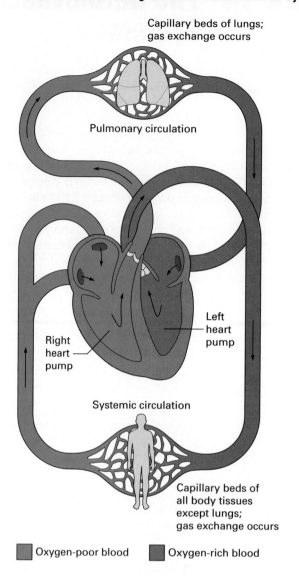

Capillary beds of lungs;
gas exchange occurs

Pulmonary circulation

Left
heart
pump

Right
heart
pump

Systemic circulation

Capillary beds of
all body tissues
except lungs;
gas exchange occurs

⬛ Oxygen-poor blood   ⬛ Oxygen-rich blood

Figure 13.3 shows the details of circulatory system function. The blood is temporarily stored within the heart, a four-chambered pump (Figure 13.3A). There are two superior smaller chambers, the **right** and **left atria** (**AY**-tree-ah), and two inferior larger chambers, the **right** and **left ventricles**. Contraction of the muscle in the heart wall creates a **blood pressure** (Figure 13.3B). This blood pressure pushes the blood out of the heart and into several major **arteries** (**AR**-ter-eez). These large vessels subdivide into several smaller branches, the **arterioles** (ar-**TEER**-ee-ohlz). The resistance of the walls of the arteries and arterioles makes the blood pressure higher. Blood circulates under pressure from the arterioles into the **capillaries** (**KAP**-ih-lahr-eez). Some of the components of the blood are then filtered out (pushed across the thin wall of the capillaries by pressure). There is also a diffusion of gases, wastes, and various nutrients across the thin capillary walls. From the capillaries in the body tissues, the blood enters the **venules** (**VEH**-nyoolz). These are small branches of the veins. Several huge veins, the **venae cavae** (**VEE**-nee **KAY**-vee), finally return the blood to the heart.

Along the way, the blood is filtered and cleansed by the **spleen**. The spleen is usually considered a member of the **lymphatic** (lim-**FAT**-ik) **system** as well as the blood circulatory system. The importance of the blood and **lymph (LIHMF)** will be considered in Chapter 14.

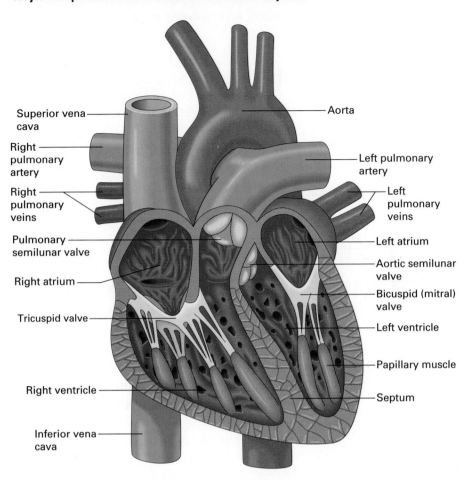

Superior vena cava

Right pulmonary artery

Right pulmonary veins

Pulmonary semilunar valve

Right atrium

Tricuspid valve

Right ventricle

Inferior vena cava

Aorta

Left pulmonary artery

Left pulmonary veins

Left atrium

Aortic semilunar valve

Bicuspid (mitral) valve

Left ventricle

Papillary muscle

Septum

(A) Internal Heart Anatomy

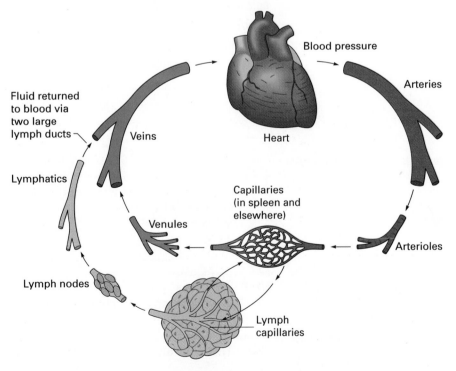

Blood pressure

Arteries

Heart

Fluid returned to blood via two large lymph ducts

Veins

Lymphatics

Venules

Capillaries (in spleen and elsewhere)

Arterioles

Lymph nodes

Lymph capillaries

(B) Blood Pressure and Blood Flow

This chapter highlights the terms of normal cardiovascular anatomy and physiology, the terms of cardiovascular diseases, the terms for lab tests and diagnoses of cardiovascular disorders, and the terms associated with the surgery and therapy for circulatory problems.

CHAPTER OBJECTIVES

By the end of this chapter, you should be able to:

1 Identify major prefixes, roots, suffixes, and abbreviations related to the cardiovascular system.

2 Dissect cardiovascular terms into their component parts.

3 Translate cardiovascular terms into their common English equivalents.

4 Build new terms associated with the cardiovascular system.

Normal A & P

Word Parts Associated with Normal Anatomy and Physiology of the Cardiovascular System

The following is a list of word parts and abbreviations associated with normal anatomy and physiology of the cardiovascular system. Use this list to help you complete **frames 1505 to 1587**.

angi/o	vessel	**cardi/o**	heart	**sept/o**	wall or partition
aort/o	lifting up	**cholesterol/o**	bile solid	**sin/o**	large vein storing blood
apic/o	the apex	**diastol/o**	relaxation		
arter/i	air passage; arteries	**lumin/o**	open space	**SL**	semilunar
arteriol/o	little artery	**lun/o**	moon	**systol/o**	contraction
atri/o	room; chamber	**mitr/o**	a bishop's mitre	**vas/o**	vessel
AV	atrioventricular	**phleb/o**	vein	**ven/o**	vein
capill/o	tiny hair	**SA**	sinoatrial	**venul/o**	tiny vein

---

vascul

vascular

1505 The "heart" itself is represented by the root **cardi** (**KAR**-dee). Recall that "vessels" in general are denoted by the root _____ **(frame 1114)**. This root combines with the appropriate "referring to" suffix to create _____ ("referring to vessels," **frame 1115**).

---

cardi/o/vascul/ar

1506 Therefore _____ / _____ / _____ / _____ is a term that literally means, "pertaining to the heart and (blood) vessels."

---

cardiovascular

1507 The heart and blood vessels are structures in the body's _____ system.

angi (**AN**-jee) **vas** (**VAS**)	**1508** Scan the word list and find two other roots meaning "vessel." These are _____ and _____.
vas/o/dilat/ion (**vas**-oh-digh-**LAY**-shun) **vas/o/constrict/ion** (**vas**-oh-kun-**STRIK**-shun)	**1509** Dilat/**ion** (**frame 419**) is "a process of widening," while constrict/**ion** is "a process of narrowing." Use these facts and the second root cited in the above frame to create: _____ /_____ /_____ /_____ "a process of vessel widening" _____ /_____ /_____ /_____ "a process of vessel narrowing"
vasoconstriction vasodilation	**1510** The "narrowing," or _____, of blood "vessels" generally causes the blood pressure to rise. Conversely, the "widening," or _____, of blood "vessels" usually causes the pressure to fall.
Information Frame	**1511** Both vasoconstriction and vasodilation affect the size of a vessel's **lumen** (**LOO**-men)—its "open space." **Lumin** is the root generally used for lumen.
lumin/al (**LOO**-mih-nul)	**1512** Lumin can take the ending in laryngeal (**frame 1320**). The result is _____ /_____, "referring to a lumen or open space."
luminal	**1513** Vasoconstriction reduces the _____ ("open space") diameter of a blood vessel, while vasodilation increases it.
lumen	**1514** An **artery** (**AR**-ter-**ee**) usually has a large _____ ("open space"). **Arteries** are vessels that carry blood away from the heart.
arter (**AR**-ter)	**1515** The root of artery is _____. The suffix here is identical to that in anatomy (**frame 318**). This root generally takes **i** as its combining vowel.
arter/i/es	**1516** Arteries is subdivided as _____ /_____ /_____.
artery arteries **arter/i/al** (ar-**TEER**-e-al)	**1517** Arter, the root in _____ (singular) and _____ (plural), takes the same suffix for "pertaining to" as does lumin. Create, therefore, _____ /_____ /_____, "pertaining to arteries."
arterial	**1518** Arter actually means "air passage" or "windpipe." So _____ literally "pertains to an air passage or windpipe." This root was used because of the mistaken notion of the early Greeks that the arteries carried air rather than blood.

1519 Arteries subdivide into smaller branches, the **arterioles**. A term related to arterioles is **arteriolar** (**ar-TEER**-ee-**OH**-lar). The **ol** fragment generally denotes something "little."

arteriol/**es**
arteriol/**ar**
arteriol (**ar-TEER**-ee-ohl)

1520 From the common stem found in the two terms, you can probably guess that arterioles is dissected as _____ /_____ and that arteriolar is dissected as _____ /_____. Observe that the common root in both is _____, "little artery."

arterioles
arteriolar

1521 The literal meaning of _____ is "little air passages," while _____ "refers to little air passages."

arterioles
arteriolar

1522 In reality, _____, like their larger cousins, the arteries, carry blood. Eventually, _____ blood flows into even tinier blood vessels, the **capillaries**.

capill/ary (**KA**-pil-ayr-ee)

1523 The singular form of capillaries is _____ /_____, which contains the same "pertaining to" suffix as ovary **(frame 1392)**.

capill (**KA**-pil)
capill/o
pertains to tiny hairs

1524 The root in capillary is _____, "tiny hair." The combining form is _____/_____. Capillary therefore "_____ ____ _____ _____," just as ovary "pertains to eggs."

capillaries
luminal

1525 The _____ are tiny, hairlike blood vessels with minute _____ ("open space," **frame 1512**) diameters.

1526 Veins are large-diameter blood vessels that carry blood away from the heart. **Ven/o** (**VEE**-noh) is a combining form for "vein." **Venul/o** (**VEHN**-yoo-loh) is a combining form for "tiny vein" much as

arteriol

_____ **(frame 1520)** is a root for "little artery."

venul/es
venul/ar (**VEHN**-yoo-lar)

1527 In the same manner as arteriol/**es** are "little arteries present," _____ /_____ are "tiny veins present." And just as arteriol/**ar** "refers to little arteries or air passages," _____ /_____ "refers to tiny veins."

venules
venular

1528 The _____ are actually "tiny" branches of the "veins." They receive blood from the capillaries, and then the _____ ("tiny vein") blood passes into the much larger veins.

ven/a (**VEE**-nah)
ven/ous (**VEE**-nus)

1529 Ven commonly takes the "presence of" ending in medulla **(frame 1086)** and the "pertaining to" suffix in osseous **(frame 770)**. This knowledge allows us to build _____ /_____ ("presence of a vein") and _____ /_____ ("pertaining to veins"), respectively.

vena

venous

1530 The superior _____ **cava** (**KAY**-vah), for instance, is a very large "cave vein present" above the heart. This vessel contains a large amount of _____ ("vein") blood.

---

arterial

venous

venae

1531 Blood that starts out on the _____ ("pertaining to arteries," **frame 1517**) side of the circulation passes through much smaller types of vessels and eventually flows into the _____ ("pertaining to veins") side. The largest of these veins are the **superior** and **inferior** _____ **cavae**. Figure 13.4 shows some of the major blood vessels attached to the heart.

FIGURE 13.4   **Major Vessels Attached to the Heart**

Superior vena cava
Aorta
Right pulmonary artery
Left pulmonary artery
Right pulmonary veins
Left pulmonary veins
Right auricle (attached to right atrium)
Left auricle (attached to left atrium)
Right coronary artery
Left coronary artery
Right coronary vein
Left coronary vein
Right ventricle
Left ventricle

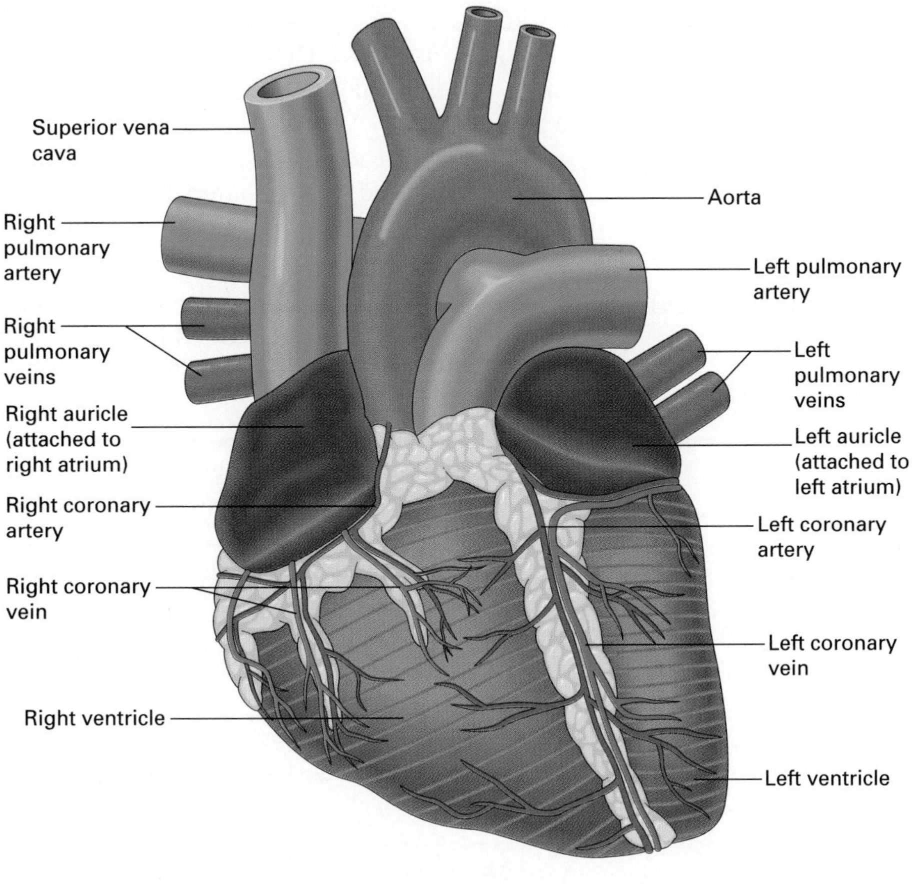

a/vascul/ar (a-**VAS**-kyoo-lar)

1532 Recall that vascular (**frame 1505**) "refers to vessels or little vessels." Extract the "without" prefix from atrophy (**frame 141**) and create ____ /_____ /____, "a condition without vessels."

---

avascular

1533 Structures that are _____ ("without vessels") can provide no storage of blood. On the other hand, **sin (SIGHN)** suggests blood storage because it means "curved bay."

---

sin/us (**SIGH**-nus)

1534 Employ the suffix in thalamus (**frame 1127**) to help you construct _____ /____, a large "curved bay" vein in which blood is "present."

---

sinus	**1535** A venous _____ is a vein that resembles a large "curved bay." Such veins store considerable quantities of blood.
Information Frame	**1536** One notable example of a venous sinus is the superior vena cava. It returns blood to a particular **atri** (**AY**-tree), or "chamber," at the top of the heart.
atri/um (**AY**-tree-um)	**1537** The name of the chamber in the above frame is the **right** _____ /_____, where the ending is the same as in tympanum **(frame 1268)**.
right atrium	**1538** The _____ _____ receives blood from the superior vena cava. Then the blood is squirted down into the right ventricle, a "little belly," or cavity **(frame 1112)**.
atri/al (**AY**-tree-al)	**1539** Add the suffix of arterial **(frame 1517)** to the root of atrium. This yields _____ /_____, "referring to a chamber."
atrial	**1540** The _____ (upper "chamber") region of the heart forms a broad base where several major arteries and venous sinuses attach.
sin/o/atri/al curved bay chamber	**1541** In the wall of the right atrium is the **sinoatrial** (**sigh**-noh-**AY**-tree-al) **node**. Sinoatrial is properly subdivided as _____ /_____ /_____ /_____. This term literally means "pertaining to a _____ _____ and _____ ."
sinoatrial sinus	**1542** The _____ area is the medial wall of the right atrium, just below the entrance of the superior vena cava, a major _____ ("curved bay", **frame 1534**). (See Figure 13.5.)
SA **sin** **atri** **sin/o** **atri/o**	**1543** Sinoatrial is abbreviated as _____ _____, for its two roots, _____ and _____. The combining forms are _____ /_____ and _____ /_____.
SA	**1544** There is a sinoatrial, or _____ _____, node of tissue located within the sinoatrial region.
sinoatrial node	**1545** The _____ _____ (SA node) is the major **cardiac** (**KAR**-dee-ak) **pacemaker**. This small oval area in the heart wall contains self-exciting cells that start the heartbeat. Figure 13.5 shows this area and its spread of cardiac excitation.

Chapter 13 The Cardiovascular System

FIGURE 13.5   The Sinoatrial Region

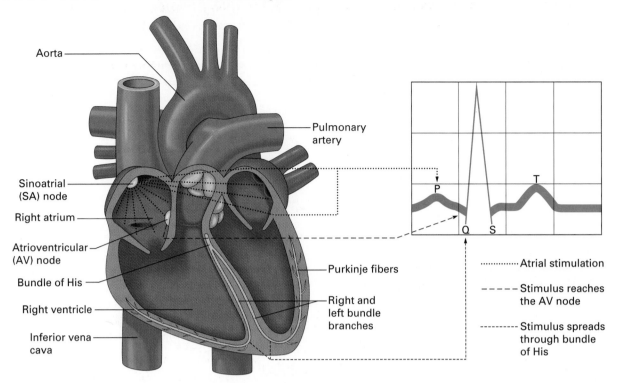

- Aorta
- Pulmonary artery
- Sinoatrial (SA) node
- Right atrium
- Atrioventricular (AV) node
- Bundle of His
- Right ventricle
- Inferior vena cava
- Purkinje fibers
- Right and left bundle branches

P Q S T

············ Atrial stimulation
------ Stimulus reaches the AV node
-------- Stimulus spreads through bundle of His

---

cardi/ac

1546 Cardiac is dissected as _____ /____, with its root for "heart" being the same as in cardiovascular **(frame 1505)** and its suffix being **-ac (frame 91)** rather than -ic. Two closely related words are **cardial** (**KAR**-dee-al) and **cardium** (**KAR**-dee-um).

---

cardi/al
cardi/um

1547 Cardial is dissected as _____ /____, cardium as _____ /____.

---

cardiac
cardial
cardium

1548 By now you may know that both _____ and _____ are adjectives that "refer to the heart," while _____ is a noun that denotes "presence of the heart."

---

sinoatrial
cardiac
cardial
cardium

1549 The SA (_____) node is present in the right _____ or _____ ("heart") wall. Starting from this area, nerve impulses travel throughout the heart, or _____.

1550 Adopt the root in myoma **(frame 1010)**, the "around" prefix in periosteum **(frame 786)**, and use cardial and cardium to build four new terms:

my/o/cardi/um
(my-oh-**KAR**-dee-um)
my/o/cardi/al (my-oh-**KAR**-dee-al)
peri/cardi/um
(peh-rih-**KAR**-dee-um)
peri/cardi/al (peh-rih-**KAR**-dee-al)

____ /____ /_____ /____   "presence of heart muscle"
____ /____ /_____ /____   "referring to heart muscle"
_____ /_____ /____   "presence of (something) around the heart"
_____ /_____ /____   "referring to (something) around the heart"

myocardium pericardium	**1551** The _____, or "heart muscle," is "present" within the heart wall, while the _____ is a serous membrane located outside, being "present around the heart."
myocardial pericardial	**1552** We use the term _____ when we are "referring to the heart muscle," but use _____ when we are "referring to" the membranous sac "around the heart."
apic/o	**1553** The pericardium covers the entire heart, from its broad upper base to its inferior pointed tip, or **apex** (**AY**-peks). **Apic** (**AY**-pik) is the root for apex and _____ /_____ is the combining form.
apic/al (AY-pik-al)	**1554** The term _____ /_____ ("referring to apex") is built the same as myocardial or pericardial.
apical	**1555** A nursing student usually learns how to use a stethoscope to take the _____ pulse of a patient by placing the bell upon the chest, over the apex of the heart.
Information Frame	**1556** **Sept** is a root meaning "wall or partition." This root takes the same "presence of" ending found in cardium and the same "pertaining to" suffix as cardial and apical.
sept/um (SEP-tum) **sept/al (SEP**-tal)	**1557** A _____ /_____ is a "wall present" between both the right and left atria and the ventricles. This _____ /_____ ("partitioning") wall extends downward into the apical area.
septum septal	**1558** Blood in the right atrium is prevented from flowing directly into the adjacent left atrium by the _____, or "wall present" between them. A _____ defect is a hole or breakage in this "wall."
atri ventricular	**1559** Within each side of the heart, the atrium above is separated from its ventricle below by a connective tissue valve. We need to review several word parts here. Remember that _____ **(frame 1536)** means "chamber" and that _____ **(frame 1115)** "refers to a little belly."
atri/o/ventricul/ar (**ay**-tree-oh-ven-**TRIK**-yoo-lar)	**1560** Adopting the pattern for building cardiovascular **(frame 1506)**, construct _____ /_____ /_____ /_____, "referring to a chamber and little belly."
atrioventricular	**1561** There are two _____, or AV valves, one separating the "atrium" from its underlying "ventricle" on the left side of the heart, and another doing the same on the right.

AV	**1562** Each _____ _____, or atrioventricular, valve opens and allows the blood in its atrium above to empty into the ventricle beneath.
atrioventricular **AV**	**1563** The **left** _____ **(AV) valve** is also known as the **bicuspid** (**BIGH**-kus-pid), or **mitral** (**MIGH**-tral) valve. The right atrioventricular (_____ _____) valve is also known as the tricuspid (**TRY**-kus-pid) valve.
2 3	**1564** You should be able to deduce that the bicuspid valve has _____ (give the number) "cusps," or flaps, while the tricuspid valve has _____ (give the number).
mitr/al	**1565** Note from **frame 1563** that the left AV, or bicuspid, valve is also known as the _____ /_____ valve, with the same suffix as septal **(frame 1557)**.
mitral	**1566** Figure 13.6 provides a close-up view of two of the four heart valves. Note that the _____ valve is imaginatively named for its resemblance to an inverted **mitr/e** (**MIGH**-ter), or "bishop's hat."

FIGURE 13.6   **Detailed Views of Bicuspid (Mitral) and Left Semilunar Valves**

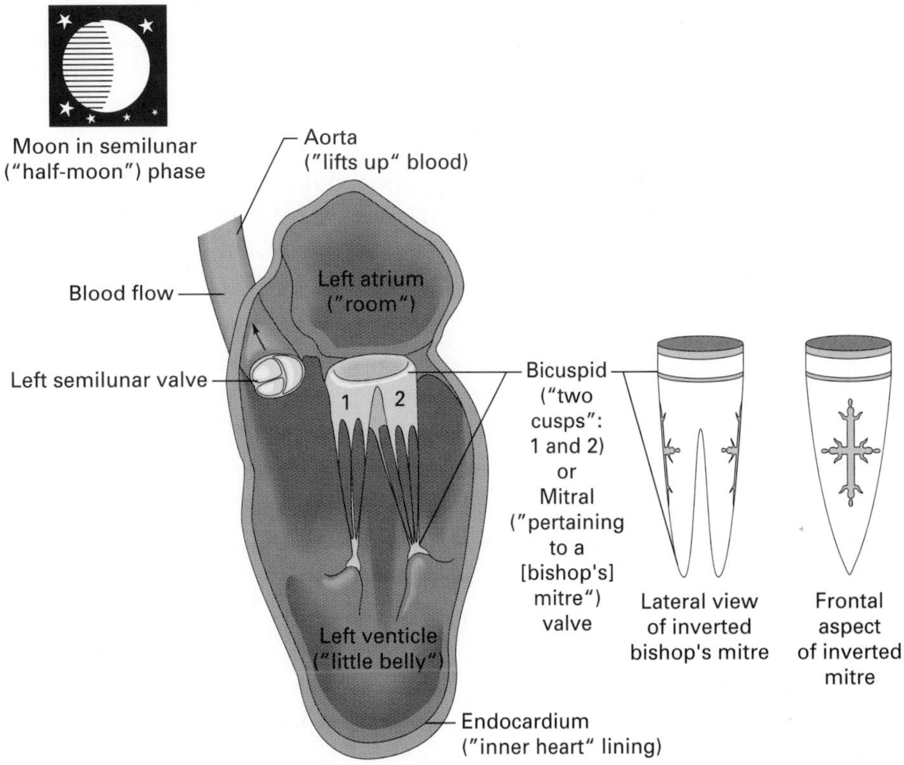

Moon in semilunar ("half-moon") phase

Aorta ("lifts up" blood)

Blood flow

Left semilunar valve

Left atrium ("room")

Bicuspid ("two cusps": 1 and 2) or Mitral ("pertaining to a [bishop's] mitre") valve

Lateral view of inverted bishop's mitre

Frontal aspect of inverted mitre

Left venticle ("little belly")

Endocardium ("inner heart" lining)

mitral	**1567** The _____ ("pertaining to mitre") valve has two flaps. Observe that the left semilunar (**sem**-ee-**LOON**-ar) valve, which lies immediately above it, has valve flaps with half-moon shapes. **Lun (LOON)** is a root for "moon."

lun/ar (LOO-nar)

semi-

1568 We can build _____ /____ for "referring to the moon" just as we built venular **(frame 1527)** for "referring to little veins." A useful prefix for this term is _____, as found in semicircular **(frame 1276)**, meaning "half or partial."

---

semi/lun/ar

SL

1569 The left _____ /_____ /____ valve has flaps that "refer to half or partial moons." This name is abbreviated by the two letters ____ ____.

SL
semilunar

1570 Blood is pushed through the right and left ____ ____, or _____ ("half-moon") valves when the wall of each ventricle contracts. A root for "contraction" is **systol (SIS-**tohl). One for "relaxation" is **diastol (DIGH-**ah-stohl).

---

systol
diastol

1571 Both _____ ("contraction") and _____ ("relaxation") take the "presence of" ending in venule **(frame 1527)** and the "pertaining to" ending in pancreatic **(frame 1412)**.

---

systol/e (SIS-toh-lee)
diastol/e (digh-**AS-**toh-lee)
systol/ic (sis-**TAHL-**ik)
diastol/ic (digh-ahs-**TAHL-**ik)

1572 Employ your word-building skills and create:
_____ /____ "presence of contraction"
_____ /____ "presence of relaxation"
_____ /____ "pertaining to contraction"
_____ /____ "pertaining to relaxation"

---

systole

diastole

1573 During ventricular _____ (systole/diastole) the semilunar valves are pushed open by the force of myocardial "contraction." During ventricular _____ (systole/diastole), however, they snap shut because of myocardial "relaxation."

---

systolic

diastolic

1574 The _____ blood pressure is large and pushes the semilunar valves open. During the resting phase of the ventricles, however, the associated _____ blood pressure is low.

Information Frame

1575 **Aort (**ay-**ORT)** means "lifting up." This root takes the noun-forming suffix of vena **(frame 1529)** and the same adjective-forming ending as diastol **(frame 1571)**.

---

aort/a (ay-**OR-**tah)
aort/ic (ay-**OR-**tik)

1576 Construct _____ /____ for "presence of a lifting up" and _____ /____ for "pertaining to lifting up."

---

aorta

1577 The _____ is the major systemic artery, serving to "lift" blood "up" out of the heart and send it on its way toward most of the individual body systems.

---

aortic	**1578** All of the _____ ("lifting up") blood eventually reaches other points in the **systemic** ("body system") **circulation**.
systemic	**1579** The _____ ("body system") circulation serves the heart itself, as well as the heart's broad top or "crown." It does not serve the lungs, however.
coron	**1580** Recall that _____, the root in coronal **(frame 326)**, means "crown." **Pulmon** (**PUL**-mahn) is a root for "lungs."
Information Frame	**1581** Remember that the suffix -**ary**, as in capillary **(frame 1523)**, means "pertaining to."
coron/ary (**KOR**-uh-nayr-ee) **pulmon/ary**	**1582** Now use the information from **frame 1580** and the suffix -**ary** to help you synthesize _____ /_____ ("pertaining to a crown") and _____ /_____ ("pertaining to the lungs").
coronary	**1583** The _____ ("pertaining to crown") circulation arises as branches from the aorta, wraps like a "crown" around the superior end of the heart, and is chiefly responsible for supplying blood to the myocardium.
pulmonary	**1584** The _____ circulation is that which supplies blood to both "lungs." It follows a path separate from that of the systemic circulation.
coronary	**1585** **Cholesterol** (koh-**LES**-ter-ahl), or "bile solid," is a lipid substance that often accumulates in the lumens of blood vessels, especially those in the systemic circulation. The _____ ("crown") arteries feeding the heart muscle, being extremely narrow, are very susceptible to clogging with this material. 
cholesterol pulmonary	**1586** Too much _____ in the blood of any vessel, whether systemic or _____ ("lung"-supplying), can greatly reduce luminal diameter.
angi/o ven/o	**1587** Cholesterol blockage or other problems associated with the heart and vessels will be discussed in the next section. An **a**-beginning combining form for "vessel" **(frame 1508)**, _____ /_____, and **phleb** (**FLEB**), which like _____ /_____ **(frame 1526)** denotes "vein," are often used with other word parts associated with cardiovascular diseases.

Word Parts Associated with Diseases of the Cardiovascular System

The following is a list of word parts and abbreviations associated with diseases of the cardiovascular system. Use this list to help you complete **frames 1589 to 1660**.

aneurysm/a	wideness	**CHF**	congestive heart failure	**MVP**	mitral valve prolapse
angin/o	tightness with pain			**occlus/o**	shut off
ather/o	fat	**infarct/o**	tissue death	**pector/o**	chest
CAD	coronary artery disease	**ischem/o**	keep back blood	**PVC**	premature ventricular contraction
		MI	myocardial infarction		
CHD	coronary heart disease			**sten/o**	narrow
		MS	mitral stenosis		

Information Frame

1588 Diseases of the cardiovascular system (especially those involving the heart) are still the major cause of death and disability in the developed countries of the world today.

-oma

1589 **Ather** (**ATH**-er) is a root for "fat." Recall that _____, the suffix in glioma **(frame 1167)**, means "tumor."

---

ather/oma (**AH**-ther-**oh**-ma)

1590 Therefore an _____ /_____ is a "fatty tumor."

---

atheromas

1591 "Fatty tumors," or _____, tend to develop whenever the blood cholesterol level becomes excessive.

---

hyper-

1592 Remember that _____, as in hyperchromatic **(frame 740)**, means "above normal or excessive." A particular suffix, **-emia** (**EE**-mee-ah), denotes a "blood condition of."

---

hyper/cholesterol/emia (**high**-per-koh-**LES**-ter-ahl-**EE**-mee-ah)

1593 A "blood condition of excessive cholesterol" is constructed as _____ /_____ /_____.

---

hypercholesterolemia

atheromas

1594 An excessive blood cholesterol, or _____, seems to contribute to the deposition of cholesterol crystals onto the lining of arteries. Along with high circulating blood fats, such deposition appears to trigger the formation of _____ ("fatty tumors," **frame 1590**).

---

hypertrophy

-megaly

1595 Remember that another hyper- state is described by _____ ("a process of excessive nourishment or stimulation"). Commonly associated with such above-normal tissue stimulation is a "condition of enlargement," indicated by the **m**-beginning suffix, _____ **(frame 138)**.

---

cardi/o/megaly (**kar**-dee-oh-**MEG**-uh-lee)	**1596** Extract the "heart" root from cardium **(frame 1547)** and synthesize a new term, _____ /____ /_____, a "condition of heart enlargement."
cardiomegaly	**1597** Cardiac hypertrophy, or overstimulation, may lead to _____ ("heart enlargement").
-pathy **angi/o/pathy** (an-jee-**AH**-pah-thee) **cardi/o/pathy** (kar-dee-**AH**-pah-thee)	**1598** The suffix in myopathy **(frame 1006)** is _____. Using angi for "vessel" and the appropriate root for "heart," construct the following: _____ /____ /_____ "disease of vessels" _____ /____ /_____ "disease of the heart" Note the pronunciation of cardi/o (**KAR**-dee-oh) and path/**y** (**PATH**-ee). Now note the change in pronunciation when these two word parts are combined. Say cardiopathy and angiopathy several times. Observe that the accent shifts to the combining vowel in each of the terms.
cardiopathy	**1599** Cardiomegaly is a type of _____ (angiopathy/cardiopathy), since it is the "heart" that is enlarged.
cardi/o/path/ies (kar-dee-**AH**-pah-theez) **angi/o/path/ies** (an-jee-**AH**-pah-theez)	**1600** There are many _____ /____ /_____ /_____ ("heart diseases") as well as _____ /____ /_____ /_____ ("vessel diseases"). Because vessel disease often precedes heart disease, we will discuss it first.
-sclerosis **arteri/o/sclerosis** **o** arteri/o	**1601** Perhaps you recollect that _____, as found in arteriosclerosis **(frame 148)**, is an "abnormal condition of hardening." Arteriosclerosis is dissected as _____ /____ /_____, where the root is **arteri** (ar-**TEER**-ee), the combining vowel is ____, and the combining form is _____ /____.
angiopathy arteriosclerosis	**1602** The _____ (angiopathy/cardiopathy) called _____ denotes an "abnormal condition of hardening of the arteries."
arteriosclerosis	**1603** The most common type of _____ ("arterial hardening") is called **atherosclerosis** (**ath**-er-oh-skleh-**ROH**-sis).
ather/o/sclerosis	**1604** Atherosclerosis is analyzed with slashes as _____ /____ /_____.
atherosclerosis	**1605** Technically speaking, _____ represents an "abnormal condition of fatty hardening" of the arteries. It occurs because of the build-up of atheromas within the arterial lumen.

atherosclerosis	**1606** The condition of _____ ("fatty hardening") can be a serious problem. The hardening process is largely due to the laying down of calcium crystals onto the fatty deposits. Hard atheromas present on the inner arterial wall then partially shut off the flow of blood through the lumen. **Occlus/o** (uh-**KLOOZ**-oh) is a combining form for "shut off."
occlus/ion (uh-**KLOO**-zhun)	**1607** Extract the "process of" suffix from concussion **(frame 1149)** and build a new term that translates as, "the process of shutting (something) off": _____ /_____.
occlusion	**1608** When atherosclerosis gets very extensive, the atheromas may become so large that _____ ("shutting off") of the diseased arteries results.
Information Frame	**1609** When the lumens of many arteries narrow, the total resistance to blood flow, hence the blood pressure, increases. **Tens/ion** is "a condition of tension or pressure."
hyper/tens/ion (high-per-**TEN**-shun) **hypo/tens/ion** (high-poh-**TEN**-shun)	**1610** Use the information in the frame above and the prefix of hypercholesterolemia **(frame 1593)** to create _____ /_____ /_____, a "condition of excessive (blood) pressure." The prefix of hypodermis **(frame 637)** leads to _____ /_____ /_____, a "condition of below normal (blood) pressure."
hypertension hypotension	**1611** Occlusion, by partially or totally shutting off the arterial lumen, tends to contribute to a state of _____ (hypertension/hypotension). On the other hand, _____ may involve such "low" pressure that fainting or syncope occurs.
hypertension arteriosclerosis	**1612** High blood pressure, or _____, if severe and prolonged, gradually destroys the elastic fibers in arterial walls and contributes to _____ ("arterial hardening").
CAD **CHD**	**1613** The coronary arteries, having such narrow lumens, are especially susceptible to arteriosclerosis and atherosclerosis. This problem is usually called either **coronary artery disease**, abbreviated as ____ ____ ____, or coronary heart disease, which is abbreviated as ____ ____ ____.
coronary artery disease coronary heart disease	**1614** The problem of _____ _____ _____ (CAD), or _____ _____ _____ (CHD), is by far the greatest killer in the United States today. A major crisis is the great reduction in blood flow to the pumping tissue—the myocardium.

occlusion atherosclerosis	**1615** **Ischem** (is-**KEEM**) is a root indicating "keeping back blood," that is, a deficiency of blood flow. This condition is generally due to a partial or total _____ ("shutting off") of vessel lumens by _____ ("fatty hardening").
ischem/ia (is-**KEE**-mee-uh) **ischem/ic** (is-**KEE**-mik)	**1616** Use the "(abnormal) condition" suffix in phobia **(frame 1178)** to build _____ /_____, "a condition of keeping back blood," and the "referring to" suffix in systolic **(frame 1572)** to build _____ /_____, "referring to keeping back blood."
ischemia ischemic	**1617** Persons suffering _____ have an inadequate flow of blood to particular tissue areas. We say that these blood-deficient tissues are _____.
acute **myocardial ischemia**	**1618** Recollect that acute **(frame 134)** means "sudden" and that myocardial **(frame 1550)** "refers to the heart muscle." Employ this information to help you build a phrase that indicates "a condition of sudden keeping back of blood from the heart muscle": _____ _____ _____.
acute myocardial ischemia	**1619** An _____ _____ _____ is caused by a partial or total occlusion of the lumens of the coronary arteries. You will remember that these vessels provide nutrients to the myocardium, or heart muscle.
ischemic	**1620** Acute myocardial ischemia results in a sudden bout of _____ ("referring to keeping back blood") heart pain. The victim tends to experience both tightness and pain sensations in the chest area. **Angin** (an-**JIGHN**) means "tightness with pain."
angin/a (an-**JIGH**-nah) pector	**1621** The root **angin** commonly takes **-a** as its "presence of" suffix. Thus _____ /_____ means "presence of tightness with pain." Its occurrence in the "chest" involves the root _____, a shorter version of the root in pectoralis **(frame 987)**.
pector/is (**PEK**-tor-is)	**1622** Extract the "presence of" suffix from pectoralis **(frame 987)** and build _____ /_____, "presence of the chest."
angina pectoris	**1623** Now, using the information from the last two frames, create the phrase _____ _____, "presence of tightness with pain in the chest."
angina pectoris	**1624** Myocardial ischemia due to occlusion of the coronary arteries by atheromas usually results in _____ _____ ("chest tightness and pain") as a warning.

Information Frame	**1625** This pain is a warning of impending **infarction** (in-**FARK**-shun). The ending of this term is the same as in hypotension **(frame 1610)**.
infarct/ion	**1626** The term _____ /_____ denotes the "process of having an infarct" (an area of tissue death).
infarction myocardial	**1627** An _____ is the "process of tissue dying," in the heart or elsewhere. The major cause of such death is a choking off of oxygen and other vital nutrients during tissue ischemia. In the heart, the death is due to occlusion of the coronary arteries that feed the heart muscle. Recall that _____ **(frame 1550)** "refers to heart muscle."
myocardial infarction	**1628** We can therefore describe _____ _____ as a "process of tissue dying (affecting) the heart muscle."
myocardial infarction **MI**	**1629** The process of _____ _____ results from severe acute myocardial ischemia. If a large amount of myocardium becomes necrotic (dead), the heart is no longer able to pump sufficient amounts of blood, and the patient dies. Figure 13.7 illustrates the natural history of coronary heart disease, leading to a myocardial infarction (abbreviated as ____ ____).
myocardial infarction cardiopathy	**1630** An MI (_____ _____) is a type of _____ (angiopathy/cardiopathy), since the heart itself is damaged. However, the underlying reason for the heart damage is severe vessel damage involving atherosclerosis and occlusion of one or more branches of the coronary arteries.
Information Frame	**1631** Another possible feature of arteriosclerosis is **aneurysm** (**AN**-yoo-rizm), an unnatural "widening" of a vessel that is accompanied by a destructive thinning of its wall.
aneurysm aortic aneurysm	**1632** Chronic hypertension may result in _____ or "widening," thinning, and ballooning out of the wall of a major blood vessel. Rupture of an _____ ("pertaining to lifting up," **frame 1576**) _____ ("widening"), for instance, may be fatal within a few minutes, because of extensive loss of blood.
Information Frame	**1633** Other types of problems involve too much blood rather than too little. Take, for example, **congestion**, or "stuffing up," of a damaged heart with blood.
congestion	**1634** If one side of the heart is severely damaged, it can no longer pump out the blood returning to it. The damaged heart undergoes _____, or "stuffing up," with blood. The patient then runs the risk of going into **congestive heart failure**.

FIGURE 13.7

The Natural History of Coronary Heart Disease

Cross sections through a coronary artery
undergoing progressive atherosclerosis
and arteriosclerosis

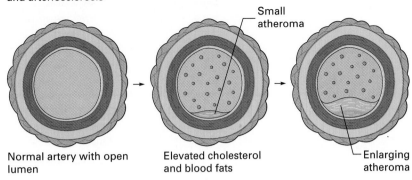

Normal artery with open lumen

Elevated cholesterol and blood fats

Small atheroma

Enlarging atheroma

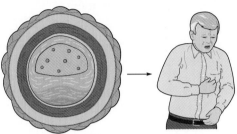

Moderate atherosclerotic narrowing of lumen

Moderate myocardial ischemia

Angina pectoris

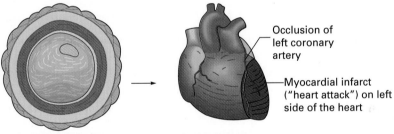

Complete/almost complete occlusion, with hardening due to calcium deposition

Severe acute myocardial ischemia and infarction

Occlusion of left coronary artery

Myocardial infarct ("heart attack") on left side of the heart

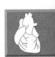

CHF

1635 Congestive heart failure, abbreviated as _____ _____ _____, is a failure of the heart to pump because it has become too stuffed **(congested)** and swollen with blood to operate.

---

congestive heart
failure
myocardial
infarction

1636 The affliction called _____ _____
_____ (CHF) is often the end-state after a severe "heart attack"—a massive occurrence of _____
_____ (MI).

-o/rrhexis
cardi/o/rrhexis
(**kar**-dee-oh-**REK**-sis)

1637 The congested heart may balloon out so far that it actually ruptures. Remember that the suffix ____ / _____ **(frame 147)**, means "a rupture." Therefore _____ / ____ / _____ **(frame 148)** denotes "a rupture of the heart."

cardiorrhexis	**1638** Heart rupture, or _____, occurs when the heart wall has become overstretched to the point of tearing.
card/itis	**1639** Search your memory and bring back the suffix for "inflammation of" along with the root for "heart." The result is _____ /_____ ("inflammation of the heart," **frame 152**).
peri/card/itis (**peh**-rih-kar-**DIGH**-tis) **phleb/itis** (fleh-**BIGH**-tis)	**1640** Build two more terms involving inflammation. Extract the "around" prefix from pericardium **(frame 1550)** for one. For the other, use phleb as the root. This gives us: _____ /_____ /_____ "inflammation of (the area) around the heart" _____ /_____ "inflammation of veins"
carditis pericarditis phlebitis	**1641** Both _____ ("heart inflammation") and _____ ("inflammation" of the sac "around" the "heart") are examples of cardiopathy, while _____ reflects angiopathy.
Information Frame	**1642** The inflammatory changes of carditis, if severe enough, may have a disturbing effect on the heart's rhythm of excitation and contraction. One potentially dangerous effect is **arrhythmia** (ay-**RITH**-mee-ah).
a/rrhythm/ia	**1643** Arrhythmia contains the same prefix as avascular **(frame 1532)** and the same suffix as ischemia **(frame 1616)**. Arrhythmia is consequently subdivided as ____ /_____ /____.
arrhythmia	**1644** An _____ is literally an "abnormal condition of lack of rhythm."
arrhythmias **PVC**	**1645** Some _____ ("conditions lacking rhythm") are very serious. A potentially dangerous example is **premature ventricular contraction**, abbreviated as ____ ____ ____.
premature ventricular contraction	**1646** A _____ _____ _____ (PVC) occurs when the ventricles are abnormally excited before the atria.
PVCs arrhythmia	**1647** Too many premature ventricular contractions, or ____ ____ ____ over a short time period may result in a fatal heart _____ ("absence of rhythm").

brady- tachy-	**1648** Alterations in the speed of the beat or rhythm of the heart are not always disease-related. For example, when the heart has too much "slowness," as indicated by the prefix _____ **(frame 149)**, or when it contracts too "fast," as indicated by the prefix _____ **(frame 149)**, disease is not necessarily present.
brady/**card**/ia (**brahd**-e-**KAR**-dee-ah) tachy/**card**/ia (**tach**-e-**KAR**-dee-ah)	**1649** Employ the prefixes above, the suffix in arrhythmia **(frame 1643)**, and the root in carditis **(frame 1639)** to build _____ / _____ / ____ ("condition of heart slowness") and _____ / _____ / ____ ("condition of heart fastness").
tachycardia bradycardia	**1650** The "rapid" heartbeat of _____ occurs normally during heavy exercise, while _____ is a normal finding among well-trained endurance athletes with strong, "slow" heart contractions.
Information Frame	**1651** Other cardiopathies are directly linked to the heart valves. In general, **murmurs** are abnormal heart sounds related to turbulent flow through valves. Another name for murmur is **bruit** (**BROO**-it).
murmur bruit	**1652** One common cause of _____ or _____ (abnormal heart sound) is **stenosis** (steh-**NOH**-sis).
sten/o/**sis**	**1653** Stenosis is properly dissected as _____ / ____ / _____, with the same "condition of" suffix as in dermatosis **(frame 670)**.
sten condition of abnormal narrowing	**1654** The root in stenosis, _____, means "narrowing." Stenosis therefore translates as a "_____ ____ _____ _____."
stenosis	**1655 Mitral** _____, for example, is an "abnormal narrowing of the mitral" valve.
MS	**1656** Mitral stenosis, abbreviated as ____ ____, may occur after bacterial infection damages the valve flaps, causing an abnormal narrowing of its opening.
mitral stenosis	**1657** Besides MS (_____ _____), the mitral valve may also be affected by **prolapse** (**PROH**-laps), a "falling downward" or reversal.

1658 In **mitral valve prolapse**, abbreviated as ____ ____ ____, the mitral valve flaps "fall downward" in the sense of reversing their usual direction.

mitral valve prolapse

1659 In MVP, or _____ _____ _____, the valve flaps that normally open downward into the left ventricle below, now open upward into the left atrium above. This means that there is a back-leak of blood from the left ventricle up into the left atrium.

mitral valve prolapse

1660 Auscultation with a stethoscope can reveal a heart murmur that may be associated with _____ _____ _____ (MVP).

1661 Now let us examine some aspects of diagnosis for the cardiovascular system.

Lab Tests and Diagnoses

Word Parts Associated with Lab Tests and Diagnoses for the Cardiovascular System

The following is a list of words, word parts, and abbreviations associated with lab tests and diagnoses of cardiovascular problems. Use this list to help you complete **frames 1662 to 1691**.

cardiac MRI	cardiac magnetic resonance imaging	**electr/o**	electric current
ECG	electrocardiogram	**-graphy**	process of recording
EKG	electrocardiogram		

-gram
-graph

1662 There are a number of important procedures for determining the state of health of the heart and vessels. One of these is by making records of various kinds. Recall that _____, the suffix in radiogram **(frame 191)**, as well as _____, the suffix in radiograph **(frame 193)**, can mean "a record."

angi/o/gram (**AN**-jee-oh-gram)
angi/o/graph (**AN**-jee-oh-graf)

1663 Now remove the root from angiopathy **(frame 1598)** and create two terms that mean "(x-ray) record of a vessel":
_____ /____ /_____
_____ /____ /_____

angiogram
angiograph

1664 An _____ or _____ record reveals whether any occlusion of a vessel lumen has occurred. Such a record is displayed in Figure 13.8.

FIGURE 13.8

Example of an Angiogram (Angiograph) (From R. Carlton and A. Adler, *Principles of Radiographic Imaging: An Art and a Science*, Albany, NY: Delmar Publishers Inc, 1992)

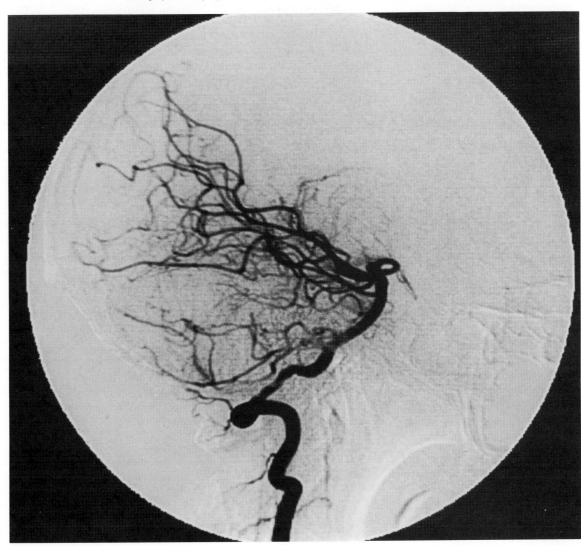

---

cine
-graphy

1665 You may remember that _____, a root in cineradiography **(frame 202)**, means "movies." In addition, remember that _____, a suffix in this same term, denotes "the process of recording."

---

cine/angi/o/cardi/o/graphy
(sin-ee-**an**-jee-oh-**kar**-dee-**AH**-grah-fee)

1666 Build a single long term that means, "the process of recording movies of the vessels and heart":
_____ / _____ / _____ / _____ / _____ / _____.

---

cineangiocardiography

1667 The technique of _____ can reveal, by "moving pictures," the flow of blood through the "heart" and major "vessels."

1668 Other techniques involve the insertion of **catheters** (**KATH**-eh-ters). These are long thin flexible tubes. Catheterization (**kath**-eh-ter-ih-**ZAY**-shun) is the process of inserting a catheter.

cardiac catheterization

1669 If it "pertains to the heart," then this procedure is called

_____ _____.

cardiac catheterization

angiogram
angiograph

1670 The specific process of _____ _____ involves the insertion of a catheter into a vein or artery. The catheter tip is then fed back into a chamber of the heart. This setup allows dyes to be injected. An _____ or _____ ("vessel record") then reveals patterns of blood flow through the coronary arteries.

nuclear magnetic resonance

MRI

1671 Do you remember the diagnostic use of magnetic waves in

_____ _____ _____, or NMR **(frame 214)**? This imaging technique is also called **magnetic resonance imaging**, abbreviated as ____ ____ ____.

magnetic resonance
imaging
**cardiac magnetic resonance
imaging**

1672 If MRI (_____ _____

_____) "pertains to the heart," it is then called

_____ _____

_____, or **cardiac MRI**.

1673 Other means of heart visualization include the **cardiac scan** and **echocardiography** (ek-oh-**kar**-dee-**AH**-grah-fee).

cardiac scan

echo/cardi/o/graphy

1674 The _____ _____ follows the flow of radioactively labeled material through the heart vessels. On the other hand, _____ /_____ /_____ /_____ "records echoes" of sound waves bounced off "cardiac" structures.

cardiac scan
echocardiography

1675 The _____ _____ can help to detect blockage of blood flow radioactively. In _____, gross defects in heart structure can be "recorded" because of the way they deflect sound echoes.

electr/o

1676 Remember that a graph is also an "instrument used to record (something)." Consider _____ /_____ **(frame 216)**, a combining form for "electrical current or activity."

electr/o/cardi/o/graph
(ee-**lek**-troh-**KAR**-dee-oh-graf)

1677 Refering to **frame 190**, build

_____ /_____ /_____ /_____ /_____, an "instrument used to record the electrical activity of the heart."

electrocardiograph	**1678** An _____ machine creates visible waves that indirectly represent the pattern of "electrical" excitation and relaxation of the "myocardium."
electr/o/cardi/o/gram (ee-**lek**-troh-**KAR**-dee-**oh**-gram)	**1679** Employ the suffix in angiogram **(frame 1663)** to build _____ /____ /_____ /____ /_____, "a record of the electrical activity of the heart."
electrocardiogram	**1680** The _____ can be abbreviated as either **EKG** or **ECG**.
E K C G	**1681** The ____ in the abbreviation stands for "electrical activity," the ____ or ____ for "heart," and the ____ for "record." (The **k** derives from the German form of the root for "heart," **kardi**.)
electrocardiogram	**1682** The _____ contains waves of varying size, direction, and duration. These waves can help in the diagnosis of problems affecting heart electrical activity, such as arrhythmias.
EKG ECG	**1683** The ____ ____ ____ or ____ ____ ____ (electrocardiogram) pattern is more likely to reveal arrhythmias during a so-called **stress test**.
stress test	**1684** In the _____ _____, the patient is subjected to the physiological stress of vigorous exercise. If the blood flow to the myocardium is blocked, wave abnormalities may appear.
Information Frame	**1685** The electrocardiogram can be watched continuously by use of a **Holter** (**HOHL**-ter) monitor.
Holter monitor	**1686** The _____ _____ is a compact electrocardiograph strapped to the body.
cardi/o/logy (**kar**-dee-**AHL**-oh-jee) **cardi/o/logist** (**kar**-dee-**AHL**-oh-jist)	**1687** All of these tools are used in the medical science involving the heart. Utilizing the word-synthesizing mode of endocrinology **(frame 1486)** and endocrinologist **(frame 1488)**, build two new heart-related terms: _____ /____ /_____ "study of the heart" _____ /____ /_____ "heart specialist"
cardiology cardiologist	**1688** In _____ ("heart study"), the EKG has come to be an invaluable tool. Any competent _____ ("heart specialist") should be well schooled in its interpretation.

1689 The cardiologist may also do blood chemical evaluations, such as **serum (SEE**-rum) **enzyme tests**.

---

serum enzyme tests

1690 These _____ _____ _____ evaluate the levels of various enzymes released into the bloodstream from dying cardiac muscle.

---

serum enzyme

1691 Use of _____ _____ tests and other means of cardiovascular diagnosis ultimately point to various treatments to alleviate the problems.

Surgery and Therapies

Word Parts Associated with Surgery, Pharmacology, and other Therapies for the Cardiovascular System

The following is a list of word parts and an abbreviation associated with surgery and other therapies for the cardiovascular system. Use this list to help you complete **frames 1692 to 1731**.

fibrill/o	little fiber	**-ive**	pertaining to
nitr/o	nitrogen	**PTCA**	percutaneous transluminal coronary angioplasty
per-	through		

---

hypertension

1692 Both chemotherapy and surgery are often indicated in the treatment of cardiovascular problems. There are millions of people with _____, or "excessive blood pressure" **(frame 1610)**, for example, where chemotherapy is the treatment of choice.

---

hyper/**tens/ive**

1693 The suffix **-ive**, like **-ate**, means "pertaining to (something)." Create a term that "pertains to excessive (blood) pressure": _____ / _____ / _____.

---

hypertensive

1694 Persons with _____ ("high blood pressure") conditions are more likely to suffer from strokes, or cerebrovascular accidents, than are persons with normal blood pressure.

---

anti/hyper/**tens/ive**
(**an**-tee-high-per-**TEN**-siv)

1695 Use **anti-** and produce a new term that "pertains to something against excessive (blood) pressure": _____ / _____ / _____ / _____.

---

antihypertensive

1696 Drugs with _____ properties reduce the blood pressure enough to limit the danger of vessel aneurysms rupturing.

Information Frame	**1697** Various blockers work to reduce excitation of already overstimulated muscle cells. Areas called **beta** (**BAY**-tah) **sites** are present on many cells and serve as receptor sites for epinephrine.
beta-blockers **calcium** **channel blockers**	**1698** Certain drugs, called _____ _____, literally act to "block" the "beta" sites for epinephrine. Further, _____ _____ _____ literally are "blockers" of the "calcium channels."
beta calcium channel	**1699** Both _____-blockers and the _____ _____ blockers serve to relax the smooth muscle fibers in the walls of blood vessels. This relaxation acts to promote the vasodilation of many vessels, causing the blood pressure to fall.
vas/o/dilat/or (**vas**-oh-digh-**LAY**-tor)	**1700** Remove the suffix from abductor **(frame 965)** and consult the word parts of vasodilation **(frame 1509)**. Use these to build _____ / _____ / _____ / _____, "one that widens vessels."
vasodilator	**1701** Any drug that blocks beta sites or otherwise relaxes vascular smooth muscle can be classified as a _____, because it causes "vessels" to "widen."
nitr/ate	**1702** **Nitr/o** (**NIGH**-troh) is the combining form for the element nitrogen. When the root is combined with the suffix **-ate**, _____ / _____ is formed.
nitrates vasodilators	**1703** The nitrogen-containing substances, or _____, are potent vessel wideners, or _____.
nitr/ic	**1704** **Nitric** (**NIGH**-trik) is subdivided as _____ / _____. It literally "refers to nitrogen."
nitric	**1705** The nitrates, being compounds of nitrogen, are all chemically derived from _____ ("referring to nitrogen") **acid**. One especially prominent vasodilator in this group is nitroglycerin (**nigh**-troh-**GLIHS**-er-in).
beta-blockers	**1706** A final important cardiac drug is **digitalis** (**dij**-ih-**TAL**-is). Unlike _____ _____ (blockers of beta sites), digitalis has an excitatory effect. It stimulates the heart to contract without need for additional oxygen.

digit/al (DIJ-ih-tal)	**1707** **Digit** (**DIJ**-it) means "finger." Therefore, _____ / _____ "refers to fingers," where the ending is that in septal **(frame 1557)**.
digitalis digital	**1708** The drug name, _____, is closely related to _____ ("referring to fingers"). The reason is that the drug is named after its plant source—the purple foxglove, or "ladies' fingers" plant.
Information Frame	**1709** Sometimes electrical shocks rather than drugs are employed to correct abnormal heart rhythms. A relevant root in this case is **fibrill** (**FIH**-bril), which means "(contraction of) little fibers." The heart muscle fibers normally contract in unison, many hundreds at a time, as if they were a single fiber—not a bunch of independent "little fibers."
fibrill/a/tion (fih-brih-**LAY**-shun)	**1710** Following the pattern of hallucination **(frame 1176)**, create _____ / _____ / _____, "a process of little fibers (contracting)."
fibrillation	**1711** In _____, many "little fibers" within the myocardium are "contracting" independently, in a chaotic and uncoordinated manner. If severe, a fatal arrhythmia may ensue.
fibrillation de-	**1712** When a person's heart goes into a chaotic _____, it is important to get the heart away from this state. Recall that _____, the prefix in deoxyribose **(frame 507)**, means "away from."
de/fibrill/a/tion (dee-**fih**-brih-**LAY**-shun)	**1713** Therefore, _____ / _____ / _____ / _____ is "the process of (moving) away from (contraction) of little fibers."
defibrillation	**1714** In the emergency room, electrical paddles can be used to apply shock to a patient's chest. The shock may cause a _____ and return the heart to its coordinated rhythm.
angi/o/plasty (**AN**-jee-oh-**plas**-tee)	**1715** Sometimes surgical intervention is required to unplug the lumens of occluded vessels. Remember that keratoplasty **(frame 1355)** is "surgical repair of the cornea." Using the root in angiogram **(frame 1663)**, create _____ / _____ / _____, "surgical repair of the vessels."
angioplasty	**1716** One type of _____ ("vessel repair") is **arterectomy** (**ar**-ter-**EK**-toh-mee).

arter/**ectomy** removal artery	**1717** Referring to **frame 1491**, dissect arterectomy as _____ / _____. It indicates the "_____ of an _____."
arterectomy	**1718** In _____, either all or just a part of an artery is removed. Sometimes, however, just atheromas or other material within an artery can be removed, rather than the artery itself.
end/**arter**/**ectomy** (**end**-ar-ter-**EK**-toh-mee)	**1719** Borrow the prefix from endoplasmic **(frame 519)** and drop its last letter. Now construct a new term, _____ / _____ / _____, the "removal of (material) within an artery."
endarterectomy	**1720** Atheromas may sometimes be removed by _____ from the inner lining of arterial walls.
endarterectomy	**1721** An alternative to _____ ("removal" of material from "within arterial" lumens) is flattening of the occluding material against the inner arterial wall.
Information Frame	**1722** A technique called **balloon catheter dilation** or **percutaneous** (per-kyoo-**TAY**-nee-us) **transluminal** (trans-**LOO**-mih-nuhl) **coronary angioplasty** can be performed.
percutaneous transluminal coronary angioplasty	**1723** The operation of _____ _____ _____ _____ is abbreviated as **PTCA.**
percutaneous per/**cutane**/ous	**1724** The **P** in PTCA stands for _____. This term is subdivided as _____ / _____ / _____, an extension of cutaneous **(frame 621)**.
per-	**1725** The prefix in percutaneous is _____. It means "through."
through skin	**1726** Percutaneous denotes something that moves "_____" unbroken "_____." It indicates that a catheter is fed into an artery or vein to reach a chamber of the heart, rather than breaking the skin over the heart itself.
transluminal **trans**/lumin/**al**	**1727** The **T** in PTCA denotes _____. This term is dissected as _____ / _____ / ____. It is an extension of luminal **(frame 1512)**, with the prefix **trans-**, meaning "across," added.

transluminal	**1728** Within PTCA, _____ indicates that a balloon is inflated from the tip of the inserted catheter, moving "across the lumen" of an occluded coronary artery.
transluminal coronary angioplasty	**1729** After the _____ ("across-the-lumen") balloon is inflated, the atheromas are flattened out against the inner arterial wall. There is thus a _____ ("crown," **frame 1583**) artery _____ ("vessel repair"), indicated by the **CA** in PTCA.
Information Frame	**1730** If the atherosclerosis is too widespread or severe, however, the most drastic solution must be tried: **coronary bypass surgery**.
coronary bypass surgery bypassing	**1731** In _____ _____ _____, vessels from other body areas are grafted onto the affected coronary arteries. Blood then flows into the myocardium by simply _____ or moving around the occluded sections of coronary artery.

Multiple Choice

1. Ather/o refers to

   a. arteries   b. veins   c. joint   d. fat

2. The root for "tiny hair" is

   a. papill   b. capill   c. vascul   d. fibril

3. The term for abnormal "widening" is

   a. stenosis   b. ischemia   c. aneurysm   d. megaly

4. Angina is a direct result of

   a. ischemia   b. cardiomegaly   c. cardiorrhexis   d. aneurysm

5. Another name for "murmur" is

   a. stenosis   b. bruit   c. prolapse   d. angina

6. Surgical repair of the vessels is

   a. venopathy   b. adenoplasty   c. phlebopathy   d. angioplasty

Meanings of Selected Roots

Add the correct combining vowel (cv) after each root. Then write the definition of each root in the space provided.

ROOT/CV	DEFINITION
1. arteri/_____	_____
2. cardi/_____	_____
3. phleb/_____	_____
4. capill/_____	_____
5. angin/_____	_____
6. ather/_____	_____
7. lun/_____	_____
8. systol/_____	_____
9. ven/_____	_____
10. sin/_____	_____

Word Dissection and Translation

Analyze the following terms by dissecting them with slashmarks and identifying their word parts. To the right of each term, write its correct English translation.

Key: R (root), cv (combining vowel), P (prefix), S (suffix)

1. angiogram

_____/_____/_____
       R   cv   S   _____

2. hypercholesterolemia

_____/_____/_____
   P   R   S   _____

3. cineangiocardiography

_____/_____/_____/_____/_____/_____
   R   R   cv   R   cv   S

_____

4. avascular

_____/_____/_____
   P   R   S   _____

5. myocardium

_____/_____/_____/_____
      R   cv   R   S   _____

6. stenosis

_____/_____/_____
      R   cv   S   _____

7. vasodilation

_____/_____/_____/_____
      R   cv   R   S   _____

8. semilunar

_____/_____/_____
   P   R   S   _____

9. electrocardiogram

_____/_____/_____/_____/_____
      R   cv   R   cv   S   _____

10. atherosclerosis

_____/_____/_____
      R   cv   S   _____

11. cardioasthenia

_____/_____/_____
      R   cv   S   _____

12. cardiomalacia

_____/_____/_____
      R   cv   S   _____

Terms and Their Abbreviations

In the list below, when the term is given, write its abbreviation in the space provided. When the abbreviation is given, write its corresponding term.

TERM	ABBREVIATION
1. electrocardiogram	_____
2. _____	CAD
3. atrioventricular	_____
4. _____	MI
5. _____	CHD
6. _____	PVC
7. cardiac magnetic resonance imaging	_____
8. percutaneous transluminal coronary angioplasty	_____

Word Spelling

Look at each of the terms listed below. Identify those that are misspelled by circling Y for "Yes." Write the correct spelling in the blank.

WORD	MISSPELLED?	CORRECT SPELLING
1. tackycardia	Y/N	_____
2. defibrilation	Y/N	_____
3. plhebitis	Y/N	_____
4. arthymia	Y/N	_____
5. paricarditis	Y/N	_____
6. atrioventricular	Y/N	_____
7. cardiologist	Y/N	_____
8. angiapathy	Y/N	_____
9. anuerysm	Y/N	_____
10. infarction	Y/N	_____
11. iscemia	Y/N	_____
12. myokardial	Y/N	_____
13. angiahpathies	Y/N	_____
14. vasoconstriction	Y/N	_____

New Word Synthesis

Using word parts that appear in this and previous chapters, build new terms with the following meanings:

1. _____ process of relaxing around (something)

2. _____ an abnormal narrowing of the heart

3. _____ relating to deficient curved bays

4. _____ pertaining to tissue death

5. _____ rupture of the veins

6. _____ pertaining to a male-producing heart

7. _____ the process of lifting up eggshells

8. _____ abnormal vessel widening

9. _____ removal of little vessels (from) the glands

10. _____ presence of chamber muscle

C ASE S TUDY

Read through the following partial risk assessment for heart disease. Note the terms in bold print. A series of multiple choice questions probes your knowledge of these terms.

Heart Disease Risk Assessment

A young (8-year-old) Caucasian male sought risk assessment from the mobile **cardiology** clinic, accompanied by his mother. The mother was concerned because the father, age 34, had recently suffered **acute myocardial infarction**. A family history revealed a pattern of severe **hypercholesterolemia** and early death from **CAD** for a large number of related males.

Case Study Questions

1. The mobile **cardiology** clinic must have been set up to

   (a) search out reasons for the current AIDS epidemic.

   (b) detect those persons with high risk or early signs of heart disease.

   (c) carry out coronary bypass surgery upon randomly selected clients.

   (d) immunize local children against communicable diseases.

2. The father suffering **acute myocardial infarction** would likely have experienced what preceding symptoms?

   (a) angina pectoris

   (b) gross dermatitis

   (c) femoral atherosclerosis

   (d) facial erythema

3. A pattern of **hypercholesterolemia** is one involving a

   (a) malignancy of blood pressure.

   (b) disease of the skeleton.

   (c) disorder of blood lipid balance.

   (d) deficiency of fat in the blood.

4. Early death from **CAD** is early death because of

   (a) deficiency of calcium.

   (b) chronic artery disease.

   (c) disease of circulating antibodies.

   (d) occlusion of coronary arteries.

CHAPTER 14 The Blood and Lymphatic-Immune Systems

INTRODUCTION

Chapter 13 considered the heart and blood vessels and mentioned the lymphatic system. Chapter 12 provided just a few facts about the immune system and antibodies. Now Chapter 14 looks at the blood and lymph. It also considers the terms of the immune system in much more depth.

The **blood** is a red, sticky, fluid connective tissue that circulates under pressure within the blood vessels. It has a volume of about 5–6 **liters** (**LEE**-ters) or quarts in an average-sized adult. The blood has two major types of components: **formed elements** plus the **blood plasma** (Figure 14.1). The formed elements are fairly large, solid objects in the blood that have a definite shape, or "form." Specifically, these are the blood cells of various kinds and the fragments of the blood cells. Plasma is the watery extracellular fluid of the blood. It surrounds the formed elements and carries them along through the blood vessels.

FIGURE 14.1   **Major Components of the Blood**

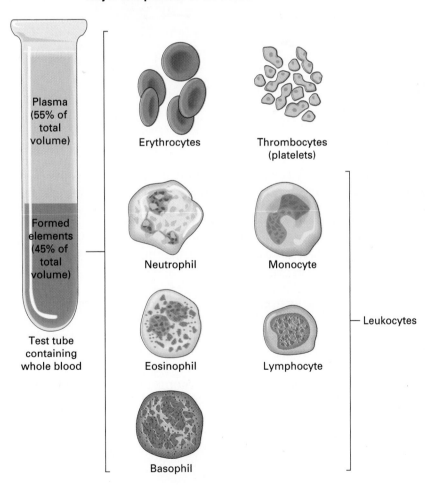

Plasma (55% of total volume)

Formed elements (45% of total volume)

Test tube containing whole blood

Erythrocytes

Thrombocytes (platelets)

Neutrophil

Monocyte

Eosinophil

Lymphocyte

Basophil

Leukocytes

Blood is under continuous pressure from the pumping action of the heart. When the pressure pushes straight ahead, it creates blood flow. Simultaneously, however, the blood pressure exerts force against the walls of the blood vessels. The tiniest blood vessels, the capillaries, have walls that are only one-cell-layer thick. Much fluid escapes out, across the thin walls, every day. The leaked (filtered) material enters the surrounding extracellular fluid. Parallel to the blood capillaries are the lymphatic capillaries. Leaked blood capillary fluid enters the lymphatic capillaries and becomes **lymph (LIMF)**. (See Figure 14.2.)

FIGURE 14.2   **Relationship Between Blood Capillaries and Lymphatic Capillaries**

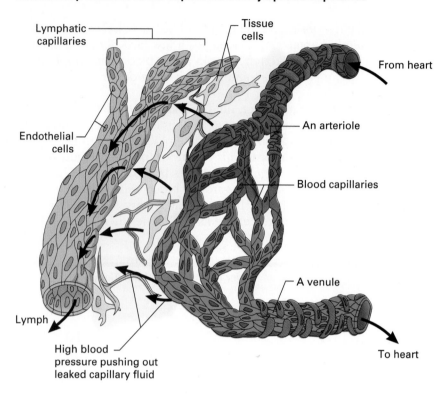

Lymph means "clear spring water," reflecting its watery appearance. This fluid circulates through the lymph nodes and spleen. The **lymph nodes** are small beanlike structures scattered throughout the body. They are especially concentrated in certain areas, such as the cervical, inguinal, and breast regions. With the spleen, the lymph nodes act to filter and cleanse the lymph. Bacteria, cancer cells, or other threatening factors that have leaked out of the bloodstream are usually destroyed and removed by the lymphatic system. Antibodies chemically destroy these factors, and moving macrophages devour them and cell debris. The lymphatic vessels then circulate the cleansed lymph back toward the heart, where it eventually spills into the blood veins. Figure 14.3 provides an overview of the lymphatic circulation.

In summary, the **lymphatic system** includes the lymph, lymphatic vessels, lymph nodes, spleen, and an endocrine gland called the **thymus (THIGH-mus)**. Because this system produces antibodies and includes many macrophages, it is a major part of the body's **immune**, or **self-defense**, **system** against foreign invaders.

This chapter presents terms associated with the normal structure and function, diseases, lab tests and diagnoses, and surgery and other therapies for the blood, lymphatic, and immune systems.

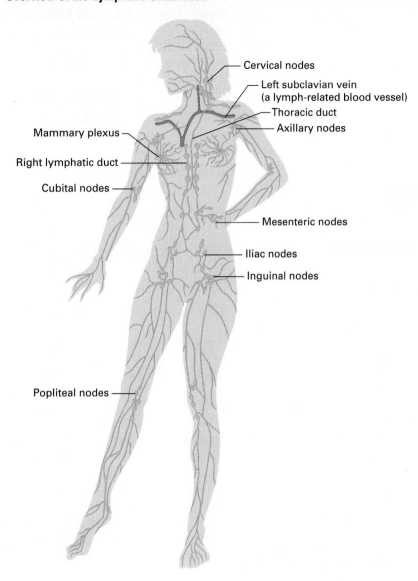

- Cervical nodes
- Left subclavian vein (a lymph-related blood vessel)
- Thoracic duct
- Axillary nodes
- Mammary plexus
- Right lymphatic duct
- Cubital nodes
- Mesenteric nodes
- Iliac nodes
- Inguinal nodes
- Popliteal nodes

CHAPTER OBJECTIVES

By the end of this chapter, you should be able to:

1 Identify major prefixes, roots, suffixes, and abbreviations related to the blood, lymphatic, and immune systems.

2 Dissect blood, lymphatic, and immune terms into their component parts.

3 Translate blood, lymphatic, and immune terms into their common English equivalents.

4 Build new terms associated with the blood, lymphatic, and immune systems.

Word Parts Associated with Normal Structure and Function of the Blood, Lymphatic, and Immune Systems

The following is a list of word parts associated with normal anatomy and physiology of the blood, lymphatic, and immune systems. Use this list to help you complete **frames 1732 to 1787**.

glob/o	globe	**hemat/o**	blood	**-poiesis**	formation of
globul/o	little globe	**lymph/o**	clear spring water	**thromb/o**	clot
hem/o	blood	**lymphat/o**	clear spring water		

---

hem (HEEM)
hemat (HEE-mat)

1732 "Blood" is denoted by two roots on the word list, _____ and _____.

---

hemat/o/poiesis
(**he**-mah-toh-poy-**EE**-sis)

1733 The suffix **-poiesis** (**poy-EE**-sis) indicates the "formation of (something)." Use this fact and the longer root in the preceding frame to help you build _____ /_____ /_____, "formation of blood."

---

hematopoiesis

1734 The process called _____ is responsible for forming both red blood cells and white blood cells.

---

hematopoiesis

1735 The blood cells created by _____ can appear "red," indicated by a root in erythrocyte (eh-**RITH**-roh-**sight**), or "white," denoted by a root in **leukocyte** (**LOO**-koh-**sight**).

---

erythr/o/cyt/e
erythr (eh-RITH-er)
cyt
-e

1736 Erythrocyte is subdivided as _____ /____ /_____ /____, with _____ being a root for "red," _____ a root for "cell," and _____ a one-letter "presence of" suffix. The "cell" root is that found in cytoplasm **(frame 489)**, while the suffix is that in microscope **(frame 427)**.

---

leuk/o/cyt/e
erythrocyte
leuk (LOOK)

1737 Similarly, leukocyte is subdivided as _____ /____ /_____ /____. It contains the same "cell" root and suffix as _____. Its root for "white" is _____.

---

erythrocytes
leukocytes

1738 "Red (blood) cells," or _____, are far more numerous than the _____, or "white (blood) cells."

---

erythrocyte
leukocyte

1739 Each _____ owes its "reddish" appearance to the occurrence of a particular substance. Each _____ appears "whitish" when viewed under the microscope because it has a fairly clear cytoplasm.

---

glob/in (GLOH-bin)

1740 **Glob (GLOHB)** is a root meaning "globe." The term _____ /____ means "a substance that" is a "globe," much as myelin **(frame 1081)** means "a substance that (resembles) marrow."

Chapter 14 The Blood and Lymphatic-Immune Systems

globin **hem/o/glob/in** (**HEE**-moh-**gloh**-bin)	**1741** The term _____ ("globe-substance") can be combined with the shorter root for "blood" in **frame 1732**. The result is _____ /____ /_____ /____, "a substance that" is a "globe" in the "blood."
hemoglobin	**1742** Molecules of _____ are large and "globe"-shaped and carry oxygen in the erythrocytes of the "blood."
hemoglobin	**1743** The approximately 250 million _____ molecules contained within an erythrocyte turn a bright cherry red when they combine with oxygen. These molecules basically give blood its red appearance.
little	**1744** A **globul** (**GLAHB**-yool) is a "_____ globe," much as vascul (**frame 1114**) is a "little vessel."
globul/in (**GLAHB**-yoo-lin)	**1745** Create a new term for "a substance that" is a "little globe": _____ /____.
globulins	**1746** The _____ are a group of **plasma proteins** (proteins outside blood cells, in the surrounding plasma). They are named for their fairly globular shape.
globulins	**1747** One group of these proteins, the **gamma** (**GAH**-muh) _____, act as important antibodies against foreign bacteria and other invaders.
anti- -gen	**1748** Recall that _____, the prefix in antibody, means "against." The suffix _____, as in estrogen (**frame 1403**), means "produce."
anti/gen (**AN**-tih-jen)	**1749** Now build _____ /_____, which means "produced against."
antigen	**1750** An _____ is a chemical marker on the surface of a cell. It serves to identify cells as either familiar to the body or foreign to it. If the immune system identifies cells as foreign, then antibodies are "produced against" them.
antigens	**1751** When a person is exposed to certain _____ and produces antibodies against them, protection is often acquired. Recall that immun (**frame 1473**) means "not serving (disease)."
immun/ity (ih-**MYOO**-nih-tee)	**1752** Using -ity for "condition of," construct _____ /_____, "a condition of not serving (disease)."
immunity	**1753** The condition called _____ does "not serve disease" in the sense that it represents a large degree of protection.

immunity	**1754** Resistance, or _____, to a particular disease is often acquired when one develops antibodies against the antigens on the cells of the invaders.
lysis	**1755** When antigens are attacked, the cells carrying them may be "broken down." Remember that _____ **(frame 539)** is "a breakdown," as of cells.
hem/o/lys/is (hee-**MAHL**-ih-sis)	**1756** Adopting one of the roots in hemoglobin allows us to construct _____ /_____ /_____ /_____, "a breaking down of blood (cells)."
hemolysis	**1757** Although _____ literally denotes a "breaking down of blood" in general, in practical use it indicates the breaking down of erythrocytes, which are so common.
hemolysis	**1758** When erythrocytes not compatible with a person's blood type are transfused, the recipient's antibodies will attack their antigens. This attack results in _____ of the transfused erythrocytes. The red blood cells break down as their surface antigens are being destroyed.
Information Frame	**1759** Where do the attacking antibodies come from? They are produced by the plasma cells. These **plasma** cells are highly specialized derivatives of the **lymphocytes** (**LIM**-foh-sights), or "clear spring water cells."
lymph/o/cyt/e	**1760** Lymphocyte is dissected as _____ /_____ /_____ /_____, similar to the dissection of erythrocyte **(frame 1736)**.
lymphocytes	**1761** As their name indicates, the _____ are often found within the lymph. These cells are actually a particular type of leukocyte.
mono-	**1762** Try to retrieve the **m**-beginning prefix, _____, which, like uni- **(frame 80)**, means "single" or "one."
mono/cyt/e (**MAHN**-oh-sight)	**1763** A _____ /_____ /_____ is a type of white blood "cell" that has a "single," large nucleus.
monocyte	**1764** The single nucleus of the _____ may have the shape of a horseshoe.
lymphocytes monocytes	**1765** Both _____ and _____ are types of leukocytes that are either directly or indirectly involved with protecting the body from foreign invaders.

lymph	**1766** **Lymphat** (lim-**FAT**), like _____ , denotes "clear spring water."
lymphat/ic	**1767** The term _____ /_____ "refers to lymph" much as aortic **(frame 1576)** "refers to lifting up."
lymphatic	**1768** It was mentioned in the Introduction to this chapter that the capillaries of the _____ system largely travel parallel to the capillaries of the cardiovascular system.
lymphatic	**1769** The _____ ("referring to lymph") tissue contains lymphocytes, monocytes, and other cell types.
Information Frame	**1770** Certain lymphatic tissue occurs in masses at the posterior wall of the nose and throat. One good example, the **tonsils** (**TAHN**-sils), are literally "little stakes" located within this body area.
tonsils	**1771** As Figure 14.4 reveals, however, the _____ are actually oval, almond-shaped masses of lymphatic tissue.
tonsils	**1772** The ancient Arabs, in fact, called the _____ the "almonds of the throat"!

FIGURE 14.4 **The Tonsils**

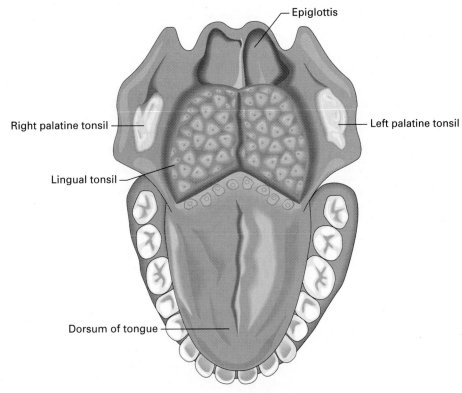

aden thyroid	**1773** Hypertrophy of lymphatic tissue produces a "glandlike" appearance. Chapter 12 told you that _____ **(frame 1458)** is "gland," and you probably remember the suffix in _____ ("shield-like," **frame 1383**).
aden/**oid** (**AD**-eh-noyd)	**1774** Use the appropriate word parts from the above frame to help you construct _____ /_____ , "glandlike."
adenoids	**1775** The _____ are enlarged, "gland-resembling" masses of lymphatic tissue in the back of the throat, posterior to the nose.
adenoids	**1776** Hypertrophy of the _____ in young children may become so great that it actually interferes with their breathing.
Information Frame	**1777** Besides having lymphatic tissue in various places to promote immunity, the body protects itself from uncontrollable bleeding by forming clots. **Thromb (THRAHMB)** is a root for "clot."
thromb/in (**THRAHM**-bin)	**1778** Following the word-constructing pattern of globin **(frame 1740)** results in _____ /_____ , "a substance that" is involved in "clots."
thrombin	**1779** The active clotting substance in the bloodstream is called _____.
thromb/o/cyt/es (**THRAHM**-boh-sights)	**1780** Also involved in forming clots are the _____ /_____ /_____ /_____ or "clot cells present" within the blood.
thrombocytes	**1781** The _____ ("clot cells") are actually just small fragments of certain large, disintegrated bone marrow cells. Their alternate name is **platelets** (**PLAYT**-lets), since they look like "little plates."
thromb/us (**THRAM**-bus)	**1782** Thromb generally takes the "presence of" suffix in sinus **(frame 1534)**. The result is _____ /_____ , "a clot."
thrombus	**1783** Thrombocytes, thrombin, and various other clotting factors interact to produce a _____ , or "clot present" within a vessel.
thrombus	**1784** A _____ is technically a stationary blood clot. It usually serves to plug a hole in the wall of a broken blood vessel. This plug stops any further blood loss.

serous	**1785** Retrieve the knowledge that _____ (**frame 665**) is an **s**-beginning word that means "watery." The root in this term commonly takes -um rather than -us as its noun-forming ending.
ser/um (**SEER**-um)	**1786** Create _____ /_____ for "presence of (something) watery."
serum	**1787** We can describe _____ as the clear "watery" portion of the plasma that remains after a thrombus has been formed.

Diseases

Word Parts Associated with Diseases of the Blood, Lymphatic, and Immune Systems

The following is a list of word parts and abbreviations describing disease states of the blood, lymphatic, and immune systems. Use this list to help you complete **frames 1788 to 1860**.

AIDS	acquired immunodeficiency syndrome	**embol/o**	plug	**-ile**	relating to (something)
		febr/o	fever		
		hemorrhag	bleed	**phil/i**	abnormal attraction or fondness
edem/o	swelling	**HIV**	human immunodeficiency virus		
edemat/o	swelling				

hem/o/rrhag/e	**1788** Clotting is useful in that it stops **hemorrhage** (**HEM**-eh-rij). This term can be dissected as _____ /_____ /_____ /_____, where the suffix is the same as in lymphocyte (**frame 1760**).
-o/rrhagia	**1789** It will be helpful to recall that _____ /_____ (**frame 147**) is a suffix for "a bursting forth."
hemorrhage	**1790** It is then quite easy to translate _____ as "a bursting forth of blood." It contains a word element closely related to -o/rrhagia.
hemorrhage	**1791** The problem of _____ can be life-threatening if too much blood is lost.
hem/o/rrhag/ic (hem-oh-**RAJ**-ik)	**1792** Borrow the suffix in lymphatic (**frame 1767**) and construct _____ /_____ /_____ /_____, "relating to bursting forth of blood."
hemorrhage hemorrhagic	**1793** A person with _____ is undergoing bleeding from ruptured vessels. This person is obviously suffering from a _____ (bleeding) condition.

phil/ia (**FIL**-ee-ah)	**1794** **Phil (FIL)** is a root for "attraction" or "fondness." If we add the ending in phobia **(frame 1178)** we obtain _____ / _____ .
philia	**1795** Opposite to the way in which phobia denotes "an abnormal condition of insane fear," _____ denotes "an abnormal condition of attraction or fondness."
hem/o/phil/ia (**hee**-moh-**FIL**-ee-ah)	**1796** Extract an appropriate root from hemorrhage and construct _____ / _____ / _____ / _____ for "an abnormal condition of fondness for bleeding."
hemophilia	**1797** The disease called _____ involves extensive and uncontrolled bleeding.
phil/i/ac (**FIL**-ee-ak)	**1798** Use **phil/i** (**FIL**-ee) rather than phil and append the suffix of cardiac **(frame 1546)**. The result is _____ / _____ / _____ , which "refers to fondness or attraction (for something)."
philiac **hem/o/phil/i/ac** (**hee**-moh-**FIL**-ee-ak)	**1799** Just as we added to philia to produce hemophilia, add to _____ ("referring to fondness") to get _____ / _____ / _____ / _____ / _____ , "referring to a fondness for bleeding."
hemophilia hemophiliac	**1800** A person afflicted with _____ ("abnormal fondness for bleeding") can be called a _____ .
hemophiliac hemophilia	**1801** Although labeling someone as a _____ , (one with a "fondness" for "bleeding") may seem cruel, the name is appropriate in a certain sense. The person with _____ , on the face of it, appears to be very "fond" of bleeding! If not, then why does such a person keep bleeding and bleeding after suffering only minor cuts?
-penia	**1802** The real reason for uncontrolled bleeding is a lack or deficiency of certain clotting factors. Search in your memory for the **p**-beginning suffix _____ **(frame 143)** for "poverty," or a deficiency of something.
platelets thrombocytes	**1803** Recall that _____ ("little plates," **frame 1781**) or _____ ("clot cells," **frame 1780**) are cell fragments necessary for clot formation.
thromb/o/cyt/o/penia (**thram**-boh-sight-oh-**PEE**-nee-ah)	**1804** A new term, _____ / _____ / _____ / _____ / _____ , denotes a "poverty of clot cells."

leukocyte

leuk/o/cyt/o/penia
(**loo**-koh-**sigh**-toh-**PEE**-nee-ah)
leuk/o/penia (**loo**-koh-**PEE**-nee-ah)

1805 Briefly return to _____, or "white blood cell" (**frame 1737**). Create two other related terms:

_____ / _____ / _____ / _____ / _____ a "poverty of white cells"

_____ / _____ / _____, a "poverty of white (things)"

---

leukocytopenia
leukopenia
thrombocytopenia

1806 Both _____ and _____ indicate a "deficiency" of "white" blood "cells," while _____ indicates a "deficiency" of "thrombocytes," or platelets.

---

leukocytopenia
leukopenia

1807 Leukocytes are involved in the body's immune response. Therefore _____ or _____ will likely result in a diminished immunity to disease.

---

thrombocytopenia
hemorrhaging

1808 Thrombocytes are important in the process of blood clotting. Therefore _____ may well result in a diminished ability of the blood to clot and stop _____ (bleeding).

---

thromb/o/sis (thrahm-**BOH**-sis)

1809 Regardless of the number of white cells, a thrombus can usually form. Adopt the ending in stenosis (**frame 1653**) and synthesize _____ / _____ / _____, "a condition of clotting."

---

thrombosis

1810 A "condition of clotting," or _____, can be helpful, if it staunches severe hemorrhaging. It can be harmful, however, if the resulting clot partially or totally occludes a vessel lumen.

---

thrombosis

1811 The clotting process of _____ can also be associated with an inflammation of the veins.

---

phlebitis

1812 Remind yourself that _____ (**frame 1640**) is an "inflammation of the veins."

---

thromb/o/phleb/itis
(**thram**-boh-flee-**BIGH**-tus)

1813 Use the information of **frames 1809** and **1812** to create _____ / _____ / _____ / _____, "inflammation of a vein (that involves) a clot."

---

thrombophlebitis

1814 President Nixon was said to suffer from a bad case of _____ ("inflammation of veins with clots").

---

thrombophlebitis

1815 The pathology of _____ ("inflamed veins with clots") is especially common in the great veins of the lower leg.

Information Frame

1816 **Embol** (**EM**-bul) is a root meaning "plug." It implies a moving or dislodged plug of material that passes through blood vessels until it gets stuck again.

embol/us (**EM**-boh-lus)

1817 An _____ /_____ is "a plug" just as a thrombus is "a clot."

---

embolus

1818 Technically, an _____ is "a plug" (blood clot, air bubble, clump of bacteria) that travels through the bloodstream until it occludes a narrow vessel.

---

embol/ism (**EM**-boh-lizm)

1819 Adopt the ending of hyperthyroidism **(frame 1447)** and make _____ /_____, a "condition of (having) a plug."

---

embolus
embolism

1820 Note that _____ is an actual moving "plug" in the bloodstream, while _____ denotes the "condition" of having such a "plug."

---

embolism

embol/i (**EM**-boh-ligh)

1821 The disease of _____ can be very dangerous, if essential vessels become "plugged" by one or more dislodged _____ /_____ (the plural of embolus, which forms like the plural of bacillus, **frame 546**).

Information Frame

1822 If lymphatic vessels become blocked, then the fluid spilling out of the blood capillaries continues to pool and accumulate in the surrounding tissues. The result is **edem/a** (eh-**DEE**-mah), "a swelling."

---

edem (eh-**DEEM**)
edemat (eh-**DEM**-at)

1823 The word list provides two similar roots for "swelling." One is _____, the other, _____.

---

edema

1824 An _____ ("swelling present") in the arms and legs is a common complication of lymph vessel blockage or removal.

---

edemat

edemat/ous (eh-**DEM**-ah-tus)

1825 The longer root for "swelling," _____, usually assumes the "pertaining to" suffix of venous **(frame 1529)**. The result is _____ /_____, "pertaining to swelling."

---

edema
edematous

1826 The term _____ is a noun indicating "a swelling," while _____ is an adjective that "refers to" such a "swelling."

---

edematous

1827 Blockage of lymphatic vessels by a tumor can sometimes result in an _____ ("swollen") condition of the affected area.

---

lymph

lymph/oma (limf-**OH**-mah)

1828 Use the shorter _____ rather than longer lymphat **(frame 1766)** root, plus the suffix in adenoma **(frame 1461)**, to write out _____ /_____, "a tumor of clear spring water."

---

hemat **hemat/oma** (**hee**-mah-**TOH**-mah)	**1829** Use the longer root for "blood," _____, rather than hem (**frame 1732**) to create _____ / _____, "a tumor of blood."
lymphoma hematoma	**1830** A _____ is an actual neoplasm of lymphatic tissue. A _____, however, is not really a tumor of blood. Rather, it is a partially clotted, tumorlike mass of blood that has hemorrhaged out of a vessel.
sarcoma	**1831** Lymphatic tissue is considered a type of connective tissue. You may remember that a _____, or "fleshy tumor" (**frame 573**) is a malignant neoplasm of connective tissue.
lymph/o/sarc/oma (**limf**-oh-sar-**KOH**-mah)	**1832** Build _____ / ____ / _____ / _____, a "fleshy tumor of clear spring water."
lymphoma lymphosarcoma	**1833** A _____ is really a benign tumor of lymphatic tissue, while a _____ is a malignant one.
lymphosarcoma -emia	**1834** A _____ is a type of malignant neoplasm afflicting lymph rather than blood. Recall that _____, the suffix in hyper-cholesterolemia (**frame 1593**), means a "blood condition of."
leuk/emia (loo-**KEE**-mee-ah)	**1835** Borrow the root from leukopenia (**frame 1805**) and synthesize _____ / _____, an "(abnormal) condition of white blood."
leukemia	**1836** The disease called _____ is actually a malignant neo-plasm of the bone marrow. Highly accelerated abnormal hematopoiesis (formation of blood) in the marrow results in way too many leukocytes. Therefore the disease is named after "white blood."
leukemia	**1837** The "blood" of a person with _____ contains excessive "leukocytes" with grossly abnormal structure and function.
an/emia (ah-**NEE**-mee-ah)	**1838** There are many abnormal conditions of the blood besides leukemia. Some of these involve a lack of particular things. Extract the "without" prefix from anesthesia (**frame 265**) and, using the "blood condition" suffix of leukemia (**frame 1835**), construct ____ / _____, "a con-dition without blood."
anemia	**1839** In _____, blood is still present, but there is a reduction in certain factors associated with the blood.
anemia	**1840** In iron-deficiency _____, for instance, there is not enough iron consumed in the diet. The result is a great lack of iron-containing hemoglobin in all the erythrocytes produced.

1841 Weakness is one common symptom of anemia. It is also a symptom of **infectious mononucleosis (mahn-oh-noo-klee-OH-sis)** and of **acquired immunodeficiency (im-yoo-noh-dee-FISH-en-see) syndrome.**

---

acquired immunodeficiency syndrome

1842 **AIDS** is the familiar abbreviation for the dreaded disease called

_____ _____ _____ _____ .

AIDS

1843 Acquired immunodeficiency syndrome (____ ____ ____ ____) is becoming a much more common cause of death.

---

mononucleosis

1844 **Infectious** _____, though generally not fatal, can cause the victim to experience temporary weakness.

---

mono/**nucle**/o/sis

1845 When you realize that it contains the same suffix as thrombosis **(frame 1809)**, you should be able to dissect mononucleosis as

_____ / _____ / _____ / _____ .

---

mononucleosis

1846 Infectious _____ is an enlargement of the spleen and lymph nodes accompanied by excessive numbers of "monocytes" with atypical cell "nuclei" in the blood. It is "infectious," or "catching."

---

febr (FEE-ber)
pyr
pyret

1847 A frequent symptom of mononucleosis is fever. An **f**-beginning root on the word list, _____, like the two **p**-beginning roots _____ and _____ **(frame 153)**, means "fever." A new suffix, **-ile (IGHL)**, means "relating to (something)."

---

febr/ile (FEHB-ril)

1848 Take advantage of the above facts to construct _____ / _____, an **f**-beginning term that "relates to fever."

---

febrile

1849 A _____ ("feverish") state is characteristic of many infectious diseases.

---

febrile
febr/is (FEE-bris)

1850 The root of _____, febr, usually takes the same "presence of" ending as pectoralis **(frame 987)**. The result is _____ / ____, "presence of fever."

---

febris

1851 The "presence of a fever" (_____) suggests mononucleosis or some other type of infection or inflammation.

---

febris
acquired immunodeficiency syndrome

1852 Chronic _____ ("fever") is frequent among

_____ _____ _____

(AIDS) patients, because their greatly weakened immunity leaves them susceptible to many infections.

---

viral	**1853** Both AIDS and mononucleosis are _____ ("pertaining to poison," **frame 535**) in origin. AIDS is caused by infection with the **human immunodeficiency virus**.
human immunodeficiency virus	**1854** The AIDS-causing organism, _____ _____ _____, is the subject of much intense worldwide study.
HIV	**1855** The human immunodeficiency virus, abbreviated by the three letters ____ ____ ____, attacks and progressively destroys the effectiveness of a person's immune system.
HIV	**1856** The chief problem in AIDS, caused by the ____ ____ ____ organism, is a dramatic decline in protective antibodies. The patient is simply no longer able to chemically protect him- or her- "self."
auto- immunity	**1857** The **a**-beginning prefix _____, if you remember **(frame 85)**, means "self" or "own." Also recall that _____ **(frame 1752)** is "a condition of not serving (disease)."
auto/**immun**/ity (**aw**-toh-ih-**MYOO**-nih-tee)	**1858** Putting the above word elements together yields _____ / _____ / _____.
autoimmunity	**1859** In diseases of _____, the problem is not lack of antibodies. Rather, the difficulty is that we mistakenly manufacture antibodies against our "own" tissues or "self."
autoimmunity	**1860** Certain arthritic conditions, for example, result when _____ causes production of antibodies that attack one's own synovial membranes.
	1861 Lab tests can quickly reveal autoimmunity or other abnormalities in our immune apparatus.

Lab Tests and Diagnoses

Word Parts Associated with Lab Tests and Diagnoses for the Blood, Lymphatic, and Immune Systems

The following is a list of word parts and abbreviations related to diagnoses and lab tests for disorders involving the blood, lymphatic, and immune systems. Use this list to help you complete **frames 1862 to 1894**.

CBC	complete blood count	**-crit**	separation	**ESR**	erythrocyte sedimentation rate
centrifug/o	fleeing from the center	**ELISA**	enzyme-linked immunosorbent assay	**PT**	prothrombin time

biopsy	**1862** There are various ways to extract and examine the cells in the lymph and blood. One technique is called **bone marrow** _____ ("vision of life," **frame 582**).
bone marrow biopsy	**1863** In the technique of _____ _____ _____, the sternum or some other bone is punctured. A needle is inserted, and a sample of marrow is aspirated out.
bone marrow biopsy	**1864** The sample extracted by _____ _____ _____ is examined and a determination is made of the types and number of leukocytes present within the bone marrow. Another blood cell assessment is the **complete blood count**.
CBC	**1865** A complete blood count, abbreviated as ____ ____ ____, is a tally of all major cell types occurring in a certain volume of blood.
complete blood count	**1866** The CBC, or _____ _____ _____, involves an identification and counting of all the different cell types as they occur together in the blood.
Information Frame	**1867** It may be desirable for the different types of blood cells to be physically separated from one another for analysis. The suffix -**crit** (**KRIT**) means "separation."
hemat/o/crit (hee-**MAT**-uh-krit)	**1868** Employ the root in hematopoiesis **(frame 1733)** to help you synthesize _____ /____ /_____, a "separation of blood."
hematocrit	**1869** The _____ is technically defined as the volume of erythrocytes spun out and packed down from whole blood. It is usually expressed as the percentage of the total blood volume that consists of erythrocytes.
hematocrit	**1870** Average values of the _____ at sea level are 42% for women and 47% for men.
Information Frame	**1871** **Centrifug** (**SEN**-trih-fyooj) means "fleeing from the center." This root commonly takes the "presence of" ending in monocyte **(frame 1763)**.
centrifug/e (**SEN**-trih-fyooj)	**1872** Thus _____ /____ is "a fleeing from the center."
centrifuge	**1873** A _____ is a revolving machine that spins solid materials in solution "away from the center" of the machine and out into test tubes.

centrifuge	**1874** The _____ allows one to separate out erythrocytes from leukocytes according to their differing weights. This procedure makes it possible to measure the hematocrit (erythrocytes alone).
erythrocyte	**1875** Another useful measure is the _____ ("red cell") **sedimentation rate**.
erythrocyte sedimentation rate	**1876** The _____ _____ _____ indicates the rate at which erythrocytes "settle out," or **sediment**, after whole blood is spun around in a centrifuge.
ESR **hemat**/o/**logy** (hee-mah-**TAHL**-oh-jee)	**1877** Such measures as the CBC and _____ _____ _____ (erythrocyte sedimentation rate) are useful topics for clinical "study of the blood." Just as cardiology **(frame 1687)** is "study of the heart," _____ / _____ / _____ is "study of the blood."
hemat/o/**logist** (hee-mah-**TAHL**-oh-jist)	**1878** Just as a cardiologist **(frame 1687)** is "one who specializes in the study of the heart," a _____ / _____ / _____ is "one who specializes in the study of the blood."
Hematology hematologists	**1879** Some hospitals have a Department of _____, where _____ are employed doing blood work.
hematology hematologists	**1880** The discipline of _____ ("blood study") and its professional practitioners, the _____, have some concern with antibodies—at least as they appear in the bloodstream.
immunity	**1881** Antibodies elsewhere fall under a different specialization of study. They are closely connected to body _____ **(frame 1752)**, "a condition of not serving (disease)."
immun/o/**logy** (**im**-yoo-**NAHL**-oh-jee) **immun**/o/**logist** (**im**-yoo-**NAHL**-oh-jist)	**1882** Technically speaking, _____ / _____ / _____ is the "study of (factors) not serving (disease)," while an _____ / _____ / _____ is "one who specializes in the study of (factors) not serving (disease)."
hematology hematologist immunology immunologist	**1883** An analysis of blood clotting is more likely to fall under the discipline of _____ (hematology/immunology) and be studied by a(n) _____ (hematologist/immunologist). An analysis of antigen-antibody reactions within areolar connective tissue is more likely to fall under the discipline of _____ (hematology/immunology) and be evaluated by a(n) _____ (hematologist/immunologist).

1884 One aspect of hematology is an examination of the ability of the blood to clot. **Prothrombin** (proh-**THRAHM**-bin) time is one such measure.

---

thrombin

pro/thromb/in

1885 Recall that _____ **(frame 1778)** is "a substance that clots." This information should help you subdivide prothrombin as _____ /_____ /_____.

---

pro-
prothrombin

1886 Since it incorporates _____, or "before" **(frame 82)** as its prefix, _____ translates as "a substance that (is present) before a clot."

---

prothrombin

1887 Another way of looking at _____ is that it is the substance present in the bloodstream "before thrombin" appears. It is this substance that is converted to the active clotting enzyme, thrombin, after a tear in a blood vessel wall.

---

prothrombin time

1888 We can speak of _____ _____ **(PT)** as the amount of "time" required "before a clot" appears, after the addition of calcium to a blood sample. The faster this time, the greater the clotting ability of the blood.

---

serum

1889 Recall that the _____ **(frame 1786)** is the "watery" portion of the blood plasma remaining after a clot has been formed.

---

hematology
ser/o/logy (see-**RAHL**-oh-jee)

1890 Much as _____ is the "study of blood" as a whole, _____ /____ /_____ is "the study of" blood "serum" and its components.

---

serology

1891 The discipline of _____ includes the study of blood antibodies, since these remain after a clot has developed.

ELISA

1892 One special test on the serum is called **enzyme-linked immunosorbent** (ih-**myoo**-noh-**SOR**-bent) **assay**. The five-letter abbreviation for this test is _____ _____ _____ _____ _____.

---

enzyme-linked immunosorbent
assay

1893 The _____-_____ _____ _____ or ELISA, is a test for the presence of antibodies to the HIV organism in persons suspected of being infected with AIDS.

ELISA
immunology
immunology

1894 The enzyme-linked immunosorbent assay (_____ _____ _____ _____ _____) and other measures are carried out in the science of _____, or "the study of not serving (disease)," **(frame 1882)**. The discipline of _____ actually is the "study of the immune" system and its problems. The next set of frames looks at some terms describing treatments for such problems.

Word Parts Associated with Surgery, Pharmacology, and Other Therapies for the Blood, Lymphatic, and Immune Systems

The following is a list of word parts and an abbreviation associated with surgery, pharmacology, and other therapies for the blood, lymphatic, and immune systems. Use this list to help you complete **frames 1895 to 1927**.

-ant one that

AZT azidothymidine; drug used to treat AIDS

coagul/o curdle

splen/o spleen

---

immune

1895 A deficiency in the _____ **(frame 1477)** or "not serving (disease)" system can be somewhat corrected by various drugs.

AZT

1896 One helpful immune-boosting drug is called **azidothymidine** (ah-**zid**-oh-**THIGH**-mih-deen), abbreviated by the three letters ____ ____ ____ .

---

azidothymidine

1897 The drug _____ (AZT) is often administered in the treatment of AIDS.

AZT
leukemia

1898 Azidothymidine, or ____ ____ ____ , is not very effective, however, in the treatment of _____ ("abnormal condition of white blood," **frame 1835**). For this disease, a **bone marrow transplant** may be performed.

---

bone marrow transplant

1899 The operation of _____ _____ _____ removes malignant bone marrow and replaces it with healthy marrow from a compatible donor.

Information Frame

1900 Rather than being transplanted, diseased or damaged lymphatic or cardiovascular structures sometimes must be removed. Do you remember the suffix used for "removal of"?

---

splen (SPLEN)

1901 Take, for example, the "spleen," which is represented by the **s**-beginning root _____ on the word list.

---

splen/ectomy (splee-**NEK**-toh-mee)

1902 The correct term for "removal of the spleen" is _____ / _____.

---

aden

adenectomy

1903 Now consider the lymph nodes. In a sense, these nodes are very much like "glands," indicated by the root _____ **(frame 1458)**. Remember that "removal of glands" is denoted by _____ **(frame 1491)**.

---

lymph/aden/ectomy (**limf**-ah-den-**EK**-toh-mee)	**1904** Now create a new term, one that means "removal of lymph glands": _____ / _____ / _____.
lymphadenectomy splenectomy	**1905** The operation of _____ may be performed to remove tumorous lymph nodes. In contrast, _____ is an operation for removing a spleen that is ruptured and dangerously hemorrhaging.
Information Frame	**1906** A great many terms describe treatments for clotting disorders. **Coagul** (koh-**AG**-yool) means "curdle." The "curdling" of milk, blood, or any other substance is the process of changing a liquid into a soft, lumpy, jelly-like solid. This process is part of what happens during blood clotting.
coagul/a/tion (koh-**ag**-yoo-**LAY**-shun)	**1907** Adopting trephination **(frame 1213)** as your model, create _____ / ____ / _____, the "process of curdling."
coagulation	**1908** The "curdling process," or _____, is a synonym (word with similar meaning) for clotting.
coagulation	**1909** In _____ (clotting), the fluid blood "curdles" into a jelly-like, semisolid blob—a thrombus.
Information Frame	**1910** There is always something that is doing the coagulation or clotting. The suffix **-ant (ant)** denotes "one that."
coagul/ant (koh-**AG**-yoo-lant)	**1911** A _____ / _____ literally is "one that curdles."
coagulants	**1912** The blood "curdlers," or _____, promote clotting.
coagulants coagulation	**1913** The administration of _____ ("curdlers") to promote _____ ("curdling or clotting") is justified when the patient might otherwise experience excessive hemorrhaging.
coagulants	**1914** Quite often, however, any promotion of clotting is dangerous. In atherosclerosis of the coronary arteries, for instance, administration of _____ may cause abnormal thrombi to form, totally occluding the already narrowed arterial lumens.
anti/coagul/ant (**an**-tigh-koh-**AG**-yoo-lant)	**1915** Extract the prefix from antigen **(frame 1749)** and build _____ / _____ / _____, "one that (is) against curdling."

anticoagulant	**1916** Whereas a coagulant substance promotes blood clotting, an _____ substance acts "against clotting."
anticoagulant	**1917** The _____ drugs inhibit new clot formation or dissolve old clots.
Information Frame	**1918** Anticoagulant drugs come in two basic types: **direct-acting anticoagulants** and **indirect-acting anticoagulants**.
direct-acting indirect-acting	**1919** As their name clearly states, the _____-_____ anticoagulants prevent activation of clotting factors by "acting directly" upon the blood itself. The _____-_____ anticoagulants, in contrast, do not act directly upon the blood. Rather, they operate by preventing the synthesis of clotting factors within the liver, before they ever reach the bloodstream.
indirect-acting	**1920** **Coumadin** (**KOO**-mah-din) acts primarily on the processes of protein synthesis within the liver. Therefore, it is an example of the _____-_____ (direct-acting/indirect-acting) anticoagulants.
direct- acting	**1921** **Heparin** (**HEP**-ar-in) interferes with the initiation of the blood-clotting process itself. Hence, it is an example of the _____-_____ (direct-acting/indirect-acting) anticoagulants.
lys/is **thromb/o/lys/is** (thrahm-**BAHL**-ih-sis)	**1922** A large thrombus already blocking the lumen of a vessel may be broken down and dissolved before it causes severe tissue necrosis downstream. Recall that _____ /____ **(frame 539)** is "a breaking down." Build _____ /____ /_____ /____, "a breaking down of clots or thrombi."
thrombolysis	**1923** Anticoagulants that speed up _____ ("breaking down of thrombi") may work in time to spare the life of a heart attack victim.
adjective	**1924** **Lyt/ic** (**LIT**-ik) is a(n) _____ (noun/adjective) that "pertains to breaking down."
thromb/o/lyt/ic (**thrahm**-boh-**LIT**-ik)	**1925** Consequently, _____ /____ /_____ /____ "pertains to breaking down clots."
thrombolytic	**1926** A technique called _____ **therapy** involves the use of medications to quickly dissolve stubborn blood clots.
thrombolytic therapy	**1927** Examples of specific agents employed in _____ _____ are **tissue plasminogen** (plas-**MIN**-oh-jen) **activator**, abbreviated as **tPA**, and a drug called **streptokinase** (strep-toh-**KIGH**-nays).

Multiple Choice

1. A suffix meaning "formation of" is

   a. -poiesis   b. penia   c. -ity   d. -o/rrhagia

2. A combining form for "white" is

   a. leuk/o   b. erythr/o   c. thromb/o   d. embol/o

3. A term that means "clot cell" is

   a. coagulocyte   b. embolocyte   c. thrombocyte   d. lymphocyte

4. An expert in the "watery portion of blood" is a

   a. pathologist   b. immunologist   c. dermatologist   d. serologist

5. Edema means

   a. nodal tissue   b. gland-like   c. tissue swelling   d. half lymph

6. A traveling clot is an example of

   a. embolism   b. thrombosis   c. thrombophlebitis   d. phlebitis

Meanings of Selected Roots

Add the correct combining vowel (cv) after each root. Then write the definition of each root in the space provided.

ROOT/CV	DEFINITION
1. lymph/_____	_____
2. ser/_____	_____
3. phil/_____	_____
4. leuk/_____	_____
5. hemat/_____	_____
6. coagul/_____	_____
7. febr/_____	_____
8. thromb/_____	_____
9. erythr/_____	_____
10. glob/_____	_____

Word Dissection and Translation

Analyze the following terms by dissecting them with slashmarks and identifying their word parts. To the right of each term, write its correct English translation.

Key: R (root), cv (combining vowel), P (prefix), S (suffix)

1. immunity

    _____/_____   _____
         R   S

2. serology

    _____/_____/_____   _____
         R   cv   S

3. thrombin

    _____/_____   _____
         R   S

4. leukocytopenia

    _____/_____/_____/_____/_____   _____
         R   cv   R   cv   S

5. mononucleosis

    _____/_____/_____/_____   _____
       P   R   cv   S

6. hematocrit

    _____/_____/_____   _____
         R   cv   S

7. lymphadenectomy

    _____/_____/_____   _____
         R   R   S

8. coagulation

    _____/_____/_____   _____
         R   cv   S

9. febrile

    _____/_____   _____
         R   S

10. autoimmunity

    _____/_____/_____   _____
       P   R   S

11. centrifuge

    _____/_____   _____
         R   S

12. embolectomy

    _____/_____   _____
         R   S

Terms and Their Abbreviations

In the list below, when the term is given, write its abbreviation in the space provided. When the abbreviation is given, write its corresponding term.

TERM	ABBREVIATION
1. complete blood count	_____
2. _____	HIV
3. acquired immunodeficiency syndrome	_____
4. enzyme-linked immunosorbent assay	_____
5. azidothymidine	_____

Word Spelling

Look at each of the terms listed below. Identify those that are misspelled by circling Y for "Yes." Write the correct spelling in the blank.

WORD	MISSPELLED?	CORRECT SPELLING
1. airithrohsite	Y/N	_____
2. hematopoiesis	Y/N	_____
3. hematology	Y/N	_____
4. antigen	Y/N	_____
5. hemoreage	Y/N	_____
6. thrombosis	Y/N	_____
7. emballous	Y/N	_____
8. heatmatoma	Y/N	_____
9. immunology	Y/N	_____
10. glabyoulens	Y/N	_____
11. auntiecoagulants	Y/N	_____
12. hemophiliac	Y/N	_____
13. lymphosarcoma	Y/N	_____
14. thrombolitic	Y/N	_____

New Word Synthesis

Using word parts that appear in this and previous chapters, build new terms with the following meanings:

1. _____ a substance that is a little globe of clots
2. _____ a breaking down of glands
3. _____ white-producer
4. _____ a bursting forth of clear spring water
5. _____ a condition of abnormal fondness for plugs
6. _____ pertaining to breakdown of the heart
7. _____ a fleshy tumor of whiteness
8. _____ pertaining to fleeing from the center
9. _____ formation of red blood cells
10. _____ hemorrhage of the spleen

C ASE S TUDY

Read through the following partial report for hematology. Note the terms in bold print. A series of multiple choice questions probes your knowledge of these terms.

Hematology Report

A 35-mL specimen of **coagulated** blood was brought down to the lab this morning. A large **thrombus** was extracted and the remaining **serum** analyzed. No significant numbers of **autoantibodies** could be detected.

Case Study Questions

1. By **coagulated**, it was meant that the blood was

   (a) lacking in erythrocytes.

   (b) already clotted.

   (c) undergoing rapid hemolysis.

   (d) frozen to preserve its integrity.

2. A large **thrombus** means that

   (a) vessel occlusion in the body must have occurred.

   (b) extensive hemorrhaging was present.

   (c) prothrombin was converted into thrombin.

   (d) streptokinase was unusually active.

3. Analysis of the **serum** suggests that

   (a) a determination of blood hemoglobin concentration was carried out.

   (b) no monocytes could ever have been present in the whole blood.

   (c) cardiology rather than serology was the major focus.

   (d) the watery material around the clot was investigated.

4. No significant numbers of **autoantibodies** probably indicates that

   (a) no blood-borne autoimmune diseases were present.

   (b) the patient was having a severe transfusion reaction.

   (c) a mild form of leukemia was afflicting the patient.

   (d) antibodies were directly attacking many of the patient's own body tissues.

8

CHAPTER 15 The Respiratory System

INTRODUCTION

The **respiratory** (**RES**-pir-ah-**toh**-ree) **system** is a collection of organs that together regulate the acid-base balance in the bloodstream, provide oxygen for cellular energy, and remove carbon dioxide produced by cellular metabolism. Its major organs include the lungs, nose, throat, and the so-called **respiratory tree**. This respiratory tree somewhat resembles an inverted (upside down) olive tree—or so Hippocrates, the Father of Modern Medicine, thought! Look at Figure 15.1 and see if you agree. Note that the olive tree is composed of branches, which in the respiratory tree are the air passageways of varying diameters. At the end of the narrowest branches are olives. On the respiratory tree, one finds **alveoli** (al-**VEE**-oh-ligh)—rounded air sacs—instead.

One might well ask what this inverted respiratory tree is doing. Most of the passageways can be compared to the ventilation shafts in a building. That is, they bring fresh oxygen-rich air into the lungs and carry stale oxygen-poor air out of the lungs. The key to the whole process is shown in Figure 15.2. It reveals that **respiration**, or gas exchange, goes on between the air in the alveoli and the blood in the pulmonary capillaries. The **pulmonary capillaries** are extremely thin-walled members of the pulmonary circulation (mentioned in Chapter 14). The walls of the alveoli are also remarkably thin. Because of the very close proximity of the alveoli and pulmonary capillaries, there is a net diffusion of gases between them. Specifically, there is a net diffusion of oxygen molecules out of the oxygen-rich air in the alveoli into the blood of the pulmonary capillaries. When these oxygen molecules combine with hemoglobin in the erythrocytes, the blood turns a bright reddish color. The red blood circulates to other body tissues. There oxygen diffuses out of the blood into the tissue cells. There is a net diffusion of carbon dioxide out of the tissue cells and into the blood of the systemic capillaries. The blood of the systemic capillaries turns a dark bluish color. Finally, the blue blood from the systemic capillaries circulates back to the lungs and enters the pulmonary capillaries. Many carbon dioxide molecules diffuse across their walls and enter the alveoli. When the person exhales, some of this carbon dioxide-rich air is expelled into the external environment.

This chapter looks further at some of the structural and functional characteristics of the respiratory system. Terms describing its anatomy, physiology, diseases, lab tests, diagnoses, and therapies are examined.

The Respiratory Tree

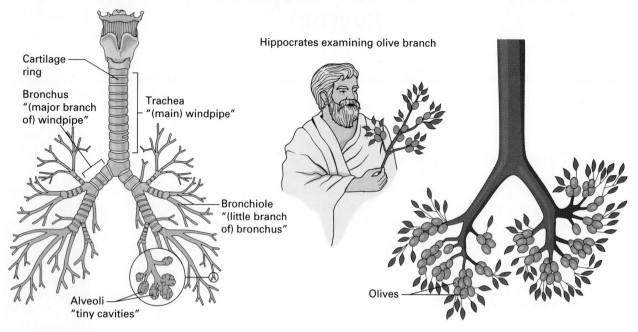

Cartilage ring

Bronchus "(major branch of) windpipe"

Trachea "(main) windpipe"

Bronchiole "(little branch of) bronchus"

Alveoli "tiny cavities"

Hippocrates examining olive branch

Olives

Respiratory ("characterized by breathing again") tree

Inverted olive tree

The Process of Respiration

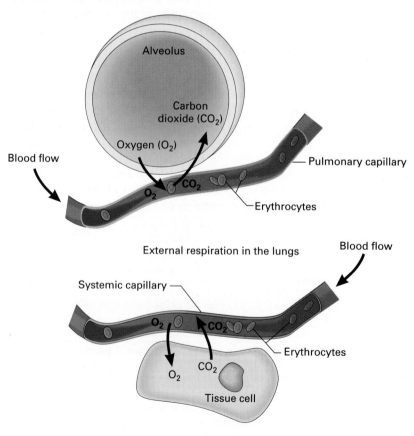

Alveolus

Carbon dioxide (CO_2)

Oxygen (O_2)

Blood flow

Pulmonary capillary

O_2 CO_2

Erythrocytes

External respiration in the lungs

Blood flow

Systemic capillary

O_2 CO_2

O_2 CO_2

Tissue cell

Erythrocytes

Internal respiration at the cell

By the end of this chapter, you should be able to:

1 Identify major prefixes, roots, suffixes, and abbreviations related to the respiratory system.

2 Dissect respiratory terms into their component parts.

3 Translate respiratory terms into their common English equivalents.

4 Build new terms associated with the respiratory system.

Normal A & P	

Word Parts Associated with Normal Structure and Function of the Respiratory System

The following is a list of word parts associated with normal anatomy and physiology of the respiratory system. Use this list to help you complete **frames 1928 to 1994**.

acid/o	sour	**bronchiol/o**	little (branch of) bronchus	**pneumon/o**	lung
alkal/i	ashes of plants			**pulmon/o**	lung
alveol/o	tiny cavity	**nas/o**	nose	**rhin/o**	nose
bas/o	base; foundation or stepping	**pharyng/o**	throat	**spir/o**	breathe
		pharynge/o	throat	**trache/o**	(main) windpipe
bronch/o	(major branch of) windpipe	**pleur/o**	rib	**ventil/o**	fan; blow
		pneum/o	air; lungs		

---

nas/o (NAY-zoh)
rhin/o (RIGH-noh)

1928 For breathing of air, it is only natural to start with the "nose." This structure is denoted by two combining forms on the word list, _____ /_____ and _____ /_____.

---

nas/al (NAY-zal)
rhin/al (RIGH-nal)

1929 Both roots for "nose" assume the "pertaining to" ending in digital **(frame 1707)**. This suffix results in two terms that "pertain to the nose," _____ /_____ and _____ /_____.

---

nasal
rhinal

1930 External _____ or _____ (nose) anatomy is essentially that of a pointed box of cartilage, covered with skin and adipose tissue, and graced with a pair of nostrils.

---

pharyng (fahr-INJ)
pharynge (fahr-IN-jee)

1931 Posterior to the nose and the mouth lies the "throat," indicated by the two roots _____ and _____.

1932 Both of these roots are the basis of the entire term **pharynx** (fahr-**INKS**)—"throat."

---

pharynx

1933 The _____ ("throat") is a common passageway for food, liquid, and air, since it lies dorsal to both the nose and the cavity of the mouth.

---

pharynge/al (fah-**RIHN**-jee-al)

1934 Using the longer root for "throat" **(frame 1931)**, adopt the suffix of nasal and create _____ /____, "referring to the throat."

---

pharyngeal
larynx

1935 The basic _____ ("throat") anatomy is that of a large tapered tube that leads downward to the _____, or "voicebox" **(frame 1317)**.

---

larynx

1936 The _____ ("voicebox") is a boxlike collection of nine carti-lage plates interlinked by connective tissue fibers. This box contains the **vocal cords** for making speech and other voice sounds.

---

thyroid
thyroid

1937 The _____ ("shield-resembling") **cartilage** of the larynx, like each major lobe of the _____ gland **(frame 1383)**, has a shape resembling a shield. Refer to Figure 2.1. (In this case the shield is a single, large, doorlike one.)

Information Frame

1938 The thyroid cartilage of the larynx was named after its resemblance to a long doorlike shield used by ancient Greek soldiers. (Even earlier, doors themselves were used as shields!) This shield covered the soldier from his neck all the way down to his legs, and it bore a deep notch for his chin at its top. You can see the resemblance in Figure 2.1.

---

edema

1939 Caudal to the larynx is the **trachea** (**TRAY**-kee-uh), or "main wind-pipe." This term contains the same "presence of" suffix as _____ ("a swelling," **frame 1822**).

---

trache/a

1940 Trachea is properly dissected as _____ /____.

---

trachea
trache

1941 The noun _____ denotes "presence of the main wind-pipe." Its root, _____, can combine with the "referring to" ending in pharyngeal **(frame 1934)**, to create an adjective.

---

trache/al (TRAY-kee-al)	**1942** Create a new term, _____ /_____, that "refers to the main windpipe."
trachea tracheal	**1943** The _____ (main "windpipe") bears a number of **U**-shaped _____ rings composed of cartilage.
tracheal	**1944** These _____ rings continue down onto the right and left **bronchi** (**BRAHN**-kigh), the two smaller "windpipes" that are branches of the trachea.
bronch/us (BRAHNG-kus) embol/us	**1945** The singular of bronch/i is _____ /_____, just as the singular of embol/i ("plugs") is _____ /_____ **(frame 1817)**.
bronchus	**1946** Each _____ penetrates the medial wall of a lung.
bronchi	**1947** Together, the two _____ carry air directly into and out of the right and left lungs.
bronchus	**1948** Within a lung, each _____ subdivides into a series of smaller branches, the bronchioles (**BRAHNG**-kee-ohls).
bronchiol/es arterioles	**1949** Bronchioles is analyzed as _____ /_____, the same way as the _____, or "little (branches) of the arteries" **(frame 1520)**.
bronchioles	**1950** The _____ are the "little (branches) of the bronchi."
bronchioles	**1951** The trachea and bronchi have rigid walls. But the walls of the _____ ("little bronchi") are flexible, because they mostly lack the rigid cartilage rings.
bronchiol (BRAHNG-kee-ohl)	**1952** The root of bronchioles, _____, usually assumes the "pertaining to" suffix in arteriolar **(frame 1520)**.
bronchiol/ar (brahng-kee-OH-lar)	**1953** We can therefore write _____ /_____ for "pertaining to little (branches) of the bronchi."

bronchiolar	**1954** Tracheal diameter is inflexible, while _____ ("little bronchi") diameter can vary considerably.
bronch	**1955** The flexibility of the bronchioles allows them to constrict at some times, dilate at others. The bronchi have a limited ability to change their diameters as well. The root for bronchus, _____, is often used in naming processes of narrowing and widening.
bronch/o/constrict/ion (**brahng**-koh-kun-**STRIK**-shun) **bronch/o/dilat/ion** (**brahng**-koh-digh-**LAY**-shun)	**1956** Use the above information to help you build two new terms: _____ / ____ / _____ / _____, a "process of narrowing of the bronchi" _____ / ____ / _____ / _____, a "process of widening of the bronchi" Appropriate models for word-building are vasoconstriction and vasodilation (**frame 1509**), respectively.
bronchodilation bronchoconstriction	**1957** During exercise, _____ ("widening of the bronchi") occurs, allowing more air to enter the lungs. When a nonsmoking person is forced to inhale cigarette smoke or some other toxic material, _____ ("narrowing of the bronchi") occurs.
alveoli bronchoconstriction bronchodilation	**1958** You may remember from the Introduction that the _____ are the rounded air sacs in the lungs. The bronchioles, and indirectly, the bronchi, lead down into these tiny air sacs. Therefore, _____ (bronchoconstriction/bronchodilation) reduces air flow into these tiny sacs, while _____ (bronchoconstriction/bronchodilation) increases air flow into them.
alveol/us (al-**VEE**-oh-lus) bronchus	**1959** The singular of alveol/i is _____ / ____, just as the singular for bronchi is _____ (**frame 1945**).
alveol (al-**VEE**-ohl)	**1960** The root in alveolus, _____, means "tiny cavity."
alveolus alveoli	**1961** Each _____ is a microscopic, thin-walled air sac. These _____ ("tiny cavities") form the terminal portion of the respiratory tree.
alveol/ar (al-**VEE**-oh-lar)	**1962** Borrow the suffix from bronchiolar (**frame 1953**) and construct _____ / ____, "pertaining to tiny cavities."

alveolar	**1963** The major _____ ("tiny cavity") function is respiration.
re/**spir**/**a**/**tion**	**1964** **Spir (SPIR)** is a root for "breathe." **Re- (REE)** is a prefix for "again." Use these facts to help you dissect respiration as _____ / _____ / _____ / _____. The combining vowel and suffix appeared earlier in amputation **(frame 950)**.
respiration	**1965** The literal translation of _____ is the "process of breathing again."
respiration	**1966** The term _____ indicates that breathing is a repetitive process, occurring again and again (**re-**).
Information Frame	**1967** **Ventil (VEN**-til) is a root meaning "fan" or "blow." In modern usage, it is more correct to say that we "fan" or "blow" air into and out of the lungs as we breathe.
ventil/**a**/**tion** (ven-tih-**LAY**-shun)	**1968** Adopting respiration as your word-building model, create _____ / _____ / _____, the "process of fanning or blowing."
ventilation respiration	**1969** Technically, _____ is the process of sucking air into the lungs or "blowing" air out of the lungs. (Think of a ventilation system in a modern office building.) "Breathing again" (_____), however, is considered the process of gas exchange between different body compartments.
respiration	**1970** The alveoli, being extremely thin-walled, have _____ (ventilation/respiration) as their primary function. That is, oxygen gas molecules within each alveolus diffuse into a different compartment, the blood in a pulmonary capillary. The carbon dioxide molecules within the pulmonary capillary blood diffuse in the opposite direction, entering the alveolus. Thus, oxygen and carbon dioxide gas molecules are exchanged between the alveolar and blood compartments.
ventilation	**1971** The rest of the respiratory tree (the trachea, bronchi, and bronchioles) has _____ (ventilation/respiration) as its key function. The reason is that these passageways are simply too thick-walled to permit effective gas exchange to occur. (Respiration and ventilation are diagrammatically compared in Figure 15.3.)

FIGURE 15.3   **Respiration versus Ventilation**

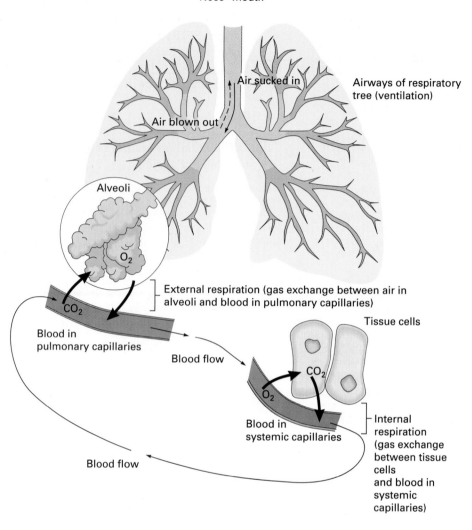

Nose–mouth

Airways of respiratory tree (ventilation)

Air sucked in

Air blown out

Alveoli

O_2

CO_2

External respiration (gas exchange between air in alveoli and blood in pulmonary capillaries)

Blood in pulmonary capillaries

Blood flow

Tissue cells

CO_2

O_2

Blood in systemic capillaries

Internal respiration (gas exchange between tissue cells and blood in systemic capillaries)

Blood flow

---

out

1972 We know that **in-** is a prefix for something going "into," while **ex-** is a prefix denoting something going "_____."

---

in/**spir**/a/**tion** (**in**-spir-**AY**-shun)
ex/**pir**/a/**tion** (**eks**-pir-**AY**-shun)

1973 This knowledge helps us build two new terms, again using respiration as our model:

____ /_____ /____ /_____   the "process of breathing in"
____ /_____ /____ /_____   the "process of breathing out"
Note that in the second term, the initial **s** of spir has been dropped.

---

inspiration
expiration

1974 "Breathing in," or _____ and "breathing out," or
_____ are actually aspects of ventilation rather than respiration!

---

inspiration
expiration

1975 You can think of _____ as the sucking of air "into" the lungs and of _____ as the blowing of air "out" of the lungs. Each process is a different phase of ventilation.

1976 Respiration affects the **acid-base balance** of the bloodstream. An **acid** is something "sour," as in lemon juice. A **base**, or **alkal/i** (**AL**-kah-ligh), is a substance originally derived from the "ashes of plants" that had been burned! The root, **bas** (**BAYS**), denotes a "foundation" or "stepping."

---

acid/ic (ah-**SID**-ik)
bas/ic (**BAYS**-ik)
alkal/ine (**AL**-kah-lin)

1977 Use the suffix in thrombolytic **(frame 1925)** to help you synthesize _____ /____, or "referring to (something) sour," and _____ /____, or "referring to a foundation or stepping." Employ **-ine** to create _____ /_____, "a substance (in) the ashes of plants."

---

acidic
bases
alkali

1978 Chemically speaking, _____ substances are those that may taste "sour," but also donate H^+ (hydrogen) **ions**. The _____ ("foundations") or _____ ("ashes of plants") are substances that donate **hydroxyl** (high-**DRAHKS**-ul), or OH^- ions.

---

basic
alkaline

1979 The human blood is considered to be slightly _____, or _____, in that it has a fairly high proportion of OH^- ions.

---

acid

alkali

1980 The substance H_2CO_3 is an example of an _____ (alkali/acid) because it gives off H^+ ions. The substance **NaOH**, in contrast, is classified as an _____ (alkali/acid) because it gives off hydroxyl ions.

---

respiration

1981 Carbon dioxide (CO_2) in the bloodstream reacts with water to produce H_2CO_3 **(carbonic acid)**. When CO_2 leaves the blood and enters the alveoli during _____ (ventilation/respiration), the production of this acid in the body falls.

---

expiration

1982 When _____ ("breathing out") occurs, this exchanged (CO_2) is released from the body.

---

pneumon/o (**NOO**-mah-noh)
pulmon/o (**PUL**-mah-noh)
pneum/o (**NOO**-moh)

1983 Processes of both respiration and ventilation take place within the lungs. According to the word list, two **p**-beginning combining forms for "lung" are _____ /____ and _____ /____. The combining form for "air" is _____ /____.

---

pulmonary

1984 You have seen the second of these "lung" roots (when listed in alphabetical order) plus the suffix in coronary **(frame 1582)** before. You may remember the phrase _____ ("pertaining to the lung," **frame 1584**) circulation.

pulmonary	**1985** Proper _____ ("lung") function is necessary if acid-base balance in the body is to be maintained.
rib	**1986** When the lungs expand, they press against the internal surfaces of the ribs. **Pleur/o (PLOO-roh)**, like cost **(frame 855)**, means "_____."
pleur/a (PLOO-rah)	**1987** Create _____ /____ for "a rib," just as you wrote out trachea **(frame 1940)** for "a (main) windpipe."
pleuras (PLOO-rahs)	**1988** Remember that terms ending in -a can form plurals by adding an -s Therefore we can say that the _____ are serous membranes associated with the "ribs."
pleur/al (PLOO-ral)	**1989** The root in pleura can take the ending of costal **(frame 856)** for its "relating to" suffix. This combination results in _____ /____, "relating to the ribs."
pleural	**1990** The _____ ("rib") **cavity** is the area within the thoracic cavity that contains the lungs.
viscera pariet	**1991** The lungs are examples of _____, that is, "guts" or internal organs **(frame 405)**. When the lungs inflate, they press against the "wall" of the thoracic cavity. Recall that _____ **(frame 404)** is a **p**-beginning root for "wall."
visceral **parietal**	**1992** You may also remember **(frame 404)** that _____ "pertains to guts," while _____ "pertains to a wall."
parietal pleura **visceral pleura**	**1993** Combine the information from **frames 1987, 1988,** and **1992** and name two related body structures: _____ _____ the serous membrane lining the interior "wall" of the "ribs" _____ _____ the serous membrane covering the lungs and some other "guts or internal organs" within the thoracic cavity
visceral pleura parietal pleura	**1994** When the lungs inflate during inspiration, the _____ _____ covering the lungs comes very close to the _____ _____ lining the ribs and chest wall.
	1995 Even though the parietal and visceral pleuras provide some protection, along with the ribs, the components of the respiratory system are not immune to disease or injury.

Word Parts Associated with Diseases of the Respiratory System

The following is a list of word parts and an abbreviation related to diseases of the respiratory system. Use this list to help you complete **frames 1996 to 2026**.

catarrh/o	running down; a runny nose	**emhysem/o**	blowing up (with air)
COPD	chronic obstructive pulmonary disease	**emhysemat/o**	blowing up (with air)
		-pnea	breathing

1996 The word list at the beginning of the chapter contains roots that can be combined with the suffix from thrombophlebitis **(frame 1813)** to indicate "inflammation of" various respiratory structures. See how many of these terms of "inflammation" you can create:

rhin/itis (righ-**NIGH**-tis)

_____ /_____ "inflammation of the nose" (using rhin in **frame 1928**)

bronch/itis (brahng-**KIGH**-tis)
pleur/itis (ploo-**RIGH**-tis)
pneumon/itis (noo-mah-**NIGH**-tis)

_____ /_____ "inflammation of bronchi"
_____ /_____ "inflammation of the pleuras"
_____ /_____ "inflammation of the lungs," using pneumon

sinus/itis (sigh-nus-**IGH**-tis)

_____ /_____ "inflammation of a sinus" (using sinus itself)

1997 Several of the **-itis** terms in the preceding frame have alternative names. "Inflammation of the pleuras," _____, is also called **pleurisy** (**PLOO**-rih-see). "Inflammation of the lungs," _____, is more commonly referred to as **pneumonia** (noo-**MOHN**-yuh). Remember that **-ia** is a suffix meaning "(abnormal) condition of" **(frame 1616)**.

pleuritis

pneumonitis

1998 A refinement of pneumonia is _____ /_____ /_____ /_____, a compound term that adds the root in bronchus to "abnormal condition (inflammation) of the bronchi and lungs."

bronch/o/pneumon/ia
(**brahng**-koh-noo-**MOHN**-yuh)

1999 "Inflammation of the nose," or _____, is often called **coryza** (kor-**EE**-zuh), "head cold."

rhinitis

2000 **Catarrh** (kah-**TAR**) translates as "running down." In modern usage, however, it generally indicates a "runny" nose. This is a frequent symptom of rhinitis, or _____ ("head cold").

coryza

2001 A _____ ("runny" nose) or stuffed-up nose can make it very hard to breathe. An adjective using this term takes the ending in pleural **(frame 1989)**.

catarrh

2002 A _____ /_____ inflammation of the lining of the nose results in a flow or "running down" of mucus from the nostrils.

catarrh/al (kah-**TAR**-al)

2003 Such _____ ("running down") symptoms may also occur during _____ ("inflammation of" the nasal "sinuses").

catarrhal
sinusitis

pleuritis pleurisy	**2004** Taking a swim in extremely cold water can result in _____ **(frame 1996)**, "inflammation of the pleuras." This condition is also called _____ **(frame 1997)**.
bronchitis	**2005** Chronic irritation of the bronchi from the particles in cigarette smoke is a major cause of _____ ("inflammation of the bronchi," **frame 1996**).
pneumonitis pneumonia bronchopneumonia	**2006** Potentially much more serious is _____ ("inflammation of the lungs"), also called _____ ("abnormal condition of the lungs," **frame 1997**). When bronchitis is also present, a state of _____ ("abnormal condition of the bronchi and lungs," **frame 1998**) is said to exist.
COPD	**2007** A bad case of bronchitis or bronchopneumonia may create bulky mucous plugs that block the airways. This blockage sometimes results in **chronic obstructive pulmonary disease**, abbreviated as ____ ____ ____ ____.
chronic obstructive pulmonary disease	**2008** Like a case of coryza, a case of _____ _____ _____ (COPD) can severely interfere with normal breathing.
Information Frame	**2009** The noun suffix (root + suffix), **-pnea** (puh-**NEE**-uh), indicates "breathing." Certain prefixes are used with it to describe different states of breathing.
-pnea a/pnea (**AP**-nee-uh) dys/pnea (**DISP**-nee-uh) brady/pnea (**brad**-ip-**NEE**-uh) tachy/pnea (**tak**-ip-**NEE**-uh)	**2010** Some examples using _____ ("breathing") are ____ /_____ "lack of breathing" (using the prefix in avascular, **frame 1532**) _____ /_____ "difficult breathing" (using the prefix in dysplasia, **frame 558**) _____ /_____ "slowness of breathing" (using the prefix in bradycardia, **frame 1649**) _____ /_____ "fastness of breathing" (using the prefix in tachycardia, **frame 1649**)
dyspnea	**2011** "Difficult breathing," or _____, occurs with COPD.
apnea	**2012** Sleep _____ is a halting ("lack") "of breathing" during sleep.
tachypnea brachypnea	**2013** Emotional overexcitement may lead to _____ ("fastness of breathing"), while extreme mental depression may be associated with _____ ("slowness of breathing").
pneum thorax hem	**2014** Various other problems involving the lungs can lead to dyspnea or apnea. Recall that _____, a shorter version of pneumon, is a root for "lungs" or "air." Also remember that the _____ **(frame 396)** is the "chest." Remind yourself that the root for "blood" in hemoglobin **(frame 1741)** is _____.

pneum/o/thorax
(**noo**-moh-**THOH**-raks)
hem/o/thorax
(**hee**-moh-**THOH**-raks)

2015 Employ the facts in the previous frame to help you build two new terms: _____ / ____ / _____ , or "air (in) the chest," and _____ / ____ / _____ , or "blood (in) the chest."

pneumothorax

hemothorax

2016 The problem of _____ is that air trapped within the chest, but outside the lungs, tends to compress the lungs and make them difficult to inflate. (See Figure 15.4.) Similarly, _____ is a condition where blood external to the lungs tends to push them flat.

FIGURE 15.4   **An Example of Pneumothorax** (From R. Carlton and A. Adler, *Principles of Radiographic Imaging: An Art and a Science,* Albany, NY: Delmar Publishers Inc., 1992)

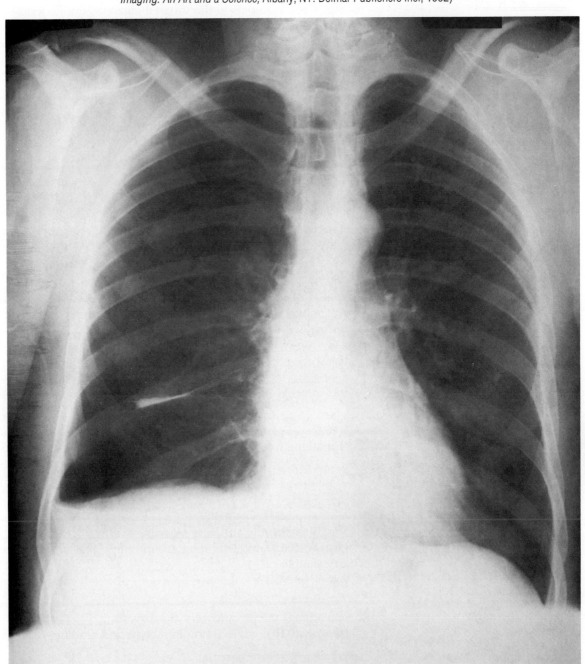

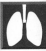

alveoli

2017 Another problem interfering with normal breathing is an excessive dilation, or "blowing up," of the _____ ("tiny cavities," **frame 1961**). Two roots, **emphysem** (em-fih-**SEEM**) and **emphysemat** (em-fih-**SEE**-mat), denote a "blowing up" with air.

emphysem/a (**em**-fih-**SEE**-mah)
emphysemat/ous
(**em**-fih-**SEHM**-ah-tus)

2018 Borrow the ending from pleura (**frame 1987**) and add it to emphysem, and borrow the ending from venous (**frame 1529**) and add it to emphysemat. The results are _____ /_____ and _____ /_____ , respectively.

emphysema

emphysematous

2019 The disease of _____ is an excessive "blowing up" or dilation of the alveoli. This often happens as a result of chronic smoking. Toxic materials in the inhaled cigarette smoke tend to break down the connective tissue fibers in the walls of the alveoli. This breakdown causes _____ changes, inducing the alveoli to overfill and remain "blown up." Expiration of this accumulated air is difficult.

tachypnea

2020 Emphysema may contribute to _____ (**frame 2010**) or "abnormally fast (and shallow) breathing."

ventilation

hyper-
hypo-

2021 After heavy exercise, breathing rapidly and deeply is normal. Recall that _____ (**frame 1968**) is the "process of fanning or blowing," that is, breathing. Now if something is "excessive," as in hypertension (**frame 1610**), we indicate that by the prefix _____. If something is "deficient," as in hypotension (**frame 1610**), we indicate that by the prefix _____.

hyper/ventil/a/tion
(**high**-per-ven-tih-**LAY**-shun)
hypo/ventil/a/tion
(**high**-poh-ven-tih-**LAY**-shun)

2022 Assemble the information from the above frame and create two new terms:
_____ /_____ /_____ /_____ ,
the "process of excessive fanning or blowing"
_____ /_____ /_____ /_____ ,
the "process of deficient fanning or blowing"

hyperventilation
hypoventilation

2023 "Breathing excessively" for current metabolic needs is called _____. "Breathing deficiently" for such needs is called _____.

bradypnea

hypoventilation

2024 "Breathing" softly and very "slowly," with _____ (**frame 2010**), after running around the block at break-neck speed, is an example of _____.

tachypnea

hyperventilation

2025 "Breathing" deeply and very "fast," with _____ (**frame 2010**), while sitting in a chair and reading, is an example of _____.

hyperventilation
hypoventilation

2026 Either _____, which "blows" off "too much" CO_2, or _____, which "blows" off "too little" CO_2, can disturb acid-base balance and produce a morbid state.

Word Parts Associated with Lab Tests and Diagnoses for the Respiratory System

The following is a list of word parts and an abbreviation associated with lab tests and diagnoses for respiratory problems. Use this list to help you complete **frames 2028 to 2046**.

ral/o	rattle	**SOB**	shortness of breath
respir/o	breathing again	**sput/o**	spit
rhonch/o	snore		

Information Frame

2027 There are special instruments and processes for examining and measuring various aspects of the respiratory system.

---

arthroscope

arthroscopy

bronch/o/scop/e
(**BRAHNG**-koh-skohp)
laryng/o/scop/e
(lah-**RIHN**-goh-skohp)
bronch/o/scopy
(brahng-**KAHS**-koh-pee)
laryng/o/scopy
(lah-rihn-**GAHS**-koh-pee)

2028 For instance, using the suffixes from _____ ("an instrument used to examine joints," **frame 923**) and _____ ("the process of examining joints," **frame 925**) and the appropriate roots from bronchus (**frame 1945**) and otolaryngology (**frame 1318**), build these terms:

_____ /____ /_____ /____ "an instrument used to examine a bronchus"

_____ /____ /_____ /____ "an instrument used to examine the voicebox"

_____ /____ /_____ "the process of examining a bronchus"

_____ /____ /_____ "the process of examining the voicebox"

---

bronchoscope

bronchoscopy

2029 A _____ is a type of endoscope that can be fed down into a bronchus to examine it. The technical name for the procedure in which this is done is _____.

---

laryngoscope

laryngoscopy

2030 A _____ is an endoscope that can be slid down into the larynx to examine it or perform surgery on it. The technical name for this procedure is _____.

Information Frame

2031 Deeper structures within the lungs may have to be visualized indirectly. A **lung scan**, for instance, produces images after radioactive materials are inhaled into the lungs.

---

lung scan

angi/o/graphy (**an**-jee-**AH**-grah-fee)

2032 A _____ _____ is not the only means for imaging deep structures in the respiratory system. You learned the term cineangiocardiography in **frame 1666**. This term can be shortened to _____ /____ /_____, "the process of recording (x-ray images) of the vessels."

pulmonary **pulmonary angiography**	**2033** Recall that _____ **(frame 1582)** "pertains to the lungs." Using this fact and that discussed previously, allows us to construct the phrase _____ _____, "the process of recording (x-ray images) of the vessels (in) the lungs."
pulmonary angiography	**2034** From a technical standpoint, _____ _____ is the use of dyes to take radiograms of the blood vessels in the lungs. In this way, any occlusion or rupture may be noted.
rhonch/us (RAHNK-us) **ral/es (RALS)**	**2035** Partial or total occlusion of respiratory passageways can result in loud snoring or rattling sounds during auscultation. **Rhonch (RAHNK)** takes -**us** and **ral (RAL)** takes -**es**, yielding _____ / ____ ("presence of snoring") and _____ / ____ ("rattling"), respectively.
rhonchus rales	**2036** "Snoring," or _____ and "rattling," or _____ during respiration, may suggest the presence of mucous plugs in the airways.
sput/um (SPYOO-tum)	**2037** Upper respiratory mucus can be "spit out" with some effort. **Sput (SPYOOT)** means "spit." Therefore, _____ / ____, denotes "presence of spit" where the suffix is -**um**.
sputum	**2038** The "spit," or _____, is mainly mucous-containing material that has been coughed up from the respiratory tree. Too much of this material often indicates the presence of respiratory disease.
sputum	**2039** The _____ can be analyzed for infecting bacteria and other abnormal components after the patient "spits" into a collecting jar.
respir **respir/o/meter (res-pir-AH-meh-ter)**	**2040** Rather than respiratory structures or secretions themselves, respiratory functions may be measured. Using _____ ("breathing again," **frame 1964**) as a single root, we can combine it with -**meter (frame 1330)** and create _____ / ____ / _____, "an instrument used to measure (the process of) breathing again."
spir/o/meter (spir-AH-meh-ter)	**2041** Let us change the term in the preceding frame to mean "an instrument used to measure (the process of) breathing." The result is _____ / ____ / _____ .
respir/o/metry (res-pir-AH-meh-tree) **spir/o/metry (spir-AH-meh-tree)**	**2042** With the same approach, build two related terms, using optometry **(frame 1331)** as a model: _____ / ____ / _____ "the process of measuring breathing again" _____ / ____ / _____ "the process of measuring breathing" These terms are interchangeable.

respirometry spirometry respirometer spirometer	**2043** The technique of _____ (_____) applies scientific measurement to various pulmonary function tests. A _____ (_____) is the machine gen- erally used to conduct such breathing trials.
respirometer spirometer respirometry spirometry	**2044** A _____ or _____ might be used, for instance, to assess a person's **vital capacity**—the total amount of air moved into and out of the lungs. This procedure is an aspect of _____ or _____, that is, lung func- tion measurement.
SOB	**2045** A very low vital capacity might reinforce a patient's complaints about suffering from **shortness of breath**, abbreviated as ____ ____ ____.
shortness of breath	**2046** Assessment of SOB, or _____ ____ _____, may lead to treatment interventions.

Surgery and Therapies

Word Parts Associated with Surgery, Pharmacology, and Other Therapies for the Respiratory System

The following is a list of word parts and an abbreviation associated with surgery, pharmacology, and other therapies for respiratory problems. Use this list to help you complete **frames 2048 to 2075**.

-centesis	surgical puncture and tapping of	**IPPB**	intermittent positive pressure breathing	**lob/o**	lobe (as of a lung)
dilat/o	widen	**laryng/o**	larynx	**thorac/o**	chest

	2047 Starting with the nose and working caudally, let us define surgical and other treatment procedures for the respiratory system.
nas/o/plasty (**NAYS**-oh-**plas**-tee) **rhin/o/plasty** (**RIGH**-noh-**plas**-tee)	**2048** Remove the roots from nasal and rhinal **(frame 1929)**. Attach them to the suffix in arthroplasty **(frame 305)**. The two resulting products are _____ / ____ / _____ and _____ / ____ / _____, "surgical repair of the nose."
nasoplasty rhinoplasty	**2049** The operation of _____ or _____ is rather crudely nicknamed a "nose job."
thorac laryng trache	**2050** The thorax, represented by the root _____ **(frame 397)**; the larynx, represented by _____ **(frame 1318)**; and the trachea, represented by _____ **(frame 1940)**, may also be surgically repaired.

2051 All of the structures in the preceding frame may be "cut into," and then have a "permanent opening made" in them. One appropriate word-model is arthrotomy **(frame 294)**. Another is osteostomy **(frame 297)**.

---

thorac/o/tomy
(thor-ah-**KAHT**-oh-mee)
thorac/o/stomy
(thor-ah-**KAHS**-toh-mee)
laryng/o/tomy
(lahr-in-**GAHT**-oh-mee)
laryng/o/stomy
(lahr-in-**GAHS**-toh-mee)
trache/o/tomy
(tray-kee-**AHT**-oh-mee)
trache/o/stomy
(tray-kee-**AHS**-toh-mee)

2052 Take the preceding information and use it to build:

_____ /____ /_____ "incision into the thorax"
_____ /____ /_____ "forming a permanent opening in the thorax"
_____ /____ /_____ "incision into the voicebox"
_____ /____ /_____ "forming a permanent opening in the voicebox"
_____ /____ /_____ "incision into the (main) windpipe"
_____ /____ /_____ "forming a permanent opening in the (main) windpipe"

---

thoracotomy

thoracostomy

2053 Any surgery of the lungs or heart will generally require a _____ to enter the chest, first. If this "chest incision" is to be a fairly "permanent" one, it is correctly called a _____.

---

laryngotomy

2054 Gulping down large chunks of meat that have not been thoroughly chewed may sometimes block the entrance to the larynx. The person may suffocate or die of a so-called cafe coronary due to choking. If the well-known **Heimlich (HIGHM**-lik) **maneuver** is unsuccessful in dislodging the laryngeal obstruction, then _____ ("cutting into the larynx") may be the only hope.

---

laryngostomy

2055 Smokers with cancer of the larynx may have their vocal cords removed. They then have to speak through a _____, a "permanent hole" made in the "larynx."

---

tracheotomy

tracheostomy

2056 A physician may perform an emergency _____ to let air into the "(main) windpipe" if the passage is blocked with some obstruction. If necessary, the original incision can be modified and made into a permanent _____.

---

tracheal
endo-

2057 Recall that _____ **(frame 1942)** "refers to the (main) windpipe" and that _____, the prefix in endoplasmic **(frame 519)**, means "within."

---

endo/trache/al
(**en**-doh-**TRAY**-kee-al)

2058 Therefore, _____ /_____ /_____ "refers to (something) within the (main) windpipe."

---

endotracheal intubation	**2059** **Intubation** (in-too-**BAY**-shun) is the "process of inserting a tube." Use this fact plus the preceding frame to help you build the phrase _____ _____ ("the process of inserting a tube into the (main) windpipe").
endotracheal intubation	**2060** The procedure of _____ _____ may accompany tracheotomy or tracheostomy, if a tube needs to be inserted deeper into the airways to suck out excessive mucus.
IPPB	**2061** External assistance with breathing may also be required. A technique called **intermittent positive pressure breathing**, abbreviated as ____ ____ ____ ____, can be quite helpful.
intermittent positive pressure breathing	**2062** In IPPB, or _____ _____ _____ _____, a machine with a tube is placed into either the mouth or the tracheostomy. Air under "positive" (high, forceful) pressure is then delivered into the patient's lungs.
Information Frame	**2063** A person may have dyspnea if excessive mucus is being secreted, as during bronchitis. The natural body chemical **histamine** (**HIS**-tah-**meen**) promotes fluid secretion.
anti/histamine (**an**-tih-**HIS**-tah-meen)	**2064** Recall that an anticoagulant **(frame 1915)** is something that is "against curdling." In similar fashion, an _____ /_____ is a drug that literally acts "against histamine."
antihistamines	**2065** The _____ commonly occur in over-the-counter drugs. They help dry out the respiratory passageways by inhibiting mucus secretion.
vasodilator **bronch/o/dilat/or** (**brahng**-koh-**DIGH**-lay-ter)	**2066** Remember that a _____ **(frame 1700)** is "one that widens vessels." Replace vas with the root in bronchitis **(frame 1996)** and build _____ /____ /_____ /____, "one that widens the bronchi."
bronchodilator	**2067** The _____ drugs help relax and open the bronchioles, permitting breathing to occur freely and easily once again. A good example is provided by epinephrine (adrenalin). If a person is barely breathing after surgery, then **respiratory stimulants** may be given. An example here is the drug **doxapram** (**DAHKS**-ah-pram).
respiratory stimulants	**2068** Giving _____ _____ to accelerate breathing may do little or no good if the patient's chest is filled with fluid.

thora/centesis
(thor-ah-sen-**TEE**-sis)

2069 "Surgical puncture and tapping of" fluid from the chest may be required. Following the same pattern as used in osteocentesis **(frame 299)**, create _____ /_____, "surgical puncture and tapping of the chest." Note here that the terminal **c** in the root for "chest" has been left out.

thoracentesis

2070 Performance of _____ may be necessary, for instance, to remove the excessive blood pressing against the lungs in hemothorax.

-ectomy

2071 If the problem is carcinoma of the lung, then surgical removal of the cancerous tissue may be required. The appropriate terms involve the suffix _____, as in endarterectomy **(frame 1719)**. Either an entire "lung," indicated by the root in pneumonitis **(frame 1996)**, or just a lung "lobe," **lob (LOHB)**, may have to be removed.

lob/ectomy (**loh-BEK**-toh-mee)

pneumon/ectomy
(**noo**-mah-**NEK**-toh-mee)

2072 Less extensive cancer may need _____ /_____, "removal of a lobe" in the affected lung. Widespread cancer, however, could require _____ /_____, "removal of a lung."

lobectomy
pneumonectomy
laryng/ectomy (**lar**-in-**JEK**-toh-mee)

2073 If a "lobe" is removed, _____ is performed. If a "lung" is removed, _____ is performed. If the "voice-box" is removed, then a _____ /_____ is performed.

laryngectomy
larynx

2074 The operation of _____ may be appropriate if one is suffering from cancer of the _____ ("voicebox," **frame 1317**).

laryngectomy

2075 The surgical procedure of _____ ("voicebox removal") is most commonly done in chronic smokers.

Multiple Choice

1. A combining form for air sacs in the lungs is
   a. alkal/i   b. pleur/o   c. alveol/o   d. bronchiol/o

2. Which of these roots means "throat"?
   a. trache   b. laryng   c. pharyng   d. rhin

3. The singular form of bronchi ends in _____ rather than **i**.
   a. -ae   b. -um   c. -oles   d. -us

4. Which of these denotes "breathing"?
   a. -pnea   b. pneum/o   c. pneumon/o   d. pleur/a

5. To indicate "blowing up with air," use the medical term
   a. emphysema   b. ventilation   c. respiration   d. catarrh

6. "Presence of spit" is indicated by the term
   a. sputum   b. sputal   c. catarrh   d. catarrhal

Meanings of Selected Roots

Add the correct combining vowel (cv) after each root. Then write the definition of each root in the space provided.

ROOT/CV	DEFINITION
1. spir/_____	_____
2. bronch/_____	_____
3. pneumon/_____	_____
4. emphysem/_____	_____
5. ventil/_____	_____
6. catarrh/_____	_____
7. rhin/_____	_____
8. sput/_____	_____
9. trache/_____	_____
10. bronchiol/_____	_____

Word Dissection and Translation

Analyze the following terms by dissecting them with slashmarks and identifying their word parts. To the right of each term, write its correct English translation.

Key: R (root), cv (combining vowel), P (prefix), S (suffix)

1. bronchoscope

_____ / ____ / _____ / _____
R   cv   R   S

_____

2. dyspnea

_____ / _____
P   S

_____

3. endotracheal

_____ / _____ / _____
P   R   S

_____

4. respirometry

_____ / ____ / _____
R   cv   S

_____

5. bronchodilators

_____ / ____ / _____ / _____
R   cv   R   S

_____

6. laryngectomy

_____ / _____
R   S

_____

7. pulmonary

_____ / _____
R   S

_____

8. tachypnea

_____ / _____
P   S

_____

9. thoracentesis

_____ / _____
R   S

_____

10. rhonchus

_____ / _____
R   S

_____

11. laryngocatarrhal

_____ / ____ / _____ / _____
R   cv   R   S

_____

12. pneumocephalus

_____ / ____ / _____ / _____
R   cv   R   S

_____

Terms and Their Abbreviations

In the list below, when the term is given, write its abbreviation in the space provided. When the abbreviation is given, write its corresponding term.

TERM	ABBREVIATION
1. _____	COPD
2. intermittent positive pressure breathing	_____
3. _____	SOB

Word Spelling

Look at each of the terms listed below. Identify those that are misspelled by circling Y for "Yes." Write the correct spelling in the blank.

WORD	MISSPELLED?	CORRECT SPELLING
1. bronchocunstrikchen	Y/N	_____
2. pneumoneyetus	Y/N	_____
3. hyperventilation	Y/N	_____
4. guittarhal	Y/N	_____
5. alkaline	Y/N	_____
6. angeahgrahfee	Y/N	_____
7. respeerahmuhtar	Y/N	_____
8. alveolar	Y/N	_____
9. railes	Y/N	_____
10. nasoplastie	Y/N	_____
11. pleural	Y/N	_____
12. pneumothoraks	Y/N	_____
13. antihistamine	Y/N	_____
14. coreezuh	Y/N	_____

New Word Synthesis

Using word parts that appear in this and previous chapters, build new terms with the following meanings:

1. _____ surgical repair of the voicebox
2. _____ widening of the arteries
3. _____ process of breathing and blowing
4. _____ pertaining to the ribs and the lungs
5. _____ removal of the major windpipe
6. _____ surgical puncture and tapping of the vessels and lungs
7. _____ relating to the heart and lungs
8. _____ an instrument used to measure circulation
9. _____ one which narrows the bronchi
10. _____ referring to spit
11. _____ pertaining to the voicebox
12. _____ inflammation of the nose and throat

C A S E   S T U D Y

Read through the following partial report for respiratory therapy. Note the terms in bold print. A series of multiple choice questions probes your knowledge of these terms.

Respiratory Therapy Report

The patient, a 55-year-old white male suffering from **dyspnea** and **COPD**, was given 15 minutes of **IPPB** treatment after performance of **respirometry**.

Case Study Questions

1. "Suffering **dyspnea**" indicates that the patient was bothered by

   (a) angina pectoris.

   (b) cerebral aneurysm.

   (c) difficult and labored breathing.

   (d) myocardial ischemia.

2. The **COPD** mentioned tells you that the

   (a) bronchial tubes were partially blocked.

   (b) extreme bronchodilation was bringing too much air into the lungs.

   (c) pulmonary vessels were examined radiographically.

   (d) alveoli were all dilated and emphysematous.

3. Fifteen minutes of **IPPB** provided

   (a) enhanced blood flow to the myocardium.

   (b) sputum for cytological examination.

   (c) forced air to help further inflate the lungs.

   (d) radioactive images of lung physiology.

4. **Respirometry** resulted in

   (a) a useful tracing of pulmonary blood flow.

   (b) radiographs of the heart and lung.

   (c) the same thing as angiography of the pulmonary tree.

   (d) precise measurement of lung volumes and capacities.

CHAPTER 16 The Digestive System

INTRODUCTION

The digestive system essentially consists of a long tube that extends from the mouth at one end of the body to the **anus** (**AY**-nus) at the other. The main organs are shown in Figure 16.1.

FIGURE 16.1   **The Digestive System**

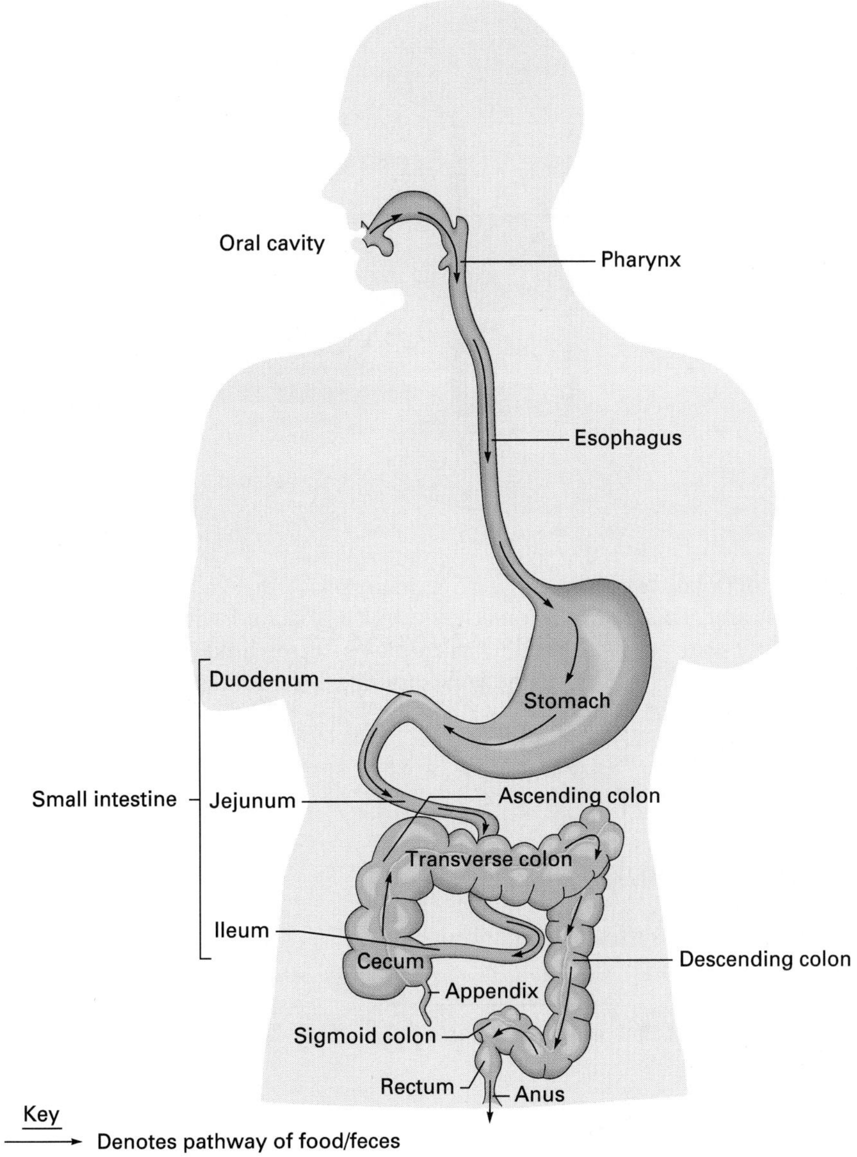

Key
→ Denotes pathway of food/feces

The five main processes carried out by the digestive system are **ingestion** (**in-JEST**-shun), **diges-tion, secretion, absorption,** and **egestion** (**ee-JEST**-shun), or **defecation** (**def**-eh-**KAY**-shun). Ingestion is simply taking food or liquid into the mouth. Digestion is the physical and chemical breakdown of food. Secretion is the release of useful products (such as acid and enzymes) that aid the digestive process. Absorption is the movement of digested material out across the wall of the digestive tube and into the bloodstream. Finally, egestion, or defecation, is the release of unusable residue from the anus.

Special accessory digestive organs are attached to the main digestive tube. These organs include the **salivary** (**SAL**-ih-**vahr**-ee) **glands**, pancreas, gallbladder, and liver. They are all called "accessory" because they are not part of the digestive tube itself—no food or feces passes through them. Rather, they are connected to the sides of the tube and add their important secretions to it. These secretions often promote better digestion of foodstuffs. The liver and gallbladder, for instance, secrete bile into the small intestine. The bile helps break down large globules of fat into tiny fatty droplets. Thus the digestion and eventual absorption of fatty material is enhanced.

FIGURE 16.2   **The Five Main Processes of the Digestive System**

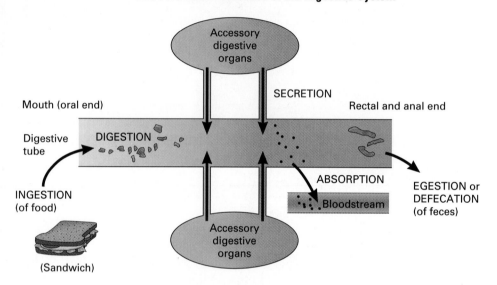

Figure 16.2 provides a functional overview of the five main processes carried out by the digestive tube and its accessory organs. This chapter considers terms associated with the normal structure and function of the digestive system, terms related to its diseases, terms linked to lab tests and diagnoses of digestive problems, and terms of surgery and other therapies for digestive disorders.

CHAPTER OBJECTIVES

By the end of this chapter, you should be able to:

1 Identify major prefixes, roots, suffixes, and abbreviations related to the digestive system.

2 Dissect digestive terms into their component parts.

3 Translate digestive terms into their common English equivalents.

4 Build new terms associated with the digestive system.

Word Parts Associated with Normal Structure and Function of the Digestive System

The following is a list of word parts and an abbreviation associated with normal anatomy and physiology of the digestive system. Use this list to help you complete **frames 2077 to 2158**.

aliment/o	food; nourishment	**col/o**	colon (large intestine)	**intestin/o**	intestine
an/o	ring	**cyst/o**	bladder	**jejun/o**	jejunum (empty)
append/o	attachment; appendix	**dent/o**	tooth	**lapar/o**	abdominal wall
		dont/o	tooth	**lingu/o**	tongue
appendic/o	attachment; appendix	**duoden/o**	duodenum (twelve)	**or/o**	mouth
bili/o	bile	**esophag/o**	esophagus	**proct/o**	straight; rectum
cec/o	(something) blind	**gastr/o**	stomach	**pylor/o**	gatekeeper; pylorus
cheil/o	lips	**GI**	gastrointestinal	**rect/o**	straight; rectum
chil/o	lips	**gingiv/o**	gums	**saliv/o**	spit
chol/e	bile; gall	**gloss/o**	tongue	**sigm/o**	S
cholecyst/o	gallbladder	**hepat/o**	liver	**-stalsis**	a constriction
		ile/o	ileum (twisted)	**ton/e**	strength; stretch

2076 **Aliment** (**AY**-lih-ment) means "food" or "nourishment." Recall that pulmonary **(frame 1582)** "relates to the lungs."

aliment/ary (ay-lih-**MEN**-tah-ree)

2077 The digestive system is also called the _____ / _____ system, since it "relates to food or nourishment."

alimentary

2078 Another name for the digestive system or tube is the _____ tract. This name reflects its important role in the ingestion, digestion, and absorption of "foods."

Information Frame

2079 It will be helpful to learn the roots for digestive or alimentary structures in their logical order—from the top to the bottom of the digestive tube. Pronounce the terms and roots listed in Table 16.1. They all represent structures at the top of the tube. Specifically, they name structures associated with the mouth and throat.

T A B L E   1 6 . 1   **Some Names and Roots for Structures in the Mouth and Throat Area**

Structure Name and/or Root	Meaning
oral (OR-al) **cavity; or (OR)**	mouth
cheil (KIGHL); chil	lips
gingiva (JIN-jih-vah); **gingivae (JIN**-jih-vee); **gingiv (JIN**-jiv)	gums
dent (DENT); dont (DAHNT)	teeth
gloss (GLAHS); lingu (LING-gwah)	tongue
salivary (SAL-ih-**vahr**-ee) **glands; saliv (SAH**-liv)	spit

Now work with these words and word parts in the next series of frames.

or or/al	**2080** You can see from Table 16.1 that _____ is the root for "mouth." Just as tracheal **(frame 1942)** "pertains to the main windpipe," ____ /____ "pertains to the mouth."
oral cheil chil	**2081** Before food is ingested into the _____ (mouth) **cavity**, it is grasped by the "lips." The two roots for "lips" are _____ and _____.
dent dont	**2082** After the lips, food is usually gripped by the "teeth," denoted by either of the two roots _____ and _____.
dent/al **(DEN**-tal)	**2083** Use dent and the pattern of oral to create _____ /____, "pertaining to the teeth."
dental gloss lingu	**2084** The _____ ("toothy") gripping and tearing of food is assisted by the "tongue," which is denoted by either the root _____ or the root _____. Both roots for "tongue" take the "referring to" suffix of dental.
gloss/al **(GLAHS**-al) **lingu**/al **(LING**-gwal)	**2085** The _____ /____ or _____ /____ ("pertaining to the tongue") actions roll the food about as it is being chewed.
gingiv gingiv/a **gingiv**/al **(JIN**-jih-val)	**2086** Table 16.1 cites _____ as a root for "gum." This root takes the "presence of" suffix found in trachea **(frame 1940)** and the "referring to" ending of lingual. The results are _____ /____ ("presence of the gum") and _____ /____ ("referring to the gums"), respectively.
gingival	**2087** The roots of the teeth are implanted in the _____ (gum) surface.
gingiva **gingiv**/ae	**2088** We know that many words whose singular ends in **-a** form plurals using **-ae**. The plural of _____ ("the gum"), for instance, is _____ /____.
gingivae	**2089** The _____, or "gums," are the soft fleshy pads that help support the teeth.
salivary	**2090** Note in Table 16.1 the _____ **glands**, which secrete "spit."

saliv/**ary** saliv	**2091** Salivary takes the same "referring to" suffix as alimentary **(frame 2077)** and is properly dissected as _____ / _____. Its root, _____, denotes "spit."
saliv/**a** (sah-**LIGH**-vah)	**2092** Saliv forms its "presence of" ending as gingiv does. The result is _____ / ____, or "presence of spit."
saliva	**2093** The _____, or "spit," is really a solution of several important enzymes that begin the chemical digestion of carbohydrates.
pharynx	**2094** When chewed food is well mixed with the saliva, the tongue flips it into the back of the _____, or "throat" **(frame 1932)**.
larynx	**2095** The pharynx subdivides into two branches as it descends into the neck. The more anterior branch becomes the _____, or "voicebox" **(frame 1317)**. The more posterior branch is the **esophagus** (eh-**SAHF**-uh-**gus**), or "gullet."
esophag/**us**	**2096** Esophagus is subdivided as _____ / ____, the same way as bronchus **(frame 1945)**.
esophagus	**2097** The _____ ("gullet") is the tube that carries swallowed food and liquid from the pharynx down into the "stomach," or gastr/o (**GAS**-troh).
gastr **gastr/ic** (**GAS**-trik)	**2098** The _____ ("stomach") root generally takes the "referring to" ending in acidic **(frame 1977)**. The result, _____ / ____, "refers to the stomach."
gastric	**2099** The _____ ("stomach") secretions include powerful acid and enzymes.
gastric	**2100** Part of _____ ("stomach") physiology is storing food temporarily, then being a "gatekeeper" that allows partially digested food to pass into the small intestine. **Pylor** (pigh-**LOR**) means "gatekeeper."
-us **pylor/us** (pigh-**LOR**-us)	**2101** Pylor, like esophag, assumes _____ as its "presence of" ending. Consequently, _____ / ____ denotes "a gatekeeper."

pylor/ic (pigh-**LOR**-ik)

2102 Just as gastric "pertains to the stomach," _____ / ____ "pertains to the gatekeeper."

pylorus
pyloric

2103 The _____ is the narrow terminal pouch at the inferior end of the stomach. It contains the _____ **sphincter**—a muscular ring of tissue that regulates the emptying of material from the stomach into the small intestine.

pylorus

2104 Figure 16.3 provides a detailed view of the stomach and small intestine. Note that the _____ is "a gatekeeper" in that its sphincter opens and closes, somewhat like a gate. This sphincter regulates the movement of partially digested material from the stomach into the small intestine.

F I G U R E   1 6 . 3   **Detailed View of the Stomach and Small Intestine Area**

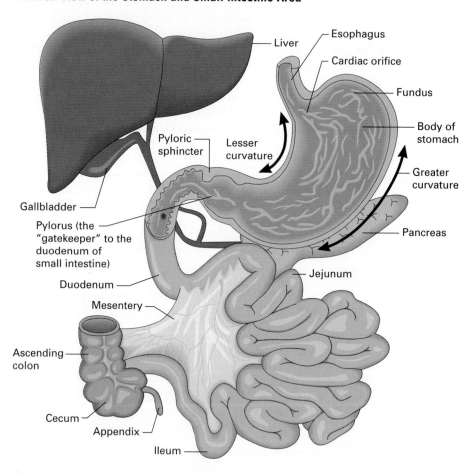

gastr

2105 As Figure 16.3 makes clear, the "stomach," denoted by the root _____, and the "intestine," denoted as **intestin** (in-**TES**-tin), are very closely related.

gastr/o/intestin/al
(gas-troh-in-**TES**-tih-nal)

2106 Adopt the "referring to" suffix in gingival **(frame 2086)** and create _____ /____ /_____ /____, "relating to the stomach and intestine."

---

gastrointestinal

2107 The digestive system is sometimes called the _____ tract, in that a large portion of it is composed of the "stomach" and "intestines."

---

gastrointestinal

2108 The upper _____ (GI) tract is displayed in Figure 16.3.

GI

2109 Along with the upper gastrointestinal, or ____ ____, tract, Figure 16.3 shows three major digestive accessory organs—the liver, pancreas, and gallbladder—that are directly or indirectly attached to the small intestine.

Information Frame

2110 Table 16.2 provides a listing of intestinal structures and related accessory organs. Pronounce these terms or roots and look at their meanings.

T A B L E   1 6 . 2   **Some Names and Roots for Structures Related to the Small Intestine**

Structure Name and/or Root	Meaning
duodenum (doo-**AH**-deh-num); **duoden** (doo-**AH**-den)	twelve
jejunum (jeh-**JOO**-num); **jejun** (jay-**JOON**)	empty
ileum (**IL**-ee-um); **ile** (**IL**-ee)	twisted
hepat (he-**PAT**)	liver
cholecyst (**KOH**-lee-sist)	gallbladder

Now work with these words and word parts in the next series of frames.

---

duoden/**um**

2111 The small intestine is narrow (small) in diameter, but it is over 20 feet long. The most proximal part of the small intestine, the _____ /____, means "presence of twelve," much as sputum **(frame 2037)** means "presence of spit."

---

duodenum

jejun/**um**

2112 The _____ ("presence of twelve") connects directly to the pylorus. In the middle of the small intestine is the _____ /____, which denotes the "presence of (something) empty."

jejunum	**2113** The _____ derives its name from the fact that ancient scholars observed that it was usually "empty" after death.
ile/**um**	**2114** The term _____ /_____ indicates a "twisted presence."
ileum	**2115** The _____ is the terminal, "twisted" or engorged, portion of the small intestine. Unlike the jejunum, this part was seen by the ancients to be full and swollen with liquid waste matter, giving it a "twisted" appearance.
duodenum jejunum ileum **duoden/al** (doo-**AH**-den-al) **jejun/al** (jeh-**JOO**-nal) **ile/al** (**IL**-ee-al)	**2116** All three parts of the small intestine—the _____, _____, and _____—take the same "pertaining to" suffix as gastrointestinal **(frame 2106)**. This combination yields _____ /_____ ("pertaining to twelve"), _____ /_____ ("pertaining to emptiness"), and _____ /_____ ("pertaining to twisted-ness"), respectively.
duodenal	**2117** The _____ ("referring to twelve") term is especially interesting. Visualize in your mind a group of early scholars, working on a **cadaver** (kah-**DAH**-ver), or "dead body." This "dead body" may be that of an animal. The scholars bend over its open abdominal cavity and place their fingers side-by-side along the length of the duodenum. They find the duodenum to be approximately "twelve" finger-breadths long—hence its name!
duodenal	**2118** The _____ ("twelve" finger-breadths) area is the site where secretions from some of the accessory digestive organs flow in. Three such organs are the pancreas, liver, and gallbladder.
pancreat hepat cholecyst	**2119** Recall that _____ **(frame 1411)** is a root for the pancreas, or "all flesh" gland. Table 16.2 cites _____ as a root for "liver" and _____ as an entire term for "gallbladder."
chole/**cyst** **chole** (**KOH**-lee)	**2120** Since cyst **(SIST)** is a "bladder," cholecyst must be subdivided as _____ /_____. The other root in cholecyst, _____, denotes "bile" or "gall."
chole	**2121** Like _____ **(frame 2120)**, **bili** (**BIL**-ee) is a root for "bile."

bili

2122 The liver produces bile continuously. Its brownish-green color is due to the addition of an orange pigment called **bilirubin** (**BIL**-ee-**roo**-bin). In this term you can see one of the two "bile" roots, _____, included.

---

cholecyst

2123 The bile produced by the liver is stored temporarily in the _____ ("gallbladder").

---

bili/ary (**BIL**-ee-**ay**-ree)
hepat/ic (heh-**PAT**-ik)
cholecyst/ic (**koh**-lee-**SIS**-tik)

2124 Bili takes the same "referring to" ending as salivary (**frame 2091**), while hepat and cholecyst assume the suffix in pancreatic (**frame 1412**). Use that information to synthesize:
_____ / _____   "referring to bile"
_____ / ____   "referring to the liver"
_____ / ____   "referring to the gallbladder"

---

hepatic
cholecystic

biliary

2125 A major _____ ("liver") function is bile production. A major _____ ("gallbladder") function is storage of bile and its release during digestion of a fatty meal. The chief _____ ("bile") function is the breaking down of large globules of ingested fat into tiny fatty droplets that are much more digestible.

Information Frame

2126 After fats are thoroughly digested, their particles pass into the large intestine. Two roots, **col** (**KOHL**) and **cec** (**SEEK**), are closely associated with this body area. Col means "large intestine," while cec denotes "(something) blind."

---

col

col/on (**KOH**-lun)
col/ic (**KAHL**-ik)

2127 The _____ ("large intestine") root takes the "presence of" suffix in myelencephalon (**frame 1083**) and the "relating to" ending in hepatic (**frame 2124**). This information should allow you to build _____ / ____ ("the large intestine") and _____ / ____ ("relating to the large intestine").

---

cec

cec/um (**SEE**-kum)
cec/al (**SEE**-kal)

2128 The _____ ("blind") root assumes the "presence of" suffix in duodenum (**frame 2111**) and the "relating to" ending in duodenal (**frame 2116**). This information should permit you to build _____ / ____, or the "presence of (something) blind" and _____ / ____, or "relating to (something) blind."

---

cecum
colon

2129 The _____ is a "blind," that is, dead-ended pouch that forms the proximal portion of the _____ ("large intestine"). The detailed anatomical relationships of this area are displayed in Figure 16.4.

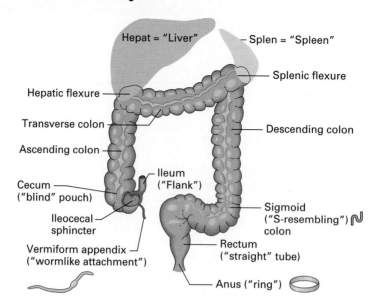

2130 Take the root for ileum, or "twisted" **(frame 2114)**, and combine it with cecal. The result is _____ /____ /_____ /____, "relating to the ileum and cecum."

ile/o/cec/al (**il**-ee-oh-**SEE**-kal)

2131 Take the root for ileum and combine it with colic. The result is _____ /____ /_____ /____, "relating to the ileum and colon."

ile/o/col/ic (**il**-ee-oh-**KAHL**-ik)

2132 Now use each of the terms in the preceding two frames to name a sphincter. It is called the _____ or _____ **sphincter**. This sphincter is a ring of muscle that regulates the emptying of the ileum into the cecum of the large intestine.

ileocecal
ileocolic

2133 At the inferior tip of the cecum is an "attachment." A quick review of the skeletal system (Chapter 8) may refresh your mind about the _____ skeleton, which is attached to the axial skeleton. Two roots in this chapter, **append** (ah-**PEND**) and **appendic** (ah-**PEN**-dik), denote the **appendix** (ah-**PEN**-diks)

appendicular

2134 The _____ is a thin, wormlike "attachment" to the caudal tip of the cecum. It probably plays some minor role in the body's immune system, since it contains lymphatic tissue.

appendix

2135 The "attachment" root ending in **c**, _____, is the one most often combined with other word parts to represent the appendix.

appendic

appendic/eal (ah-**pend**-ih-**SEEL**)	**2136** Using -**eal** (**EEL**) as a "relating to" suffix, for instance, permits us to build _____ / _____, "relating to the appendix or attachment."
appendiceal	**2137** Attached to the base of the cecum is an _____ structure.
Information Frame	**2138** Occurring in sequence after the cecum and appendix are the ascending colon, transverse colon, and descending colon. These are followed by the **sigmoid** (**SIG**-moyd) **colon**.
sigm/oid	**2139** Sigmoid, containing the same "resembling" ending as thyroid (**frame 1383**), is properly dissected as _____ / _____.
sigm (**SIG**-im) **S**-resembling	**2140** The root in sigmoid, _____, means **S**. The whole term, sigmoid, therefore translates as "____-_____."
sigmoid colon	**2141** The _____ _____ is the final "S-shaped" or "S-resembling" portion of the "large intestine" (**frame 2127**).
rect	**2142** After the sigmoid colon comes a straight tube. Recall that _____, the root in rectus (**frame 993**), indicates something "straight." An alternative root with this meaning is proct (**PRAHKT**).
rect/um (**REKT**-um)	**2143** Remove the suffix from rectus and replace it with the "presence of" ending in ileum (**frame 2114**). The outcome is _____ / _____, "the presence of (something) straight."
rectum	**2144** The _____ is a "straight" tube leading from the sigmoid colon. It terminates at the **anus** (**AY**-nus)—a "ring" of muscle surrounding the hole through which one defecates.
an/us	**2145** Anus is dissected as ____ / ____, with the same ending as rectus (**frame 993**).
rect proct an **rect/al** (**REK**-tal) **proct/al** (**PRAHK**-tal) **an/al** (**AY**-nal)	**2146** All three roots, _____ or _____ ("straight," **frame 2142**) and ____ ("ring") assume the "pertaining to" ending in ileocecal (**frame 2130**). Now create three terms: _____ / _____ or _____ / _____ "pertaining to the rectum or (something) straight" ____ / _____ "pertaining to the anus or ring"

rectal proctal anal	**2147** When the muscle in the _____ or _____ ("straight") wall contracts, it creates pressure that pushes fecal material onward toward the anus. The resulting _____ pressure forces feces out of the hole.
abdomin	**2148** It is not the wall of the abdominal cavity itself that constricts. **Lapar** (**LAP**-ar), by the way, like _____, the root in abdominal **(frame 379)**, is a root for "abdomen" or "abdominal wall."
lapar/al (**LAP**-ar-al)	**2149** Just as abdominal "pertains to the abdomen," _____ / _____ does as well.
laparal	**2150** The _____, or abdominal, walls enclose the caudal portion of the digestive tube. This part of the tube undergoes constriction during defecation. **-Stalsis** (**STAL**-sis), a noun suffix, denotes "a constriction" or "a contraction."
peri/stalsis (**peh**-rih-**STAL**-sis)	**2151** Extract the "around" prefix from periosteum **(frame 786)** and construct _____ / _____, "a constriction around (something)."
peristalsis laparal	**2152** The action of _____ creates "a constriction around" the caudal part of the GI tract. This narrowing pushes food or fecal material toward the anus. The abdominal (_____) muscles can assist forceful defecation by pressing on the exterior wall of the digestive tube.
ton	**2153** Both the interior wall of the abdominal cavity and the exterior wall of the digestive tube have serous membranes that in a sense are stretched around them. Recall that _____, as in tonic **(frame 468)**, is a root for "strength." It can also denote "stretching" and is followed by an **e** as combining vowel.
peri/ton/e/um (**peh**-rih-toh-**NEE**-um)	**2154** Take advantage of the preceding facts to help you build _____ / _____ / _____ / _____, "a stretching around (something)." The ending reflects that in duodenum.
peritoneum	**2155** A _____ is a type of serous membrane that is literally "stretched around" various structures.
peri/ton/e/al (**peh**-rih-toh-**NEE**-al)	**2156** Borrow the adjectival ending from laparal and create _____ / _____ / _____ / _____, which "pertains to stretching around (something)."

peritoneal	**2157** There are two kinds of _____ membranes within the abdominal cavity, just as there are two kinds of pleuras within the thoracic cavity. Remember that the _____ pleura **(frame 1993)** lines the "wall" of the thoracic cavity. In similar fashion, the _____ _____ is a serous membrane that lines the "wall" of the abdominal cavity.
parietal	
parietal peritoneum	

visceral	**2158** Remember that the _____ pleura **(frame 1993)** covers the "guts" within the thoracic cavity. In parallel manner, the _____ _____ is a serous membrane that covers the "guts" within the abdominal cavity.
visceral peritoneum	

2159 Even though the internal organs of the digestive system are protected somewhat by the parietal and visceral peritoneum, they are still vulnerable to disease and injury.

Word Parts Associated with Diseases of the Digestive System

The following is a list of word parts associated with diseases of the digestive system. Use this list to help you complete **frames 2160 to 2224**.

calcul/o	little rock	**herni/o**	rupture	**lith/o**	stone
-cele	rupture, swelling	**hiat/o**	hole	**phag**	eat, swallow
choledoch/o	bile duct	**jaundic/o**	yellow (appearance)	**py/o**	pus
cirrh/o	reddish yellow			**splen/o**	spleen
diverticul/o	off-shoot or by-path				

	2160 It is convenient to look at diseases of the digestive system according to their broad types. Take, for example, the "inflammation of" various structures, denoted by the suffix _____.
-itis	

	2161 If necessary, review earlier frames describing normal structures of the digestive system. Then build some inflammatory conditions related to the mouth, stomach, and accessory digestive organs:
gingiv/itis (jin-jih-**VIGH**-tis)	_____ / _____ "inflammation of the gums"
cheil/itis (**kigh-LIGH**-tis)	_____ / _____ or
chil/itis	_____ / _____ "inflammation of the lips"
gastr/itis (**gas-TRIGH**-tis)	_____ / _____ "inflammation of the stomach"
hepat/itis (hep-ah-**TIGH**-tis)	_____ / _____ "inflammation of the liver"
cholecyst/itis (koh-lee-sist-**IGH**-tis)	_____ / _____ "inflammation of the gallbladder"

gingivitis	**2162** "Inflammation of the gums," or _____, may especially affect the gum area around the base of the teeth.

peri/**o**/**dont**/**itis**
(**peh**-ree-oh-**dahn**-**TIGH**-tis)

2163 Employ dont as a root for "teeth" and apply the "around" prefix in peristalsis **(frame 2151)** to help you construct a new term, _____ / _____ / _____ / _____, "inflammation of the (area) around the teeth." Using **o** as a combining vowel helps to smooth out pronunciation.

---

periodontitis

2164 **Caries** (**KAHR**-ees) is Latin for "dry rot." It especially affects the bony structure of the teeth, and it is not directly related to _____ ("inflammation" of the area "around" the "teeth").

---

caries

2165 "Dry rot," or **dental** _____ is the more scientific term for **dental cavities**, which result from the "rot" of bony tooth tissue.

---

periodontitis
dental caries

2166 It is claimed that _____ ("inflammation around the teeth"), rather than _____ _____ ("tooth dry rot"), is the major cause of tooth loss in most adults.

Information Frame

2167 **Plaque** (**PLAK**) is a sticky "plate." It consists of a film of bacteria that adheres to the teeth and releases corrosive acids.

---

plaque

periodontitis
gingivitis

2168 The acids associated with _____ (sticky "plate") can wear away the hard white tooth **enamel**, resulting in dental caries. Irritation along the gumline can also result in _____ around the teeth and _____ ("gum inflammation") in general.

Information Frame

2169 Old plaque hardens into **calculus** (**KAL**-kyoo-lus), or **tartar** (**TAR**-ter). Tartar originally meant the hard sediment that naturally forms in the bottom of aged wine casks!

---

calcul/**us**
calcul (**KAL**-kyool)

2170 Calculus contains the same "presence of" suffix as esophagus **(frame 2096)**. This term is therefore dissected as _____ / _____. Its root, _____, means "little rock."

---

calculus

plaque

2171 Dental _____ is a "little rock present" on the bases and sides of the teeth. It is actually a thin, rocklike, hardened deposit of _____ (sticky "plate," **frame 2167**).

---

dent/**algia** (den-**TAL**-jee-uh)

2172 Recall that the suffix in arthralgia **(frame 901)** denotes "pain." Extract the root from dental and use it to build _____ / _____, "tooth pain."

---

dentalgia	**2173** When the hard enamel of the teeth has been breached by bacterial acids, dental nerves can be severely irritated, resulting in _____, or "toothache."
gingiv/algia (jin-jih-**VAL**-jee-ah)	**2174** If the gums are all red and inflamed, then their nerves will also be extremely irritated, resulting in _____ /_____, "gum pain."
dentalgia gingivalgia gastritis **gastr/algia** (gas-**TRAL**-jee-ah)	**2175** Although _____ ("tooth pain") and _____ ("gum pain") affect the mouth, _____ ("inflammation of the stomach") often causes _____ /_____, "stomach pain."
gastralgia	**2176** The technical word for "stomachache" is _____.
enter/o	**2177** Areas associated with the intestines can also be inflamed and painful. Like intestin/o, _____ /_____ **(frame 277)** denotes the "intestine."
duoden/itis (doo-**wah**-den-**IGH**-tis) **enter/itis** (**en**-ter-**IGH**-tis) **gastr/o/enter/itis** (gas-troh-**en**-ter-**IGH**-tis) **col/itis** (koh-**LIGH**-tis) **appendic/itis** (ah-**pen**-dih-**SIGH**-tis)	**2178** Keep the above information in mind as you build some more intestine-related terms having "inflammation of" suffixes: _____ /_____, "inflammation of the duodenum" _____ /_____, "inflammation of the intestine" _____ /_____ /_____ /_____, "inflammation of the stomach and intestines" _____ /_____, "inflammation of the large intestine or colon" _____ /_____, "inflammation of the appendix"
gastroenteritis	**2179** "Inflammation of the stomach and intestines," or _____ is often wrongly called the "flu." Actually, it consists of vomiting and diarrhea due to an inflammation of the stomach and intestines.
enteritis colitis appendicitis duodenitis	**2180** "Inflammation of the intestine" alone is properly called _____. "Inflammation of the large intestine" only is termed _____. Just the "appendix being inflamed" is called _____; just the duodenum, _____.
duoden/algia (doo-**wah**-den-**AL**-jee-uh)	**2181** Severe duodenitis may give rise to _____ /_____, "duodenal pain."

duodenitis	**2182** Severe gastritis or _____ ("duodenal inflammation") may cause a **reflux** (**REE**-fluks) or "back-flow" of stomach acid up into the esophagus. This back-flow creates a painful burning sensation.
pyr	**2183** Gastric pain can be so bad that the stomach feels as if it's on fire! Remember that _____ and pyret **(frame 153)** are two roots for "fever." They can also be interpreted as "burn" or "fire."
pyr/o/sis (pigh-**ROH**-sis)	**2184** Use the "condition of" suffix in thrombosis **(frame 1809)** to create _____ /_____ /_____, a "condition of burning or fire."
pyrosis	**2185** "Heartburn" is technically called _____. There is no direct involvement of the heart. Gastric acid flows back up into the esophagus during indigestion. This strong acid irritates the lining of the esophagus and causes a burning sensation near the heart.
Information Frame	**2186** Two major sites for **ulcers** (abnormal holes or sores) are the esophagus and duodenum. These sites are vulnerable because of their frequent contact with stomach acid, which can burn through their relatively unprotected linings. Another site for ulcers is the colon. **Ulcerative** (**UL**-ser-ah-tiv) "pertains to holes or sores," which can occur in these body areas.
ulcerative **colitis**	**2187** Inflammation of the large intestine is frequently accompanied by ulcers. The technical phrase is _____ _____, "inflammation of the large intestine" accompanied by "holes and sores."
ulcerative duodenitis duodenalgia	**2188** A similar phrase, _____ _____, refers to "inflammation of the duodenum" accompanied by "holes and sores." Such a condition can result in severe _____ ("duodenal pain," **frame 2181**).
diverticul/itis	**2189** Inflammations occur in other unusual or abnormal body sites as well. Take, for instance, **diverticulitis** (**digh**-ver-tik-yoo-**LIGH**-tis). This term is subdivided as _____ /_____.
diverticul (digh-ver-**TIK**-yool)	**2190** The root in diverticulitis, _____, means an "off-shoot" or "by-path."

diverticulitis	**2191** The disease of _____ is literally an "inflammation of off-shoots or by-paths." Such structures are named **diverticul/a** (digh-ver-**TIK**-yoo-lah).
diverticula **diverticul/um** (digh-ver-**TIK**-yoo-lum)	**2192** The term _____ is the plural form of _____ /____, "presence of an offshoot or by-path," where the suffix is that in cecum **(frame 2128)**.
diverticulum diverticula diverticulitis	**2193** Each _____ is an abnormal outpouching along the wall of the small intestine. When several _____ ("off-shoots") become "inflamed," _____ is the result.
Information Frame	**2194** The body wall can also pouch out when something internal ruptures. **Herni/a** (**HER**-nee-ah) denotes "a rupture" or "protrusion," specifically of an internal organ through a breach in a body wall or gross membrane. **Abdominal hernias**, where loops of intestine outpouch through ruptures in the front of the abdominal wall, are quite common.
hernias	**2195** "Ruptures," or _____, are outpouchings that occur at spots of weakness in the body wall. They are not actually holes. **Hiat** (high-**AYT**), however, is a root for "hole" commonly associated with "ruptures."
hiat/al (high-**AYT**-al)	**2196** Build _____ /____ for "relating to a hole" just as you built gastrointestinal **(frame 2106)** for "relating to the stomach and intestines."
hiatal hernia	**2197** A _____ _____ is "a rupture that (involves) a hole." Specifically, an abnormal hole forms in a weakened, ruptured spot on the diaphragm muscle. Part of the stomach or small intestine then protrudes cranially through this hole and into the thoracic cavity above. This condition often causes **dysphagia** (dis-**FAY**-juh).
dys/phag/ia phag **dys-**	**2198** Dysphagia is subdivided as _____ / _____ /____. You may well recognize _____, the root for "eat" or "eating." It also means "swallowing." The prefix _____, for "bad or difficult," may also be familiar. And you have encountered the suffix **-ia** for "(abnormal) condition of."
dysphagia	**2199** The problem of _____ is literally "an abnormal condition of difficult eating."

-cele (SEEL)	**2200** Hernias can, indeed, interfere with swallowing or other digestive system functions. A suffix on the word list with a meaning very close to that of hernia is _____. It represents "a swelling or rupture of (something)."
rect/o/cele (**REK**-toh-seel) **proct/o/cele** (**PRAHK**-toh-seel)	**2201** Referring to the two roots for "straight" **(frame 2142)**, you can build _____ / _____ / _____ and _____ / _____ / _____. Both terms denote "a swelling or rupture of the rectum."
rectocele proctocele	**2202** A _____ or _____ stems from a "rupture" in the posterior wall of the **vagina** (vah-**JIGH**-nah), or birth canal, in females. Part of the wall of the rectum then protrudes into the vagina through this rupture.
rectocele proctocele	**2203** A _____ or _____ ("rectal rupture") forms a tumorlike swelling at the anus. Other problems around the anus include **hemorrhoids** (**HEM**-or-oyds).
hemorrhoids	**2204** The term _____ literally means "veins likely to bleed."
hemorrhoids	**2205** The _____ are actually **varicose** (**VAR**-ih-kohs) **veins** around the anus. These veins are "abnormally dilated and twisted," that is, varicose.
Information Frame	**2206** Being dilated is close in meaning to being enlarged. Remember that the ending in **acromegaly (frame 1452)** indicates an "enlargement of." Sometimes the "liver," indicated by the root in hepatic **(frame 2124)**, and the "spleen," denoted by the root in splenectomy **(frame 1902)**, both become enlarged.
hepat/o/splen/o/megaly (heh-**pat**-oh-**splen**-oh-**MEG**-ah-lee)	**2207** The above facts help us construct _____ / _____ / _____ / _____ / _____, an "enlargement of the liver and spleen."
hepatosplenomegaly	**2208** The abnormal "enlargement" of _____ may occur in cases where toxic substances have been ingested, triggering the immune factors in the "liver" and "spleen" to work overtime.
col/o/rect/al (koh-loh-**REK**-tal)	**2209** Much more serious than hepatosplenomegaly is _____ / _____ / _____ / _____ cancer. This type of cancer "pertains to the large intestine" and the "rectum." Its adjective-creating suffix is identical to that in hiatal **(frame 2196)**.

colorectal cancer	**2210** The disease of _____ _____ is a malignant neoplasm of the digestive tract that may be fatal if not diagnosed and treated promptly.
reddish yellow	**2211** The liver (not the colon or rectum) has a tendency to turn color when diseased. **Cirrh (SER)**, for example, means "_____ _____," according to the word list. **Jaundice (JAWN**-dis), similarly, indicates "yellowness." Both word elements are commonly applied to diseased liver.
cirrh/o/sis (sir-**OH**-sis)	**2212** Borrow the suffix from pyrosis **(frame 2183)** and build _____ /____ /_____, a "condition of reddish yellowness."
cirrhosis jaundice	**2213** A "reddish-yellow condition," or _____, reflects a fatty degeneration of the liver. It is accompanied by hardening and a change in color from the normal brown to an abnormal reddish yellow. This fatty hepatic hardening goes along with a _____, or "yellowing," of the skin due to bile spilling over into the bloodstream.
chole	**2214** Stones are, of course, hard. **Lith (LITH)** is a root for "stone." Recall that _____ **(frame 2120)** is a root for "gall" or "bile." The root for "bile duct" is **choledoch (KOH**-leh-dahk).
chole/lith (KOH-leh-lith) **choledoch/o/lith** (koh-**LED**-ah-koh-**lith**)	**2215** Make use of the preceding information to construct _____ /_____, which is a term for "gallstone" or "bile stone." Similarly, _____ /____ /_____ is a "gallstone" in the "bile duct."
cholelith choledocholith	**2216** A _____ ("gallstone") or _____ ("bile duct stone") is usually the result of too much cholesterol in the bile. The excess cholesterol settles out in the liver, bile ducts, or gallbladder, serving to stimulate formation of stones.
-iasis	**2217** The term for "gallstone" frequently takes _____, the suffix in hypochondriasis **(frame 114)**, as an "abnormal condition of" ending.
chole/lith/iasis (**koh**-lee-lih-**THIGH**-ah-sis) **choledoch/o/lith/iasis** (koh-**led**-oh-koh-lih-**THIGH**-ah-sis)	**2218** We therefore have _____ /_____ /_____ for an "abnormal condition of gallstones." Likewise, _____ /____ /_____ /_____ denotes an "abnormal condition of bile duct stones."

cholelithiasis	**2219** The general "gallstone condition of" _____, may also be called **choledocholithiasis**, if there are choleliths or **choledocholiths** large enough to block the **common bile duct**. The bile dams up behind this blockage, spills into the bloodstream, and creates jaundice.
-o/rrhea	**2220** While cholelithiasis may prevent a flow of bile, other digestive upsets involve an excessive flow of materials. Recall that ____ / _____, the suffix in otorrhea **(frame 1298)**, means "flow" or "discharge." Such a discharge may be abnormal or excessive in certain cases. **Py (PIGH)**, for instance, denotes "pus," which is always abnormal.
py/o/**rrhea** (**pigh**-or-EE-uh)	**2221** Synthesize ____ / ____ / _____, a term for "flow of pus."
pyorrhea	**2222** Severe gingivitis complicated by the presence of **abscesses** (**AB**-ses-ehz), or pus-filled sacs, may result in _____ ("discharge of pus") when the gums and teeth are brushed.
dia/rrhea	**2223** A related term is diarrhea. Subdivide this term by inserting slashmarks: _____ / _____.
diarrhea dia-	**2224** Since _____ contains the prefix _____, for "through," it denotes an excessive "flowing through" of liquid fecal matter out of the anus.
	2225 A patient afflicted with uncontrolled diarrhea must be carefully studied and tested. A number of possible causes must be considered for diagnosis.

Lab Tests and Diagnoses

Word Parts Associated with Lab Tests and Diagnoses for the Digestive System

The following is a list of word parts and abbreviations associated with lab tests and diagnoses of digestive diseases. Use this list to help you complete **frames 2226 to 2257**.

ALK PHOS	alkaline phosphatase	**enem/o**	inject	ortho-	straight
colon	large intestine	**nas/o**	nose	**ped/o**	child
-clysis	washing out of	**NG tube**	nasogastric tube	**SGOT**	serum glutamic oxalacetic transaminase

dont	**2226** Some particular specialties of dentistry are able to help diagnose digestive difficulties that may start with the mouth. Most of them contain _____ rather than dent **(frame 2082)** as their root for "teeth."
dont/ist (**DAHN**-tist)	**2227** Remember that -**ist** means "one who specializes in." Consequently _____ /_____ (like dentist) denotes "one who specializes in the teeth."
Information Frame	**2228** Dontist, however, is generally seen only in combination with other word parts. Take **ortho-** (**OR**-thoh), for instance, a prefix for "straight." Another example is **ped (PEED)**, which means "child" as well as "foot." Finally, remember that the prefix in periodontitis **(frame 2163)** means "around."
ortho/**dont**/**ist** (or-thoh-**DAHN**-tist) **ped**/**o**/**dont**/**ist** (**pee**-doh-**DAHN**-tist) **peri**/**o**/**dont**/**ist** (**pahr**-ee-oh-**DAHN**-tist)	**2229** Now employ the information provided in the preceding two frames to help you build the following terms for dental specialists: _____ /_____ /_____ "one who specializes in straightening the teeth" _____ /____ /_____ /_____ "one who specializes in the teeth of children" _____ /____ /_____ /_____ "one who specializes in (problems) around the teeth"
pedodontist orthodontist periodontist	**2230** A small child would most likely visit a(n) _____ to get her teeth checked. If her teeth were crooked, she might be referred to a(n) _____ to get them straightened. If she had severe gum problems around her teeth, she might be taken to a(n) _____.
-graphy	**2231** We know that dentists of all types rely heavily on x-rays for diagnosis. Radiography, however, is also performed on various alimentary organs by other types of specialists. Recall that _____, the suffix of radiography **(frame 194)**, denotes "the process of recording."
cholecyst/o/graphy (**koh**-lee-sis-**TAH**-grah-fee)	**2232** Build _____ /____ /_____, "the process of recording (x-ray images) of the gallbladder."
cholecystography	**2233** "X-raying of the gallbladder," a process called _____, may reveal the presence of gallstones.
cholecystography	**2234** Gallbladder x-raying, or _____, is only one type of digestive organ x-raying. Organs lying directly in the lower GI tract are often x-rayed after the patient swallows a mixture of the substance **barium (BAH**-ree-um).

barium	**2235** A white chalky substance, _____ **sulfate** (**SUHL**-fayt), is useful to mark the outline of various digestive passages because it is not penetrated by x-rays.
Information Frame	**2236** Barium gets into the body by being, in a sense, "injected." This concept is named **enem** (**EH**-nem).
enem/a (**EH**-neh-mah)	**2237** Borrow the suffix from saliva **(frame 2092)** and write out a new term, _____ /____ , "an injection."
enema	**2238** An _____ is technically the "injection" of some material into the rectum and intestine.
barium enema	**2239** A _____ _____ is "an injection of barium" into the rectum. The barium creates a white shadow on x-ray film that allows easy inspection of lower intestinal structures.
Information Frame	**2240** Some enemas are merely cleansing. The suffix **-clysis** (**KLIGH**-sis), for instance, means "washing out of."
enter/o/clysis (**en**-ter-**AHK**-lih-sis) **proct/o/clysis** (**prahk-TAHK**-lih-sis)	**2241** Employing the **e**-beginning root for "intestine" **(frame 2177)** yields _____ /____ /_____ , "washing out of the intestine." Using the **p**-beginning root for "rectum" **(frame 2201)** results in _____ /____ /_____ , "washing out of the rectum."
enteroclysis proctoclysis	**2242** Either an _____ or a _____ is an enema of the intestines and rectum. Such enemas may consist of nothing more than soapy water.
thoracentesis **abdomin/o/centesis** (ab-**dahm**-ih-noh-sen-**TEE**-sis)	**2243** While enemas add fluid to the digestive tube, other diagnostic techniques draw fluid off. For the thoracic cavity, the procedure called _____ **(frame 2069)** surgically punctures and taps fluids from the chest. Using abdomin as the root, name the comparable procedure for the abdominal cavity: _____ /____ /_____ .
abdominocentesis	**2244** The "surgical puncture and tapping" of fluids from the "abdominal" cavity is termed _____ . An alternative term is **paracentesis** (**pahr**-ah-sen-**TEE**-sis).

abdominocentesis paracentesis	**2245** The technique of _____ or _____ is a convenient means of sampling the serous fluid bathing organs in the abdominal cavity.
nas gastric	**2246** Tubes or needles can also be inserted into other areas, such as the nose and stomach. Remind yourself that _____, like rhin **(frame 1928)**, means "nose," and that _____ **(frame 2098)** "refers to the stomach."
nas/o/gastr/ic (**nay**-soh-**GAS**-trik)	**2247** Create _____ /_____ /_____ /_____, which "refers to the nose and stomach."
nasogastric	**2248** A _____ **tube** is one that is inserted into the "nose" and then fed down into the "stomach."
NG	**2249** A nasogastric tube (abbreviated as _____ _____ **tube**) can help suck out a sample of gastric contents for analysis.
-o/scopy **colon/o/scopy** (**koh**-lahn-**AHS**-koh-pee) **esophag/o/scopy** (eh-**sah**-fah-**GAHS**-koh-pee) **lapar/o/scopy** (**lap**-ar-**AHS**-koh-pee)	**2250** Endoscopy of various kinds can be performed by inserting endoscopes into digestive structures. Write the following terms for the "process of examining," employing the suffix _____ /_____ **(frame 180)**, plus the appropriate roots: _____ /_____ /_____ "process of examining the large intestine" _____ /_____ /_____ "process of examining the esophagus" _____ /_____ /_____ "process of examining the abdomen (lapar)"
colonoscopy laparoscopy esophagoscopy	**2251** Tumors within the large intestine would most likely be revealed by _____. In contrast, _____ might find such growths externally covering the intestinal wall. Problems within the tube leading into the stomach can be located by _____.
Information Frame	**2252** Many chemical tests are performed on digestive tube contents and secretions. The liver is a prime target of such tests, for two reasons. It produces the bile, and it is a great **detoxifier** (dee-**TAHKS**-ih-figh-er), or "de-poisoner," of many harmful substances.
scan	**2253** Just as a lung scan **(frame 2031)** tracks radioactive particles after they are inhaled, a **liver** _____ tracks radioactive ingested chemicals as they concentrate within the liver. **Liver enzyme tests** may also be conducted.

enzyme	**2254** Liver _____ tests look at the levels of specific liver enzymes that are related to disease. Examples include **alkaline phosphatase** (**FAHS**-fah-tays), abbreviated as **ALK PHOS**, and **serum glutamic** (gloo-**TAM**-ik) **oxalacetic** (ahks-al-ah-**SEE**-tik) **transaminase** (trans-**AM**-ih-nays). The second tongue-twisting enzyme name is conveniently abbreviated with four letters as ____ ____ ____ ____.
SGOT	

ALK	**2255** Elevated blood serum levels of alkaline (____ ____ ____) phos-
PHOS	phatase (____ ____ ____ ____) and _____
serum	_____ _____ _____
glutamic oxalacetic transaminase	(SGOT) are often characteristic of liver disease.

Information Frame	**2256** Sometimes the microbial contents of the stools or feces are analyzed.

stool	**2257** A common type of procedure is preparing _____ **cultures**. Feces (stools) are placed into a growth medium, which is later tested for the presence of various microbes.

	2258 Procedures for treating digestive infections and surgically correcting alimentary disorders have been in use since ancient times.

Surgery and Therapies

Word Parts Associated with Surgery, Pharmacology, and other Therapies for the Digestive System

The following is a list of word parts associated with surgery, pharmacology, and other therapies for digestive problems. Use this list to help you complete **frames 2259 to 2301**.

anastom/o	to furnish with a mouth	**cathart/o**	purification; cleansing; purging
ant-	against	**laxativ/o**	slacken; relax
cathars/o	purification; cleansing; purging	non-	not

ant- (ANT)	**2259** Various drugs have proven effective in treating digestive problems. Some drugs work "against" such problems. Take the **a**-beginning prefix for "against" and remove its terminal **i** to get _____.

ant/acids (ant-**ASS**-ids)	**2260** Now build _____ /_____, substances that work "against acids."

system/ic	**2261** You may remember the _____ /_____ (Chapter 13) circulation, which supplies blood to all major body "systems" except for the lungs.

systemic antacids	**2262** We can combine the facts from the preceding two frames and create a phrase. This phrase is _____ _____, that is, "antacids (that affect all body) systems."
systemic antacids	**2263** The _____ _____ are those absorbed directly into the "systemic" circulation after being consumed. Examples of this group include **Alka Seltzer** and **sodium bicarbonate (bicarbonate of soda)**.
non-	**2264** If a psychiatric patient is _____ /violent, this term means that he or she is "not violent."
non/system/ic (**nahn**-sis-**TEM**-ik)	**2265** Similarly, _____ / _____ / ____ "refers to (something) that is not (associated) with (many body) systems."
nonsystemic antacids	**2266** We can therefore coin the phrase _____ _____, "antacids not (associated) with (many body) systems."
nonsystemic antacids	**2267** More precisely, the _____ _____ are those that neutralize acid locally, remaining within the GI tract after being consumed. This broad chemical group includes **Gelusil, Maalox,** and **Mylanta**.
cathars (kah-**THARS**) **cathart** (kah-**THART**)	**2268** Other drugs are often administered to relieve constipation or otherwise stimulate defecation. Glancing back at the word list, you will note that two roots, _____ and _____, mean "purification, cleansing, or purging."
cathars/is (kah-**THAR**-sis)	**2269** Using cathars and the "presence of" suffix in pectoralis **(frame 987)**, construct _____ / ____, "a purging."
catharsis	**2270** By _____ is usually meant a thorough "purging," either of the mind or of the bowels!
cathart/ic (kah-**THAR**-tik)	**2271** Using cathart and the ending in systemic, build _____ / ____, "pertaining to purging."

cathartic catharsis	**2272** The _____ drugs are those that stimulate _____, or "purging" of the bowels.
cathart/ics (kah-**THAR**-tiks)	**2273** If a cathartic is "a purger," then _____ /_____ are "purgers."
cathartics	**2274** As a group, the _____, or "purgers," exert an extremely powerful stimulation for defecation. An example of this group is **Colace** (**KOH**-lays). A related group is described by the root **laxativ** (**LAKS**-ah-tiv), "slacken" or "relax."
laxativ/e (**LAKS**-ah-tiv)	**2275** Adding the suffix in leukocyte **(frame 1738)** results in _____ /_____, "a slackening or relaxing."
laxatives (**LAKS**-ah-**tivs**)	**2276** The _____ ("slackeners or relaxers") provide mild stimulation for defecation, by "slackening or relaxing" the bowels.
laxative	**2277** A well-known _____ ("relaxer") that can be purchased over-the-counter is **milk of magnesia**.
Information Frame	**2278** As with other body systems, surgical interventions are sometimes necessary. A surgically related root is **anastom** (ah-nah-**STOHM**). It means "to furnish with a mouth," that is, an opening.
anastomos/is (ah-**nas**-tah-**MOH**-sis)	**2279** Adding the suffix in catharsis results in _____ /_____, "a furnishing with a mouth."
anastomosis	**2280** An _____ is a natural "mouthlike" connection between two body structures, or the surgical creation of such a connection.
anastomosis -o/stomy	**2281** Making a mouthlike _____, or any "permanent opening," is represented by the ending _____ /_____ **(frame 296)**.
gastr/o/jejun/o/stomy (**gas**-troh-**jay**-joo-**NAHS**-toh-mee)	**2282** Build a single term that means "making a permanent opening (between) the stomach and the jejunum." (Use the appropriate root for each.) The term is _____ /_____ /_____ /_____ /_____. Quite a mouthful, or anastomosis, isn't it?

gastrojejunostomy	**2283** A _____ may be performed to directly connect the stomach to the jejunum when the duodenum is damaged or diseased.
duoden/o/jejun/o/stomy (dew-**wah**-den-oh-**jay**-joo-**NAHS**-toh-mee)	**2284** Another long word indicating a surgical anastomosis is _____ / ____ / _____ / ____ / _____. This term indicates the "making of a permanent (new) opening (between) the duodenum and jejunum."
duodenojejunostomy	**2285** In actuality, a _____ is the creation of a permanent artificial channel between the duodenum and the jejunum, since the duodenum already leads into the jejunum naturally.
gastr/o/stomy (**gas-TRAHS**-toh-mee) **ile/o/stomy** (il-ee-**AHS**-toh-mee) **col/o/stomy** (koh-**LAHS**-toh-mee)	**2286** Have some fun "making permanent new openings in": the "stomach": _____ / ____ / _____ the "ileum": _____ / ____ / _____ the "large intestine": _____ / ____ / _____
-o/tomy	**2287** Making any new opening first requires "cutting into" or an "incision into," denoted by the combining form ____ / _____.
lapar/o/tomy (**lap**-ar-**AHT**-oh-mee) **enter/o/tomy** (**en**-ter-**AHT**-oh-mee) **cholecyst/o/tomy** (**koh**-leh-sist-**AHT**-oh-mee)	**2288** Create surgical "incision into" terms for each of the following structures: "abdomen" (using lapar): _____ / ____ / _____ "intestine" (using enter): _____ / ____ / _____ "gallbladder" (using cholecyst) _____ / ____ / _____
cholecystotomy choleliths choledocholiths	**2289** The surgery of _____ ("incision into the gallbladder") is often done to remove _____ ("gallstones") or _____ ("bile duct stones," **frame 2215**).
lith/o/tomy (lith-**AHT**-oh-mee)	**2290** Employ the "stone" root in cholelith **(frame 2215)** and build _____ / ____ / _____, "incision (to get at) a stone."
lithotomy **chole/lith/o/tomy** (**koh**-leh-lith-**AHT**-oh-mee)	**2291** A _____ ("stone-incision") is more precisely called a _____ / _____ / ____ / _____, or "incision (to get at) a gallstone."

lithotomy cholelithotomy cholecyst	**2292** If a cholelith is too huge to be removed by _____ (_____), then removal of the _____ ("gallbladder," **frame 2119**) may be required.
	2293 Extract the suffix from laryngectomy **(frame 2073)** and use it to build the following terms: _____ / _____, "removal of the gallbladder" _____ / _____, "removal of the stomach" _____ / _____, "removal of the large intestine" _____ / _____, "removal of the appendix" _____ / _____, "removal of hemorrhoids"
cholecyst/ectomy (**koh**-lee-sist-**EK**-toh-mee) **gastr/ectomy** (**gas-TREK**-toh-mee) **col/ectomy** (koh-**LEK**-toh-mee) **append/ectomy** (**ah**-pen-**DEK**-toh-mee) **hemorrhoid/ectomy** (**hehm**-or-oyd-**EK**-toh-mee)	
cholecystectomy hemorrhoidectomy	**2294** The operation of _____ takes away a painful, stone-filled gallbladder, while _____ gets rid of painful hemorrhoids.
colectomy	**2295** Colorectal cancer may require _____, full or partial removal of the large intestine, to save a patient's life.
gastrectomy	**2296** Similarly, _____ can remove a cancerous stomach.
appendectomy	**2297** Severe appendicitis may prompt an _____, before the swollen, bacteria-filled appendix ruptures and contaminates the abdominal cavity.
Information Frame	**2298** Finally, defects may just require "surgical repair" (as in rhinoplasty, **frame 2048**), rather than complete removal of a body structure.
cheil/o/plasty (kigh-loh-**PLAS**-tee) **pylor/o/plasty** (pigh-**LOR**-oh-plas-tee)	**2299** Take, for instance, cheil as a root for "lips" **(frame 2079)** and the root for "gatekeeper" **(frame 2100)**. Combining them with **-plasty** results in _____ / _____ / _____ ("surgical repair of the lips") and _____ / _____ / _____ ("surgical repair of the gate-keeper").
cheiloplasty	**2300** A _____ may improve the looks of a person's face after being in a severe car accident.
pyloroplasty	**2301** A _____ may allow the contents of the stomach to properly drain from the pylorus into the duodenum.

Multiple Choice

1. The physical and chemical breakdown of food is

    a. egestion   b. secretion   c. digestion   d. absorption

2. Which of these combining forms means "blind"?

    a. chol/e   b. cec/o   c. cheil/o   d. chil/o

3. Which of these is the combining form for the first part of the small intestine?

    a. ile/o   b. duoden/o   c. jejun/o   d. cec/o

4. Which of the following combining forms denotes the serous membrane of the abdominal cavity?

    a. pylor/o   b. proct/o   c. cholecyst/o   d. periton/e

5. "Relating to the appendix" uses the adjectival suffix

    a. -al   b. -ic   c. -iac   d. -eal

6. To build a term meaning "flow of pus" use

    a. -orrhagia   b. -orrhea   c. -orrhaphy   d. -orrhexis

Meanings of Selected Roots

Add the correct combining vowel (cv) after each root. The write the definition of each root in the space provided.

ROOT/CV	DEFINITION
1. esophag/_____	_____
2. hepat/_____	_____
3. appendic/_____	_____
4. col/_____	_____
5. rect/_____	_____
6. enem/_____	_____
7. gastr/_____	_____
8. lapar/_____	_____
9. bili/_____	_____
10. laxativ/_____	_____

Word Dissection and Translation

Analyze the following terms by dissecting them with slashmarks and identifying their word parts. To the right of each term, write its correct English translation.

Key: R (root), cv (combining vowel), P (prefix), S (suffix)

1. gastrectomy

_____ / _____   _____
R   S

2. dysphagia

_____ / _____ / _____   _____
P   R   S

3. hiatal

_____ / _____   _____
R   S

4. hepatosplenomegaly

_____ / ___ / _____ / ___ / _____   _____
R   cv   R   cv   S

5. cholelith

_____ / _____   _____
R   R(S)

6. enteroclysis

_____ / ___ / _____   _____
R   cv   S

7. sigmoid

_____ / _____   _____
R   S

8. rectocele

_____ / ___ / _____   _____
R   cv   S

9. cholecystography

_____ / ___ / _____   _____
R   cv   S

10. laparoscopy

_____ / ___ / _____   _____
R   cv   S

Terms and Their Abbreviations

In the list below, when the term is given, write its abbreviation in the space provided. When the abbreviation is given, write its corresponding term.

TERM	ABBREVIATION
1. gastrointestinal	_____
2. _____	NG
3. alkaline phosphatase	_____
4. serum glutamic oxalacetic transaminase	_____

Word Spelling

Look at each of the terms listed below. Identify those that are misspelled by circling Y for "Yes." Write the correct spelling in the blank.

WORD	MISSPELLED?	CORRECT SPELLING
1. hehpatic	Y/N	_____
2. pearastalsis	Y/N	_____
3. cirrhosis	Y/N	_____
4. cholelithiasis	Y/N	_____
5. colunoscopy	Y/N	_____
6. antacids	Y/N	_____
7. cathartic	Y/N	_____
8. gastrostomy	Y/N	_____
9. esawphagoscopy	Y/N	_____
10. hernia	Y/N	_____
11. enteritis	Y/N	_____
12. kolonoscopie	Y/N	_____
13. orthodontist	Y/N	_____
14. abdominocentesis	Y/N	_____

New Word Synthesis

Using word parts that appear in this and previous chapters, build new terms with the following meanings:

1. _____ pertaining to stones

2. _____ surgical repair of the liver

3. _____ removal of an off-shoot or by-path

4. _____ inflammation of the gatekeeper, stomach, and abdomen

5. _____ a process of recording (images) of hemorrhoids

6. _____ referring to a reddish yellow voicebox

7. _____ the presence of (something) against a constricting around

8. _____ surgical repair of the lips

9. _____ pertaining to the tongue and throat

10. _____ pertaining to the large intestine and rectum

C ASE S TUDY

Read through the following partial laparoscopic evaluation. Note the terms in bold print. A series of multiple choice questions probes your knowledge of these terms.

Laparoscopic Evaluation

A 15-year-old female was examined **laparoscopically** to detect possible causes of recurrent **ileocolic** spasms. Upon examination, a **laparal** stricture was seen over the **ileocecal sphincter**.

Case Study Questions

1. The evaluation was performed **laparoscopically** by

   (a) means of an ophthalmoscope.

   (b) inserting an endoscope through a small slit in the abdominal wall.

   (c) crushing and removing painful bile stones.

   (d) extracting the colon from the abdominal cavity.

2. The **ileocolic** spasms kept occurring in

   (a) the area where the large and small intestines join.

   (b) the distal third of the esophagus.

   (c) waves of constriction around the oral cavity.

   (d) the area where the stomach and small intestine join.

3. The **laparal** stricture ("narrowing") mainly involved the

   (a) heart.

   (b) laryngeal wall.

   (c) aortic lumen.

   (d) abdominal wall.

4. The stricture was seen over the **ileocecal sphincter**, the ring of muscle between the

   (a) pharynx and esophagus.

   (b) esophagus and stomach.

   (c) stomach and small intestine.

   (d) small intestine and large intestine.

CHAPTER 17 The Urinary System

INTRODUCTION

The **urinary** (**YOO**-rih-**nayr**-ee) **system** shares many things in common with both the cardiovascular system and the digestive system. By definition, the urinary system involves **urine**. Urine is a yellowish, salty, highly acidic derivative of the blood plasma.

Figure 17.1 outlines four major processes involved with forming and releasing urine. First, there is **filtration**. Filtration is the pressure-driven movement of a fluid across a semipermeable membrane. For urine formation, there is a relatively high blood pressure within certain kidney vessels, the **glomeruli** (gloh-**MEHR**-yoo-ligh). This high pressure pushes fluid out of the blood, across the semipermeable membranes of the cells that line the vessel walls. The pushing process is filtration. (The operation here is similar to what we saw in Chapter 14 for formation of lymph from blood.) Closely associated with the glomeruli is a series of microscopic kidney tubules. Fluid filtered out of the blood in the glomeruli enters these tubules. This fluid is called the **urinary filtrate** (**FIL**-trayt).

The urinary filtrate within the kidney tubules is the starting fluid for the urine. The next step is tubular **secretion**—the release of additional material into the filtrate by special mechanisms in the kidney cells. Then comes tubular **reabsorption**, the movement of certain selected solutes and water out of the kidney tubules and back into the bloodstream. By tubular reabsorption, a deficiency in blood sodium or other particles is corrected by mechanisms that move more sodium out of the urinary filtrate and back into the plasma.

After filtration, tubular secretion, and tubular reabsorption, the final act is **urination**—the excretion of urine from the body. This excretion process somewhat parallels that in the digestive tube, because waste matter is discarded. In the urinary system, however, the waste is mainly fluid, while for the digestive system, the waste is primarily solid (feces).

FIGURE 17.1

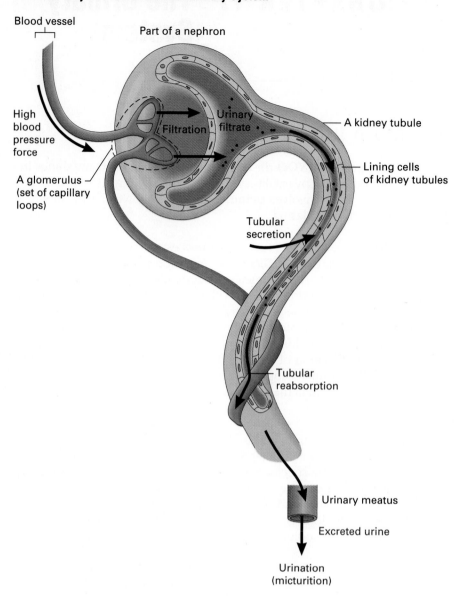

Figure 17.2 shows the major anatomical features of the **nephron** (**NEF**-rahn). It is the major structural and functional unit of urine formation within the kidneys. Each kidney contains millions of microscopic nephrons. The processes associated with urine formation and release all occur within each of these tubular structures.

Figure 17.3 reveals the interior of the kidney and the rest of the gross anatomy of the urinary system. Note that urine collects within the funnel-shaped **renal** (**REE**-nal) **pelvis**, which receives the urine from all the nephrons. From the renal pelvis, the urine is carried out of each kidney by a **ureter** (**YOO**-reh-ter). The right and left ureters both connect to the urinary bladder. From the base of the **urinary bladder**, a long **urethra** (yoo-**REE**-thrah) finally conducts the urine out to the **urinary meatus**—the hole through which one urinates.

This chapter discusses terms associated with normal anatomy and physiology of the urinary system. Terms describing urinary diseases, related lab tests and diagnostic procedures, and surgery and other therapies for urinary problems are likewise considered.

The Anatomy of a Nephron

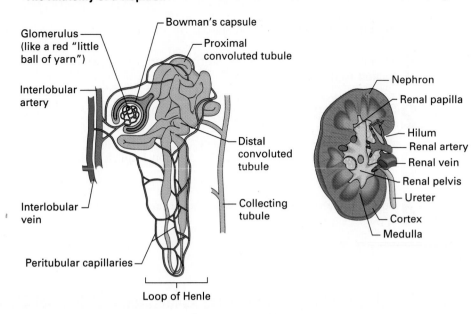

Glomerulus (like a red "little ball of yarn")

Bowman's capsule

Proximal convoluted tubule

Interlobular artery

Distal convoluted tubule

Collecting tubule

Interlobular vein

Peritubular capillaries

Loop of Henle

Nephron

Renal papilla

Hilum

Renal artery

Renal vein

Renal pelvis

Ureter

Cortex

Medulla

Gross Anatomy of the Urinary System

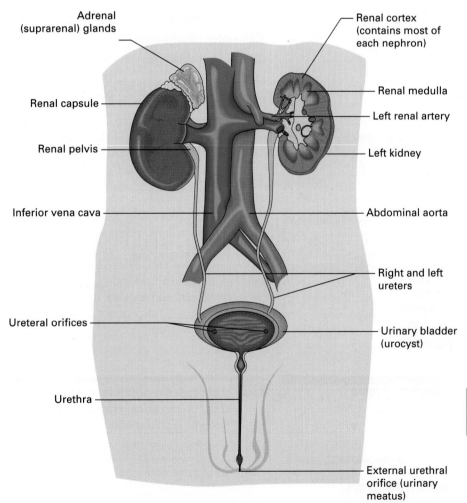

Adrenal (suprarenal) glands

Renal cortex (contains most of each nephron)

Renal capsule

Renal medulla

Left renal artery

Renal pelvis

Left kidney

Inferior vena cava

Abdominal aorta

Right and left ureters

Ureteral orifices

Urinary bladder (urocyst)

Urethra

External urethral orifice (urinary meatus)

CHAPTER OBJECTIVES

By the end of this chapter, you should be able to:

1 Identify major prefixes, roots, suffixes, and abbreviations related to the urinary system.

2 Dissect urinary terms into their component parts.

3 Translate urinary terms into their common English equivalents.

4 Build new terms associated with the urinary system.

Normal A & P

Word Parts Associated with Normal Structure and Function of the Urinary System

The following is a list of word parts and an abbreviation associated with normal anatomy and physiology of the urinary system. Use this list to help you complete **frames 2302 to 2356**.

genit/o	produce	**pyel/o**	pelvis; the renal pelvis	**uret/o**	urine
glomerul/o	little ball of yarn			**ureter/o**	urinary tube
GU	genitourinary	**ren/o**	kidney	**urethr/o**	to make water
mictur/i	urine	**ur/o**	urine	**urin/a**	urine
nephr/o	kidney	**ure/o**	urine	**urocyst/o**	the urinary bladder

---

urin/**ary**

2302 The Introduction talked about the urinary system. Borrowing the same approach as used for biliary **(frame 2124)**, we can dissect urinary as _____ / _____.

---

urinary

2303 Just as biliary "refers to bile," _____ "refers to urine."

---

urin (**YOO**-rin)
ur (**YUR**)
ure (**YOO**-ree)
uret (**YOO**-reht)
mictur (**MIK**-ter)

2304 The root in urinary, _____, denotes "urine." According to the word list, three other **u**-beginning roots, _____, _____, and _____, also denote "urine." A fifth root _____, has the same meaning.

Information Frame

2305 Although the suffix **-ate**, has been defined **(frame 92)** as "something that," it can also assume a meaning as a verb: "to do" or "to pass." The second verbal meaning is often attached to urin and mictur.

---

urin/ate (**YOO**-rih-nayt)
mictur/ate (**MIK**-too-rayt)

2306 Using the above information, create two new terms, _____ / _____ and _____ / _____, both of which mean, "to pass urine." The ending **-s** is often added to indicate present tense.

---

urinates micturates urinary	**2307** A person "passes urine," that is, _____ or _____, by voiding some or all of the contents of the _____ ("referring to urine") bladder.
urin/a/tion **mictur/i/tion** (mik-too-**RIH**-shun)	**2308** The roots in urinate and micturate can be used with the ending in ven- tilation **(frame 1968)**, to build _____ /_____ /_____ and _____ /_____ /_____, respectively. Both terms indicate the "process of (excreting) urine." The combining vowel for urin is **a**; for mictur, it is **i**.
urination micturition	**2309** The kidney is the primary organ tied to _____ or _____ ("urine excretion").
nephr **ren**	**2310** The word list cites two roots, _____ and _____, for "kidney." The former root occurred in epinephrine **(frame 1419)**, the latter in adrenal **(frame 1368)**.
nephr/**on**	**2311** Nephr takes the same "presence of" ending as colon **(frame 2127)**. This combination results in _____ /_____, or "presence of the kidney."
ren/**al**	**2312** Ren takes the "relating to" ending of colorectal **(frame 2209)**. The product is _____ /_____, "relating to the kidney."
nephron renal	**2313** Although _____ literally means "the (whole) kidney," as stated in the Introduction, it is actually a microscopic functional unit of the kidney. In contrast, _____, both in theory and in practice, does "relate to the (whole) kidney."
nephrons **renal** **renal**	**2314** Most of the _____, the main structural and functional units of the kidney, are located in the more peripheral _____ ("relating to kidney") **cortex** rather than the more central _____ ("relating to kidney") **medulla**.
glomerul/us (gloh-**MEHR**-yoo-lus) alveolus	**2315** The kidney contains many **glomerul/i**. You may surmise that the sin- gular of glomeruli is _____ /_____, just as the singular of alveoli **(frame 1959)** is _____.
glomerul (gloh-**MEHR**-yool)	**2316** The root in glomerulus, _____, means "little ball of yarn." This name is owing to the resemblance of this set of blood-con- taining capillary loops to a little ball of red yarn.

glomerulus	**2317** Each _____ is the starting point of a nephron. Filtration of blood plasma occurs across the thin, leaky walls of this structure's capillaries.
pyel (**PIGH**-el)	**2318** All of the nephrons in the kidney eventually dump their filtrate into the renal pelvis. According to the word list, a root for pelvis is _____.
renal pelvis	**2319** The _____ _____ is a large, funnel-shaped sac embedded within the "kidney." It gets its name because it collects urine as "a bowl" would.
pyel/ic (pigh-**EH**-lik)	**2320** Borrow the ending from pyloric **(frame 2102)** and create _____ /_____, "referring to the (renal) pelvis."
pyelic	**2321** The _____ ("referring to pelvis") sac eventually drains its collected urine out of the kidney and into a ureter.
uret/**er**	**2322** Ureter is dissected as _____ /_____. It contains the suffix, **-er**, which has the same meaning as **-or (frame 99)**.
ureter	**2323** The _____ is a hollow, muscular-walled tube that conducts urine out of the renal pelvis and emerges from the medial wall of the kidney. Eventually, the urine within this tube is carried into the urinary bladder.
cyst	**2324** Ur is one of several roots that denotes "urine." This root can be combined with _____, the "bladder" portion of cholecyst **(frame 2120)**.
ur/o/cyst (**YOO**-roh-sist)	**2325** Integrate the two word fragments in the above frame: _____ /_____ /_____. Of course, the usual combining **o** will have to be added to make it sound right!
urocyst	**2326** The rough translation of _____ is the "urinary bladder."
urocyst ureters	**2327** The _____ ("urinary bladder") is a large muscular pouch that receives urine draining through the _____ **(frame 2323)**, the tubes attached to the kidneys.

ureter urocyst	**2328** Interestingly enough, both _____ (urinary tube) and _____ (urinary bladder), although complete terms in themselves, can also be used as roots.
ureter/al (yoo-**REE**-ter-al) **urocyst/ic** (**yoo**-roh-**SIS**-tik)	**2329** Ureter, for instance, can be combined with the suffix in renal **(frame 2312)**, while urocyst can take the ending in pyelic **(frame 2320)**. The results are _____ /_____ ("pertaining to the urinary tube") and _____ /_____ ("pertaining to the urinary bladder"), respectively.
ureteral urocystic	**2330** The diameter of the _____ (urinary tube) lumen determines to some extent the _____ (urinary bladder) volume of urine.
urethr (yoo-**REE**-ther)	**2331** Hippocrates was the first to use the root _____. According to the word list, this root means, "to make water." This root takes the same "presence of" ending found in gingiva **(frame 2086)**.
urethr/a (yoo-**REE**-thrah)	**2332** Now write _____ /_____, "the making of water" (a noun).
urethra urocyst	**2333** The _____ is a single long tube that empties urine out of the _____ (urinary bladder). In a very real sense, then, it actually does help us "to make water"!
urethr/al (yoo-**REE**-thral) -al	**2334** Just as renal **(frame 2312)** "relates to the kidney," _____ /_____ "relates to making water." You can see that the suffix in both is _____.
urethral	**2335** At the end of the urethra is a tiny hole, the _____ **orifice**—a hole for "making water."
urethral orifice	**2336** One releases urine out of the body through the _____ _____ ("hole for making water").
meatus **urinary meatus**	**2337** Remind yourself that a _____ (as in external auditory meatus, **frame 1266**) is "a passageway." Therefore the urethral orifice is alternatively named the _____ _____, or "passageway relating to urine."
urinary meatus	**2338** The urethral orifice, or _____ _____, is the opening or passageway through which one urinates.

2339 When urine leaves the body through this hole, it often has a strong, ammonialike odor. **Urea** (yoo-**REE**-ah) is the name of the substance that mainly causes this odor.

ure/a

2340 Urea is subdivided as _____ /_____, with the same "presence of" ending as urethra **(frame 2332)**.

ure
presence of
urine

2341 Quickly reviewing the meaning of _____ (the root in urea, **frame 2304**), allows you to translate urea as the "_____ ____ _____."

urea

2342 The substance _____ is a major nitrogen-containing waste product "present" in the "urine."

ur/ic (**YOO**-rik)

2343 The smallest "urine" root is that in urocyst **(frame 2325)**. To form an adjective denoting presence of urine use the adjectival suffix **-ic**. The result is _____ /_____, meaning "pertaining to urine."

uric

2344 Occurring along with urea is _____ ("pertaining to urine") **acid**.

uric acid

2345 The name _____ _____ derives from the fact that this chemical was first isolated in "urine"-soaked bladder stones!

2346 Another name for uric acid is **lithic** (**LITH**-ik) **acid**. From your knowledge of medical terminology, why would you say this alternate name is appropriate?

urea
uric acid

produce

2347 Urine, along with its two major chemical components, _____ and _____ _____, are excreted from the tip of the **penis** (**PEE**-nis) in males. Yet the penis is also a reproductive structure, in that it releases sperm. **Genit** (**JEN**-it), like genet **(frame 500)**, means "_____."

genit/o/urin/ary
(**jen**-ih-toh-**YOO**-rih-nayr-ee)

2348 Combine genit with urinary to obtain a new term, _____ /_____ /_____ /_____.

genitourinary

2349 The long term _____ literally "pertains to urine and the production of (something)."

genitourinary	**2350** The penis is a _____ structure, because it releases both sperm and urine.
GU	**2351** Genitourinary, abbreviated as ____ ____, can be restated as another word.
genit/al (**JEN**-ih-tal)	**2352** Extract the ending from urethral (**frame 2334**) and build _____ /____, "referring to the production of (something)."
genital	**2353** The penis is the main _____ organ in the male, ejaculating sperm cells by the thousands.
ur/o/genit/al (**yoo**-roh-**JEN**-ih-tal)	**2354** Employing the "urine" root in uric and placing this before genital, results in a new term, ____ /____ /_____ /____.
urogenital GU	**2355** This word, _____, like genitourinary (____ ____), "pertains to urine and the production of (something)."
genitourinary urogenital	**2356** The penis can be described as either a _____ (GU) or a _____ structure, owing to its dual roles.

Diseases

Word Parts Associated with Diseases of the Urinary System

The following is a list of word parts associated with diseases of the urinary system. Use this list to help you complete **frames 2357 to 2394**.

glycos/o	glucose; sugar	**noct/o**	night
hydr/o	water	**poly-**	many

-ia	**2357** You may recall that _____, the suffix in bronchopneumonia (**frame 1998**), means "abnormal condition of (something)."
ur/ia (**YOO**-ree-ah)	**2358** Extract the appropriate root from urogenital (**frame 2354**) and create ____ /____, an "abnormal condition of the urine."
uria	**2359** Let us create some terms with _____ ("abnormal condition of urine") as the trailing word element. The first group concerns the presence of various substances or materials in the urine:
glycos/ur/ia (**gligh**-koh-**SOO**-ree-ah) **glycos** (**GLIGH**-kohs)	_____ /____ /____ "abnormal condition of glucose (in) the urine" (using _____ as a root for "glucose")
hemat/ur/ia (**hee**-mah-**TOO**-ree-ah)	_____ /____ /____ "abnormal condition of blood (in) the urine" (uses "blood" root in hematopoiesis, **frame 1733**)
py/ur/ia (pigh-**YOO**-ree-ah)	____ /____ /____ "abnormal condition of pus (in) the urine" (uses "pus" root in pyorrhea, **frame 2221**)

noct/ur/ia (nahk-**TOO**-ree-ah)

dys/ur/ia (dis-**YOO**-ree-ah)

poly/ur/ia (**pah**-lee-**YOO**-ree-ah)
poly-

2360 Now build several terms describing abnormal conditions of the urine that are associated with particular times or sensations:

_____ /_____ /_____ "abnormal condition of urine (in) the night" (employing same "night" root as noctambulism, **frame 1171**)

_____ /_____ /_____ "abnormal condition of painful or difficult urination" (uses same prefix as in dysphagia, **frame 2198**)

_____ /_____ /_____ "abnormal condition of too many (times) urinating" (adopts _____ as a prefix for "many," **frame 80**)

---

dysuria
hematuria
pyuria

2361 The trauma of _____ ("painful urination") may be accompanied by both _____ ("bloody urine") and _____ ("urine with pus").

---

glycosuria
polyuria
nocturia

2362 A "sugary urine," or _____, however, often occurs simultaneously with _____ ("many times urinating"), especially as reflected by _____ ("urinating" during the "night"), when one would normally be sleeping.

---

ur/emia (yoo-**REE**-mee-ah)

2363 If you take **ur** and combine it with the "blood condition of" suffix in leukemia **(frame 1835)**, you get _____ /_____.

---

uremia

2364 "A blood condition of" too much "urea" is called _____.

---

uremia

2365 Symptoms of _____ appear when the kidneys fail to function in their job of excreting urea.

---

uremia
uric/emia (yoo-rih-**SEE**-mee-ah)

2366 Both urea and uric acid largely give the urine its characteristic ammonialike smell. Just as _____ denotes "a blood condition of urea," _____ /_____ denotes "a blood condition of uric" acid.

---

uricemia

2367 Too much uric acid in the blood, that is, a condition of excessive _____, is one of the primary signs of **gout (GOWT)**.

---

hyper/uric/emia
(**high**-per-**yoo**-rih-**SEE**-mee-ah)

2368 Parallel to the way that hyperglycemia **(frame 1429)** indicates "a condition of excessive blood sugar," _____ /_____ /_____ indicates "a condition of excessive blood uric" acid.

---

uremia
hyperuricemia

2369 The conditions of _____ (too much "blood urea") and _____ ("too much blood uric" acid) are often associated with decreased or abnormal function of the kidneys.

---

nephr/itis (nef-RIGH-tis)

2370 Other problems of the urinary system involve some type of inflammation. Using nephr and the suffix in hepatitis **(frame 2161)**, for example, we can create _____ / _____ for "inflammation of the kidneys."

---

nephritis

2371 "Kidney inflammation," or _____, often affects the glomeruli.

---

glomerul/o/nephr/itis
(gloh-MEHR-yoo-loh-nef-RIGH-tis)

2372 Extract the root from glomeruli and attach it to "kidney inflammation." The result is _____ / ____ / _____ / _____, "inflammation of the kidney glomeruli."

---

glomerulonephritis

2373 The disease of _____ is essentially the same thing as nephritis. This is true because if millions of glomeruli in the kidney are inflamed, then practically the whole kidney is affected.

---

nephritis
glomerulonephritis

2374 The condition of _____, or _____, is just one of many types of inflammation affecting the urinary system.

---

pyel/itis (pigh-eh-LIGH-tis)

2375 Pull out the root from pyelic **(frame 2320)**, for instance, and synthesize _____ / _____, "inflammation of the pelvis."

---

pyelitis

2376 You may see a problem with the term _____ ("pelvic inflammation"). It might be mistaken for an osteitis or osteomyelitis involving the bony pelvis of the hips!

---

pyel/o/nephr/itis
(pigh-eh-loh-neh-FRIGH-tis)

2377 To prevent this problem, excise the "kidney" root from glomerulonephritis and produce _____ / ____ / _____ / _____, or "inflammation of the renal pelvis."

---

pyelitis
pyelonephritis

2378 Either term, _____ or _____, correctly names a bacterial inflammation of the kidney and its renal pelvis.

---

pyel/o/cyst/itis
(pigh-eh-loh-sis-TIGH-tis)

2379 Integrate the root for "bladder," as found in urocyst **(frame 2325)**. Create a single long term for "inflammation of the pelvis and bladder": _____ / ____ / _____ / _____.

---

cyst/itis (sis-TIGH-tis)

2380 "Inflammation of the bladder" alone is _____ / _____.

cystitis pyelocystitis	**2381** While _____ results from bacterial infection of the urinary "bladder," _____ may develop from an infection of the "pelvis and bladder."
nephr/o/lith (**NEF**-roh-lith)	**2382** Such types of inflammatory reactions can also be associated with irritating stones. Remove the "stone" from cholelith **(frame 2214)** and the "kidney" from pyelonephritis **(frame 2377)**. Put them together as _____ / _____ / _____, or "kidney stone."
nephrolith	**2383** Just as a cholelith is a stone in the bile, a _____ is a "stone" in the "kidney."
nephr/o/lith/iasis (**nef**-roh-lith-**IGH**-ah-sis)	**2384** Returning again to Chapter 16 **(frame 2218)**, we see that cholelithiasis for "abnormal condition of gallstones" is akin to _____ / _____ / _____ / _____, "an abnormal condition of kidney stones."
nephrolithiasis	**2385** A patient with _____ ("kidney stone condition") may suffer from blockage of the ureter.
hydr	**2386** We know that most of the urine consists of "water," whose **h**-beginning root is _____. This root can be used in combination with several word parts, including another "abnormal condition" or "condition of" suffix, **-o/sis**
hydr/o/nephr/o/sis (**high**-droh-nef-**ROH**-sis)	**2387** Transpose the "kidney" root from nephrolithiasis and create _____ / _____ / _____ / _____ / _____, an "abnormal condition of the kidney (involving) water" build-up.
hydronephrosis	**2388** Blockage of the ureter due to nephrolithiasis can cause _____, the accumulation of large amounts of "watery" urine within the "kidneys."
hydronephrosis -sclerosis	**2389** If _____ is severe enough, so much dammed, aqueous fluid may build up within the kidneys that their tissue is destroyed and hardened. Recall that _____, as in otosclerosis **(frame 1300)**, is an "abnormal condition of hardening."
nephr/o/sclerosis (**nef**-roh-skleh-**ROH**-sis)	**2390** Employ the above information to build _____ / _____ / _____, an "abnormal condition of kidney hardening."

nephrosclerosis
hypertension

2391 A "kidney hardening condition" of _____ is one possible cause for renal _____, or "condition of excessive (blood) pressure" **(frame 1610).**

renal hypertension

2392 The disease of _____ _____, or high blood pressure due to problems in the kidney, may be caused by such things as nephrosclerosis or a narrowing of the **renal artery** feeding into the kidney.

carcinoma

2393 One kidney disease not related to hypertension is **renal cell** _____ ("crab tumor," **frame 571**).

renal cell
carcinoma

2394 "Kidney cell crab tumor," or _____ _____ _____, like most cancers, can be deadly if not diagnosed promptly.

Lab Tests and Diagnoses

Word Parts Associated with Lab Tests and Diagnoses Involving the Urinary System

What follows is a list of some word parts and abbreviations associated with lab tests and diagnoses involving the urinary system. Use this list to help you complete **frames 2396 to 2415.**

BUN	blood urea nitrogen	**-opsy**	vision of
IV	intravenous	**ven/o**	vein
IVP	intravenous pyelogram		

2395 Diagnostic procedures often look at the urinary structures or examine the urine itself.

pyel/o/gram (PIGH-eh-loh-gram)

2396 Indirect methods of examining urinary structures include the usual x-ray procedures. Employ the root in pyelitis **(frame 2375)** and the suffix in angiogram **(frame 1663)** to build _____ / ____ / _____, an x-ray "record of the (renal) pelvis."

pyelogram

venous

2397 In reality, a _____ is an x-ray record of the entire kidney, including the renal pelvis. Dye is circulated into the kidney to make its soft structures visible on x-ray. An arm vein serves as the usual injection site. Recall from **frame 1529** that _____ "pertains to a vein."

intramuscular
intra/ven/ous (in-trah-VEE-nus)

intravenous

2398 Just as _____ **(frame 1057)** "pertains to (something) within muscle," the term _____ / _____ / _____ "pertains to (something) within a vein." The abbreviation for _____ is IV.

IV	**2399** A pyelogram is usually done **intravenously** (**in**-trah-**VEE**-nus-lee), that is, by an ____ ____ ("within vein") route.
intravenous pyelogram	**2400** An _____ _____, abbreviated as IVP, literally is an x-ray "record of the pelvis that pertains to (injection) within a vein."
IVP	**2401** An intravenous pyelogram (or ____ ____ ____) uses the blood circulation to provide a record of the interior of the kidney.
biopsy	**2402** Direct visualization of living kidney tissue is possible. Recall that a _____ **(frame 582)** literally is a "vision of life."
biopsy	**2403** The technique of **renal** _____ obtains a "vision of living kidney" samples.
renal biopsy	**2404** The endoscopic technique of _____ _____ is employed for extracting plugs of living kidney tissue.
cyst	**2405** Endoscopes are often given particular names corresponding to the word roots of the structures they examine. Take for example, the _____ **(frame 2120)**, or "bladder."
cyst/o/scop/e (**SIST**-oh-skohp) **cyst/**o/**scopy** (sis-**TAHS**-koh-pee) bronchoscope bronchoscopy	**2406** A _____ /____ /_____ /____ is "an instrument used to examine the (urinary) bladder." Further, _____ /____ /_____ is "the process of examining the (urinary) bladder." Parallels in word synthesis here are provided by _____ and _____ **(frame 2028)**, which denote "an instrument used to examine a bronchus" and "the process of examining a bronchus," respectively.
cystoscopy cystoscope	**2407** The procedure of _____ using a _____ can be quite helpful in locating bladder stones.
ur/o/**logy** (yoo-**RAHL**-oh-jee)	**2408** Such instruments and techniques are an important part of ____ /____ /_____, "the study of the urinary" system. The appropriate "urinary" root in this case is the one found in urocyst **(frame 2325)**.
urology	**2409** The discipline of _____ studies both the urine and its sources—especially the kidneys and urinary bladder.

ur/o/logist (yoo-**RAHL**-oh-jist)
cardiologist

2410 A ____ / ____ / _____ is a specialist in urology, much as a _____ **(frame 1687)** is a specialist in cardiology.

---

urologist

2411 A _____ may interpret the results of a **urinalysis** (**yoo**-rih-**NAL**-ih-sis).

---

urinalysis

2412 The technical name for an analysis of the urine is _____. Related to such an examination is the **urine specific gravity**.

---

urine specific gravity

2413 The _____ _____ _____ is a measure of the density of a sample of urine compared with that of pure water. This measure reveals how concentrated or dilute the urine has become.

BUN

2414 Since urine is formed from the blood plasma, it is logical to look at the chemical composition of the blood. One important factor is **blood urea nitrogen**, abbreviated as ____ ____ ____.

---

blood urea nitrogen

2415 The _____ _____ _____ (BUN) reflects the concentration of urea in the blood. The greater the amount of this waste product in the blood, the greater the concentration of it in the urine.

2416 Once disease etiology and characteristics have been determined, the course is set for treatment.

Surgery and Therapies

Word Parts Associated with Surgery, Pharmacology, and Other Therapies Involving the Urinary System

The following is a list of word parts associated with surgery, pharmacology, and other therapies for urinary disorders. Use this list to help you complete **frames 2417 to 2437**.

lys/o	breakdown	**-pexy**	surgical fixation of
meat/o	opening	**ton/o**	stretching

---

nephr/o/tomy (neh-**FRAHT**-oh-mee)

urocyst/o/tomy (**yoo**-roh-sis-**TAH**-toh-mee)

urethr/o/tomy (yoo-ree-**THRAHT**-oh-mee)

meat/o/tomy (mee-ah-**TAHT**-oh-mee)

2417 Various urinary structures may be cut into during surgery. Use the suffix for "incision into," as in enterotomy **(frame 2288)**, and the roots representing the structures involved to build:

_____ / ____ / _____ "incision into the kidney" (using nephr)

_____ / ____ / _____ "incision into the urinary bladder"

_____ / ____ / _____ "incision into the urethra"

_____ / ____ / _____ "incision into the (urinary) meatus"

nephr/o/stomy
(neh-**FRAHS**-toh-mee)
urocyst/o/stomy
(**yoo**-roh-sis-**TAHS**-toh-mee)

2418 Employing the suffix for "making permanent new openings in," as in gastrostomy **(frame 2286)**, create:

_____ /_____ /_____ "making permanent new openings in the kidney"

_____ /_____ /_____ "making permanent new openings in the urinary bladder"

---

urocystotomy
urocystostomy

2419 The operation of _____ must be performed before _____, because the "urinary bladder" must be "cut into" before any "permanent new openings" can be created.

---

nephrotomy
nephrostomy

2420 In the same sense, _____ is done before _____, because the "kidney," too, must be incised before new long-term holes are created.

---

urethrotomy

2421 A _____ involves "cutting into the urethra," specifically to remove a stricture—a narrowing or kinking.

---

meatotomy

2422 The surgery in _____ involves "cutting into" the urinary "meatus," as for enlarging its opening.

-pexy

2423 Other surgical operations are commonly performed on the kidney. One type is described by the suffix _____, as in arthropexy **(frame 302)**, "surgical fixation of a joint."

---

nephr/o/pexy (**NEF**-roh-peks-ee)

2424 "Surgical fixation of the kidney" is given by the term _____ /_____ /_____.

---

nephropexy

2425 A dislodged kidney may be anchored to the abdominal wall by means of _____.

---

nephr/ectomy (neh-**FREK**-toh-mee)

2426 Extract the ending from appendectomy **(frame 2293)** and construct _____ /_____, "removal of the kidney."

---

nephrectomy

2427 A _____ may be done if a kidney has been badly damaged in a car accident.

Information Frame

2428 If the kidneys have been severely damaged or removed, then their vital job of filtering and cleansing the blood must be accomplished by artificial means. The technique is called **dialysis** (digh-**AL**-ih-sis).

---

dia/lys/is
dia-

2429 If you remember similar terms, such as hemolysis **(frame 1756)** and lysis **(frame 539)**, you should be able to subdivide dialysis as _____ /_____ /_____. Its prefix, _____, means "through," and its root means "breakdown."

---

breakdown through

2430 Dialysis translates as "a _____ _____."

---

dialysis

2431 The literal definition is somewhat clumsy, but _____ is a procedure whereby certain substances "break down" and move "through" a semipermeable membrane.

---

dialysis

2432 The procedure of _____ is very useful medically, because substances in the blood that break down into smaller particles can be artificially separated from other particles that do not break down, hence cannot cross a membrane.

---

hem/o/dia/lys/is
(**hee**-moh-digh-**AL**-ih-sis)

2433 Borrow the appropriate root from hemolysis **(frame 1756)** and create a compound word with dialysis:
_____ /_____ /_____ /_____ /_____, "dialysis of the blood."

---

hemodialysis

2434 The technique of renal dialysis is usually a form of _____ employing an artificial membrane for removing kidney wastes from the blood.

---

peri/ton/e/al

2435 The visceral peritoneum and parietal peritoneum within the abdominal cavity can also be tapped for removing body wastes. Remember _____ /_____ /_____ /_____ **(frame 2156)**, which "refers to the peritoneum" or to "stretching around (something)."

**peritoneal
dialysis**

2436 We can therefore coin the phrase _____ _____, "dialysis referring to the peritoneum."

---

peritoneal dialysis

2437 The procedure of _____ _____ involves the insertion of a catheter into the abdominal cavity. The walls of this catheter are semipermeable. Consequently, chemical wastes diffuse out of blood vessels in the peritoneum, cross into the catheter, and are then carried out of the body.

Multiple Choice

1. The combining form for urethra is

   a. ureter/o   b. urethr/i   c. urethr/o   d. ur/o

2. The combining form for "bowl" or "pelvis" is

   a. pyel/o   b. nephr/o   c. genit/o   d. ren/o

3. All of the following mean "urine" except for

   a. uro   b. ureo   c. micturo   d. urethro

4. The prefix necessary to form "much" urine is

   a. dys-   b. an-   c. poly-   d. py-

5. The root for "nightly" urine is

   a. glyc/o   b. pyel   c. pyo   d. noct

6. The combining form for a "little ball of yarn" is

   a. nephr   b. pyel/o   c. glomerul/o   d. cyst/o

Meanings of Selected Roots

Add the correct combining vowel (cv) after each root. Then write the definition of each root in the space provided.

ROOT/CV	DEFINITION
1. nephr/_____	_____
2. ure/_____	_____
3. pyel/_____	_____
4. ren/_____	_____
5. mictur/_____	_____
6. glomerul/_____	_____
7. uret/_____	_____
8. urethr/_____	_____
9. genit/_____	_____
10. ur/_____	_____

Word Dissection and Translation

Analyze the following terms by dissecting them with slashmarks and identifying their word parts. To the right of each term, write its correct English translation.

Key: R (root), cv (combining vowel), P (prefix), S (suffix)

1. polyuria

_____ / _____ / _____   _____
   P   R   S

2. cystoscopy

_____ / _____ / _____   _____
   R   cv   S

3. dialysis

_____ / _____ / _____   _____
   P   R   S

4. genitourinary

_____ / _____ / _____ / _____   _____
   R   cv   R   S

5. glomerulonephritis

_____ / _____ / _____ / _____   _____
   R   cv   R   S

6. nephrotomography

_____ / _____ / _____ / _____ / _____   _____
   R   cv   R   cv   S

7. renal

_____ / _____   _____
   R   S

8. intravenous

_____ / _____ / _____   _____
   P   R   S

9. cystostomy

_____ / _____ / _____   _____
   R   cv   S

10. ureter

_____ / _____   _____
   R   S

11. renopathy

_____ / _____ / _____   _____
   R   cv   S

12. pyeloplasty

_____ / _____ / _____   _____
   R   cv   S

Terms and Their Abbreviations

In the list below, when the term is given, write its abbreviation in the space provided. When the abbreviation is given, write its corresponding term.

TERM	ABBREVIATION
1. intravenous	_____
2. _____	GU
3. blood urea nitrogen	_____
4. _____	IVP

Word Spelling

Look at each of the terms listed below. Identify those that are misspelled by circling Y for "Yes." Write the correct spelling in the blank.

WORD	MISSPELLED?	CORRECT SPELLING
1. uremia	Y/N	_____
2. urethra	Y/N	_____
3. nefrohstuhmy	Y/N	_____
4. nocturia	Y/N	_____
5. pyelonephritis	Y/N	_____
6. hydronephroosis	Y/N	_____
7. glomerulis	Y/N	_____
8. urocyst	Y/N	_____
9. ureea	Y/N	_____
10. urinalysis	Y/N	_____
11. urolgenital	Y/N	_____
12. nephrolith	Y/N	_____
13. micturition	Y/N	_____
14. nephrosclerosis	Y/N	_____

New Word Synthesis

Using word parts that appear in this and previous chapters, build new terms with the following meanings:

1. _____ removal of a little ball of yarn

2. _____ surgical fixation of the urethra

3. _____ a condition of pus (in) the blood

4. _____ inflammation of the producers

5. _____ condition of hardening of the urinary bladder

6. _____ surgical fixation of the nose and stomach

7. _____ an abnormal condition of the kidney and abdomen

8. _____ referring to the tongue and pelvis

9. _____ a blood condition of the gall bladder and urinary bladder

10. _____ presence of a liver breakdown

C A S E S T U D Y

Read through the following partial urologic exam. Note the terms in bold print. A series of multiple choice questions probes your knowledge of these terms.

Urologic Exam

A 36-year-old Hispanic female showing signs of **chronic renal failure** was admitted to the hospital for workup. **Renohematologic** findings included severe **hyperuricemia** and marked **hematuria**.

Case Study Questions

1. The **urologic** exam considered the

   (a) status of blood alcohol level.

   (b) structure and function of digestive organs.

   (c) diameter of the larynx.

   (d) status of the urinary system structures.

2. **Chronic renal failure** suggests that the patient

   (a) had very little urine output for a long time.

   (b) recently experienced bedwetting incidents.

   (c) was experiencing coronary arteriosclerosis.

   (d) was visiting medical facilities too frequently for her problems.

3. **Renohematologic** findings are those involving the

   (a) blood and liver.

   (b) blood and kidneys.

   (c) blood and digestive structures.

   (d) glands and kidneys.

4. **Hyperuricemia** tells you that the patient

   (a) had an excessive blood glucose concentration.

   (b) suffered from extreme edema.

   (c) may be afflicted with gouty arthritis.

   (d) has experienced a cerebral infarction.

5. Marked **hematuria** could be quickly detected by

   (a) microscopic exam of a blood sample.

   (b) radiography of the urogenitals.

   (c) gross naked-eye examination of the urine.

   (d) inserting bile into the duodenum.

CHAPTER 18   The Reproductive System

INTRODUCTION

Chapter 17 introduced the term genitourinary. This term reflects the fact that the **generative** (**JEN**-er-ah-tiv), or **reproductive, system**, which produces new human beings, shares much in common with the urinary system. Simply put, many of the reproductive organs are involved in the excretion of urine. This fact is especially true for the male reproductive organs. Note from Figure 18.1, for instance, that the urethra carries both **ejaculated** (ee-**JAK**-yoo-**lay**-ted) sperm from the testes and urine from the bladder. In the female (Figure 18.2), the genital and urinary structures are largely separate from one another. These differences are reflected in the terms used to describe the reproductive organs.

The chief reproductive function of the male testes is **spermatogenesis** (**sper**-mat-oh-**JEN**-eh-sis)—the production of living sperm cells. Figure 18.3 provides an internal view of a testis and its **seminiferous** (**sem**-ih-**NIF**-er-us) **tubules**, the sperm-making machinery.

The main reproductive function of the female ovaries is **oogenesis** (oh-oh-**JEN**-eh-sis)—the production of living **ova** (**OH**-vah), or egg cells. Figure 18.4 shows an internal view of an ovary and its monthly cycle of **ovum** (**OH**-vum) production.

As noted in Chapter 12, the testes and ovaries also have glandular functions, secreting several important hormones. Some terms related to these hormones (testosterone, estrogen, and progesterone) were previously considered.

This chapter considers the terms of normal anatomy and physiology of the human reproductive system, terms related to reproductive diseases, lab tests and diagnosis of reproductive problems, and surgery and other therapies for reproductive disorders.

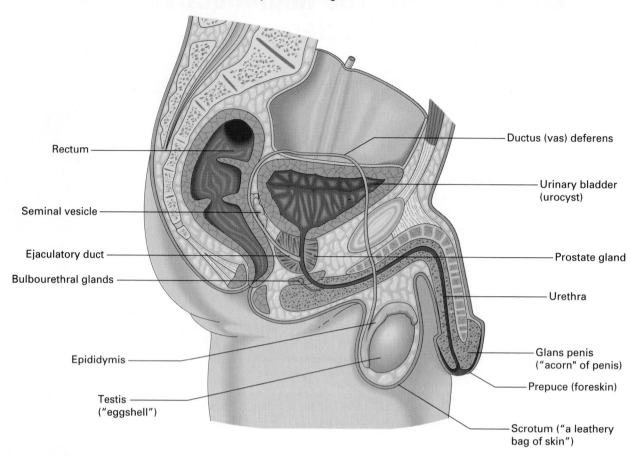

Rectum

Seminal vesicle

Ejaculatory duct

Bulbourethral glands

Epididymis

Testis
("eggshell")

Ductus (vas) deferens

Urinary bladder
(urocyst)

Prostate gland

Urethra

Glans penis
("acorn" of penis)

Prepuce (foreskin)

Scrotum ("a leathery
bag of skin")

F I G U R E   1 8 . 2   **The Female Reproductive Organs**

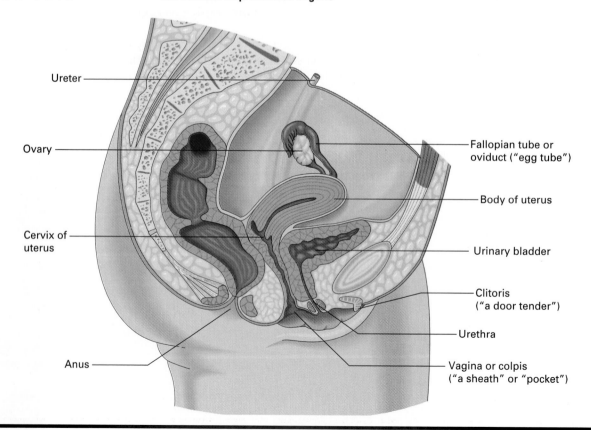

Ureter

Ovary

Cervix of
uterus

Anus

Fallopian tube or
oviduct ("egg tube")

Body of uterus

Urinary bladder

Clitoris
("a door tender")

Urethra

Vagina or colpis
("a sheath" or "pocket")

FIGURE 18.3

An Internal View of the Testis and Its Neighbors

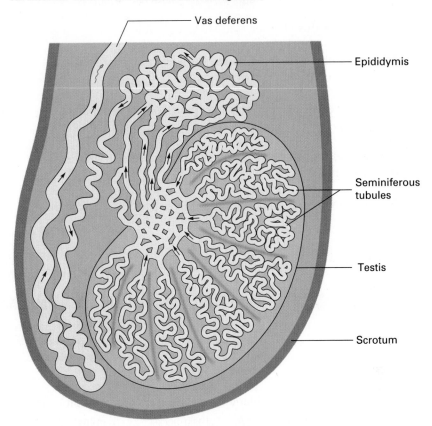

- Vas deferens
- Epididymis
- Seminiferous tubules
- Testis
- Scrotum

FIGURE 18.4

An Internal View of the Ovary and Its Neighbors

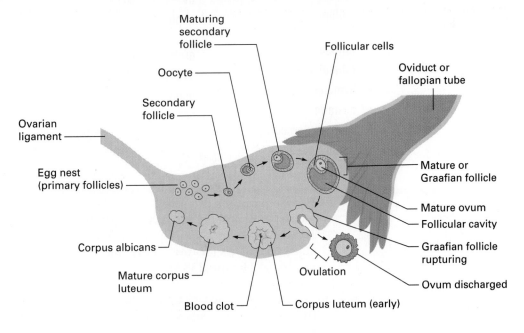

- Maturing secondary follicle
- Follicular cells
- Oviduct or fallopian tube
- Oocyte
- Secondary follicle
- Ovarian ligament
- Egg nest (primary follicles)
- Mature or Graafian follicle
- Mature ovum
- Follicular cavity
- Graafian follicle rupturing
- Corpus albicans
- Mature corpus luteum
- Ovulation
- Ovum discharged
- Blood clot
- Corpus luteum (early)

By the end of this chapter, you should be able to:

1 Identify major prefixes, roots, suffixes, and abbreviations related to the reproductive system.

2 Dissect reproductive terms into their component parts.

3 Translate reproductive terms into their common English equivalents.

4 Build new terms associated with the reproductive system.

Normal A & P

Word Parts Associated with Normal Anatomy and Physiology of the Reproductive System

The following is a list of word parts associated with normal anatomy and physiology of the reproductive system. Use this list to help you complete **frames 2439 to 2537**.

clitor/o	door-tender; clitoris	**mens/o**	month, monthly	**pudend/o**	feel ashamed; pudendum
colp/o	sheath; pocket; vagina	**menstru/o**	month, monthly		
		metr/o	uterus; womb	**salping/o**	trumpet; Fallopian tube or oviduct
didym/o	eggshell	**o/o**	egg		
episi/o	vulva	**ov**	egg	**scrot/o**	bag; scrotum
Fallopi/o	Gabriel Fallopius, Italian anatomist	**oophor/o**	egg-bearing; ovary	**semin/o**	seed; sperm; semen
				sperm/o	sperm
follic/o	bag	**orchid/o**	testis	**spermat/o**	sperm
follicul/o	little bag	**ovul/o**	little egg	**stat/o**	standing
hymen/o	membrane	**pen/o**	tail; penis	**uter/o**	uterus; womb
hyster/o	uterus; womb	**perine/o**	to swim around a thing; perineum	**vagin/o**	sheath; vagina
-ine	pertaining to			**vulv/o**	wrapper; vulva or pudendum
labi/o	lips				

2438 For the purposes of reproduction, the penis in the male, which ejaculates sperm, and the **vagina** (vah-**JIGH**-nah) in the female, which can receive the sperm, are of primary importance. Penis contains the same suffix as dialysis **(frame 2429)**, and vagina contains the same ending as urethra **(frame 2332)**.

---

pen/is
vagin/a

2439 Therefore, penis is analyzed as _____ /_____, and vagina is subdivided as _____ /_____.

---

pen (PEEN)

2440 The root in penis, _____, means "tail." It ultimately derives from the Latin **pendere**—"to hang down."

---

penis	**2441** The term _____ thus means "a tail" or "a hanging down" (like a tail). The organ is obviously named for its position when in a nonerect state.
vagin (**VA**-jin)	**2442** The root in vagina, _____, means "sheath" (as for a sword). A closely related root, **colp** (**KOHLP**), denotes "pocket."
vagina	**2443** The _____, or **colpis** (**KOHL**-pis), consequently, is "a sheath" or "a pocket."
vagina	**2444** Reproductively speaking, the _____ is "a sheath"—a long tapered inlet that receives the penis.
Information Frame	**2445** To the ancient Romans, a vagina was a sheath for "a sword" (in Latin, *gladius*). **Gladius** (**GLA**-dee-us) was also a common name for the penis.
pen/ile (**PEE**-nighl) **vagin/al** (**VAJ**-ih-nal)	**2446** Pen usually takes the "relating to" ending in febrile **(frame 1848)**, and vagin assumes the ending in ureteral **(frame 2329)**. The results are _____ / _____ ("relating to the penis") and _____ / _____ ("relating to the vagina"), respectively.
penile vaginal	**2447** A main characteristic of _____ anatomy is its tubelike, projecting shape. A main feature of _____ anatomy is its indented, sheathlike nature.
vaginal	**2448** In virgin females, the _____ ("sheath") **orifice** is at least partially blocked by the **hymen** (**HIGH**-men)—a "membrane."
hymen	**2449** The _____ is the vaginal membrane. It forms a thin vascular coating over the vaginal opening.
hymen	**2450** The _____ is generally ruptured as the penis is inserted into the vagina.
Information Frame	**2451** In early Greece, Hymen was the god of marriage, and the **hymenaeus** (**high**-men-**AY**-us) was a song sung at marriages.

hymen	**2452** The vaginal orifice and its covering _____ are hidden between the **labia** (**LAY**-bee-ah), or genital "lips" of the female.
labi/a	**2453** Labia is properly subdivided as _____ / _____, with the same ending as bacteria **(frame 541)**. Labia, like bacteria, is a plural form.
labia	**2454** Just as bacteria is the plural of bacterium **(frame 543)**, _____ is the plural of **labium** (**LAY**-bee-um).
labia vaginal	**2455** Between the _____ ("lips") and superior to the _____ orifice **(frame 2448)**, one finds the **clitoris** (klih-**TOH**-ris).
clitor/is	**2456** Clitoris is subdivided as _____ / _____, the same way as penis **(frame 2439)**.
clitoris	**2457** The _____ is, in fact, remarkably similar to the penis in both structure and function. It is a fairly long, tubular, **erectile** (eh-**REK**-tighl) stalk of spongy tissue.
penis clitoris	**2458** During sexual arousal in the male, the _____ becomes stiff, erect, and engorged with blood. During sexual arousal in the female, a similar mechanism of erection occurs with the _____.
clitoris	**2459** The term _____ derives from the ancient Greek for "door-tender."
clitoris	**2460** The _____ functions somewhat like "a door-tender," standing guard just anterior to the vaginal orifice.
clitor (**KLIH**-tor) **clitor/al** (**KLIH**-tor-al)	**2461** The root in clitoris, _____, often takes the same "pertaining to" ending found in vaginal **(frame 2446)**. The result is _____ / _____, "pertaining to the clitoris or door-tender."
clitoral	**2462** When stimulated, the highly sensitive _____ **stalk** provides sexual pleasure for the female. After this "door-tender" has been properly stimulated, the vagina is fully lubricated and ready for full insertion of the penis.

clitoral	**2463** The clitoris (including its _____ stalk) and labia are part of the **vulva** (**VUL**-vah), or **pudendum** (pyoo-**DEN**-dum).
vulv/**a** pudend/**um**	**2464** Vulva contains the same "presence of" ending as vagina **(frame 2439)**, so is dissected as _____ / ____. Pudendum includes the same ending as labium **(frame 2454)**, so is dissected as _____ / ____.
vulv pudend	**2465** The root in vulva, _____, means "wrapper," and _____, the root in pudendum, means "to feel ashamed." An alternative root for that in vulva is **episi** (eh-**PEE**-zee).
vulva pudendum	**2466** The _____ is the external "wrapper present" around the female genitals. Its basic anatomy is shown in Figure 18.5. Apparently, its alternative name of _____ **(frame 2463)** derived from the notion that it was proper to cover these genitals, or else "feel ashamed."

FIGURE 18.5   **The Vulva (Pudendum)**

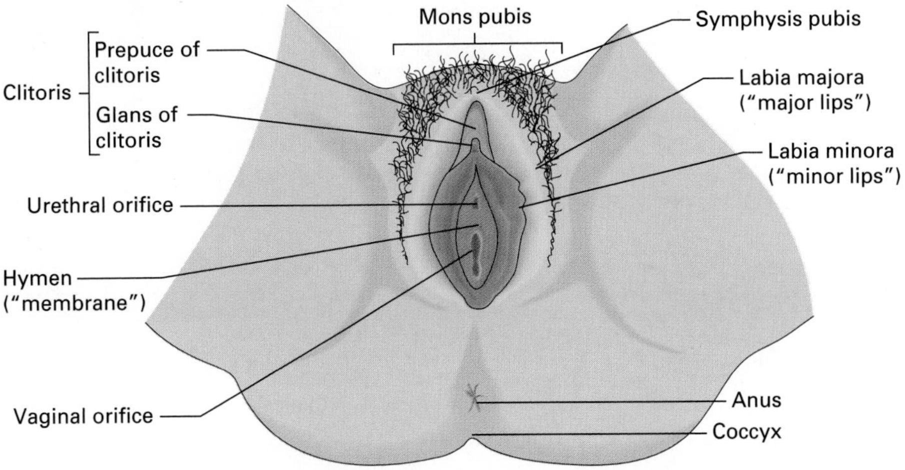

pudend/al (pyoo-**DEN**-dal)	**2467** Pudend assumes the same "referring to" ending as clitor **(frame 2461)**. Create _____ / ____, then, which "refers to feeling ashamed."
pudendal	**2468** How interesting it is to discover that terms such as _____ are related to feeling ashamed of one's own reproductive organs, reflecting the Puritanical attitudes of a bygone age!
pudendal	**2469** An area called the **perineum** (peh-rih-**NEE**-um) is located just inferior to the _____ ("feeling ashamed") region in females, just inferior to the **scrotal** (**SKROH**-tal) sac in males. (See Figure 18.6.)

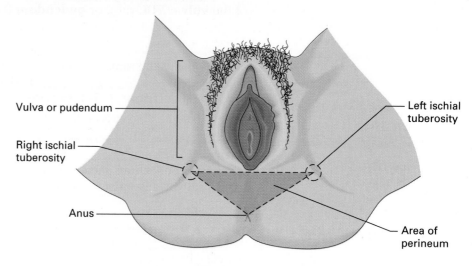

Vulva or pudendum

Right ischial tuberosity

Anus

Left ischial tuberosity

Area of perineum

The Perineum in Females
(Clinical Definition: Area Between Vulva and Anus)

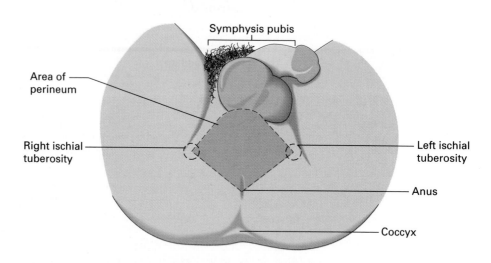

Symphysis pubis

Area of perineum

Right ischial tuberosity

Left ischial tuberosity

Anus

Coccyx

The Perineum in Males
(Clinical Definition: Area Between Scrotum and Anus)

---

perine/**um**	**2470** Perineum is analyzed like pudendum **(frame 2464)**: _____ /_____, with **-um** as its "presence of" suffix.
scrot/**al**	**2471** Scrotal is analyzed like pudendal: _____ /_____, with **-al** as its "pertaining to" suffix.
scrot (SKROHT) **perine** (peh-rih-**NEE**)	**2472** The root in scrotal, _____, denotes "leathery bag of skin." The root in perineum, _____, denotes "swimming around a thing."
scrot/um (SKROHT-um)	**2473** Extract the suffix from perineum **(frame 2470)** and use it to build _____ /_____, "a leathery bag of skin."

scrotum testes	**2474** The _____ is actually a hairy external "bag of skin" that contains the two _____ ("eggshells," **frame 1400**). Another root for these structures is **orchid** (**OR**-kid), reflecting their resemblance to the roots of those flowers.
scrotum perineum	**2475** The _____ encloses both testes. Since this external "sac" is filled and heavy, it drapes down over the _____ ("swimming around a thing," **frame 2472**).
perine/al (**peh**-rih-**NEE**-al)	**2476** Perine takes the "pertaining to" ending in scrotal, allowing us to create _____ /_____ , "pertaining to swimming around a thing."
perineum perineal	**2477** The strange meaning of _____ ("a swimming around") and _____ ("pertaining to swimming around") becomes obvious in the male. The heavy scrotum, being pressed against the skin, naturally causes this area to get hot and "swim around" with sweat!
perineum perineal vulva scrotum	**2478** Glancing back at Figure 18.6, you can confirm for yourself that the _____ or _____ area is clinically defined as the region between the base of the _____ ("wrapper," **frame 2466**) and anus in females, or as the region between the base of the _____ ("leathery skin bag," **frame 2473**) and anus in males.
scrotal	**2479** As mentioned, the testes within the _____ sac produce the **sperm** cells. Sperm or **spermat** (**SPER**-mat) means "seed." A young student assistant to the famous Dutch microscopist **Antonj van Leewenhoek** (**LOO**-ehn-**hoh**-ik), first observed human sperm through a primitive lens. He gave them a Latin name for "seed animals," since he saw them moving and alive. A **zoon** (**ZOH**-ahn) is one "animal," while **zoa** (**ZOH**-ah), its plural, means "animals."
genetic	**2480** The suffix **-genesis** (**frame 419**) indicates the "production of (something)," somewhat like the whole term _____ (**frame 504**), which "pertains to producing (something)."
spermat/o/genesis (**sper**-mat-oh-**JEN**-eh-sis) **spermat/o/zoon** (**sper**-mat-oh-**ZOH**-an) **spermat/o/zoa** (**sper**-mat-oh-**ZOH**-ah)	**2481** Now use spermat and the information in the two preceding frames to construct new terms: _____ /_____ /_____ "production of seed" _____ /_____ /_____ "seed animal" _____ /_____ /_____ "seed animals"

spermatogenesis spermatozoon spermatozoa	**2482** The processes of _____ ("sperm cell production") occur within the highly coiled seminiferous tubules of each testis. Each single _____ ("sperm cell"), as well as all the millions of _____ ("sperm cells") produced by an adult male every day, come from these structures.
spermatogenesis spermatozoa	**2483** After _____ produces many _____, they are stored in the **epididymis** (**eh**-pih-**DID**-ih-mus) prior to ejaculation.
eggshell **epi/didym/is**	**2484** The prefix epi- means "upon." **Didym** (**DID**-ihm), like test, is a root meaning "_____." Therefore, epididymis is subdivided as _____ / _____ / _____ and denotes something "present upon an eggshell."
epididymis	**2485** The _____ is a large, crescent-shaped pouch lying "upon" the "eggshell"-like testes.
spermatozoa epididymis	**2486** When the male reaches climax, the walls of his **vas deferens** (vas **DEF**-er-ens), or ductus deferens, rhythmically contract. This contracting action sucks the stored _____ ("sperm cells") up out of the _____ ("eggshell" pouch).
epi/didym/al (**eh**-pih-**DID**-ih-mal)	**2487** When used as an adjective, epididymis frequently takes the ending in perineal **(frame 2476)**. This combination yields _____ / _____ / _____, "referring to (something) upon the eggshell."
epididymal spermatozoon	**2488** From the _____ area, each ejaculated _____ ("sperm cell") enters the vas deferens and eventually mixes with fluid to become part of the **semen** (**SEE**-men).
semen spermatozoa	**2489** Like sperm and spermat, _____ denotes "seed." Rather than just _____ (sperm cells), however, this material also includes thick, whitish fluid that supports the sperm cells. In combination with other word parts, this "seed" is indicated by the root **semin** (**SEH**-min).
semin/al (**SEH**-mih-nal)	**2490** Adopting the ending in epididymal, create a new word, _____ / _____, that "refers to seed."

semen seminal	**2491** Several types of **accessory reproductive organs** add _____ ("seed"), that is, _____ ("seed") fluid, to the ejaculated spermatozoa.
seminal	**2492** These organs include the **prostate** (**PRAHS**-tayt) **gland** and a pair of _____ ("seed") **vesicles**.
pro- **pro/stat/e**	**2493** **Stat (STAYT)** is a root for "standing." Remember that _____ is a prefix for "in front of" or "before," and **-e** is a "presence of" suffix. It is then easy to dissect prostate as _____ / _____ / ____.
prostate	**2494** The literal meaning of _____ is "a standing before."
prostate	**2495** The _____ is a large, chestnut-shaped gland that "stands before" and encircles the base of the urethra in males.
pro/stat/ic (prah-**STAT**-ik)	**2496** The "stands before" fragment of prostate takes the "referring to" ending in urocystic **(frame 2329)**. The product of word-building is _____ / _____ / ____, which "refers to standing before (something)."
prostate prostatic	**2497** The _____ ("standing before" gland) adds its _____ fluid to the semen before ejaculation. This fluid drips out of the urinary meatus at the penile tip.
ov	**2498** To achieve fertilization, an ejaculated spermatozoon must contact and penetrate an ovum or "egg (cell) present" within an ovary. Recall that ____ **(frame 812)** is a two-letter root for "egg."
ov/um	**2499** Ovum is dissected as ____ / ____.
ovum **ov/a**	**2500** Just as the plural of bacterium **(frame 542)** is bacteria, the plural of _____ (an "egg" cell) is ____ / ____ ("egg" cells).
ovum ova	**2501** Each _____ (single "egg" cell) contains 23 chromosomes in its nucleus. All of the _____ ("egg" cells) originate within the female's ovaries.

2502 A root recognizing the "egg-bearing" function of the ovaries is **oophor** (**OH**-ahf-or). A related combining form is simply **o/o (OH-OH)**, "egg."

oophor/ic (oh-**AHF**-or-ik)

2503 Employ the longer egg-related root in **frame 2502** plus the suffix of prostatic **(frame 2496)** to construct _____ /_____ , "pertaining to egg bearing."

oophoric

2504 Both the right and left ovaries have an _____ ("egg-bearing") function in adult **premenopausal** (**pree**-men-oh-**PAW**-sal) women.

o/o/genesis

2505 Use the shorter egg-related combining form in **frame 2502** plus the suffix in spermatogenesis **(frame 2481)** to create _____ /_____ /_____ , "production of eggs."

ova
oogenesis
oophoric

2506 Production of _____ ("egg" cells) by _____ is the main _____ ("egg-bearing") function of the ovaries. A related root, **ovul** (ahv-**YOOL**), means "little egg."

ovul
ov
o
ovum

2507 The "little egg," or _____, root essentially means the same thing as both shorter roots for "egg": _____ and _____. Ovul pertains because each _____ ("egg cell") is microscopic, hence "little."

ovul/ar (**AHV**-yoo-lar)

2508 Remove the ending from alveolar **(frame 1962)** and synthesize _____ /_____ , "referring to little eggs."

ovular
oophoric
oogenesis

2509 There are several _____ ("little egg") events that occur within the ovary. The _____ ("egg-bearing") function consists of both _____ ("egg cell production") and mature ovum release.

ovul/a/tion (ahv-yoo-**LAY**-shun)

2510 Just as urination **(frame 2308)** is the "process of (releasing) urine," _____ /_____ /_____ is the "process of (releasing) a little egg."

ovulation

2511 In _____ a mature ovum explodes from the surface of the ovary and is then "released" into the surrounding abdominal cavity.

Information Frame

2512 The ovum was previously enveloped by a **follicle** (**FAH**-lih-kil), or "sac," of secreting and supporting cells. A root for "small sac" is **follicul** (fah-**LIK**-yool).

follicul **follicul/ar** (fah-**LIK**-yoo-lar)	**2513** The "small sac" root, _____, commonly assumes the same "referring to" ending found in ovular. The result of word-building is _____ /_____, "referring to a small sac."
follicle follicular	**2514** Each _____ ("sac") present around a developing ovum in the ovary has its walls composed of _____ cells.
follicle follicular ovulation	**2515** When the _____ enclosing a mature ovum ruptures, its _____ ("small sac") walls collapse and become glandular as _____ (ovum release) occurs.
Information Frame	**2516** Figure 18.4 displays a close-up of an ovary and the surrounding area during ovulation. **Gabriele Fallopius** (fah-**LOH**-pee-us), a sixteenth-century Italian anatomist, was one of the first to correctly describe the **oviducts** (**OH**-vih-dukts), or "egg tubes," attached to the sides of the female womb, or **uterus** (**YOO**-ter-us).
Fallopi/an (fah-**LOH**-pee-an)	**2517** Adjectives derived from people's names tend to have the **-us** or other ending replaced by **-an**. Using this fact create _____ /_____, "pertaining to Fallopius."
oviducts **Fallopian**	**2518** Another name for the _____ ("egg tubes," **frame 2516**) are the _____ **tubes**, named in honor of the Italian anatomist.
oviduct Fallopian tube	**2519** Fallopius compared the open, wide-mouthed abdominal end of each _____ or _____ _____ to an ancient "trumpet," or **salpinx** (**SAL**-pinks). This is represented by the root **salping** (**SAL**-pinj).
oviduct Fallopian tube salpinx	**2520** After ovulation, the mature ovum is usually swept into the open flared end of the _____ ("egg tube"), also called the _____ _____ or _____.
Information Frame	**2521** Fertilization, or conception, is the union of an ejaculated spermatozoan with a mature ovum. The most likely place for fertilization to occur is in the first third of the oviduct.
Information Frame	**2522** If fertilization does not occur, then a "monthly," or **menstrual** (**MEN**-stroo-al), cycle of changes in the blood and wall of the uterus commences.

menstrual menstru/**al**	**2523** Since _____ ("monthly") takes the ending in seminal **(frame 2490)**, it must be subdivided as _____ /____.
menstru (**MEN**-stroo)	**2524** The root in menstrual, _____, can also be placed into the form of a process, much as ovul in ovulation **(frame 2510)**. It therefore takes the suffix, **-tion**
menstrual **menstru/a/tion**	**2525** The female _____ **cycle** lasts about 28 days, or one "month." At the very beginning of this cycle, _____ /____ /_____, "the process of (doing something) monthly" occurs.
menstruation	**2526** The monthly process of _____ primarily involves the peeling off of the **endometrium** (en-doh-**MEE**-tree-um), the inner lining "present within" the "uterus."
Information Frame	**2527** Roots for the "womb" or "uterus" include **metr** (**MEE**-ter), **hyster** (**HIS**-ter), and **uter** (**YOO**-ter). You may remember **(frame 225)** that metr can also mean "measure."
endo/**metr**/i/um endo-	**2528** Considering the above frames, you should be able to dissect endometrium as _____ /_____ /____ /____, much as you dissected bacterium **(frame 543)**. The _____ ("within") prefix, however, is present.
endometrium	**2529** The fertilized ovum normally implants itself in the soft wall of the _____, which lines the uterus or womb.
endo/**metr**/i/al (**en**-doh-**MEE**-tree-al)	**2530** Endometrium can assume the same adjective form found in menstrual. This fact allows us to make _____ /_____ /____ /____, which "pertains to (something) within the uterus."
endometrial	**2531** The _____ lining of the uterus is the usual location of implantation. There is also, however, a more peripheral muscular layer within the **uterine** (**YOO**-ter-in) wall.
uter/ine uter **-ine**	**2532** Uterine is dissected as _____ /_____, since _____, like metr and hyster, is a root for "womb." The suffix in this case, _____, means "pertaining to."

uterine my	**2533** The _____ ("womb") wall includes a thick layer of smooth muscle fibers. Recall that _____, the root in myoma **(frame 1010)**, denotes "muscle."
my/o/metr/i/um (**migh**-oh-**MEE**-tree-um)	**2534** Using endometrium as the pattern, create _____ /_____ /_____ /_____ /_____, "presence of muscle (in) the uterus."
myometrium uterine	**2535** The _____ is the "muscular" portion of the _____ ("uterus") wall.
my/o/metr/i/al (**migh**-oh-**MEE**-tree-al)	**2536** Using endometrial as the pattern, write out _____ /_____ /_____ /_____ /_____, "pertaining to muscle (in) the uterus."
myometrial	**2537** It is the _____ region of the uterine wall, not the endometrial region, that contracts and helps expel the newborn child during labor.
	2538 Endometrial or myometrial diseases may interfere with proper development and delivery of the newborn infant.

Diseases

Word Parts Associated with Diseases of the Reproductive System

The following is a list of word parts and abbreviations associated with diseases of the reproductive system. Use this list to help you complete **frames 2539 to 2601**.

chet/o	flowing hair	**PID**	pelvic inflammatory disease	**syphil/o**	hog-loving; Syphilis
crypt/o	hidden			**VD**	veneral disease
gon/o	seed; (gonococcus bacteria)	**spir/o**	coiled	**venere/o**	Venus; love
men/o	month; monthly	**STD**	sexually transmitted disease		

-o/rrhea	**2539** The female uterus, even when normal, has a monthly flowing. Recall that _____ /_____, the suffix in pyorrhea **(frame 2221)**, means "flow" or "discharge." **Men (MEN)**, like menstru, is a root for "month" or "monthly."
men/o/rrhea (**men**-oh-**REE**-ah)	**2540** Build _____ /_____ /_____, "a monthly flowing."
menorrhea	**2541** There is a _____, or "monthly flowing," of material from the vagina, due to the shedding of the endometrium when fertilization has not occurred.

423

a/men/o/rrhea
(ah-**men**-oh-**REE**-ah)

2542 Extract the prefix from apnea **(frame 2010)** and construct
_____ /_____ /_____ /_____, "a lack of monthly flowing."

---

amenorrhea

2543 Certain female athletes (such as elite long-distance runners) can become so thin that they experience _____ during some months.

---

dys/men/o/rrhea
(**dis**-men-oh-**ree**-ah)

2544 Other women may experience "difficult" or "painful" **menses** (**MEN**-seez). Remove the prefix from dyspnea **(frame 2010)** and create _____ /_____ /_____ /_____, "a difficult or painful monthly flowing."

---

dysmenorrhea

2545 Women with hormonal imbalances may suffer from _____ during their monthly uterine cycles.

Information Frame

2546 A flowing can occur from the genitals of the male, as well as the female, during infection with **gonococci** (**gahn**-oh-**KAHK**-see).

---

gon/o/cocc/i

2547 Gonococci is dissected as _____ /_____ /_____ /_____, much like streptococci **(frame 550)**.

---

gon (GAHN)

2548 The root in gonococci, _____, means "seed."

---

gon/o/rrhea (**gahn**-oh-**REE**-ah)

2549 Synthesize a new term, _____ /_____ /_____, "a flowing of seed."

---

gonorrhea
gonococci

2550 The term _____ is actually a misnomer (mistaken name). Because an infection with _____ ("seed berries," **frame 547**) causes a milky discharge to occur from the urinary meatus at the tip of the penis, Aristotle and other early workers thought it was "seed" (sperm)!

-o/rrhagia

2551 Related to -orrhea is the suffix _____ /_____ **(frame 147)**, "a bursting forth." This suffix implies an excessive discharge.

---

metr/o/rrhagia (**met**-roh-**RAY**-juh)

2552 Using the **m**-beginning root for uterus results in _____ /_____ /_____ **(frame 148)**, "a bursting forth (from) the uterus."

Chapter 18 The Reproductive System

metrorrhagia	**2553** The problem of _____, in actual practice, is an irregular menstruation, probably due to some difficulty with the "uterus."
menorrhea **men/**o**/rrhagia** (**men**-oh-**RAY**-juh)	**2554** Extract the root from _____ ("monthly flowing," **frame 2540**) and create _____ /____ /_____, "a monthly bursting forth."
menorrhagia	**2555** The problem of _____ is an excessive menstruation, as if the monthly discharge were "bursting forth."
endo/metr/itis (**en**-doh-mee-**TRIGH**-tis) **endo/metr/i/o/sis** (**en**-doh-**mee**-tree-**OH**-sis)	**2556** Common problems in the uterus involve its endometrium. Use the prefix meaning "within" **(frame 2528)** and extract the suffixes found in glomerulonephritis **(frame 2372)** and hydronephrosis **(frame 2387)**. Combined with metr, they yield _____ /_____ /_____, or "inflammation of the inner (portion) of the uterus," and _____ /_____ /____ /____ /_____, or "an abnormal condition within the uterus."
endometritis endometriosis	**2557** In _____, the endometrium is inflamed. In _____, endometrial tissue occurs in abnormal places.
cervic/itis (ser-vih-**SIGH**-tis)	**2558** The **cervix** (**SER**-viks) is the tapered "neck"-like area at the base of the uterus. Its root is the same as that in cervical **(frame 827)**. With this information you can build _____ /_____, a term meaning "inflammation of the neck or cervix."
cervicitis	**2559** Women afflicted with _____ ("cervical inflammation") will display a reddened and swollen cervix upon examination.
colp para-	**2560** Recall that while vagin is a root for "sheath," _____ **(frame 2442)** is one for "pocket." Further, _____, the prefix in parasagittal **(frame 331)**, can mean "around" as well as "beside."
colp/itis (kohl-**PIGH**-tis) **para/colp/**itis (**par**-rah-kohl-**PIGH**-tis)	**2561** Employ the above information and the "inflammation" suffix to build two new terms: _____ /_____ "inflammation of the pocket (vagina)" _____ /_____ /_____ "inflammation of (the area) around the pocket (vagina)"
colpitis paracolpitis	**2562** Vaginal pain and itching may be a symptom of _____, while a noticeable redness and swelling "around" the outside of the vagina may well suggest _____.

fibr
fibr/oid (FIGH-broyd)

2563 Other problems may involve the uterus and its attachments. The uterus contains, for example, an abundant amount of fibrous tissue. The root in fibrous, _____, can be combined with the ending in thyroid **(frame 1383)**. The result is _____ / _____, "fiber-resembling."

fibroid

2564 Anything that is _____ appears or acts as if it is composed of fibers or fibrous tissue.

fibroids

2565 Uterine _____ are benign tumors that consist of fibrous tissue.

carcinoma

2566 Other uterine-related diseases, unfortunately, can be cancerous. Recall that a _____ **(frame 571)** is literally a "crab tumor."

cervical carcinoma

2567 Combine the root meaning a "neck" **(frame 2558)** and the suffix of scrotal to create _____ _____, a "crab tumor pertaining to the cervix."

cervical carcinoma

2568 A _____ _____ technically is a cancer restricted to the uterine cervix.

ovari

ovari/an (oh-VAHR-ee-an)

2569 The ovaries can also be afflicted with serious problems. The root in ovaries **(frame 1396)**, _____, can be combined with the suffix in Fallopian **(frame 2517)**. The result of word-building is _____ / _____, "referring to an egg or ovary."

ovarian
ovarian carcinoma
ovarian
cysts

2570 Let us pinpoint two particular _____ ("referring to the ovary") disorders. These are _____ _____ ("crab tumor referring to the ovary") and _____ _____ ("bladders related to the ovary"). Remember that "bladder" is found in urocyst **(frame 2325)**.

ovarian
carcinoma

2571 Because the "ovaries" are buried deep within the abdominal cavity, it is hard for physicians to diagnose _____ _____ or other cancers at this site.

ovarian cysts

2572 The _____ _____ are "bladder"-like sacs of fluid within the ovary. These may interfere with ovulation or other ovarian functions.

salpinx	**2573** Problems with the oviducts (Fallopian tubes) are quite common as well. Remember that Fallopius called the oviduct a _____ **(frame 2519)**, or "trumpet."
hemat/o/salpinx (hee-**mat**-oh-**SAL**-pinks)	**2574** Borrow the root in hematopoiesis **(frame 1733)** and construct _____ / _____ / _____, "bloody trumpet."
hematosalpinx	**2575** An accumulation of blood within the oviduct, as from some vessel rupture, is called _____.
salping **salping/itis** (**sal**-pin-**JIGH**-tis)	**2576** A root for "trumpet" is _____ **(frame 2519)**. Consequently, _____ / _____ is an "inflammation of the trumpet," just as cervicitis **(frame 2558)** is an "inflammation of the (uterine) neck."
salpingitis	**2577** Oviduct inflammation, or _____, can lead to female sterility, if the Fallopian tubes become blocked with scar tissue as a result.
PID	**2578** Both salpingitis and cervicitis combined are called **pelvic inflammatory disease**, which is abbreviated as _____ _____ _____.
pelvic inflammatory disease	**2579** The painful condition of _____ _____ _____ (PID) can be triggered by various pathogenic microbes.
orchid	**2580** Some pathogenic conditions affect the male reproductive organs only. Consider the testes, which have been compared to the roots of a particular flower, the _____ **(frame 2474)**.
orchid/ism (**OR**-kid-izm)	**2581** Extract the suffix from hyperthyroidism **(frame 1447)** and synthesize _____ / _____, an "abnormal condition of the testes."
crypt (KRIPT)	**2582** Normally, both testes descend from the abdominal cavity and enter the scrotal sac shortly before birth. If they remain undescended, they are "hidden." Note that _____ on the word list means "hidden."
crypt/orchid/ism (kript-**OR**-kid-izm)	**2583** An "abnormal condition of hidden testes" is given by the single word, _____ / _____ / _____.

cryptorchidism	**2584** A case of undescended testes, or _____, can result in sterility of the male, because the abdominal cavity is too hot for the seminiferous tubules to function properly for _____ ("sperm production," **frame 2481**).
spermatogenesis	
prostatic	**2585** Other difficulties may plague the prostate. Recall that _____ **(frame 2496)** "refers to the prostate" or to "standing before (something)." Likewise remember that _____ **(frame 139)** denotes a "process of excessive nourishment or stimulation."
hypertrophy	
prostatic hypertrophy	**2586** Thus we can coin the phrase **benign** _____ _____, "a process of excessive stimulation relating to the prostate."
benign prostatic hypertrophy	**2587** The condition of _____ _____ _____ is a noncancerous enlargement of the prostate gland. This lesion is very common in older males.
VD **STD**	**2588** Certain reproductive problems occur in both sexes. One general classification is **venereal** (veh-**NEE**-ree-al) **disease**, abbreviated simply as ____ ____. These are now often called **sexually transmitted diseases**, or ____ ____ ____s.
venere/al **venere** (veh-**NEE**-ree)	**2589** Venereal is subdivided as _____ /____, the same way as perineal **(frame 2476)**. Its root, _____, denotes "Venus," the mythical goddess of love.
venereal	**2590** The term _____ literally "pertains to love."
venereal disease	**2591** Obviously, _____ _____ (VD) "pertains to love" in a physical sense, because such a condition usually arises from sexual intercourse with an infected partner.
sexually transmitted disease gonorrhea	**2592** Two very common types of venereal disease or _____ _____ _____ (STD) are _____ ("flowing of seed," **frame 2549**) and **syphilis** (**SIF**-ih-lis).
Information Frame	**2593** Syphilis literally means "hog-lover" and was the name of an infected swineherder in a 1530 Italian poem.

syphil/**is**	**2594** Syphilis is analyzed as _____ /____, containing the same ending as clitoris **(frame 2456)**.
syphilis	**2595** The literal translation of _____ is "presence of a hog-lover."
syphil/o/genesis (**sif**-ih-loh-**JEN**-eh-sis)	**2596** Extract the suffix from oogenesis **(frame 2505)** and create _____ /___ /_____, "production of syphilis or a hog-loving (condition)."
syphilogenesis	**2597** The process of _____ ("production of syphilis") is due to the spreading of **spirochetes** (**SPIGH**-roh-keets) from an infected mucous membrane (as within the vagina or the urethra of the penis).
Information Frame	**2598** One meaning of **spir** (**SPIGH**-er) is "coiled." **Chet** (**KEET**) denotes "loose flowing hair."
spir/o/chet/e (**SPIGH**-roh-keet)	**2599** Adopting the "presence of" suffix in prostate **(frame 2493)**, construct _____ /___ /_____ /___, "presence of a coiled, loose flowing hair."
spirochetes syphilis	**2600** The _____ are long, coiled, hairlike bacteria that can infect humans and cause _____ (hog-lover's disease). These organisms are named for their individual appearance under the microscope (Figure 18.7).

FIGURE 18.7 **A Look at Spirochetes**

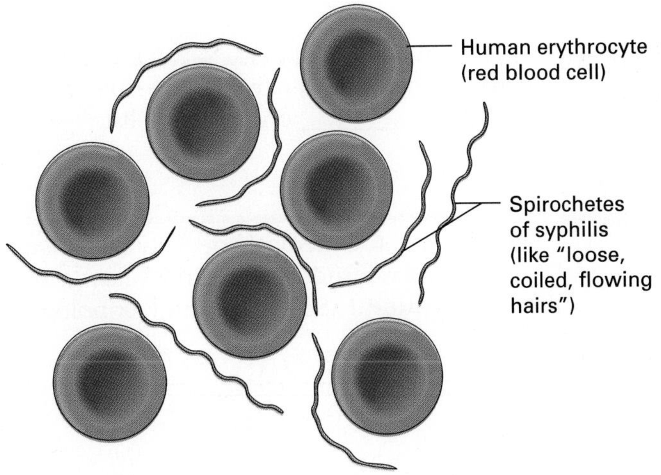

Human erythrocyte (red blood cell)

Spirochetes of syphilis (like "loose, coiled, flowing hairs")

spirochetes	**2601** The Chicago gangster Al Capone died of syphilis. His brain had been invaded by _____! Diagnosis of his problem came too late!

Word Parts Associated with Lab Tests and Diagnoses Involving the Reproductive System

The following is a list of word parts and abbreviations associated with lab tests and diagnoses of problems involving the reproductive system. Use this list to help you complete **frames 2603 to 2622**.

gynec/o women

Pap test Papanicolaou smear test

son/o sound

VDRL Veneral Disease Research Laboratory

2602 Some diagnostic tests for reproductive diseases can be performed in either sex. One good example is provided by tests for syphilis.

VDRL

2603 A major diagnostic test for syphilis is the **Venereal Disease Research Laboratory Test**, abbreviated as the ____ ____ ____ ____ Test.

Venereal Disease Research Laboratory

2604 The _____ _____ _____ _____ (VDRL) Test requires mixing of a patient's blood serum with spirochetes.

---

semen

2605 For male fertility, a _____ (sperm plus supporting fluid, **frame 2489**) **analysis** may be performed.

---

semen
analysis

2606 In order to count the number of active spermatozoa, the _____ _____ requires the man to ejaculate into a container. The number of active sperm cells per area of semen is then compared with normal values.

---

gynec (GIGH-nek)

2607 Other reproductive tests focus on "women," denoted by the root _____ on the word list.

---

gynec/o/logy
(**gigh**-neh-**KAHL**-oh-jee)
gynec/o/logist
(**gigh**-neh-**KAHL**-oh-jist)

2608 An entire medical specialty has arisen around the special problems experienced by women. Follow a pattern like that in endocrinology **(frame 1486)** and in endocrinologist **(frame 1488)** to help you build:
_____ /____ /_____   "the study of women"
_____ /____ /_____   "one who specializes in the study of women"

---

gynecology

gynecologist

2609 The specialty of _____ involves the systematic study and treatment of diseases of the female genital organs. A _____ is a physician who specializes in this area.

---

gynecology **gynec/o/log**/ical (**gigh**-neh-koh-**LAHJ**-ih-kal)	**2610** Borrow the suffix from anatomical **(frame 321)** and use it to replace the terminal **-y** in _____ ("study of women"). The word-building product is _____ / ____ / _____ / _____, "referring to the study of women."
gynecological	**2611** If problems are _____, they concern the special anatomy and physiology of the female reproductive system.
gynecological	**2612** Many general diagnostic procedures have specific _____ ("women study") applications. Some of these involve rays or waves. A particular technique using x-rays is called **hysterosalpingography** (**his**-ter-oh-**sal**-pin-**GAHG**-rah-fee).
hyster/o/salping/o/graphy	**2613** Hysterosalpingography is properly dissected as _____ / ____ / _____ / ____ / _____.
hyster salping -graphy process recording uterus oviducts	**2614** If you remember the meanings of its two roots, _____ and _____, and apply the definition of its suffix **(frame 2231)**, _____, you should be able to translate hysterosalpingography as the "_____ of _____ (x-rays involving) the _____ and _____."
hysterosalpingography	**2615** The technique of _____ may reveal definite blockages or kinks present in the oviducts.
son ultra-	**2616** Remember that _____ **(frame 216)** is a root for "sound," while _____ **(frame 218)** is a prefix for "excessive" or "beyond."
ultrasonography	**2617** The facts in the frame above allowed us previously to build _____ **(frame 218)**, the "process of recording sound (waves) beyond" the usual frequency.
pelvic ultrasonography pelvic	**2618** A specific application of this technique is _____ _____, the "process of recording sound (waves) beyond" the usual frequency as they are being bounced off various _____ ("bowl-related," **frame 398**) structures.
pelvic ultrasonography	**2619** The unborn baby within the uterus may be safely visualized using _____ _____ as the imaging technique.

Pap (PAP)

2620 Instead of looking at rays or waves, consider the **Papanicolaou** (pah-pah-**NIK**-oh-loh) **smear test**, shortened to three initial letters as the _____ test.

Papanicolaou

2621 The Pap test is named after its developer, Dr. George _____.

Papanicolaou

2622 The _____ (Pap) smear test involves the scraping of endometrial cells from the surface of the cervix. These cells are then examined and analyzed for cancer or other problems.

2623 If cervical cancer is detected by the Pap test, immediate treatment is recommended.

Surgery and Therapies

Word Parts Associated with Surgery, Pharmacology, and Other Therapies for the Reproductive System

The following is a list of word parts and an abbreviation associated with surgery, pharmacology, and other therapies for disorders of the reproductive system. Use this list to help you complete **frames 2625 to 2669**.

circumcis/o	cut around	**dilat/o**	widen	**orchi/o**	testis
curett/o	scraping; cleaning	**fung/i**	fungus; mushroom	**tub/o**	tube
D&C	dilatation and curettage	**ligat/o**	tie; bind	**vas/o**	vas deferens

---

2624 Drugs or surgery may be required to treat reproductive system disorders.

---

anti-

2625 Recall that antimicrobial drugs **(frame 608)** "pertain to" chemical agents that are given "against microbes." You can see that the prefix here is _____ for "against." Other drugs act against **fungus** (**FUN**-gus).

---

fung/us

2626 Fungus is dissected as _____ /____, with the same suffix as glomerulus **(frame 2315)**.

---

fung (FUNG)

2627 The root in fungus, _____, means "mushroom," that is, a vegetable organism that feeds on organic matter.

---

fungus
fung/i (FUN-jigh)

2628 Just as the plural of glomerulus is glomeruli **(frame 2315)**, the plural of _____ ("a mushroom") is _____ /____.

---

fungi	**2629** Pathogenic _____ ("mushrooms"), or yeast, can readily infect the warm, moist mucous membranes lining the interior of many reproductive organs.
fung/al (**FUNG**-gal)	**2630** Extract the suffix from vaginal **(frame 2446)** and build _____ /_____, "referring to fungus or fungi."
fungal	**2631** The interior of the vagina and penis are prone to _____ ("mushroom"), or yeast, infections.
fungal **anti/fung/al** (**an**-tee-**FUNG**-gal)	**2632** If _____ "pertains to fungus," then _____ /_____ /_____ "pertains to (something) against fungus."
antifungal	**2633** The _____ drugs are used to combat fungus or yeast infections, some of which occur in reproductive organs. **Mycostatin** (**migh**-koh-**STAT**-in), for example, is a drug in this group used to treat vaginal fungus infections.
tub/al (**TOO**-bul)	**2634** If fung/al "refers to fungus," then _____ /_____ "refers to tubes."
tubal	**2635** The term _____ can pertain to such particular "tubes" as the oviducts.
Information Frame	**2636** Such tubes can be tied. **Ligat** (**LIGH**-gayt) is a root meaning "tie" or "bind." It can take the same ending as found in dilation **(frame 1332)**.
ligat/ion (ligh-**GAY**-shun)	**2637** The "process of tying or binding (something)" is called _____ /_____.
tubal ligation	**2638** A phrase that "pertains to the process of tying tubes" is _____ _____.
tubal ligation	**2639** A _____ _____ is actually the tying or cutting off of the oviducts, in order to prevent future pregnancies.
Information Frame	**2640** In males, interference with the vas deferens can prevent the ejaculation of living spermatozoa. A root to indicate the vas deferens is simply **vas** (**VAS**).

vas/ectomy (vas-**EK**-toh-mee)	**2641** Apply the suffix for "removal" **(frame 1346)** and create _____ /_____ , "removal of the vas deferens."
vasectomy	**2642** The operation of _____ is really the "removal" or blocking of a portion of the "vas deferens."
vasectomy	**2643** Both _____ and tubal ligation are popular methods of birth control.
hyster/ectomy (**his**-ter-**EK**-toh-mee)	**2644** Several major female reproductive organs are frequently removed because of cancer. One of these operations is called _____ /_____ (using the **h**-beginning root for "womb"). The other is called **salpingo-oophorectomy** (sal-**ping**-goh-**oh-ahf**-oh-**REK**-toh-mee).
hysterectomy	**2645** If uterine cancer has occurred, _____ may be performed to prevent metastasis to other areas.
salpingo-oophorectomy	**2646** The operation called _____ involves a "removal of the ovaries and trumpets (Fallopian tubes)."
hysterectomy salpingo-oophorectomy	**2647** Metastasizing carcinomas in the pelvic region may make _____ ("uterine removal") and _____ ("removal of ovaries and oviducts") a necessity for survival.
hyster/o/tomy (**his**-ter-**AH**-toh-mee)	**2648** Just as nephrotomy **(frame 2417)** denotes "incision into the kidney," _____ /_____ /_____ denotes a "cutting into the uterus."
hysterotomy hysterectomy	**2649** The cutting of _____ has to be performed before the uterus can be removed by _____.
hyster/o/pexy (**HIS**-ter-oh-**peks**-ee)	**2650** Just as nephropexy **(frame 2424)** is a "surgical fixation of the kidney," _____ /_____ /_____ is a "surgical fixation of the uterus."
hysteropexy	**2651** The operation of _____ may be indicated if the uterus has broken loose from its abdominal connections.

colp	**2652** Remember that _____ **(frame 2442)**, a root for "pocket," essentially denotes the vagina.
colp/o/**tomy** (kohl-**PAH**-toh-mee)	**2653** Therefore, write _____ / ____ / _____ for "incision into the vagina."
colpotomy	**2654** The surgery called _____ involves an "incision into the vagina" to correct various problems. After surgery, the wound must be repaired by "suturing," indicated by the suffix in blepharorrhaphy **(frame 1346)**.
colp/o/**rrhaphy** (kol-**POR**-ah-fee)	**2655** Using the root in colpotomy, build a new term, _____ / ____ / _____ , "suturing of the vagina."
colporrhaphy	**2656** The procedure of _____ entails the "suturing" up of a tear in the "vagina," as after a violent rape.
hymen/o/**tomy** (**high**-men-**AH**-toh-mee)	**2657** In female virgins whose hymen is totally closed, _____ / ____ / _____ ("incision into the hymen") may have to be surgically carried out.
dilation	**2658** **Curettage** (kyoo-reh-**TAHJ**) is "a scraping." **Dilatation** (dil-ah-**TAY**-shun), like _____ **(frame 1332)**, is "a process of widening."
dilatation curettage	**2659** A minor operation called _____ ("widening") and _____ ("scraping") is often performed on the interior of the uterus.
D C	**2660** Dilatation and curettage is abbreviated as ____ & ____.
dilatation curettage	**2661** A _____ and _____ (D & C) is a widening of the cervix, followed by a scraping of its endometrium.
D C	**2662** Dilatation and curettage (____ & ____) may be recommended to remove excess endometrium that is causing menorrhagia.
curett (kyoo-**RET**)	**2663** Curettage contains _____ as a root for "scraping," while **circumcis** (**SER**-kum-sighz) is a root for "cutting around."

ligation **circumcis/ion** (**ser**-kum-**SIH**-zhun)	**2664** In the same manner that _____ **(frame 2637)** is a "process of tying or binding," _____ / _____ is a "process of cutting around."
circumcision	**2665** Technically speaking, _____ is a cutting around the head of the penis to remove the foreskin.
circumcision **orchid/ectomy** (or-kid-**EK**-toh-mee) orchid	**2666** A much more serious operation in males than _____ (foreskin removal) is _____ / _____, "removal of the testes." Here the flowery root for testes, _____ **(frame 2474)**, is adopted.
orchid	**2667** **Orchi** (**OR**-kee), like _____, means "testes."
orchi/ectomy (or-kee-**EK**-toh-mee)	**2668** Therefore, _____ / _____ is an alternative term for "removal of the testes."
orchidectomy orchiectomy	**2669** The procedure called _____ or _____ may be performed in cases of carcinoma of the testes.

Meanings of Selected Roots

Add the correct combining vowel (cv) after each root. Then write the definition of each root in the space provided.

ROOT/CV	DEFINITION
1. didym/_____	_____
2. menstru/_____	_____
3. salping/_____	_____
4. tub/_____	_____
5. vas/_____	_____
6. hyster/_____	_____
7. colp/_____	_____
8. gynec/_____	_____
9. crypt/_____	_____
10. ovul/_____	_____

Terms and Their Abbreviations

In the list below, when the term is given, write its abbreviation in the space provided. When the abbreviation is given, write its corresponding term.

TERM	ABBREVIATION
1. venereal disease	_____
2. _____	D & C
3. pelvic inflammatory disease	_____
4. Papanicolaou	_____

Word Dissection and Translation

Analyze the following terms by dissecting them with slashmarks and identifying their word parts. To the right of each term, write its correct English translation.

Key: R (root), cv (combining vowel), P (prefix), S (suffix)

1. menstrual

_____/_____   _____
       R   S

2. endometritis

_____/_____/_____   _____
   P   R   S

3. hematosalpinx

_____/____/_____   _____
       R   cv   R

4. gynecology

_____/____/_____   _____
       R   cv   S

5. antifungal

_____/_____/_____   _____
   P   R   S

6. vasectomy

_____/_____   _____
       R   S

7. hysteropexy

_____/____/_____   _____
       R   cv   S

8. circumcision

_____/_____   _____
       R   S

9. vulva

_____/_____   _____
       R   S

10. labia

_____/_____   _____
       R   S

11. cryptomenorrhea

_____/____/_____/____/_____   _____
       R   cv   R   cv   S

12. hysteropexy

_____/____/_____   _____
       R   cv   S

Word Spelling

Look at each of the terms listed below. Identify those that are misspelled by circling Y for "Yes." Write the correct spelling in the blank.

WORD	MISSPELLED?	CORRECT SPELLING
1. semen	Y/N	_____
2. epididymis	Y/N	_____
3. spirmatazooa	Y/N	_____
4. hystearosalpingography	Y/N	_____
5. ligation	Y/N	_____
6. colpotomy	Y/N	_____
7. salpingo-oophorectomy	Y/N	_____
8. orkeectomy	Y/N	_____
9. pudendum	Y/N	_____
10. penis	Y/N	_____
11. jihnecology	Y/N	_____
12. histerectomy	Y/N	_____
13. salpingitis	Y/N	_____
14. heematosalpinks	Y/N	_____

New Word Synthesis

Using word parts that appear in this and the previous chapters, build new terms with the following meanings:

1. _____ removal of the eggshell and trumpets

2. _____ inflammation of (the area) around the prostate

3. _____ presence of a stone (within) the womb

4. _____ process of tying the urinary bladder

5. _____ referring to (something) hidden

6. _____ removal of the tail

7. _____ production of urine and sperm

8. _____ incision into the wrapper

9. _____ suturing of ureter

10. _____ pertaining to (something) within the muscle of the uterus

11. _____ prolapse of the testes

12. _____ sperm (in) the urine

CASE STUDY

Read through the following partial surgical report. Note the terms in bold print. A series of multiple choice questions probes your knowledge of these terms.

Surgical Report

A 53-year-old female complaining of **hysteroabdominal** cramping was examined **laparoscopically** and found to have bilateral **hematosalpinx**. Consequently, R & L **salpingoligation** was performed.

Case Study Questions

1. **Hysteroabdominal** cramping means that the woman suffered from cramping of her

   (a) renal arteries.

   (b) uterus and abdomen.

   (c) pelvis and axilla.

   (d) throat and chest.

2. Examination **laparoscopically** tells you that the physician viewed the patient by a(n)

   (a) endoscope inserted into her abdominopelvic cavity.

   (b) tracheoscope fed down through the windpipe.

   (c) incision into the abdomen for direct visceral inspection.

   (d) cold-lit probe inserted into the vagina.

3. Bilateral **hematosalpinx** is a

   (a) hemorrhaging ureter on one side of the body.

   (b) lack of normal menses.

   (c) bleeding from the ureters on both sides of the body.

   (d) hemorrhaging from both Fallopian tubes.

4. **Salpingoligation** is a procedure that

   (a) ties the urinary bladder to keep it from leaking.

   (b) removes the oviducts to prevent dehydration.

   (c) binds the oviducts to prevent further hemorrhage.

   (d) scrapes and cleans the interior of the vulval chamber.

CHAPTER 19 Pregnancy and Human Development

INTRODUCTION

This final chapter looks at the results of successful reproductive activity—pregnancy, labor, birth, and the early stages of human development. Both before and after delivery, the breasts are dramatically affected. The rich terminology describing these miracles of life will be our concluding topic of discussion.

FIGURE 19.1   **The Ovum and Spermatozoon**

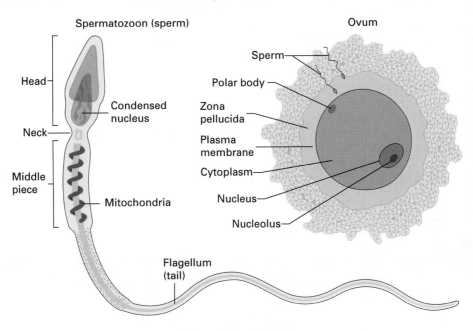

FIGURE 19.2   **Some Steps in Early Development**

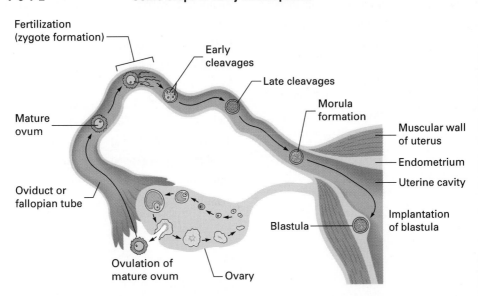

Figure 19.1 provides a microscopic view of an ovum and spermatozoon. Figure 19.2 shows some major steps of early human development, starting with fertilization of the ovum by a **spermatozoon**.

This chapter considers terms related to the normal structure and function involved in the breasts, pregnancy, and human development. Further, it examines words and word parts associated with diseases, lab tests and diagnoses, and surgery and other therapies for disorders related to pregnancy and human development.

CHAPTER OBJECTIVES

By the end of this chapter, you should be able to:

1 Identify major prefixes, roots, suffixes, and abbreviations related to the breasts, pregnancy, and early development.

2 Dissect terms of breasts, pregnancy, and development into their component parts.

3 Translate terms of breasts, pregnancy, and development into their common English equivalents.

4 Build new terms associated with breasts, pregnancy, and early development.

Normal A & P

Word Parts Associated with Normal Structure and Function of the Breasts, Pregnancy, and Early Development

The following is a list of word parts associated with the normal anatomy and physiology of the breasts, pregnancy, and development. Use this list to help you complete **frames 2670 to 2784**.

amni/o	lamb; amnion	**embryon/o**	sweller	**nat/o**	birth
amniot/o	lamb; amnion	**fet/o**	offspring	**nulli-**	none
blastul/o	little sprouter; blastula	**gastrul/o**	little stomach	**par/o**	to bring forth; to bear
		gestat/o	to bear (be pregnant)	**part/o**	to bring forth; to bear
chori/o	membrane; chorion			**per/o**	to bring forth; to bear
		lact/o	milk	**parturi/o**	to be in labor
chorion/o	membrane; chorion	**lactat/o**	to give milk	**placent/o**	flat cake
		lactif/o	milk-bearing	**puer/o**	child
coit/o	sexual intercourse	**lactifer/o**	milk-bearing	**vill/i**	tuft of hair
copulat/o	a joining	**mamm/o**	breast	**zygot/o**	yoked
embry/o	sweller	**mast/o**	breast		

copulat (**KAHP**-yoo-layt)
coit (**KOH**-iht)

2670 Before any reproductive events happen, the male and female must join together in sexual intercourse. Find two appropriate roots on the word list: _____ , for "joining," and _____ , denoting "sexual intercourse."

copulat/ion (**kahp**-yoo-**LAY**-shun)

2671 "Use the first root in the frame above to build _____ / _____ , a "process of joining," just as you built ligation **(frame 2637)**, a "process of tying."

Information Frame

2672 The suffix **-ory** (**OR**-ee) means "pertaining to." It is a close relative of **-ary (frame 91)**.

copulat/ory (**KAHP**-yoo-lah-**tor**-ee)

2673 Build a term that "pertains to joining": _____ / _____ .

copulatory

2674 Behavior is _____ if it involves the performance of sexual intercourse.

copulation

2675 The process of intercourse itself is usually called _____ .

coit/us (**KOH**-ih-tus)

2676 Now let us take the root for "sexual intercourse" in **frame 2670** and add it to the suffix of glomerulus **(frame 2315)**. The result is _____ / _____ , the "presence of sexual intercourse."

coit/al (**KOH**-ih-tal)

2677 Extract the root from coitus and combine it with the ending in seminal **(frame 2490)**. The new word is _____ / _____ , "referring to sexual intercourse."

coital
coitus

2678 Activity that is _____ relates to sexual intercourse, that is, _____ .

copulation
coitus

2679 From the last few frames we have learned that both _____ and _____ essentially indicate the same thing—sexual union between partners.

Fallopian

2680 As a result of such sexual union, a sperm may penetrate an ovum within the oviduct, or _____ **(frame 2517)** tube.

Information Frame	**2681** In such a fertilization, the sperm loses its tail and yokes, or fuses, with the ovum. **Zygot** (**ZIGH**-goht) means "yoked."
zygot/e (**ZIGH**-goht)	**2682** Adopt the "presence of" ending in prostate **(frame 2493)** and create _____ /_____, "a yoking."
zygot/ic (zigh-**GAHT**-ik)	**2683** Adopt the "referring to" ending in prostatic **(frame 2496)** and create _____ /_____, "referring to yoking (together)."
zygote zygotic	**2684** A _____ is the "yoking" together of a spermatozoon and ovum at the time of fertilization. This single new _____ ("yoked") cell contains genes from both the sperm and egg cells. It is from this single cell that an entirely new human body of trillions of cells is ultimately produced!
mono- di-	**2685** You may recall **(frame 80)** that _____ is an **m**-beginning prefix for "single" or "one," and _____ is a **d**-beginning prefix for "double" or "two."
mono/**zygot**/**ic** (**mahn**-oh-zigh-**GAHT**-ik) **di**/**zygot**/**ic** (**digh**-zigh-**GAHT**-ik)	**2686** Now build a pair of related words: _____ /_____ /_____ "referring to a single yoking" _____ /_____ /_____ "referring to a double yoking"
monozygotic	**2687** **Identical twins** are those who have identical sets of genes. Identical twins are virtually the same because they are _____, having developed from the same "single zygote" (which split in two).
dizygotic	**2688** **Fraternal** (frah-**TER**-nal) **twins** are those who were born at the same time, but were _____, each of them having developed from a separate zygote. Because there are "two zygotes," the twins are not identical.
zygote	**2689** After being created via fertilization, the _____ moves through the oviduct, toward the uterine cavity.
Information Frame	**2690** The single-celled zygote divides by mitosis into two cells. These two cells each divide to create four cells. This dividing process goes on and on, new cells continually sprouting in the process. **Blastul** (**BLAS**-tyool) is a root for "little sprouter" and takes the suffix in urethra **(frame 2332)**.

blastul/a (BLAS-tyoo-luh)	**2691** Eventually, the zygote develops into a _____ /_____ , that is, "a little sprouter."
blastula	**2692** The _____ is actually a hollow ball of cells. The ball usually implants itself in the endometrium of the uterus after fertilization. (Review Figure 19.2 if desired.)
little	**2693** **Gastrul** (GAS-trool) denotes "_____ stomach." It combines gastr **(frame 2089)** for "stomach" and the ending for "little," as in blastul, a "little sprouter."
gastrul/a (GAS-troo-lah)	**2694** The term _____ /_____ translates as "a little stomach."
gastrula	**2695** The blastula soon becomes a _____, or "a little stomach."
blastul gastrul	**2696** Both _____ (the root in blastula) and _____ (the root in gastrula) commonly take **-ar** as their "referring to" ending.
blastul/ar (BLAS-tyoo-lar) **gastrul/ar** (GAS-troo-lar)	**2697** We can therefore state that _____ /_____ "refers to a little sprouter" and that _____ /_____ "refers to a little stomach."
blastular gastrular	**2698** The simple hollow ball of cells that characterizes _____ ("little sprouter") anatomy eventually gives way to the more complex, layered _____ ("little stomach") anatomy.
gastrula	**2699** The _____ is like the real stomach in that its wall or "skin" consists of several layers.
derm	**2700** The gastrula has three so-called **germ layers**. In a way, these layers are like skins. You may recollect that _____, the root in dermis **(frame 623)**, means "skin."
gastrular	**2701** Different word parts are employed to name the various derms, or "skins," in the _____ ("little stomach") wall. These are ecto- ("outer, outside, or out of place"), mes- ("middle"), and endo- ("inside or within").

445

ecto/**derm** (**EK**-toh-derm) mes/o/**derm** (**MEZ**-oh-derm) endo/**derm** (**EN**-doh-derm)	**2702** Now let us build names for the three germ layers in the gastrula: _____ / _____ the "outer skin" _____ / ____ / _____ the "middle skin" _____ / _____ the "inner skin"

ectoderm mesoderm endoderm	**2703** The _____ eventually gives rise to such surface-related features of the body as the skin. From the _____ arise the middle areas of the developing body, including the skeletal muscles. And from the _____ come the epithelial linings of many body cavities.

ecto/**derm**/al (**EK**-toh-der-mal) mes/o/**derm**/al (**MEZ**-oh-der-mal) endo/**derm**/al (**EN**-doh-der-mal)	**2704** All three terms naming the germ layers take the "referring to" ending in coital (**frame 2677**). The results are: _____ / _____ / ____ "referring to the outer skin" _____ / ____ / _____ / ____ "referring to the middle skin" _____ / _____ / ____ "referring to the inner skin"

ectodermal mesodermal endodermal	**2705** From review of **frame 2703**, you can say that the nerves in the adult skin are mainly _____ in origin. The muscles in the arms are primarily _____ in origin. The lining of the intestine is chiefly _____ in origin.

Information Frame	**2706** After the gastrula, the ectoderm, mesoderm, and endoderm continue as parts of the **embry/o** (**EM**-bree-oh).

embry (**EM**-bree)	**2707** The root in embryo, _____, means "sweller" or "something that grows in another body." An alternative root with this same meaning is **embryon** (**EM**-bree-ahn). It usually takes **-ic** as its "pertaining to" suffix.

embryo **embryon**/**ic** (em-bree-**AHN**-ik)	**2708** An _____ is "a sweller that grows in another body." The term _____ / ____ "pertains to this sweller."

embryo embryonic	**2709** The _____, or "sweller," is the early stage of a child "growing in another body"—that of its mother. This _____ stage of human development covers the first three months after fertilization.

embryo	**2710** Even in ancient times, it was noted that the _____, which eventually "swells" greatly in size, is surrounded by several membranes. **Chorion** (**KOH**-ree-ahn) denotes "a membrane."

chorion chori/**on**	**2711** "A membrane," or _____, is dissected as _____ /_____, the same way as mitochondrion **(frame 524)**. The only difference is that in mitochondrion the **i** is a combining vowel, rather than part of the root.
chorion	**2712** The _____ is an outer "membrane present" around the embryo. (Consult Figure 19.3.)

FIGURE 19.3 **The Embryo and Its Membranes**

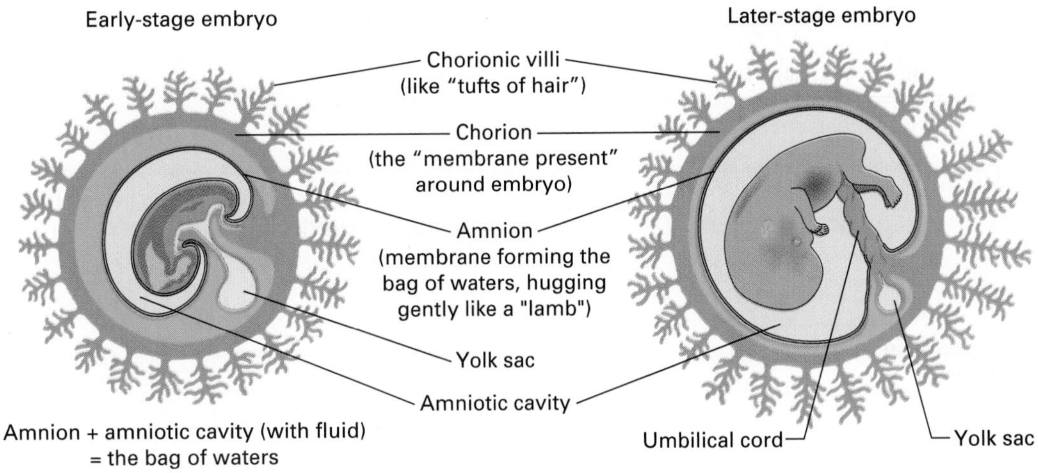

Early-stage embryo

Later-stage embryo

Chorionic villi (like "tufts of hair")

Chorion (the "membrane present" around embryo)

Amnion (membrane forming the bag of waters, hugging gently like a "lamb")

Yolk sac

Amniotic cavity

Amnion + amniotic cavity (with fluid) = the bag of waters

Umbilical cord

Yolk sac

chorion/ic (koh-ree-**AHN**-ik)	**2713** Chorion can also be used as a single root. Extract the suffix from embryonic and build _____ /_____, which "pertains to the chorion."
Information Frame	**2714** The chorion contains **vill/i** (**VIL**-igh), literally "tufts of hair."
villi	**2715** In common practice, _____ are considered hairlike projections.
chorionic villi	**2716** "Tufts of hair that pertain to the chorion" are technically known as _____ _____.
chorionic villi	**2717** The _____ _____ are, anatomically speaking, hairlike projections of the chorion that anchor the developing embryo into the endometrium of the uterus.
Information Frame	**2718** Related to the chorion is the **amnion** (**AM**-nee-ahn), or "lamb." This term contains the same suffix as chorion.

amni/**on**	**2719** Amnion is dissected as _____ /____.
amni (**AM**-nee)	**2720** The root in amnion, _____, means "lamb." An alternative root is **amniot** (**AM**-nee-aht).
amnion	**2721** The _____ is the soft, inner membrane surrounding the embryo and creating a so-called **bag of waters** around it. It apparently hugs the surface of the embryo gently, like "a lamb."
amniot/**ic** (am-nee-**AHT**-ik)	**2722** Extract the suffix from chorionic and use the alternative root for "lamb" to synthesize _____ /____, "referring to a lamb."
amniotic	**2723** The _____ **fluid** is the liquid matter within the amnion, or bag of waters, surrounding the embryo. This is true whether it is human or a "lamb."
amniotic fluid	**2724** The _____ _____ remains to bathe the unborn child throughout pregnancy.
Information Frame	**2725** **Gestat** (jehs-**TAYT**) means "to bear (be pregnant)."
gestat/**ion** (jehs-**TAY**-shun)	**2726** Just as copulat/**ion** (**frame 2671**) is a "process of joining," _____ /_____ is a "process of bearing."
gestation	**2727** The human period of _____ ("process of bearing") lasts about nine months. The first three months of this period involves the development of the embryo.
gestation **gestation**/**al** (jehs-**TAY**-shun-al)	**2728** The suffix in endodermal **(frame 2704)** can be attached to the entire term, _____ ("process of bearing"). The result of word building is _____ /____, "pertaining to the process of bearing."
gestational	**2729** The human _____ ("bearing") period is about nine months in duration.
Information Frame	**2730** Eventually, the embryo will become a full-fledged offspring of its parents. **Fet (FEET)** is a root for "offspring."

fet/us (FEE-tus)	**2731** Attach the ending in coitus **(frame 2676)** and create _____ /_____ for "an offspring."
fetus	**2732** The _____, that is, "the offspring" that will eventually be born, represents the time in gestation from the third month until birth.
fet/al (FEE-tal)	**2733** Borrow the ending from gestational and build a new adjective that "pertains to an offspring": _____ /_____.
fetal	**2734** The _____ ("offspring") bloodstream communicates indirectly with that of its mother by means of an umbilical cord in the navel region. (See Figure 19.4.)

FIGURE 19.4 **The Fetus and Placenta**

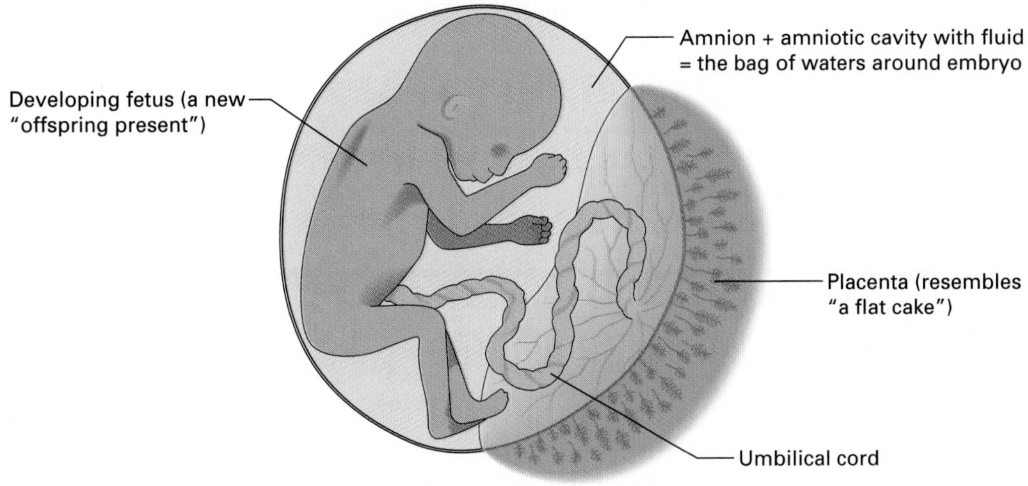

Developing fetus (a new "offspring present")

Amnion + amniotic cavity with fluid = the bag of waters around embryo

Placenta (resembles "a flat cake")

Umbilical cord

fetal	**2735** The _____ ("offspring") umbilical cord hooks into the mother's **placenta** (plah-**SEN**-tah).
placent/a	**2736** Isolate the suffix in placenta the same way you did it for gastrula **(frame 2694)**, inserting one slashmark as follows: _____ /_____.
placent (plah-**SENT**)	**2737** The root in this term, _____, denotes a "flat cake."
placenta	**2738** The _____ is an organ resembling "a flat cake."

placenta	**2739** The umbilical cord of the fetus extends into the _____ ("flat cake") present on the inner uterine wall. Nutrients and wastes from the fetal bloodstream diffuse into the mother's bloodstream at this site.
placent/al (plah-**SEN**-tal)	**2740** Attach the adjective-creating suffix in fetal **(frame 2733)** to the "flat cake" root, yielding _____ /_____ , "relating to a flat cake."
placental	**2741** The _____ ("flat cake") barrier keeps certain toxic materials in the maternal bloodstream from entering the fetal circulation.
placental	**2742** The _____ nutrition derived from this large temporary organ usually keeps the fetus alive until the time of birth arrives. **Nat (NAYT)** is one root for "birth."
nat/al (**NAY**-tal)	**2743** Take the ending from placental and write out _____ /_____ , "relating to birth."
natal gestational	**2744** The _____ process brings an end to the _____ ("pertaining to the process of bearing," **frame 2728**) period.
Information Frame	**2745** Many things must occur normally before birth, if a living infant is to result. You may remember that both pre- and ante- are prefixes meaning "before."
pre/nat/al (pree-**NAY**-tal) ante/nat/al (**an**-tee-**NAY**-tal)	**2746** Now use these facts to build _____ /_____ /_____ and _____ /_____ /_____ , two terms that both "relate to (the period) before birth."
prenatal antenatal	**2747** Good _____ , or _____ , nutrition is essential for the mother if the developing fetus is to grow normally.
par (PAR) **part (PART)** **per (PER)** **parturi** (par-**TOO**-ree)	**2748** Note that the word list contains four **p**-beginning roots related to birth and labor. These include _____ , _____ , and _____ for "to bring forth" or "to bear." A longer root, _____ , means "to be in labor."
parturi/tion (par-too-**RISH**-un)	**2749** Use the longest root in the preceding frame plus the suffix in micturition **(frame 2308)** to build _____ /_____ , the "process of being in labor."

parturition	**2750** The event of _____ results in the delivery of a new-born child. The **vertex** (**VER**-teks), or "peak," of the head usually appears first.
vertex parturition	**2751** In a _____ delivery after _____ ("labor"), the "peak" of the fetal head emerges from the vagina, or birth canal, before the rest of the body.
neo/**nat**/**e** (**NEE**-oh-nayt)	**2752** Remove the prefix from neoplasm **(frame 561)**, the root from prenatal **(frame 2746)**, and the suffix from zygote **(frame 2682)**. Put these word parts together, and you obtain _____ / _____ / ____, "presence of a newborn."
vertex neonate	**2753** Usually a _____ ("peak") delivery of the _____ ("newborn") is preferred. Less risk of birth-related complications exists.
neo/**nat**/**al** (**nee**-oh-**NAY**-tal)	**2754** Following the word-building pattern of natal **(frame 2743)**, which means "relating to birth," create _____ / _____ / ____, which means "relating to a newborn."
neonatal	**2755** The _____ (newborn) period is all about producing a viable life out of the womb.
genital	**2756** Recall that _____ **(frame 2352)** "refers to producing (something)." **Con-** is a prefix denoting "together" or "with."
con/**genit**/**al** (**kahn**-**JEN**-ih-tal)	**2757** Build _____ / _____ / ____, which "refers to (something that occurs) with producing."
congenital	**2758** When birth occurs, a neonate is "produced." In a sense, then, _____ "refers to" the conditions "produced with birth."
congenital	**2759** The neonate is born with a great many _____ conditions. It is hoped that most of them are normal.
post-	**2760** We know that the prenatal period is very important for child development. The period that occurs _____ ("after," **frame 82**) is also vital.

post/part/al (post-**PAR**-tal)	**2761** Looking at part as "birth" and **-al** as "referring to," then _____ / _____ / ____ "refers to (the period) after birth."
postpartal prenatal	**2762** To a large degree, the _____ health of the neonate after it is born depends on the _____ health of the mother before it is born.
Information Frame	**2763** **Puer (poo-EHR)** means "child." Remember that per is one of the roots for "bring forth" or "bear."
puer/per/a (**poo-EHR**-per-ah)	**2764** Take the suffix from gastrula **(frame 2694)** and synthesize _____ / _____ / ____ , "a child-bearer."
puerpera	**2765** A _____ is a woman who has just given birth to a child. The two roots in this term commonly take the "relating to" ending in postpartal.
puer/per/al (**poo-EHR**-per-al)	**2766** Synthesize _____ / _____ / ____ , "relating to a child-bearer."
puerperal postpartal	**2767** The _____ female is going through her own _____ ("after birth") adjustments —both physically and psychologically.
par/a (**PAH**-rah)	**2768** Using par rather than per, but with the same ending as in puerpera, construct _____ / ____ to denote "a bearer."
para multi- primi-	**2769** Several different prefixes of number **(frame 80)** are often attached to _____ ("a bearer"). These include _____, an **m**-beginning prefix for "many." Nulli- (**NUH**-lee), another prefix, means "none." A **p**-beginning prefix of time sequence **(frame 82)** frequently involved is _____ ("first").
nulli/**par/a** (nuhl-**IP**-ah-ruh) primi/**par/a** (prim-**IP**-ah-ruh) multi/**par/a** (mul-**TIP**-ah-ruh)	**2770** Apply the information provided in the above frame to create: _____ / _____ / ____ "a bearer of no" children _____ / _____ / ____ "a bearer of a first" child _____ / _____ / ____ "a bearer of many" children Note the change in accent when nulli-, primi-, and multi- are joined with par/a.

2771 The definitions in the preceding frame technically refer to mothers of **viable** (**VIGH**-ah-bul), that is, "living," children. A _____, for instance, is a woman who has never given birth to a viable child. Her pregnancies may all have resulted in abortions or stillborn neonates. A _____ would have one viable child; a _____, many neonates that survived.

nullipara

primipara
multipara

Information Frame

2772 Viable neonates require "milk," or **lact (LAKT)**, as from the "breast," that is, **mamm (MAM)** or **mast (MAST)**.

Information Frame

2773 The mamm root for "breast" usually takes the "presence of" ending in multipara and the "pertaining to" ending in urinary **(frame 2302)**.

---

mamm/a (MAM-ah)
mamm/ary (MAM-ah-ree)

2774 The facts in the previous frame allow us to construct _____ / _____ ("a breast") and _____ / _____ ("referring to breasts"), respectively.

---

mamma
mammary

2775 Figure 19.5 shows the internal anatomy of a _____ ("breast"). A number of _____ ("breast-related") terms are included. Note especially **lactiferous (lak-TIF-er-us)**, which "pertains to milk-bearing."

FIGURE 19.5   **Internal Anatomy of the Breast**

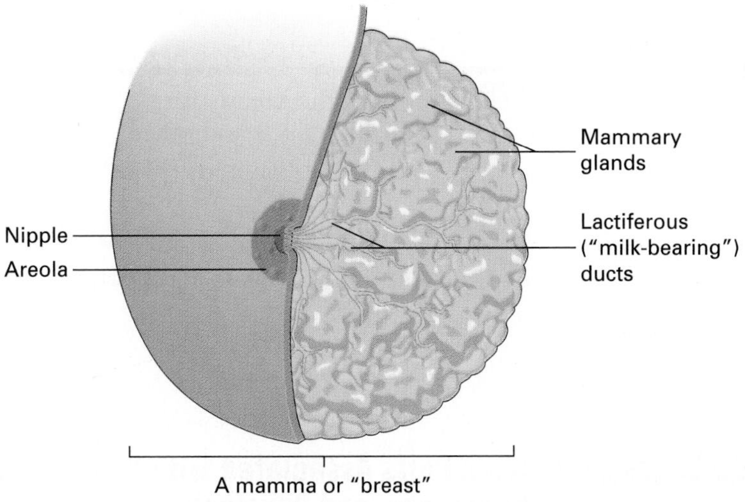

Mammary glands

Nipple

Areola

Lactiferous ("milk-bearing") ducts

A mamma or "breast"

Information Frame

2776 The breast, or mamma, derives from the infant's cry for milk from "ma-ma," which is a set of sounds common to most languages.

---

lactifer/ous
lactifer (lak-TIF-er)

2777 Lactiferous contains the same suffix as intravenous **(frame 2398)**. Therefore, this term is dissected as _____ / _____. Its root, _____, means "milk-bearing."

lactiferous	**2778** The _____ ducts within the breast are those "bearing milk" before it is ejected from the nipple.

Information Frame

2779 Lact takes the "presence of" ending in clitoris **(frame 2456)**. A closely related root, **lactat** (**LAK**-tayt), means "to give milk for sucking." This second root follows the word-building pattern in copulation **(frame 2671)**.

lact/is (**LAK**-tis)
lactat/ion (lak-**TAY**-shun)

2780 Gathering information from the preceding frame allows us to synthesize

_____ / _____   "presence of milk"
_____ / _____   "process of giving milk for sucking"

lactis
lactiferous
lactation

2781 "Milk," or _____, is "present" within the _____ ("milk-bearing") ducts of the breast because of _____, the "process of giving milk for sucking."

lactis
lactation
mammary

2782 The lactiferous ducts just carry the _____ ("milk") after _____ ("giving milk") occurs within the _____ ("pertaining to breast," **frame 2774**) glands.

lact/ic (**LAK**-tik)

2783 The root in lactis commonly assumes the "relating to" ending in monozygotic **(frame 2686)**. The result of word building is then _____ / _____, "relating to milk."

lactation
lactic

2784 Preparing the breasts for _____ ("process of giving or producing milk") and other _____ ("milk-related") functions is just one of many adjustments that the body of the puerpera makes.

2785 Either the neonate or the puerpera may be afflicted with birth-related difficulties.

Diseases

Word Parts Associated with Diseases of the Breasts, Pregnancy, and Development

The following is a list of word parts and abbreviations associated with diseases of the breasts, pregnancy, and early human development. Use this list to help you complete **frames 2787 to 2844**.

abort/o	miscarry	**emetic/o**	vomit	**NRDS**	neonatal respiratory distress syndrome
eclamps/o	a shining forth	**HDN**	hemolytic disease of the newborn	**previ/o**	in the way before (something)
ectop/o	out of place				
eme/o	vomit				

2786 Let us first consider some potential afflictions of the mother. A very serious problem is **eclampsia** (eh-**KLAMP**-see-ah).

---

eclamps/ia

2787 Eclampsia contains the same ending as nocturia **(frame 2360)**. It is subdivided as _____ /_____.

---

eclamps (eh-**KLAMPS**)

eclampsia

2788 The root in eclampsia, _____, means "a shining forth." This strange name comes from the fact that some women experiencing _____ see flashes of light "shining forth" before their eyes.

---

eclamps/ic (eh-**KLAMP**-sik)

2789 Attach the suffix in lactic **(frame 2783)** to eclamps and construct _____ /_____, "referring to a shining forth."

---

eclampsia
eclampsic

2790 A woman suffering from _____, or an _____ condition, is experiencing **toxemia of pregnancy**. This is a negative reaction of the woman's body to her own fetus. Symptoms may include edema, hypertension, convulsions, and even coma.

---

eclampsia

2791 Various signs and symptoms generally precede full-blown _____ (toxemia of pregnancy). Borrow the prefix from prenatal **(frame 2746)** to indicate "preceding" or "before."

---

pre/eclamps/ia
(**pree**-eh-**KLAMP**-see-ah)
pre/eclamps/ic
(**pree**-eh-**KLAMP**-sik)

2792 Build two related terms:
_____ /_____ /_____ "an abnormal condition (that occurs) before shining forth"
_____ /_____ /_____ "referring to an abnormal condition (that occurs) before shining forth"

---

preeclampsia
preeclampsic

2793 The nonconvulsive stage appearing "before eclampsia" is technically called _____. The _____ conditions include hypertension, edema, and **proteinuria** (**proh**-tee-in-**OO**-ree-ah)—the excretion of "proteins (in) the urine."

Information Frame

2794 Pregnant or not, women may suffer various problems with their breasts. Mast, rather than mamm, is the root for "breast" most often used to describe disease states, such as "inflammation," which is indicated by the suffix "-**itis**."

mast/itis (mas-**TIGH**-tis)	**2795** Take, for instance, _____ /_____, "inflammation of the breasts."
mastitis	**2796** When the breasts are affected by _____, they may be red, swollen, and painful to the touch.
cysts urocyst urocystic	**2797** Another common breast problem is the occurrence of fluid-filled "bladders," or _____ **(frame 2379)**. Recall the noun _____ ("urinary bladder," **frame 2326**) and the adjective _____ ("pertaining to the urinary bladder," **frame 2329**).
fibr/o/cyst (**FIGH**-broh-sist) **fibr/o/cyst/ic** (figh-broh-**SIS**-tik)	**2798** Many cysts in the breasts are filled with connective tissue "fibers," indicated by the root in fibroid **(frame 2563)**. Now build two related terms: _____ /____ /_____ a "fiber"-containing sac or "bladder" _____ /____ /_____ /____ "pertaining to" a "fiber"-containing sac or "bladder"
fibrocystic fibrocysts	**2799** A _____ breast is one that is lumpy or nodular due to the presence of _____ ("fiber"-filled sacs).
fibrocystic **breast**	**2800** The benign, noncancerous condition called _____ ("fiber-bladder") _____ is not to be confused with dangerous **carcinoma of the breast**.
carcinoma	**2801** Recall that _____ **(frame 570)** actually denotes "crab tumor," and it indicates cancer.
carcinoma breast	**2802** Therefore, "crab tumor of the breast" is technically termed _____ of the _____. This disease is very dangerous, because it can easily metastasize to the lymph nodes in the armpit region.
Information Frame	**2803** Perhaps the most well known of the afflictions related to pregnancy is "morning sickness." This hormone-associated problem is characterized by queasiness and vomiting. Two roots, **eme** (**EH**-mee) and **emetic** (eh-**MET**-ik), denote "vomiting."

eme emetic	**2804** The shorter "vomiting" root, _____, is usually attached to **-sis** rather than **-is** to denote "a condition of." The longer root, _____, is often used as an entire word that "pertains to vomiting."
eme/sis (**EH**-meh-sis) emetic	**2805** The term _____ / _____ indicates "a condition of vomiting." In contrast, an _____ condition involves "vomiting."
emesis emetic	**2806** Pregnant women with morning sickness are prone to _____ ("vomiting"). Being pregnant, then, seems to be an _____ (vomiting-promoting) experience!
hyper/eme/sis (**high**-per-**EH**-meh-sis)	**2807** Extract the prefix from hyperuricemia **(frame 2368)** and construct _____ / _____ / _____, "a condition of excessive vomiting."
hyperemesis	**2808** Pregnant women afflicted with a bad case of _____ often experience a high incidence of dental caries, due to the effect of vomited stomach acid on their tooth enamel.
hyperemesis	**2809** At the other end of the female body, **abortion** (ah-**BOR**-shun) rather than _____ (too much vomiting) is a problem.
abort/ion **abort** (ah-**BORT**)	**2810** Abortion is dissected as _____ / _____, the same way as lactation **(frame 2780)**. The root in abortion, _____, means "miscarry."
abortion	**2811** The term _____, then, literally denotes the "process of miscarrying."
abortion	**2812** The highly sensitive political issue of _____ ("miscarriage") on demand is still being hotly debated.
abortions	**2813** Natural _____ ("miscarriages") are often tied to disruption of the placenta nourishing the fetus. **Abruptio placentae** (ah-**BRUP**-tee-oh plah-**SEN**-tigh), for example, is an "abrupt," premature, tearing away of the placenta from the wall of the uterus. Another related problem is **placenta previa** (**PREE**-vee-ah). This condition is the delivery of a displaced placenta "previous" to the delivery of the fetus.

placenta previa previ/a	**2814** The previa in the _____ _____ phrase contains the same suffix as mamma **(frame 2774)**. Therefore previa is dissected as _____ /_____.
previ (PREE-vee)	**2815** The root in previa, _____, means "in the way before (something)."
placenta previa	**2816** In _____ _____, the placenta comes out "before" the fetus, "in the way" of it. This blocking threatens to cut off the vital supply of nutrients to the fetus before it is actually delivered.
abruptio placentae	**2817** In _____ _____, the "placenta" simply breaks off too "abruptly," dislodging itself from the source of the fetus' nutrients—the mother's endometrial blood vessels.
vertex	**2818** The opposite of _____ ("peak," **frame 2750**) is breech, or "britches," as in the pants covering the thighs and buttocks.
breech	**2819** In _____ delivery, there is no difficulty with the placenta. Rather, the fetus presents its thighs and buttocks first, as if showing off its covering of "britches."
Information Frame	**2820** Problems with the placenta or position of delivery may also be tied to **ectopic** (ek-**TAH**-pik), or "out of place," pregnancy. This term contains the suffix found in fibrocystic **(frame 2798)**.
ectop/ic **ectop** (ek-**TAHP**)	**2821** Ectopic is subdivided as _____ /_____. Its root, _____, means "out of place."
ectopic	**2822** Any site for fetal development is considered _____ if it lies outside the main cavity of the uterus.
ectopic	**2823** A fetus developing within one of the oviducts, for instance, would constitute an _____ pregnancy.
Information Frame	**2824** Sometimes the neonate is born successfully, but then suffers from serious congenital defects. One of the most common of these is **Down's syndrome**.

Down

2825 This syndrome, first described by Dr. John _____, is a genetic defect involving three chromosomes at the number 21 position, rather than the normal two chromosomes (Figure 19.6).

FIGURE 19.6   **Down's Syndrome and Its Chromosomes**

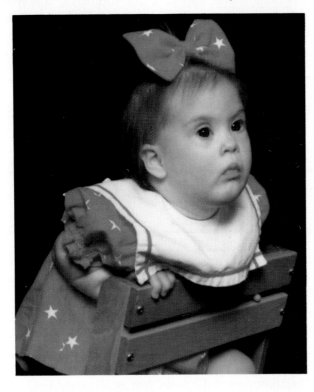
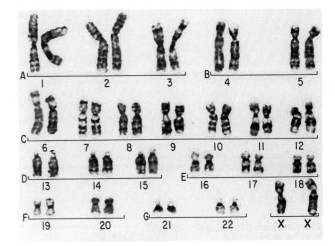

Down's syndrome

2826 A usual result of _____ _____ is moderate mental retardation of the child, along with a characteristic of narrow eyes.

Information Frame

2827 An even more disfiguring problem is **hydrocephalus** (**high**-droh-**SEF**-ah-lus), the "presence of water (in) the head."

hydr/o/cephal/us

2828 Remembering the "water" root in hydrotherapy **(frame 288)**, plus the root for "head," as in cephalic **(frame 362)**, allows us to dissect hydrocephalus as _____ /_____ /_____ /_____.

hydrocephalus

2829 An alternative phrase for _____ is "water (on) the brain." It is due to a blockage of the flow of cerebrospinal fluid (CSF). This blockage may be present at birth.

hydr/o/cephal/ic
(**high**-droh-seh-**FAL**-ik)

2830 Pull out the ending in ectopic **(frame 2821)** and modify hydrocephalus to form an adjective, _____ /_____ /_____ /_____. This adjective "pertains to water (in) the head."

hydrocephalic	**2831** A _____ infant with an enlarged head and excessive CSF may suffer irreversible brain damage due to the great intracranial pressure being exerted.
Information Frame	**2832** Other parts of the neonate's body can have developmental abnormalities. In the lung alveoli of premature infants, for instance, a **hyaline** (**HIGH**-ah-lin) **membrane** may be present.
hyal/ine **hyal** (**HIGH**-al)	**2833** Hyaline contains the same ending seen in alkaline **(frame 1977)**. It is therefore subdivided as _____ / _____. Its root, _____, means "glassy."
hyaline	**2834** The term _____ "pertains to (something) glassy."
hyaline membrane **NRDS**	**2835** In _____ _____ **disease**, a "glassy membrane" forms within the alveoli of the premature neonate. This membrane makes breathing very labored and difficult. An alternate name is **neonatal respiratory distress syndrome**, abbreviated as ____ ____ ____ ____.
erythr/o/blast (eh-**RITH**-roh-blast)	**2836** Another group of problems involves mistaken attacks of the mother's antibodies on the erythrocytes of the fetus. Just as an osteoblast **(frame 775)** is a "bone-former," an _____ / ____ / _____ is a "red (blood cell) former."
erythroblast	**2837** An _____ is simply an immature version of the erythrocyte, or mature red blood cell.
erythr/o/blast/o/sis (eh-**rith**-roh-blas-**TOH**-sis)	**2838** Remove the suffix from endometriosis **(frame 2556)** and add it to the end of erythroblast. The result is _____ / ____ / _____ / ____ / _____, an "abnormal condition of red (blood cell) formers."
erythroblastosis fetalis	**2839** Added after the large term in the above frame is **fetalis** (feh-**TAH**-lis), "a condition of the fetus." The combined phrase is _____ _____. Its rough translation is, "an abnormal condition of red (blood cell) formers (in) the fetus."
erythroblastosis fetalis hemolysis	**2840** The disease called _____ _____ causes the immature red blood cells to undergo _____ **(frame 1756)**, a "breaking down of blood (cells)."

hem/o/lyt/ic (hee-moh-**LIT**-ik)

2841 Just as thrombolytic **(frame 1925)** "pertains to breaking down clots," _____ /_____ /_____ /_____ "pertains to breaking down blood (cells)."

---

hemolytic

2842 An alternative name for erythroblastosis fetalis is _____ **disease of the newborn**, since the immature red "blood" cells are "broken down" by attacking antibodies from the mother.

---

hemolytic
disease
newborn

2843 A neonate with erythroblastosis fetalis, or _____ _____ of the _____ (abbreviated as **HDN**) may not survive. Many of its blood vessels may be plugged by clumped erythroblasts.

HDN

2844 The disease of _____ _____ _____ (hemolytic disease of the newborn) is usually due to an incompatibility between the **Rh (rhesus monkey) blood type** of the mother and her unborn fetus.

2845 If the mother's and father's blood are tested in the lab, however, many genetic incompatibilities can be predicted or detected before they even show up in the fetus.

Lab Tests and Diagnoses

Word Parts Associated with Lab Tests and Diagnoses for the Breasts, Pregnancy, and Development

The following is a list of word parts and abbreviations associated with lab tests and diagnostic procedures for the breasts, pregnancy, and early human development. Use this list to help you complete **frames 2847 to 2888**.

CVS	chorionic villi sampling	**-iatrician**	one who is a physician	**-ician**	one who specializes in
gonad/o	seed; offspring	**-iatrics**	medical treatment (by a physician)	**obstetr/o**	midwife
HCG	human chorionic gonadotrophin				

2846 Diagnostic and lab procedures may be performed on both the mother and her unborn child or neonate.

---

obstetr (ahb-STET-er)

2847 In early days a "midwife," indicated by the root _____ on the word list, would simply evaluate the pregnant woman through her past experience.

obstetr/ic (ahb-**STET**-rik)	**2848** Applying the common "pertaining to" suffix **-ic** results in _____ /_____, "pertaining to midwives."
obstetric **obstetrics** (ahb-**STET**-riks)	**2849** The modern term _____ has come to mean anything related to the childbirth condition or time period. A final **-s** is often appended to this term, resulting in _____.
Information Frame	**2850** In Latin, **obstetrix** (ahb-**STET**-riks) means "midwife." It derives from "she who stands near or before." This term indicates the position taken by the midwife near or before the laboring mother.
Information Frame	**2851** Two suffixes for "one who specializes in" are often affixed to the "midwife" root. One is found in orthopedist **(frame 939)**. The other is **-ician** (**ISH**-un).
obstetr/ist (ahb-**STET**-rist) **obstetr/ician** (ahb-steh-**TRISH**-un)	**2852** The two terms built from the above frame are _____ /_____ and _____ /_____. Both denote "one who specializes in midwifery"—that is, "standing near or before" the expectant mother.
obstetrist obstetrician	**2853** A pregnant woman usually makes frequent visits to her _____ (_____) in the final weeks before her due date.
Information Frame	**2854** Two closely related suffixes are **-iatrics** (ee-**AT**-riks), which denotes "medical treatment" by a "physician," and **-iatrician** (ee-ah-**TRISH**-un), "one who is a physician."
ped/iatrics (**pee**-dee-**AT**-riks) **ped/iatrician** (**pee**-dee-ah-**TRISH**-un)	**2855** Extract the root from orthopedist **(frame 939)** and use the preceding facts to construct _____ /_____, the "medical treatment of children," and _____ /_____, "one who is a physician for children."
pediatrician pediatrics	**2856** Although a _____ specializing in the discipline of _____ theoretically treats only children, in modern practice this care often extends up to the age of young adulthood.
pediatrics	**2857** The practice of _____ does not begin, however, until the neonate appears. Before birth, several types of diagnostic procedures of gynecology can be carried out, including "surgical puncture and tapping of the amnion."

amni/o/centesis
(AM-nee-oh-**sen-TEE**-sis)

2858 Remove the ending from thoracentesis **(frame 2069)** and add it to the root in amnion **(frame 2720)**. The result is
_____ / _____ / _____, "surgical puncture and tapping of the amnion."

---

amniocentesis

2859 The procedure for _____ generally involves the insertion of a long hypodermic needle through a tiny incision in the mother's umbilicus. A small quantity of amniotic fluid is withdrawn. Later, this fluid is analyzed. It contains epithelial cells sloughed off from the surface of the developing fetus.

---

amniocentesis
Down's

2860 The chromosome content of the cells obtained by _____ is analyzed for the genetic defects of _____ syndrome **(frame 2824)** or other errors.

---

chorionic
villi

2861 Another prenatal diagnostic procedure is _____ _____ **sampling**, that is, "sampling of the tufts of hair that pertain to the chorion **(frame 2716)**."

---

chorionic villi
sampling
CVS

2862 The procedure of _____ _____ _____, abbreviated as _____ _____ _____, involves the extraction of pieces of the chorion for analysis.

CVS

2863 The _____ _____ _____ technique is useful because the chorionic villi are fingerlike anchoring projections that must have good structural and functional integrity if the pregnancy is to go its full term.

HCG

2864 Pregnancy is detected by testing the woman's urine for the presence of **human chorionic gonadotrophin** (gahn-a-doh-**TROHF**-in), which is abbreviated as _____ _____ _____.

---

gon

2865 HCG is related to trophic **(frame 1365)**, which "pertains to nourishment or stimulation." It also relates to **gonad** (**GOH**-nad), which, like _____, the root in gonorrhea **(frame 2549)**, denotes "seed" or "offspring."

---

gonads (**GOH**-nads)

2866 The _____ are technically the "seeders," the "offspring"-producing sex glands.

gonads	**2867** The _____, or "seeders " in the male are the testes. In the female, they are the ovaries.
gonad/o/troph/in **-in**	**2868** Use the last few frames to help you dissect gonadotrophin, the **g** in HCG, as _____ /_____ /_____ /_____. Note that the "substance" suffix is _____, as found in myelin **(frame 1080)**.
gonadotrophin	**2869** The preceding facts allow us to translate _____ as "a substance that nourishes or stimulates the gonads."
gonadotrophins (**gahn**-a-doh-**TROHF**-ins)	**2870** In particular, the _____ are hormones that stimulate the ovaries in the female.
chorionic	**2871** Remembering that _____ **(frame 2713)** "pertains to the chorion," we get the **C** in HCG. The **H** means "human."
human chorionic gonadotrophin	**2872** HCG, therefore, is an abbreviation for _____ _____ _____.
HCG	**2873** Human chorionic gonadotrophin, abbreviated _____ _____ _____, stimulates the female ovaries to keep secreting estrogen and progesterone throughout the nine-month gestation period. This hormone is secreted by the placenta, so its presence in the bloodstream and urine indicates pregnancy.
fet/o/scopy (fee-**TAHS**-koh-pee)	**2874** Direct or indirect inspection of the fetus itself may be done. Just as cystoscopy **(frame 2406)** is the "process of examining the urinary bladder," _____ /_____ /_____ is the "process of examining the fetus."
fetoscopy	**2875** The procedure of _____ may reveal a fetal head that is much larger than normal.
fet/o/scop/e (**fee**-toh-skohp)	**2876** Just as a cystoscope **(frame 2406)** is "an instrument used to examine the bladder," a _____ /_____ /_____ /_____ is "an instrument used to examine the fetus."
fetoscopy fetoscope	**2877** After _____ is performed by using a _____ to examine the fetus, **pelvimetry** (pel-**VIM**-eh-tree) may be performed.

pelv/i/metry **-metry**	**2878** Subdivide pelvimetry as _____ / ____ / _____. Recall that its suffix, _____, has been seen several times earlier, as in thermometry **(frame 226)**. It means "the process of measuring."
process measuring bowl pelv	**2879** Pelvimetry translates as a "_____ of _____ a _____." The root in this term, _____ **(frame 398)**, denotes the bony "bowl" made by the two hips.
pelvimetry	**2880** The technique of _____ is the process of measuring the dimensions of the female pelvis. Such measurements help determine whether the pelvis is large enough to pass the fetal head.
fetal	**2881** As childbirth proceeds, _____ ("referring to offspring," **frame 2733**) **monitoring** is usually carried out.
fetal monitoring	**2882** In _____ _____, a machine is used to follow the heart rate of the fetus during labor.
Information Frame	**2883** **Virginia Apgar**, an American anesthesiologist, developed a rating scale of the neonate's physical condition one minute after birth.
Apgar (AP-gar)	**2884** This scale provides a reading called the _____ **score**, which is named in her honor.
Apgar score	**2885** The _____ _____ is a number from 0 to 10 that provides a summary profile of the neonate's heart rate, respiratory effort, muscle tone, reflex irritability, and color.
mamm/o/graphy (**mam-AH**-grah-fee) **mamm/o/gram** (**MAM**-oh-gram)	**2886** Some time after the mother has finished breastfeeding, an examination of her breasts is in order. Review the suffixes in hysterosalpingography **(frame 2613)** and pyelogram **(frame 2396)**. Using mamm for "breast," construct two new terms: _____ / ____ / _____ "process of recording (x-rays involving) the breasts" _____ / ____ / _____ "(an x-ray) record of the breasts"
mammography mammograms	**2887** The diagnostic process of _____ provides _____ of the breasts, which can be inspected for abnormalities.

mammography	**2888** If carcinoma of the breast or any other serious problem is detected by _____, then various forms of therapy should begin immediately.

Word Parts Associated with Surgery, Pharmacology, and Other Therapies for the Breasts, Pregnancy, and Development

The following is a list of word parts and an abbreviation associated with surgery, pharmacology, and other therapies for disorders of the breasts, pregnancy, and early human development. Use this list to help you complete **frames 2891 to 2914**.

Caesar/i	Julius Caesar	**lump/o**	a lump of breast tissue
cesar/e	cut	**radic/o**	root
C-section	Caesarian section; cesarian section		

2889 This is your last section! You have struggled mightily, as if a valiant soldier of some Roman **Caesar** (**SEE**-zer)!

Information Frame

2890 Julius Caesar, the great Roman emperor, was not delivered through the vagina of his mother. Rather, he was born by physicians making an incision into her uterus through her anterior abdominal wall.

Caesar

cesar (**SEE**-sahr)

2891 The last name of Julius _____ has now become a root representing this uterine operation. A closely related root on the word list, _____, means "cutting" (of the uterine wall).

---

cesar/o/tomy
(**seez**-ah-**ROT**-oh-mee)

2892 Using the suffix in hysterotomy **(frame 2648)**, create _____ /_____ /_____, a "cutting or incision into (the uterine wall).

---

cesarotomy

2893 A _____ is also known as a **cesarean** (see-**SAHR**-ee-an) **section**.

---

cesar

cesar/e/an

2894 The root in cesarotomy, _____, usually takes **e** as its combining vowel. This information should allow you to correctly subdivide cesarean as _____ /_____ /_____.

Caesar/i/an (see-**ZAY**-ree-an)

2895 The root representing the Roman emperor generally takes **i** as its combining vowel. Following the same pattern as used in cesarean, we can write out _____ /_____ /_____, "pertaining to (Julius) Caesar."

Caesarian section cesarotomy	**2896** A _____ _____ is exactly the same operation as a cesarean section, or _____ ("cutting into"), which incises the uterine wall to remove the fetus **nonvaginally** (nahn-**VAJ**-ih-nah-lee).
Caesarian section cesarean section	**2897** The operation of _____ _____, or _____ _____, is abbreviated as a **C-section**.
C-section	**2898** A ____-_____ (Caesarian section) is performed whenever normal vaginal delivery is either inadvisable or impossible.
Caesarian section/cesarean section	**2899** A _____ _____ (C-section) may not be required if certain **labor and delivery drugs** are employed to facilitate childbirth. These include **oxytocin** (ahk-see-**TOH**-sin), also known as **Pitocin** (pih-**TOH**-sin), and **ergonovine** (er-goh-**NOH**-vihn), also called **Ergotrate** (**ER**-goh-trayt).
labor and delivery	**2900** Such _____ _____ _____ drugs as those mentioned above tend to stimulate the uterine myometrium to contract with more force and frequency. Administration of these drugs usually speeds up delivery.
episi	**2901** As the vertex of the fetal head presents at the orifice of the vagina, great pressure in this area may cause an uneven ripping of the pudendum. Recall that _____ **(frame 2465)** is another root for the vulva, or "pudendum."
episi/o/tomy (eh-**pee**-zee-**AHT**-oh-mee)	**2902** Just as a cesarotomy is an incision into the uterine wall, an _____ /____ /_____ is an "incision into the pudendum."
episiotomy	**2903** An _____ is actually a cut through the perineum, inferior to the vaginal orifice. This incision enlarges the opening for safe passage of the fetal head.
mast/ectomy (mast-**EK**-toh-mee) **mamm/ectomy** (mam-**EK**-toh-mee)	**2904** Other types of surgery do not accompany such happy events as childbirth. Using both roots for "breast" **(frame 2772)** and the suffix in vasectomy **(frame 2641)**, construct two terms that mean "removal of the breasts": _____ /_____ _____ /_____
mastectomy mammectomy	**2905** A _____ or _____ ("breast removal") can be of several different types. For these terms, mast is typically used as the root.

mastectomy **lump/ectomy** (lump-**EK**-toh-mee)	**2906** The most conservative partial _____ is simply _____ / _____, the "removal of a (breast) lump."
lumpectomy	**2907** With the _____ procedure, only a lumpy piece of breast tissue immediately around a malignant tumor is removed.
mastectomy	**2908** A more drastic procedure is the **simple (total)** _____ ("breast removal").
simple (total) mastectomy	**2909** In the technique of _____ (_____) _____, the entire cancerous breast is excised.
radical	**2910** The exact opposite of conservative is extreme, or _____, as in "pertaining to" a "root," or **radic** (**RAH**-dik).
radical mastectomy	**2911** A _____ _____ literally "removes a breast by its roots."
lumpectomy simple (total) mastectomy	**2912** A _____ ("lump removal") or _____ (_____) _____ ("removal of a breast only") can be very helpful if the cancer has not metastasized.
radical mastectomy	**2913** If the cancer has spread to sites beyond its breast of origin, then a _____ _____ may be needed, in order to "remove" all the "roots" (adjacent nests of cancerous breast cells).
radical mastectomy	**2914** A _____ _____ is an operation wherein an entire breast, adjacent lymph nodes, and muscle tissue are removed.
Congratulations Frame	**2915** Congratulations! You did it! Now, on to the final chapter exercises!

Multiple Choice

1. A root for "yoked" is

   a. chori   b. zygot   c. puer   d. fet

2. Fraternal twins are

   a. zygotic   b. dizygotic   c. bipara   d. bichorion

3. A root meaning "to bear" is

   a. ped   b. par   c. puer   d. parturi

4. "Tufts of hair" are

   a. amnions   b. chorions   c. villi   d. gastrulas

5. A word part for "nourishment" is

   a. plasia   b. blastula   c. puerpera   d. trophy

6. A word part for "lamb" is

   a. villi   b. amni   c. embry   d. zygot

Meanings of Selected Roots

Add the correct combining vowel (cv) after each root. Then write the definition of each root in the space provided.

ROOT/CV	DEFINITION
1. par/_____	_____
2. nat/_____	_____
3. gestat/_____	_____
4. chori/_____	_____
5. part/_____	_____
6. lact/_____	_____
7. eclamps/_____	_____
8. eme/_____	_____
9. amni/_____	_____
10. obstetr/_____	_____

Word Dissection and Translation

Analyze the following terms by dissecting them with slashmarks and identifying their word parts. To the right of each term, write its correct English translation.

Key: R (root), cv (combining vowel), P (prefix), S (suffix)

1. mammography

_____/_____/_____   _____
R   cv   S

2. lumpectomy

_____/_____   _____
R   S

3. pediatrics

_____/_____   _____
R   S

4. hydrocephalus

_____/_____/_____/_____   _____
R   cv   R   S

5. mastitis

_____/_____   _____
R   S

6. preeclampsia

_____/_____/_____   _____
P   R   S

7. postpartal

_____/_____/_____   _____
P   R   S

8. congenital

_____/_____/_____   _____
P   R   S

9. antenatal

_____/_____/_____   _____
P   R   S

10. gestation

_____/_____   _____
R   S

11. episioperineorrhaphy

_____/_____/_____/_____/_____   _____
R   cv   R   cv   S

12. parturiometer

_____/_____/_____   _____
R   cv   S

Terms and Their Abbreviations

In the list below, when the term is given, write its abbreviation in the space provided. When the abbreviation is given, write its corresponding term.

TERM	ABBREVIATION
1. Caesarian section	_____
2. _____	CVS
3. human chorionic gonadotrophin	_____
4. _____	HDN

Word Spelling

Look at each of the terms listed below. Identify those that are misspelled by circling Y for "Yes." Write the correct spelling in the blank.

WORD	MISSPELLED?	CORRECT SPELLING
1. Apgar score	Y/N	_____
2. emahsis	Y/N	_____
3. fibrosistic	Y/N	_____
4. lactation	Y/N	_____
5. puerapera	Y/N	_____
6. neonate	Y/N	_____
7. fetis	Y/N	_____
8. blastula	Y/N	_____
9. copulation	Y/N	_____
10. zeyegoat	Y/N	_____
11. feetoskuhpy	Y/N	_____
12. pelvimetry	Y/N	_____
13. gonadotroofin	Y/N	_____
14. hemolitic	Y/N	_____

New Word Synthesis

Using word parts that appear in this and previous chapters, build new terms with the following meanings:

1. _____ referring to a lamb and an offspring

2. _____ inflammation of a flat cake

3. _____ pertains to (the period) after sexual intercourse

4. _____ process of (producing) milk and vomit

5. _____ surgical puncture and tapping (during) miscarriage

6. _____ presence of a first membrane

7. _____ an instrument used to examine semen

8. _____ study of swellers

9. _____ surgical incision of an offspring

10. _____ condition or disorder of pregnancy

C A S E   S T U D Y

Read through the following partial gynecological report. Note the terms in bold print. A series of multiple choice questions probes your knowledge of these terms.

Gynecological Report

An 18-year-old **nullipara** who home-tested positive for urinary **HCG** presented at the office for an **obstetrical** exam. **Preeclampsic** signs were present.

Case Study Questions

1. Being a **nullipara** tells you that the young woman had

   (a) already mothered several viable children.

   (b) never experienced rupture of the hymen.

   (c) never mothered a viable child.

   (d) frequently engaged in sexual intercourse.

2. Presence of urinary **HCG** indicates that

   (a) the patient's urine was contaminated with her blood.

   (b) placental tissue was present and releasing gonadotrophins.

   (c) premature detachment of the placenta was likely.

   (d) fertilization had occurred in an ectopic site.

3. An **obstetrical** exam must have included

   (a) an evaluation of the patient for pregnancy and motherhood.

   (b) application of an Apgar rating to the patient.

   (c) removal of several nephroliths.

   (d) cleaning of the bronchial tree.

4. The occurrence of **preeclampsic** signs hints to you that

   (a) the patient was a candidate for open heart surgery.

   (b) no incompatibility between mother and fetus was apparent.

   (c) prenatal nutrition was of high quality.

   (d) the patient is a likely candidate for future attacks of convulsions.

APPENDIX: Answers to End-of-Chapter Exercises

Answers for Chapter 1 Exercises

Word Dissection and Translation

1. ana/tom/y — process or condition of cutting (something) apart
2. physi/o/logy — study of function (or nature)
3. termin/o/logy — study of terms
4. oste/o/meter — instrument used to measure bones
5. pharmac/o/logy — study of drugs

Fill in the Blanks

1. root
2. suffix
3. suffixes
4. form
5. compound
6. prefix
7. vowel
8. suffix
9. root
10. suffix

Singular or Plural

1. (P) vertebra
2. (S) thoraces
3. (P) psychosis
4. (P) sarcoma
5. (S) mitochondria
6. (P) apex
7. (S) appendices
8. (S) cardia
9. (P) coccus
10. (S) bronchi

Answers for Chapter 2 Exercises

Multiple Choice

1. b
2. c
3. d
4. b
5. a
6. b

Meanings of Selected Roots

1. o;   time
2. o;   disease
3. i;   sensitivity to pain
4. o;   white
5. o;   nourishment
6. o;   fever
7. o;   wound, injury
8. o;   cartilage
9. o;   death
10. o;   yellow

Word Dissection and Translation

1. hyper/algesia   excessive sensitivity to pain
2. morbid/ity   condition of illness
3. syn/drom/e   a running with illness
4. traumat/ic   pertaining to wound or injury
5. hypo/algesia   deficient sensitivity to pain
6. chron/ic   pertaining to time
7. oste/o/malacia   destructive softening of bone
8. leth/al   pertaining to death
9. necr/o/tic   pertaining to death
10. osteo/o/porosis   abnormal condition of pores or holes (in) bones
11. hyper/troph/y   condition of excessive nourishment (stimulation)
12. pyret/ic   pertaining to fever

Word Spelling

1. N
2. Y   tachycardia
3. N
4. N
5. Y   hypoesthesia
6. Y   hypochondriasis
7. N
8. N
9. Y   edema
10. N
11. N
12. Y   chronic
13. N
14. Y   traumatic

New Word Synthesis

(NOTE: Additional terms are possible for some meanings.)

1. algesostasis
2. trichromatic
3. hypotrophy
4. acutoid
5. autotrophy
6. anesthesia
7. pyretopathy
8. hyperchronic
9. xanthotrauma
10. bradynecrology
11. tachyesthesia
12. melanosis

Case Study Questions

1. c
2. b
3. a
4. b

Answers for Chapter 3 Exercises

Multiple Choice

1. b
2. c
3. d
4. b
5. a
6. b

Meanings of Selected Roots

1. o; luminous (lighting up)
2. o; chest
3. a; listen
4. o; electric current
5. o; rays
6. o; heat
7. o; sound
8. o; to beat/tap
9. o; kernel
10. o; unknown

Word Dissection and Translation

1. steth/o/scop/e — instrument to examine the chest
2. radi/o/gram — record of rays (x-rays)
3. nucle/ar — pertaining to kernels
4. cine/radi/o/graphy — process of recording rays and movies
5. radi/o/logist — one who studies x-rays
6. son/o/graphy — process of recording sound
7. therm/o/meter — instrument to measure heat
8. eti/o/logy — study of cause
9. idi/o/path/ic — pertaining to unknown disease
10. dia/gnos/tic — pertaining to knowledge through

Terms and Their Abbreviations

1. intake and output — I & O
2. milliliter — ml
3. computed axial tomography — CAT
4. nuclear magnetic resonance — NMR
5. percussion and auscultation — P & A
6. free of disease — FOD
7. symptoms — Sx
8. fever of unknown origin — FUO

Word Spelling

1. Y auscultation
2. N
3. Y cineradiographer
4. N
5. N
6. N
7. Y etiology
8. N
9. Y percussion
10. Y roentgenogram
11. Y nuclear
12. N
13. N
14. Y fluoroscopy

New Word Synthesis

(*NOTE: Additional terms are possible for some meanings.*)

1. stethic
2. scintiscope
3. sonoradiography
4. fluorology
5. auscultologist
6. prognostic
7. nucleogram
8. electroradiogram
9. etist
10. laminometry
11. thyroidomalacia
12. hypochondriasis

Case Study Questions

1. b
2. a
3. d
4. b

Answers for Chapter 4 Exercises

Multiple Choice:

1. b
2. b
3. c
4. d
5. d
6. b

Meanings of Selected Roots

1. o;   water
2. o;   sleep
3. o;   sleep/numbness
4. o;   intestine
5. o;   chemical
6. o;   treatment
7. o;   life
8. o;   drug
9. o;   water
10. o;   drug

Word Dissection and Translation

1. chem/o/therapy — treatment with chemicals
2. arthr/o/desis — binding together of joints
3. par/enter/al — pertaining to (something) other than the intestines
4. anti/dot/es — against something given
5. aque/ous — pertaining to water
6. an/esthesi/o/logist — specialist in anesthesia or one who specializes in the absence of feeling
7. pharmac/ist — one who specializes in drugs
8. therapeut/ic — pertaining to treatments
9. ionto/phoresis — carry through with ions
10. physi/o/therap/ist — one who specializes in treatment with physical means

Terms and Their Abbreviations

1. nothing by mouth — NPO
2. four times a day — qid
3. immediately — stat
4. operating room — OR
5. intensive care unit — ICU
6. after meals — pc
7. when necessary — prn
8. incision and drainage — I & D

Word Spelling

1. Y arthrorrhaphy
2. N
3. N
4. Y hydrotherapy
5. N
6. Y narcotic
7. Y iontophoresis
8. N
9. Y pharmaceutical
10. Y therapeutic
11. N
12. Y physiatrics
13. N
14. N

New Word Synthesis

(NOTE: Additional terms are possible for some meanings.)

1. enterocentesis
2. narcopharmaceutic
3. iontotherapy
4. aqueochemicals
5. laminectomy
6. enteroplasty
7. hydrologist
8. stethopexy
9. enterodesis
10. traumorrhexis
11. tranquilanesthesia
12. hypertrophy

Case Study Questions

1. a
2. c
3. b
4. a
5. b

Answers for Chapter 5 Exercises

Multiple Choice

1. b
2. c
3. d
4. c
5. d
6. c

Meanings of Selected Roots

1. o; to turn
2. o; tail
3. o; back
4. a; body
5. o; side
6. o; trunk midsection
7. o; within
8. o; belly
9. i; bowl
10. o; wall

Word Dissection and Translation

1. ana/tom/ical   pertaining to cutting (something) apart
2. anter/i/or   one which is in front
3. trans/vers/e   a turning across
4. crani/al   pertaining to the skull
5. infer/i/or   one which is below
6. cyst/o/form   bladder-shaped
7. bi/o/logy   study of life
8. physi/o/log/ical   referring to the study of nature (functions)
9. viscer/al   pertaining to the guts
10. cephal/ic   relating to the head

Terms and Their Abbreviations

1. anterior   ant.
2. anatomy and physiology   A & P
3. anteroposterior   AP

Word Spelling

1. Y   medial
2. N
3. N
4. Y   midsagittal
5. Y   coronal
6. Y   thoracic
7. N
8. N
9. Y   iliac
10. Y   internal
11. N
12. Y   posterior
13. N
14. Y   biological

New Word Synthesis

(NOTE: Additional terms are possible for some meanings.)

1. proximocystal
2. ilianatomy
3. viscerology
4. peripelvic
5. diaphragmosoma
6. pharmacophysiology
7. gastroenteric
8. umbilicoform
9. anteroenteral
10. transtomothoracic

Case Study Questions

1. a
2. b
3. b
4. c

Answers for Chapter 6 Exercises

Multiple Choice

1. b
2. b
3. d
4. c
5. c
6. d

Meanings of Selected Roots

1. o; cancer/crab
2. o; poison/virus
3. o; formation
4. o; thread
5. o; little mass
6. o; eat
7. o; sugar/sweet
8. o; large
9. o; cross through
10. o; strength/concentration (of solute)

Word Dissection and Translation

1.	phag/o/cyt/o/sis	process of cell eating
2.	macr/o/scop/ic	referring to (things that) appear large or to the examination of large (things)
3.	in/organ/ic	pertaining to not having carbon
4.	electr/o/lyt/e	presence of (something that) breaks down and (conducts) an electrical current
5.	dys/plas/ia	presence of bad formation
6.	carcin/oma	tumor of crabs (cancerous tumor)
7.	bacter/i/o/logy	study of bacteria
8.	radi/o/pharmaceut/ical	pertaining to drugs and rays
9.	anti/neo/plast/ic	relating to (something) against new growths
10.	hyper/ton/ic	pertaining to excessive strength/concentration (of solute)

Terms and Their Abbreviations

1.	endoplasmic reticulum	ER
2.	diphtheria-pertussis-tetanus	DPT
3.	cancer	CA
4.	intracellular fluid	ICF
5.	deoxyribonucleic acid	DNA
6.	extracellular fluid	ECF
7.	ribonucleic acid	RNA

Word Spelling

1. Y aspiration
2. N
3. Y staphylococci
4. N
5. N
6. Y carcinogenic
7. N
8. N
9. N
10. Y pathogen
11. N
12. Y neoplasm
13. Y molecular
14. N

New Word Synthesis

(NOTE: Additional terms are possible for some meanings.)

1. streptogastric
2. hypoglycia
3. cryoaspiration
4. carcinolysis
5. microphages
6. macroscope
7. tonosomatic
8. macrophagoneoplasm
9. intracellulologist
10. mitoreticulum
11. thermolysis
12. sarcopsy

Case Study Questions

1. b
2. a
3. c
4. a
5. c

Answers for Chapter 7 Exercises

Multiple Choice

1. c
2. a
3. b
4. a
5. d
6. b

Meanings of Selected Roots

1. o; skin
2. o; sheet
3. o; red (little)
4. o; bedsore
5. o; love
6. o; skin
7. o; slime
8. o; layer
9. o; area (little)
10. o; fatty

Word Dissection and Translation

1. papill/ae   pimples/nipples
2. epi/derm/is   presence upon the skin
3. cicatric/i/al   pertaining to a connective tissue scar
4. fibr/ous   relating to fibers
5. terat/oma   monster tumor
6. decubit/us   bedsore
7. hyper/chromat/ic   pertaining to excessive color
8. hist/o/logist   one who studies tissues
9. acid/o/phil/ic   referring to love of acids
10. sub/cutane/ous   pertaining to (something) under the skin

Terms and Their Abbreviations

1. herpes simplex virus   HSV
2. hypodermic   hypo
3. subcutaneous   sc

Word Spelling

1. Y   microtome
2. N
3. Y   herpes simplex
4. Y   dermatology
5. N
6. N
7. Y   adipose
8. Y   sebaceous
9. N
10. Y   xanthosis
11. N
12. Y   subdermis
13. Y   dermatoses
14. Y   cicatricial

New Word Synthesis

(NOTE: Additional terms are possible for some meanings.)

1. dermophilia
2. histitis
3. squamorrhea
4. leukoma
5. submucia
6. lipocyte
7. sebic
8. teratochromic
9. areolitis
10. columnalopecia

Case Study Questions

1. b
2. c
3. b
4. d

Answers for Chapter 8 Exercises

Multiple Choice:

1. b
2. b
3. c
4. c
5. b
6. a

Meanings of Selected Roots

1. o; cartilage
2. o; wrist
3. o; joint
4. o; hump
5. o; painful change
6. o; ankle
7. o; bone
8. o; marrow/spinal cord
9. o; knuckle
10. o; foot

Word Dissection and Translation

1.	patell/a	kneecap; little pan; little dish
2.	clavicul/o/tomy	incision into a little key
3.	arthr/algia	joint pain
4.	kyph/o/scoli/o/sis	abnormal condition of hump back
5.	stern/al	referring to breastplate
6.	arthr/o/plasty	surgical repair of a joint
7.	bunion/ectomy	removal of a mound
8.	ortho/paed/ics	pertaining to straightening children
9.	chondr/o/cyt/e	cartilage cell
10.	intra/cartilagin/ous	relating to (something) within cartilage
11.	rheumat/o/spicul/ar	pertaining to painful change and little points
12.	sacr/o/ili/ac	pertaining to sacrum (sacred) and ilium (flank)

Terms and Their Abbreviations

1. fracture   Fx
2. fracture both bones   FxBB
3. osteoarthritis   OA

Word Spelling

1. Y fibula
2. N
3. Y synovial
4. N
5. Y endochondral
6. Y myelitis
7. N
8. Y ostectomy
9. N
10. Y arthralgia
11. N
12. Y arthrogram
13. Y amputation
14. N

New Word Synthesis

(NOTE: Additional terms are possible for some meanings.)

1. spiculoid
2. ligamentous
3. intrachondrocytes
4. chondrectomy
5. claviculoma
6. arthrodermatitis
7. femoropatellar
8. tibiotomy
9. osteohistologist
10. scoliosteoporosis

Case Study Questions

1. b
2. a
3. b
4. a

Answers for Chapter 9 Exercises

Multiple Choice

1. d
2. a
3. a
4. c
5. d
6. b

Meanings of Selected Roots

1. o; foot
2. o; little mouse (muscle)
3. o; husk
4. o; movement
5. o; hand
6. o; nerve
7. o; straight/upright/vertical
8. o; nipples/chest
9. o; move
10. o; tendon

Word Dissection and Translation

1. inter/cost/al — referring to (something) between the ribs
2. rect/us — presence of (something) straight or upright
3. neur/o/muscul/ar — referring to nerve and muscle
4. pod/iatry — diagnosing and treating problems of the feet
5. gastrocnemi/us — presence of calf/belly of leg
6. my/asthenia — weakness of muscle
7. quadri/ceps — four heads
8. electr/o/my/o/graphy — process of recording muscle electrical activity
9. my/o/ten/o/tomy — incision into a muscle and its tendon
10. ab/duct/or — one which moves away from
11. my/o/sarc/o/sis — condition of muscle flesh
12. tendin/o/plasty — surgical repair of tendons

Terms and Their Abbreviations

1. acetylcholine — ACh
2. electromyogram — EMG
3. intramuscular — IM

Word Spelling

1. Y chiropody
2. N
3. N
4. N
5. N
6. N
7. Y podiatrist
8. Y succinylcholine
9. N
10. Y diazepam
11. N
12. Y myopathies
13. Y dystrophy
14. N

New Word Synthesis

(NOTE: Additional terms are possible for some meanings.)

1. osteosarcal
2. deltotomy
3. myoextension
4. neurosupination
5. kinesiarthrography
6. tenorrhaphy
7. myochondropathy
8. myoosteomyelitis
9. arthriatrist
10. vertebroflexion
11. myoblast
12. myocele

Case Study Questions

1. b
2. c
3. a
4. d

Answers for Chapter 10 Exercises

Multiple Choice

1. c
2. c
3. d
4. b
5. c
6. c

Meanings of Selected Roots

1. o; little brain
2. o; glue
3. o; room/bedroom
4. o; mimic/imitate
5. o; brain
6. o; walk
7. o; play false/deceive
8. o; mind
9. o; wander
10. o; main brain mass

Word Dissection and Translation

1. sympath/o/mimet/ic — pertaining to imitation of sympathetic (nerves)
2. neur/o/gli/a — presence of nerve glue
3. trephin/a/tion — process of boring
4. encephal/itis — inflammation of the brain
5. schiz/o/phren/ia — abnormal condition of a split mind
6. psych/o/logist — one who studies the mind
7. ventricul/ar — pertaining to a little belly
8. thalam/o/tomy — incision into the bedroom (thalamus)
9. ambul/ism — (abnormal) condition of walking
10. quadri/plegia — paralysis of four (body limbs)
11. psych/o/therapeut/ic — pertaining to therapy for the mind
12. micr/o/cephal/us — abnormally small head

Terms and Their Abbreviations

1. somatic nervous system — SNS
2. electroencephalogram — EEG
3. central nervous system — CNS
4. peripheral nervous system — PNS
5. cerebrospinal fluid — CSF
6. autonomic nervous system — ANS
7. cerebrovasular accident — CVA
8. multiple sclerosis — MS

Word Spelling

1. Y antidepressants
2. N
3. Y encephalometer
4. Y cerebrovascular
5. N
6. N
7. N
8. Y ventricular
9. N
10. N
11. Y antiparkinson
12. N
13. Y quadriplegia
14. Y cephalalgia

New Word Synthesis

(NOTE: Additional terms are possible for some meanings.)

1. mimeta
2. cerebrosis
3. vagovascular
4. phasosyncope
5. avertigo
6. orthoneurectomy
7. myoneuritis
8. acerebral
9. cerebelloconcussion
10. schizoneurosis
11. psychogenic
12. meningomyelocele

Case Study Questions

1. b
2. a
3. c
4. c

Answers for Chapter 11 Exercises

Multiple Choice

1. b
2. c
3. b
4. d
5. b
6. b

Meanings of Selected Roots

1. o; anvil
2. o; bone
3. o; tear
4. o; dull/dim
5. o; hear
6. o; hard
7. o; cornea/tough/hornlike
8. o; widen
9. o; eye/vision
10. o; eye

Word Dissection and Translation

1. audi/o/gram — record of hearing
2. conjunctiv/itis — inflammation of the conjunctiva (eyelid lining)
3. meat/us — an opening or passage
4. ambly/op/ia — abnormal condition of dull/dim vision
5. ocul/ar — pertaining to the eyes
6. semi/circul/ar — relating to a partial circle
7. ot/itis — inflammation of the ear
8. tinnit/us — a ringing
9. ot/o/laryng/o/logy — study of the ears and voicebox
10. opt/o/metrist — one who measures vision (of eyes)
11. corne/o/blephar/on — (adhesion of) the eyelid and the cornea
12. irid/o/rrhaphy — suturing of the iris (rainbow)

Terms and Their Abbreviations

1. otitis media — OM
2. auris dextra — AD
3. auris sinistra — AS
4. eye, ear, nose, throat — EENT

Word Spelling

1. Y vestibule
2. N
3. N
4. N
5. Y myringotomy
6. Y palpebra
7. N
8. N
9. Y intraocular
10. Y ophthalmoscope
11. N
12. Y semicircular
13. N
14. Y conjunctiva

New Word Synthesis

(NOTE: Additional terms are possible for some meanings.)

1. retinectomy
2. ossimeter
3. lacrimologist
4. refractoscopy
5. myolaryngia
6. tympanoneuritis
7. pupilothalamus
8. sclerosclerosis
9. myeloiridometry
10. tympanorrhaphy
11. otorrhea
12. oculomyometer

Case Study Questions

1. c
2. a
3. b
4. d

Answers for Chapter 12 Exercises

Multiple Choice

1. c
2. d
3. c
4. c
5. c
6. b

Meanings of Selected Roots

1. o; secrete
2. o; mucus/phlegm
3. o; eggshell
4. o; siphon
5. o; body extremity
6. o; gland
7. o; little node/little knot
8. o; honey
9. o; male
10. o; cold

Word Dissection and Translation

1.	diabet/es mellit/us	honeyed siphon
2.	thryox/ine	a substance (from) the shield
3.	hypo/secret/ion	process of secreting deficiently
4.	aden/o/carcin/oma	crab tumor (cancer) of the glands
5.	endo/crin/o/logy	study of glands that secrete within
6.	hypophys/ectomy	removal of the undergrowth (hypophysis or pituitary)
7.	andr/o/gen	male-producer
8.	ad/ren/o/cortic/o/troph/ic	pertaining to nourishing (stimulating) the adrenal cortex
9.	pan/creas	presence of all flesh
10.	acr/o/megaly	enlargement of the body extremities

Terms and Their Abbreviations

1.	glucose tolerance test	GTT
2.	thyroid stimulating hormone	TSH
3.	radioimmunoassay	RIA
4.	adrenocorticotrophic hormone	ACTH

Word Spelling

1. N
2. Y diuresis
3. N
4. Y glucocorticoid
5. N
6. N
7. Y epinephrine
8. Y diuresis
9. N
10. N
11. Y steroid
12. N
13. Y endocrinology
14. Y cryohypophysectomy

New Word Synthesis

(NOTE: Additional terms are possible for some meanings.)

1. acromellitus
2. epithyroidine
3. cryoadenectomy
4. hypophysemia
5. nephritis
6. pituitotropic
7. irogenic/iridogenic
8. pansecretion
9. adenophthalmologist
10. corticitis

Case Study Questions

1. d
2. b
3. a
4. c

Answers for Chapter 13 Exercises

Multiple Choice

1. d
2. b
3. c
4. a
5. b
6. d

Meanings of Selected Roots

1. o;   artery
2. o;   heart
3. o;   vein
4. o;   hair
5. o;   tightness with pain
6. o;   fat
7. o;   moon
8. o;   contraction
9. o;   vein
10. o;   curved bay

Word Dissection and Translation

1. angi/o/gram — an (x-ray) record of a vessel
2. hyper/cholesterol/emia — blood condition of excessive cholesterol
3. cine/angi/o/ cardi/o/graphy — a process of recording movies of the heart and vessels
4. a/vascul/ar — pertaining to an absence of vessels
5. my/o/cardi/um — presence of heart muscle
6. sten/o/sis — an (abnormal) process of narrowing
7. vas/o/dilat/ion — process of vessel widening
8. semi/lun/ar — referring to half moon
9. electr/o/cardi/o/gram — a record of the electrical activity of the heart
10. ather/o/sclerosis — an abnormal condition of fatty hardening
11. cardi/o/asthenia — weakness of the heart
12. cardi/o/malacia — abnormal softening of heart (muscle)

Terms and Their Abbreviations

1. electrocardiogram	EKG (ECG)
2. coronary artery disease	CAD
3. atrioventricular	AV
4. myocardial infarction	MI
5. coronary heart disease	CHD
6. premature ventricular contraction	PVC
7. cardiac magnetic resonance imaging	cardiac MRI
8. percutaneous transluminal coronary angioplasty	PCTA

Word Spelling

1. Y   tachycardia
2. Y   defibrillation
3. Y   phlebitis
4. Y   arrhythmia
5. Y   pericarditis
6. N
7. N
8. Y   angiopathy
9. Y   aneurysm
10. N
11. Y   ischemia
12. Y   myocardial
13. Y   angiopathies
14. N

New Word Synthesis

(NOTE: Additional terms are possible for some meanings.)

1. peridiastolation
2. cardiostenosis
3. hyposinal
4. infarctal
5. venorrhexis/phleborrhexis
6. androcardiogenic
7. aortitestation
8. aneurysmosis
9. vasculadenectomy
10. myoatrium

Case Study Questions

1. b
2. a
3. c
4. d

Answers for Chapter 14 Exercises

Multiple Choice

1. a
2. a
3. c
4. d
5. c
6. a

Meanings of Selected Roots

1. o; clear spring water
2. o; watery
3. o; attraction/fondness
4. o; white
5. o; blood
6. o; curdle
7. o; fever
8. o; clot
9. o; red
10. o; globe

Word Dissection and Translation

1. immun/ity — a condition of not serving (disease)
2. ser/o/logy — the study of serum
3. thromb/in — a substances that clots
4. leuk/o/cyt/o/penia — a deficiency of white cells
5. mono/nucle/o/sis — (abnormal) condition of one nucleus
6. hemat/o/crit — separation of blood
7. lymph/aden/ectomy — removal of a lymph gland
8. coagul/a/tion — a process of curdling
9. febr/ile — relating to fever
10. auto/immun/ity — a condition of not serving your own disease
11. centrifug/e — a fleeing from the center
12. embol/ectomy — removal of plugs

Terms and Their Abbreviations

1. complete blood count — CBC
2. human immunodeficiency virus — HIV
3. acquired immune deficiency syndrome — AIDS
4. enzyme-linked immunosorbent assay — ELISA
5. azidothymidine — AZT

Word Spelling

1. Y erythrocyte
2. N
3. N
4. N
5. Y hemorrhage
6. N
7. Y embolus
8. Y hematoma
9. N
10. Y globulins
11. Y anticoagulants
12. N
13. N
14. Y thrombolytic

New Word Synthesis

(NOTE: Additional terms are possible for some meanings.)

1. thromboglobulin
2. adenolysis
3. leukogenic/leukopoietic
4. lymphorrhagia
5. embolophilia
6. cardiolytic
7. leukosarcoma
8. centrifugal
9. erythropoiesis
10. splenorrhagia

Case Study Questions

1. b
2. c
3. d
4. a

Answers for Chapter 15 Exercises

Multiple choice

1. c
2. c
3. d
4. a
5. a
6. a

Meanings of Selected Roots

1. o; breathe
2. o; windpipe/airtube
3. o; lung/air
4. o; blow up
5. o; fan/blow
6. o; running down
7. o; nose
8. o; spit
9. o; (main) windpipe
10. o; little windpipe/little bronchus

Word Dissection and Translation

1. bronch/o/scop/e — instrument used to examine a windpipe/bronchus
2. dys/pnea — difficult/painful breathing
3. endo/trache/al — pertaining to (something) within the (main) windpipe
4. respir/o/metry — the process of measuring breathing again
5. bronch/o/dilat/ors — ones which widen the bronchi (windpipe/airtubes)
6. laryng/ectomy — removal of the voicebox (larynx)
7. pulmon/ary — relating to the lungs
8. tachy/pnea — rapid breathing
9. thora/centesis — surgical puncture and tapping of the chest
10. rhonch/us — presence of snoring
11. laryng/o/catarrh/al — running down of the larynx (voicebox)
12. pneum/o/cephal/us — presence of air (in) the head

Terms and Their Abbreviations

1. chronic obstructive pulmonary disease — COPD
2. intermittent positive pressure breathing — IPPB
3. short of breath — SOB

Word Spelling

1. Y   bronchoconstriction
2. Y   pneumonitis
3. N
4. Y   catarrhal
5. N
6. Y   angiography
7. Y   respirometer
8. N
9. Y   rales
10. Y   nasoplasty
11. N
12. Y   pneumothorax
13. N
14. Y   coryza

New Word Synthesis

(NOTE: Additional terms are possible for some meanings.)

1. laryngoplasty
2. arteriodilation
3. spiroventilation
4. pneumocostal/costopneumal
5. trachectomy
6. angiopneumonocentesis/pneumoangiocentesis
7. cardiopulmonary/pulmonocardiac
8. circulometer
9. bronchoconstrictor
10. sputal
11. laryngeal
12. nasopharyngitis

Case Study Questions

1. c
2. a
3. c
4. d

Answers for Chapter 16 Exercises

Multiple Choice

1. c
2. b
3. b
4. d
5. d
6. b

Meanings of Selected Roots

1. o; esophagus/gullet
2. o; liver
3. o; appendix (attachment)
4. o; colon (large intestine)
5. o; straight/vertical
6. o; injection
7. o; stomach
8. o; abdomen
9. o; bile
10. o; slacken/relax

Word Dissection and Translation

1.	gastr/ectomy	removal of the stomach
2.	dys/phag/ia	an abnormal condition of difficult eating
3.	hiat/al	relating to a hole
4.	hepat/o/splen/o/megaly	enlargement of the liver and spleen
5.	chole/lith	gallstone
6.	enter/o/clysis	washing out of the intestines
7.	sigm/oid	resembling an s
8.	rect/o/cele	a swelling or rupture of the rectum
9.	cholecyst/o/graphy	the process of recording (x-ray images of) the gallbladder
10.	lapar/o/scopy	process of examining the abdomen

Terms and Their Abbreviations

1.	gastrointestinal	GI
2.	nasogastric	NG
3.	alkaline phosphatase	ALK PHOS
4.	serum glutamic oxalacetic transaminase	SGOT

Word Spelling

1. Y hepatic
2. Y peristalsis
3. N
4. N
5. Y colonoscopy
6. N
7. N
8. N
9. Y esophagoscopy
10. N
11. N
12. Y colonoscopy
13. N
14. N

New Word Synthesis

(NOTE: Additional terms are possible for some meanings.)

1. calculolithic
2. hepatoplasty
3. diverticulectomy
4. pylorogastrolaparitis/pylorogastroabdominitis
5. hemorrhoidography
6. cirrholaryngic
7. antiperistalsis
8. cheiloplasty/chiloplasty
9. pharyngolingual/pharyngoglossal
10. colorectal/coloproctal

Case Study Questions

1. b
2. a
3. d
4. d

Answers for Chapter 17 Exercises

Multiple Choice

1. c
2. a
3. d
4. c
5. d
6. c

Meanings of Selected Roots

1. o;   kidney
2. o;   urine
3. o;   renal pelvis
4. o;   kidney
5. o;   urine
6. o;   little ball of yarn (glomerulus)
7. o;   ureter
8. o;   urethra
9. o;   produce (genitals)
10. o;   urine

Word Dissection and Translation

1.	poly/ur/ia	abnormal condition of (too) many times urinating
2.	cyst/o/scopy	process of examining the bladder
3.	dia/lys/is	process of (something) breaking down and moving through
4.	genit/o/urin/ary	relating to urine and producing (genitals)
5.	glomerul/o/nephr/itis	inflammation of kidney and glomeruli
6.	nephr/o/tom/o/graphy	process of recording kidney sections
7.	ren/al	pertaining to the kidneys
8.	intra/ven/ous	pertaining to (something) within the veins
9.	cyst/o/stomy	making a permanent new opening in the bladder
10.	uret/er	one which is a (presence of) urinary tube
11.	ren/o/pathy	disease of the kidney
12.	pyel/o/plasty	surgical repair of the renal pelvis

Terms and Their Abbreviations

1.	intravenous	IV
2.	genitourinary	GU
3.	blood urea nitrogen	BUN
4.	intravenous pyelogram	IVP

Word Spelling

1. N
2. N
3. Y   nephrostomy
4. N
5. N
6. Y   hydronephrosis
7. Y   glomerulus
8. N
9. Y   urea
10. N
11. Y   urogenital
12. N
13. N
14. N

New Word Synthesis

(NOTE: Additional terms are possible for some meanings.)

1. glomerulectomy
2. urethropexy
3. pyemia
4. genititis
5. urocystosclerosis
6. rhinogastropexy
7. nephrolaparia
8. glossopelvic/linguopelvic
9. cholecystourocystemia/urocystocholecystemia
10. hepatolysis

Case Study Questions

1. d
2. a
3. b
4. c
5. c

Answers for Chapter 18 Exercises

Meanings of Selected Roots

1. o;   eggshell
2. o;   month/monthly
3. o;   trumpet/fallopian tube/oviduct
4. o;   tube
5. o;   vas deferens
6. o;   womb/uterus
7. o;   vagina/pocket/sheath
8. o;   woman
9. o;   hidden
10. o;   little egg

Terms and Their Abbreviations

1. venereal disease   VD
2. dilatation and curettage   D & C
3. pelvic inflammatory disease   PID
4. Papanicolaou   Pap

Word Dissection and Translation

1. menstru/al — pertaining to a month
2. endo/metr/itis — inflammation of the endometrium/inflammation of the inner (portion) of the uterus
3. hemat/o/salpinx — a bloody trumpet
4. gynec/o/logy — the study of women
5. anti/fung/al — pertaining to (something) against fungi
6. vas/ectomy — removal of the vas deferens
7. hyster/o/pexy — surgical fixation of the uterus
8. circumcis/ion — a process of cutting around (something)
9. vulv/a — presence of a wrapper
10. labi/a — presence (condition) of lips
11. crypt/o/men/o/rrhea — a hidden monthly flow
12. hyster/o/pexy — surgical fixation of the uterus (womb)

Word Spelling

1. N
2. N
3. Y   spermatozoa
4. Y   hysterosalpingography
5. N
6. N
7. N
8. Y   orchiectomy
9. N
10. N
11. Y   gynecology
12. Y   hysterectomy
13. N
14. Y   hematosalpinx

New Word Synthesis

(NOTE: Additional terms are possible for some meanings.)

1. didymosalpingectomy/testosalpingectomy
2. periprostatitis
3. hysterolith/uterolith
4. urocystoligation
5. cryptic
6. penectomy
7. urinospermatogenesis
8. vulvotomy
9. ureterorrhaphy
10. endomyometrial
11. orchidoptosis
12. spermaturia

Case Study Questions

1. b
2. a
3. d
4. c

Answers for Chapter 19 Exercises

Multiple Choice

1. b
2. b
3. b
4. c
5. d
6. b

Meanings of Selected Roots

1. o; bring forth/bear
2. o; birth
3. o; to bear (be pregnant)
4. o; membrane
5. o; bring forth/bear
6. o; milk
7. o; a shining forth
8. o; vomit
9. o; lamb (the amnion)
10. o; midwife

Word Dissection and Translation

1. mamm/o/graphy — process of recording (x-ray images) of the breasts
2. lump/ectomy — removal of a lump
3. ped/iatrics — medical treatment of children
4. hydr/o/cephal/us — presence of water (in) the head
5. mast/itis — inflammation of the breasts
6. pre/eclamps/ia — abnormal condition before a shining forth
7. post/part/al — pertaining to (the period) after birth
8. con/genit/al — referring to (something that occurs) with producing
9. ante/nat/al — pertaining to (the period) before birth
10. gestat/ion — process of bearing/process of being pregnant
11. episi/o/perine /o/rrhaphy — suturing of the vulva and perineum
12. parturi/o/meter — an instrument used to measure labor (the force of uterine contractions during birth)

Terms and Their Abbreviations

1. Caesarian section — C-section
2. chorionic villi sampling — CVS
3. human chorionic gonadotrophin — HCG
4. hemolytic disease of the newborn — HDN

Word Spelling

1. N
2. Y   emesis
3. Y   fibrocystic
4. N
5. Y   puerpera
6. N
7. Y   fetus
8. N
9. N
10. Y   zygote
11. Y   fetoscopy
12. N
13. Y   gonadotrophin
14. Y   hemolytic

New Word Synthesis

(NOTE: Additional terms are possible for some meanings.)

1. amniofetal/fetoamnial
2. placentitis
3. postcoital/postcopulatal
4. emetolactation/emeolactation
5. abortocentesis
6. primichorion
7. seminoscope
8. embryology
9. fetotomy
10. gravidism

Case Study Questions

1. c
2. b
3. a
4. d

INDEX

NOTE: Indexing is by frame number. Information in figures and tables is indexed by page numbers followed by the letter t *or* f.

Microscope, 427–428

Microscopic, 430–431

Microscopy, 585–586

Microsurgery, 613–614

Microtome, 735–736

Micturate, 2306–2307

Micturition, 2308–2309

Midsagittal, 329, 332

Midsagittal plane, 69f, 330

Midwife, 2847–2852

Milk of magnesia, 2277

Milliliter (ml), 44t

Millimeter (mm), 44t

Mimetic drugs, 1224–1225

Miscarriage, 2811–2813

Mitochondria, 88f, 524, 526

Mitochondrion, 524–525

Mitosis, 99f, 497, 499, 553

Mitral valve, 281f, 1563, 1565–1567
    prolapse of, 1657–1660
    stenosis of, 1655–1656

MODM, 1443

Molecular, 438–439

Molecule, 432, 434
    commonly found in body, 87f
    symbols and formulas for, 92t

Monocytes, 305f, 1763–1765, 1769

Mononucleosis, 1844–1846

Monozygotic, 268602687

Morbidity, 107–108, 117, 422

Morning sickness, 2803–2806

Mortality, 157–158, 422

Mouth, 2080–2093

Movement
    diagnostic study of, 1032–1040
    muscular system and, 181f,
      969–973

MRI, 43t, 1671

MS (mitral sclerosis), 1656

MS (multiple sclerosis), 1162

Mucous, 664–667

Multipara, 2770–2771

Multiple sclerosis, 1161–1163

Murmurs, 1651–1652

Muscle relaxants, 1048

Muscle stimulants, 1048

Muscular, 956

Muscular dystrophy, 1023–1026

Muscular system
    body movements involving, 181f,
      969–973
    diseases of, 1005–1029
    lab tests and diagnoses of,
      1031–1046
    major muscles in, 176f
    nervous system disorders
      involving, 1157–1163
    normal anatomy and physiology
      of, 954–1003

surgeries and therapies of,
    1048–1069

tendons and action in, 177f

types of tissue in, 175f

Musculus, 955

MVP, 1658

Myasthenia, 1016–1018

Myasthenia gravis, 1019–1020

Mycostatin, 2633

Myelencephalon, 1083–1084,
    1089–1090

Myelic, 791–793

Myelin, 203f, 1079–1082, 1092

Myelitis, 893–894, 896

Myeloma, 895–896

Myitis, 1012–1013

Mylanta, 2267

Myocardial, 1550, 1552, 1627

Myocardial infarction, 1628–1630,
    1636
    acute, 1618–1619
    natural history of, 289f

Myocardium, 1550–1551

Myogram, 1038–1039

Myography, 1035–1036

Myoma, 1010–1011

Myometrial, 2536–2537

Myometrium, 2534–2535

Myopathies, 1008–1009

Myopathy, 1006–1007

Myopia, 1290–1292

Myorrhaphy, 1068–1069

Myosarcoma, 1010–1011

Myositis, 1012–1013

Myotasis, 1066–1067

Myotenotomy, 1064–1065

Myotome, 1060–1061

Myotomy, 1062–1063

Myringotomy, 1353–1354

N

N (nitrogen), 92t, 440

Narcotics, 260, 263

Nasal, 1929–1930

Nasal cavity, 78f

Nasogastric, 224

Nasogastric tube, 2248–2249

Nasoplasty, 2048–2049

Natal, 2743–2744

Neck, 831

Necrotic, 159–160

Neonatal, 2754–2755

Neonatal respiratory distress
    syndrome, 2835

Neonate, 2752–2753

Neoplasm, 561–563, 575
    cartilage, 887

lymphatic, 1834–1838
    See also Carcinoma

Nephrectomy, 2426–2427

Nephritis, 2370–2371, 2374

Nephrolith, 2382–2383

Nephrolithiasis, 2384–2385

Nephron, 388f, 389f, 2311, 2313

Nephropexy, 2424–2425

Nephrosclerosis, 2390–2391

Nephrostomy, 2418, 2420

Nephrotomy, 2417, 2420

Nervous system, 24
    diseases of, 1140–1181
    lab tests and diagnoses of,
      1184–1200
    muscle relaxants and, 1051–1055
    normal anatomy and physiology
      of, 1070–1138
    structural organization of, 199f
    surgery and therapies involving,
      1201–1229

Neurectomy, 1218–1219

Neuroglia, 1092–1093, 1095

Neurologists, 1203, 1205

Neurology, 1202, 1205

Neuromuscular, 957–958

Neuromuscular blockers, 1053–1054

Neuromuscular junction, 1049

Neuron, 203f, 1076, 1078

Neuroradiology, 1188–1189

Neurosis, 1169–1170

Neurosurgeon, 1217

Neurosurgery, 1207–1208, 1210

Neutrophil, 305f

NG tube, 2249

Nitrate, 1702

Nitrates, 1703

Nitric, 1704

Nitric acid, 1705

Nitrogen, 92t, 440

Nitroglycerin, 1705

NMR, 214–215

Noctambulism, 1171–1172

Nocturia, 2360, 2362

Node, 1465–1467

Nodular, 1468–1469

Nodule, 1465–1467

Nonsystemic, 2265

Nonsystemic antacids, 2266–2267

Nose
    anatomy of, 1930–1931
    inflammation of, 1996,
      1999–2003

Nothing by mouth (NPO), 59t

NRDS, 2835

Nuclear, 206, 514

Nuclear magnetic resonance,
    214–215, 1671

Nuclear medicine, 204–215

INDEX OF WORD PARTS

circumcis/i, 2664
cirrh/o, 87, 2211
clavic/o, 847
clavicul/o, 847
clitor/o, 2455
-clysis, 2240
coagul/o, 1906
cocc/o, 545
coccyg/e, 832
cochle/o, 1278
coit/o, 2670
col/o, 2126
coll/a, 631
colon, 2250
colp/o, 2442
column/o, 656
con-, 83
concuss/o, 1149
condyl/o, 816
conjunctiv/o, 1243
constrict/o, 419
contra-, 83
copulat/o, 2670
cor/o, 1246, 1341
core/o, 1246
corne/o, 1244
coron/o, 326
cortic/o, 1110, 1366
cost/o, 847
crani/o, 359
creat/o, 1410
crin/o, 1482
-crit, 1867
cry/o, 615, 1495
crypt/o, 2582
curett/e, 2658
cutane/o, 620
cyan/o, 87
cyst/o, 406, 2120
cyt/o, 485, 617

D

dacry/o, 1258
de-, 507
decubit/o, 717
delt/o, 999
delus/o, 1173
demi-, 81
dent/o, 2082
deoxy-, 507
derm/o, 620
dermat/o, 620
-desis, 301, 943
dextr/o, 337
di-, 80
dia-, 162

diabet/o, 1433
diagnos/o, 162
diagnost/o, 164
diaphor/o, 677
diastol/o, 1570
didym/o, 2484
diffus/o, 481
dil/o, 1332
dilat/a, 2658
dilat/o, 419, 1332, 2066
dipl/o, 549
dist/o, 366
diures, 1436
diuret, 1436
diverticul/o, 2190
dont/o, 2082
dors/o, 350
-dot/o, 275
drom/o, 124
duct/o, 964
duoden/o, 2111
-dynia, 127
dys-, 132

E

-e, 97
eclamps/o, 2788
-ectasia, 1341
ecto-, 366
-ectomy, 307
ectop/o, 2820
edem/o, 1822
edemat/o, 1823
electr/o, 216, 464, 1676
embol/o, 1816
embry/o, 2706
embryon/o, 2707
eme/o, 2803
emetic/o, 2803
-emia, 1428
emphysem/o, 2017
emphysemat/o, 2017
en-, 366
encephal/o, 1071, 1186
endo-, 180, 518
enem/o, 2236
enter/o, 277
epi-, 366
episi/o, 2465
-erone, 1406
erythem/a, 692
erythr/o, 87
-esis, 98
esophag/o, 2095
esthes/i, 117
estr/o, 1403

eti/o, 230
eu-, 84
ex-, 366
exo-, 366
extens/o, 970
extern/o, 366
extra-, 366, 472

F

Fallopi/o, 2517
fasci/o, 633
febr/o, 1847
femor/o, 871
fet/o, 2730
fibr/o, 629
fibrill/o, 1709
fibul/o, 871
fic/a, 771
flex/o, 970
fluor/o, 183
foramen, 816
foramin/o, 823
follic/o, 2512
follicul/o, 2512
-form, 409
foss/o, 816
fung/i, 2625
furuncl/o, 702

G

gastr/o, 2097
gastrocnemi/o, 979
gastrul/o, 2693
-gen, 419
gen/o, 500
-genesis, 419
genit/o, 2347
gest/o, 1406
gestat/o, 2725
gingiv/o, 2084
glauc/o, 1310
gli/o, 1094
glob/o, 1740
globul/o, 1744
glomerul/o, 2315
gloss/o, 2084
glute/o, 979
glyc/o, 522
glycos/o, 2359
gnos/o, 162
goitr/o, 1454
gon/o, 2547
gonad/o, 2865
-gram, 191, 931

-graph, 193
-graphy, 200, 1665
gynec/o, 2607

H

hallucin/o, 1173
hem/o, 101, 1732
hemat/o, 1732
hemi-, 81
hemorrhag, 1788
hepat/o, 2124
herni/o, 2194
heter/o-, 88
hiat/o, 2195
hidr/o, 672
hist/o, 727
home/o-, 88
humer/o, 847
hydr/o, 287, 2386
hymen/o, 2448
hyper-, 121
hypn/o, 260
hypo-, 114
hypophys/o, 1131
hyster/o, 2527

I

-ia, 113
-iasis, 113
-iatrician, 2854
-iatrics, 2854
-iatrist, 1042
-iatry, 1043
-ic, 40, 91
-ical, 91
-ician, 2851
-icle, 493
icter/o, 680
idi/o, 232
-ile, 1847
ile/o, 2114
ili/o, 386
immun/o, 1473
in-, 366
inc/o, 1271
-ine, 1387, 2532
infarct/o, 1626
infer/o, 359
infra-, 359
insul/o, 1415
inter-, 366
intern/o, 366
intestin/o, 2105
intra-, 366

-ion, 98
ionto, 257
ir/o, 1249
irid/o, 1252
-is, 97
ischem/o, 1615
ischi/o, 842
-ism, 113
-ist, 208
-itis, 151
-ity, 98
-ive, 1693

J

jaundic/o, 680, 2211
jejun/o, 2112

K

kerat/o, 1244
kinesi/o, 964
kyph/o, 915

L

labi/o, 2452
lacrim/o, 1258
lact/o, 2772
lactat/o, 2779
lactif/o, 2775
lactifer/o, 2777
lamin/a, 196
lapar/o, 2148
laryng/o, 1317, 2052
later/o, 333
laxativ/o, 2274
lemm/o, 959
leps/o, 145
lept/o, 145
lesion, 106
leth/o, 156
leuk/o, 87
ligament/o, 808
ligat/o, 2636
lingu/o, 2084
lip/o, 447, 767
lith/o, 2214
lob/o, 2071
lord/o, 915
lumb/o, 383
lumin/o, 1511
lump/o, 2906
lun/o, 1567
lymph/o, 1766

lymphat/o, 1767
lys/o, 538, 2429

M

macr/o, 426
macul/o, 699
mal-, 84
malac/o, 147
malle/o, 1271
mamm/o, 2772
mandibul/o, 847
mast/o, 2772
meat/o, 1265, 2422
medi/o, 333
medull/o, 789
megal/o, 137
mei/o, 497
melan/o, 87
mellit/o, 1440
men/o, 2539
mening/o, 1119
mens/o, 2522
menstru/o, 2522
mes-, 1074
meta-, 564
metr/o, 2527
-metry, 225
micr/o, 426
microbi/o, 531
mictur/i, 2304
mimet/o, 1224
mit/o, 497
mitr/o, 1565
molecul/o, 432
mono-, 80
morbid/o, 106
mort, 1027
mortal/i, 156
muc/o, 664
multi-, 80
muscul/o, 954
my/o, 954, 1290
myet/o, 790
myos/o, 954
myring/o, 1267, 1352

N

narc/o, 260
nas/o, 1928, 2246
nat/o, 2742
necr/o, 156
neo-, 82, 561
nephr/o, 1419, 2310
neur/o, 957

Calum Colvin's Ossian · Oisein Chaluim Cholvin

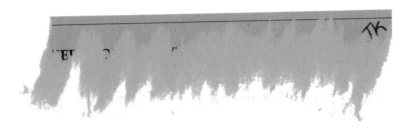

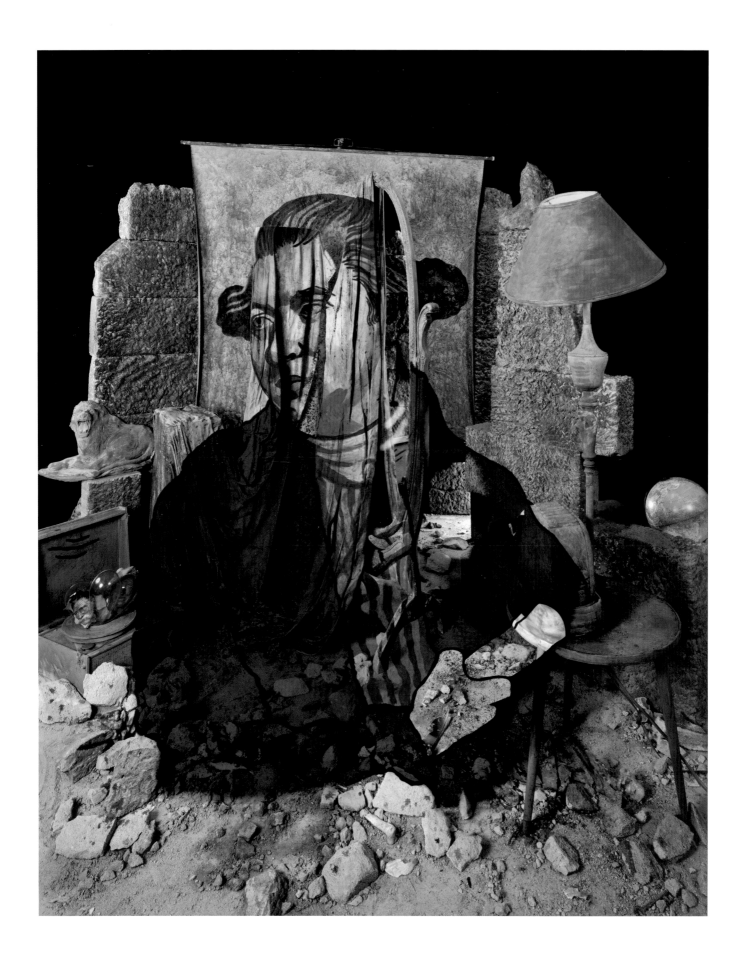

Tom Normand

OSSIAN *Fragments of Ancient Poetry*

Bloighean de Sheann Bhàrdachd OISEIN

Scottish National Portrait Gallery · Edinburgh

Galaraidh Nàiseanta Albannach nan Dealbhan Daoine
Dùn Èideann

Published by the National Galleries of Scotland
to accompany the exhibition *Ossian: Fragments of
Ancient Poetry* held at the Scottish National Portrait
Gallery, Edinburgh from 4 October 2002 to
9 February 2003

Air fhoillseachadh le Galaraidhean Nàiseanta na
h-Alba gu dhol còmhla ris an taisbeanadh *Oisein:
Bloighean de Sheann Bhàrdachd* ann an Galaraidh
Nàiseanta Albannach nan Dealbhan Daoine, Dùn
Èideann, bho 4 Dàmhair 2002 gu 9 Gearran 2003

ISBN 1 903278 35 X

Designed by Dalrymple
Deilbhte le Dalrymple

Typeset by Brian Young
Clò-shuidhichte le Brian Young

Printed by BAS Printers, Over Wallop
Clo-bhuailte le BAS Printers, Over Wallop

Front cover illustration: *Blind Ossian I* [cat. 1]
Dealbh a' chòmhdaich bheòil: *Oisein Dall I* [clàr 1]

Back cover illustration:
Portrait of Robert Burns [cat. 12]
Dealbh a' chòmhdaich cùil:
Dealbh de Raibeart Burns [clàr 12]

Frontispiece: *Portrait of James Macpherson* [cat. 22]
Tùs-dhealbh: *Dealbh de Sheumas MacMhuirich*
[clàr 22]

Chuidich Comhairle nan Leabhraichean am foillsichear
le cosgaisean an leabhair seo.

Foreword

On military campaigns, Napoleon Bonaparte took his copy of the verses of Ossian, the ancient Celtic bard. 'I like Ossian', he said, 'for the same reason that I like to hear the whisper of the wind and the waves of the sea.' These elemental evocations, which seemed to embody the romantic spirit, had been first published by James Macpherson in 1760 with the title *Fragments of Ancient Poetry*. Ossian, whom Voltaire called 'the Scottish Homer', also stood as proof that there was an indigenous culture in Scotland; one that had been eroded, and, by the middle of the eighteenth century, suppressed.

But Macpherson's *Ossian* was as controversial as it was influential. There were ferocious arguments about the authenticity of the verses and the integrity of their 'translator'. It is this theme of authenticity that is at the heart of Calum Colvin's new body of work, whose title, *Ossian: Fragments of Ancient Poetry,* is borrowed from Macpherson. Colvin's themes include the authenticity of history. How is it possible to disentangle what is historical myth from historical fact? How do we know whether what we read is an authentic utterance or a literary forgery? How do we know whether a work of art is genuine or a fake?

Calum Colvin is one of the most ingeniously innovative artists working in Scotland today. His working method is palimpsestical; the final image disguising or camouflaging what lies beneath. The resulting multi-layered 'construction' must then be deconstructed, or fragmented, by the viewer. Looking at a work by Colvin is a bit like going on an archaeological dig – in more senses than one. He seems to anticipate the future reconstructor of the 'fragments'of our modern culture.

It is appropriate that this body of work should have its first showing at the Scottish National Portrait Gallery in Edinburgh, with its core function of identifying and conserving authentic Scottish portraits. It is also singularly apt that it is subsequently to travel extensively throughout the Highlands.

This is the first book published by the National Galleries of Scotland to be printed in English and Gaelic. We are enormously grateful

Roi-Ràdha

Bhiodh Napòleon a' toirt leis a lethbhreac de rannan Oisein, an seann bhàrd Ceilteach, air na h-iomairtean cogaidh aige. "Is toil leam Oisein," ars esan, "air an aon adhbhar gura toil leam cagar na gaoithe agus tonn na mara." Chaidh na guthan eileamaideach seo – an spiorad romansach san fheòil, mar gum bitheadh – fhoillseachadh an toiseach le Seumas Bàn MacMhuirich ann an 1760 air an tiotal *Fragments of Ancient Poetry*. Bha Oisein, air an robh 'Hòmar na h-Alba' aig Voltaire, cuideachd 'na dhearbhadh gun robh cuiltear dùthchasach ann an Alba a bha a' fulang cnàmh agus (mun tàinig meadhoin an ochdamh ceud deug) ainneart.

Ach bha *Oisein* MhicMhuirich cho connspaideach 's a bha e buadhach. Bha argamaidean fiadhaich ann mu dheidhinn ùghdarrasachd nan rannan agus ionracas an 'eadar-theangair'. Tha cuspair na h-ùghdarrasachd aig cridhe an trusaidh ùir obrach aig Calum Colvin, a thug a thiotal, *Oisein: Bloighean de Sheann Bhàrdachd*, air iasad bho MacMhuirich. Am measg nan cuspairean aig Colvin tha ùghdarrasachd na h-eachdraidh. Ciamar a ghabhas uirsgeul eachdraidheil a dhealachadh ri firinn eachdraidheil? Ciamar a tha fios againn an e guth ùghdarrasach no meallsgrìobhadh litreachail a tha sinn a' leughadh? Ciamar a tha fios againn an e rud firinneach no foill a th' ann an obair ealain?

Tha Calum Colvin air aonan den luchd-ealain as innleachdaiche ùr-ghnàths a tha ag obair ann an Alba an-diugh. Tha an dòigh obrach aige pailmseisteach: tha an ìomhaigh a thig ás a' cur na tha shìos foipe fo bhreug-riochd neo fo chòmhdach meallta. Feumaidh an neach-amhairc an uair sin an 'structar' ioma-ìreach a thoirt ás a-chèile no a chur 'na bhloighean. Tha a bhith coimhead air obair Cholvin rud beag coltach ri falbh air cladhach airceòlach – ann am barrachd air aon chiall. Tha an dàrna sùil aige mar gum b' ann ris an duine san linn tha romhainn a bhios ag ath-togail 'bloighean' cuilteir an latha an-diugh.

Tha e ceart gur ann aig Galaraidh Nàiseanta Albannach nan Dealbhan Daoine an Dùn Èideann a gheibh an trusadh obrach seo a chiad shealltainn, oir tha mar bhun-dreuchd aice a bhith ag aithneachadh 's a' glèidheadh dealbhan-daoine ùghdarrasach Albannach. Tha e cuideachd air leth iomchaidh gu bheil e gu bhith a' toirt cuairt mhòr air feadh na Gaidhealtachd as dèidh sin.

Seo a' chiad leabhar a dh'fhoillsich Galaraidhean Nàiseanta na h-Alba a chaidh a chlò-bhualadh an

to the Carnegie Trust for their financial support of this publication.

We would also like to extend sincere thanks to Dr Tom Normand, Senior Lecturer in the School of Art History at the University of St Andrews, for his contribution to this publication; to Cathy Shankland, Exhibitions Officer of Highland Council Cultural and Leisure Services for her support in making the tour of the exhibition possible and to Julie Lawson who curated the exhibition.

TIMOTHY CLIFFORD
Director-General, National Galleries of Scotland

JAMES HOLLOWAY
Director, Scottish National Portrait Gallery

Gàidhlig 's am Beurla. Tha sinn fada an comain Urras Charnegie airson an taic airgid a thug iad seachad.

Bu toil leinn cuideachd taing dhùrachdach a shìneadh gu Dr Tom Normand, Àrd Òraidiche ann an Sgoil Eachdraidh na h-Ealain an Oilthigh Chill Rìmhinn, airson na thug e don leabhar seo; gu Cathy Shankland, Oifigear Thaisbeanaidhean Seirbheisean Cuiltearail agus Saor-Ùine Comhairle na Gaidhealtachd, airson a taic ann a bhith a' toirt cuairt an taisbeanaidh gu bith, agus gu Julie Lawson air a bheil uallach an taisbeanaidh fhèin.

TIMOTHY CLIFFORD
Àrd-Stiùiriche, Galaraidhean Nàiseanta na h-Alba

JAMES HOLLOWAY
Stiùiriche, Galaraidh Nàiseanta Albannach nan Dealbhan Daoine

Acknowledgements

Buidheachas

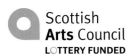

This body of work has been created with invaluable support from a number of organisations. I am particularly grateful to the Scottish Arts Council who granted a Creative Scotland Award, which I received in its inaugural year, 2000. I would also like to acknowledge the assistance given by the Leverhulme Trust (Research Fellowship, 2000–2001); Fujifilm Professional Imaging; the Carnegie Trust for the Universities of Scotland; and Fine Art Research, University of Dundee. Special thanks are due to Ewan Steel for his digital forgery; Altered Images Scotland for printing the artworks; and to Michael Windle for website design.

CALUM COLVIN

Chaidh an trusadh obrach seo a chruthachadh an cois taice luachmhor bho ghrunnan bhuidhnean. Tha mi air leth buidheach do Chomhairle nan Ealan an Alba a dheònaich dhomh Duais Alba Chruthachail, a fhuair mi sa bhliadhna thòiseachaidh aice, 2000. Bu toil leam cuideachd aithne a thoirt don chuideachadh a fhuair mi bho: Urras Leverhulme (Caidreabhachd Rannsachaidh, 2000–2001); Ìomhaigheadh Profeiseanta Fujifilm; Urras Charnegie do dh'Oilthighean na h-Alba; agus bho Rannsachadh nan Àrd Ealan, Oilthigh Dhùn Dè. Bu chòir taing air leth a thoirt do dh'Eòghan Steel airson a chuid mheallsgrìobhaidh mheuraich; do dh'Ìomhaighean Atharraichte Alba airson na h-obraichean ealain a chlò-bhualadh; agus do Mhìcheal Windle airson deilbh làraich-lìn.

CALUM COLVIN

9

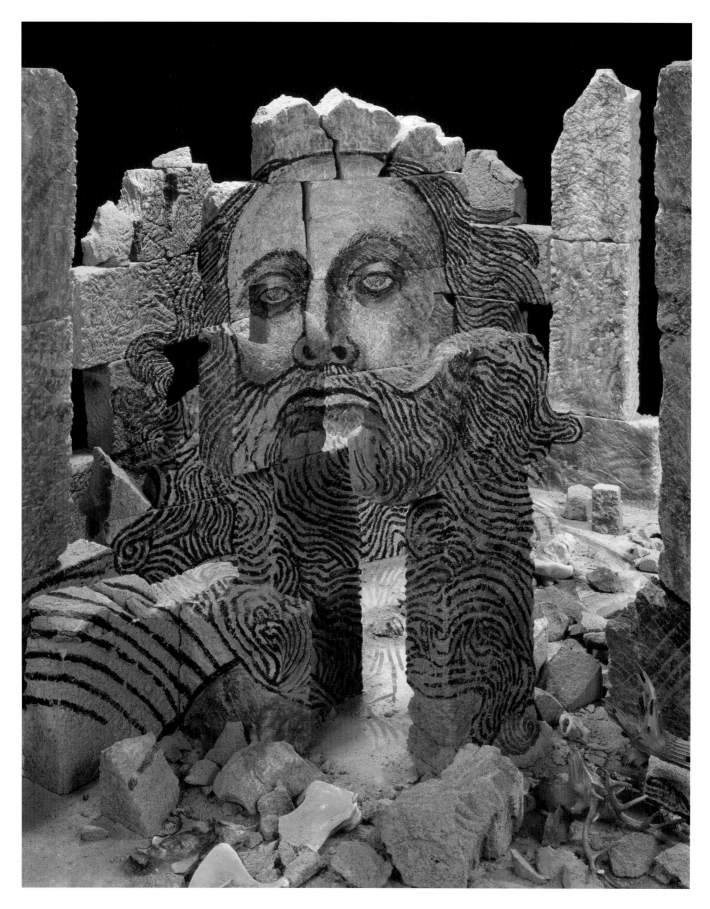

Cat.1 **Blind Ossian I** · Clàr 1 **Oisein Dall I**

Calum Colvin's Ossian

Oisein Chaluim Cholvin

Calum Colvin has prepared a group of large-scale photographs inspired by James Macpherson's eighteenth-century 'translations' of Ossian. These images are created as constructed sets, painted with iconic subjects, decorated with symbolic references, and, finally, photographed. The photographic images are subsequently digitised and presented on canvas. Sculpture, environment, collage, painting, photography, and computer-art combine in a paradoxical and fantastic vision. Here, the conundrum of Macpherson's original venture is appraised and its relevance to contemporary life assessed in the most imaginative of creative projects.

Dheasaich Calum Colvin trusadh de dhealbhan mòra camara a thàinig gu bith bho na smaointean aige mu na 'h-eadar-theangachaidhean' a rinn Seumas Bàn MacMhuirich de bhàrdachd Oisein san ochdamh ceud deug. Tha na h-ìomhaighean seo air an cruthachadh mar structaran togte, air am peantadh le cuspairean suaicheanta, air an sgeadachadh le reifreansan samhlachail agus mu dheireadh air am fotosgrìobhadh. Tha na h-ìomhaighean fotosgrìobhte an uair sin air am meurachadh agus air an cur m'ar coinneamh air canbhas. Tha snaidheadh, àrainneachd, colmadh, peantadh, fotosgrìobhadh agus ealain chompiutair air an cur ri chèile ann an lèirsinn làn paradocs agus òrachd. Tha tòimhseachan na h-iomairt a bh' aig MacMhuirich bho thùs air a mheasadh, agus a buintealas ri saoghal an latha an-diugh air a chnuasachadh, anns a' phròiseact chruthachail seo a tha a' nochdadh brod a' mhic-mheanmna.

I

I

There is an extraordinary parallel between Calum Colvin and James Macpherson that stretches across the two and a half centuries separating their art. Macpherson (1736–1796) was the 'discoverer' of Ossian, the Celtic bard and poet of the third century AD who was hailed throughout Europe and in America as a northern Homer.[1] He was, as it were, one of the first artists to exploit 'the found object', and he is known to have manipulated and transformed these finds in order to construct a unique and fascinating work of art. Likewise, Colvin is recognised as an arch-manipulator; a discoverer of objects, an appropriator of symbols, a shape-shifter who magically transforms both the commonplace and the exceptional into the most intriguing and beguiling images.

Significantly, both Colvin and Macpherson have worked with fragments. Macpherson first published his *Fragments of Ancient Poetry* in 1760.[2] Therein he declared his 'discovery' of ancient Scottish verse, collected during his sojourns in the Highlands and Islands and 'translated' from the original Gaelic and Erse languages. Acclaim for these finds was instant, and the success of Ossian was overwhelming. Encouraged, Macpherson quickly published *Fingal* in 1762

Tha co-choltas iongantach eadar Calum Colvin agus Seumas Bàn MacMhuirich a tha a' sìneadh tarsainn an dà cheud bliadhna gu leth a tha a' sgaradh an cuid ealain. B' e MacMhuirich (1736–1796) am fear a 'lorg' Oisein, am bàrd Ceilteach bhon treas linn AD a chaidh fhàilteachadh air feadh na Roinn Eòrpa 's ann an Ameireaga mar Hòmar bhon cheann a-tuath.[1] Bha MacMhuirich, mar gum bitheadh, air fear dhen chiad luchd-ealain a rinn feum den 'rud a fhuaras', agus tha fios againn gun do làimhsich 's gun do dh'ath-chruthaich e na fhuair e gus obair ealain ghramachail a chur ri chèile a tha buileach gun samhail. Air an aon dòigh, tha Colvin air aithneachadh mar làimhsichear os cionn chàich – lorgair nan rud, creachadair nan samhlaidhean, fear-mùthaidh nan cruth a tha a' cur sgilean draoidheach an sàs gus an dà chuid na tha cumanta agus na tha annasach atharrachadh gu ìomhaighean a bhios gad thàladh 's gad bhuaireadh.

Nì a tha cudromach, tha an dà chuid Colvin agus MacMhuirich a' dèiligeadh ri bloighean. 'S ann sa bhliadhna 1760 a dh'fhoillsich MacMhuirich na *Fragments of Ancient Poetry* aige an toiseach.[2] 'S ann an-siud a chuir e an cèill gun do 'lorg' e seann seann bhàrdachd Albannach a chruinnich e ann an eileanan agus tir-mòr na Gaidhealtachd 's a 'dh'eadar-theangaich' e bho na prìomh-chànanan Gàidhlig agus Gaeilge. Fhuair e moladh ann an làthair nam bonn airson na rinn e, agus shoirbhich le Oisein gu ìre a bha smaoineachail. Leis na thug seo de mhisneach dha ghrad fhoillsich e *Fingal* ann an 1762 agus *Temora* ann an 1763.[3] Nochd na duain-eachdraidh seo

and *Temora* in 1763.[3] These epics conjured a world of heroic northern warriors whose savagery was tempered by distinguished codes of honour, affectionate sentiment, and a recognisable morality.[4] Colvin, for his part, collects fragments of contemporary culture and society weaving them into patterns of elliptical associations that explore the complex character of modern life.

Recognising these parallels, Colvin selected the story of Macpherson's Ossian as a parable of his own creative endeavour in particular, and as an allegory concerning Scottish culture in general. Importantly, the story of Macpherson's Ossian is not the epic tale of the ballads and sagas in themselves. Rather it is an intriguing fable concerning cultural ambition, the problem of 'authenticity' in respect to art, and the slippery nature of a Scottish national 'tradition'.

In the final third of the eighteenth century Ossian came to represent a symbolic re-statement of Scottish cultural, and national, integrity. The idea that there had existed, with Fingal and his comrades, an heroic warrior clan noble and virtuous in its disposition asserted a sense of unique national identity in the face of incorporation into a British state. Equally, the notion that Fingal's son, the blind bard Ossian, had produced epic verse of a Homeric quality carried the implication of a deep-rooted cultural tradition that was the equivalent of the classical world. This vision became a recognised cult throughout northern Europe, and in America. It is well documented that the Ossian epics were deeply influential across the range of the arts.[5] In Scotland, Robert Burns (1759–1796) and Sir Walter Scott (1771–1832) were advocates in support of the poems, while poets as diverse as Blake, Byron, Wordsworth[6] and Yeats showed the influence of the Ossianic verses. On the Continent, Johann Goethe was to use Ossian as a model for his *The Sorrows of Young Werther*, in 1774, and a Germanic adoption of the bard extended to the music of Beethoven, Schubert, and especially Mendelssohn. It is said that Napoleon carried the verses in his knapsack throughout his European campaigns. In consequence, Ossianic subjects were much favoured by French painters, notably Ingres, Gérard and Girodet. French writers, like

saoghal de ghaisgich leòmhanta san àirde tuath a bha am buirbe air a faothachadh le codaichean suaicheanta urraim, le faireachdainnean blàth, agus le moraltachd a ghabhas aithneachadh.[4] A thaobh Cholvin, bidh esan a' cruinneachadh bloighean de chuiltear 's de dhòigh-beatha an linn againn fhìn 's gam fighe 'nam pàtrain de bhuintealasan air fiaradh a tha a' rannsachadh pearsantachd amallach saoghal an latha an-diugh.

'S e ag aithneachadh nan co-choltasan seo, thagh Colvin sgeulachd an 'Oisein' aig MacMhuirich mar chosmhalachd don iomairt chruthachail aige fhèin gu sònraichte, agus mar shamhla do chuiltear na h-Alba san fharsaingeachd. 'S e nì cudromach a th' ann nach e stòiridh 'Oisein' MhicMhuirich an stòiridh a dh'innseas na laoidhean 's na sgeulachdan annta fhèin idir ach fionnsgeul tarraingeach mu mhiann cuiltearach, mu cheist na h-ùghdarrasachd mar a bhuineas i ri ealain, agus mu nàdar sleamhnachail an 'dualchais' nàiseanta Albannaich.

Anns an trian mu dheireadh den ochdamh ceud deug thàinig Oisein gu bhith a' riochdachadh atharrais shamhlachail de dh'ionracas nàiseanta – agus cuiltearach – na h-Alba. Bha an smuain gun robh uaireigin ann, le Fionn 's a chàirdean, fine ghaisgeil de laoich uasal bheusach a' cur faireachdainn mu sgaoil de dh'ionannachd àraid nàiseanta aig an dearbh àm 's a bha Alba ga filleadh ann an stàit Bhreatannach, agus an lùib a' bheachd gun do rinn am bàrd dall Oisein mac Fhinn bàrdachd dhuan-eachdraidheil cho math 's a rinn Hòmar bha an t-amharas gun robh dualchas domhainn-fhreumhaichte ann a ghabhadh coimeas ri saoghal na Grèige 's na Ròimhe. Thàinig an sealladh seo gu bhith 'na sheòrsa de chreideamh air feadh na Roinn Eòrpa fa thuath 's ann an Ameireaga. Agus tha dearbhadh againn ann am pailteas gun robh buaidh a bha mòr agus domhainn aig na duan-eachdraidhean Oiseineach air feadh nan ealan gu lèir.[5] Ann an Alba chuir Raibeart Burns (1759–1796) agus Sir Bhàtar Scott (1771–1832) an cudrom air chùl nan dàn, agus nochd bàird cho diofraichte ri Blake, Byron, Wordsworth[6] agus Yeats buaidh nan rann Oiseineach. Air tìr-mòr na Roinn Eòrpa bha Johann Goethe a' cleachdadh Oisein mar mholltair do *Na Bròin aig Werther Òg* ann an 1774, agus lean uchd-mhacachd Ghearmailteach a' bhàird cho fada ris a' cheòl aig Beethoven, aig Schubert 's gu h-àraidh aig Mendelssohn. Thathar ag ràdh gum biodh na rannan ann an aparsaig Napòleon air feadh nan cogaidhean Eòrpach aige. Mar thoradh, bha spèis nach bu bheag aig peantairean Frangach – leithid Ingres, Gérard agus Girodet – do chuspairean Oiseineach. Bha sgrìobhaichean Frangach cleas Diderot, Madame de Staël agus Chateaubriand cuideachd fo smachd nan dàn. Rinneadh mòran mar an ceudna de bhuaidh Oisein ann an

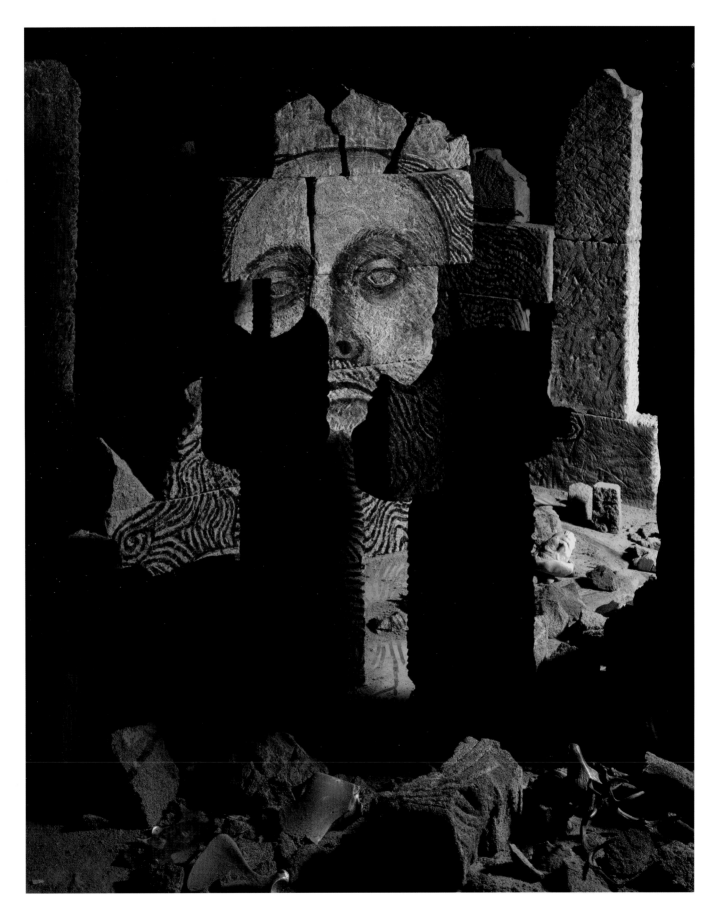

Cat.2 **Blind Ossian II** · Clàr 2 **Oisein Dall II**

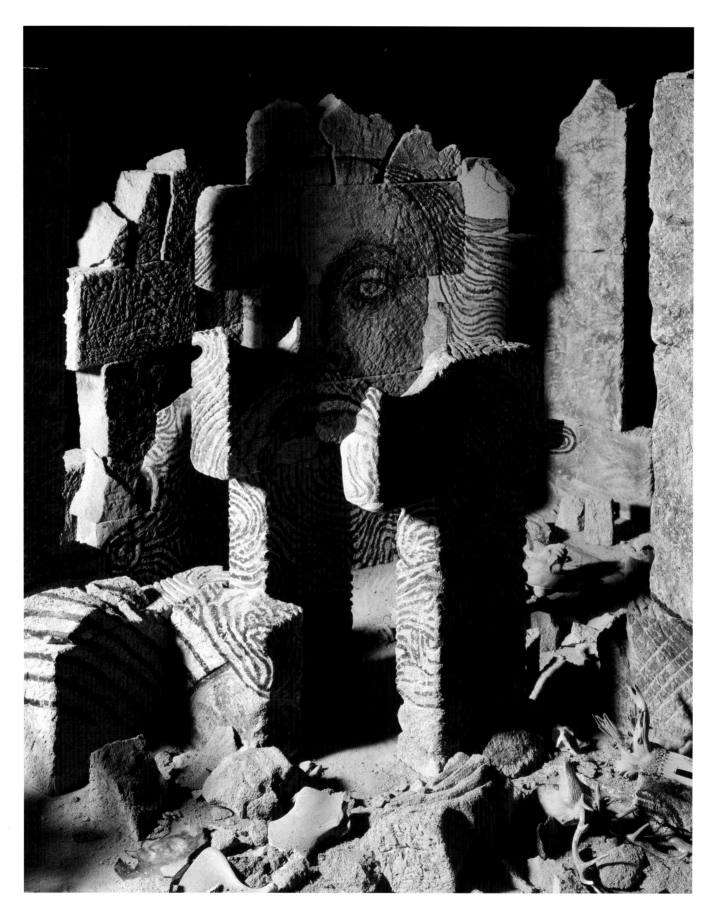

Cat.3 **Blind Ossian III** · Clàr 3 **Oisein Dall III**

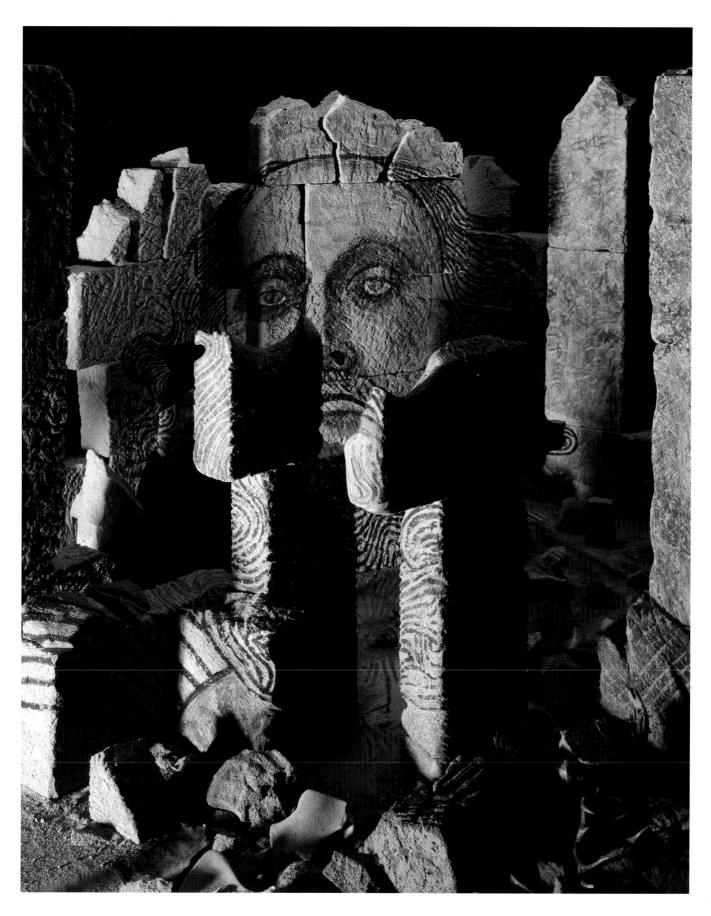

Cat.4 **Blind Ossian IV** · Clàr 4 **Oisein Dall IV**

Diderot, Madame de Staël and Chateaubriand were also in thrall to the poems. Meanwhile much has been made of the influence of Ossian in America, where James Fenimore Cooper, as well as Longfellow, were considered heirs to the language and temper of Macpherson's poems.

In truth, Ossian became a universal archetype just at the moment when Neoclassicism was suffused into Romanticism, and Ossian and his subjects bear all the characteristics of the romantic hero. But the cultural significance of the poems grew at the same time as the veracity of the 'translations' was challenged. The first, and most potent of challenges, came from that giant of late eighteenth-century letters, Samuel Johnson (1709–1784).[7] It was Johnson who, in 1775, first suggested that the poems were fraudulent and consisted wholly of manufactured verse in the 'style' of the classical epic. This challenge was inspired not so much by *Fragments of Ancient Poetry*, but by *Fingal* and *Temora*. These later works, Macpherson had suggested, were complete poems 'discovered' in the Highlands of Scotland and directly 'translated' from the Gaelic. While Johnson might accept that *Fragments of Ancient Poetry* was garnered from selections of written verse and oral renditions available in Highland culture, he refused to believe that complete epics existed in documented form. The belligerence of his attack, however, inspired Macpherson to challenge Johnson to a duel. Wisely, Macpherson made this challenge to an aged Johnson, crippled since birth, chronically infirm, deaf in one ear and blind in one eye. Not unnaturally, Johnson demurred and history was saved a piece of theatre – tragedy or farce – that would have spun a very different tale of Ossian.[8] Nevertheless, Macpherson's reluctance, or inability, to produce the original manuscripts increased the level of suspicion amongst the literati.

Given these conditions, Johnson was not alone in his reservations concerning the authenticity of Macpherson's 'translations', though voices were raised on both sides of the argument. Such was the controversy that, in the years after Macpherson's death in 1796, The Highland Society in Edinburgh commissioned a *Report on Ossian*, designed to test the veracity of Ossian's Gaelic sources. Its conclusions, that

Ameireaga, far an robh James Fenimore Cooper agus Longfellow air am meas 'nan oighrean do chànan agus nàdar nan dàintean aig MacMhuirich.

Gu firinneach, chaidh Oisein 'na phrìomh shamhla uile-choitcheann aig an dearbh ìre 's gun robh Romansachd ag èirigh á Nuachlasaigeachd – air Oisein 's a chuid chuspairean tha gach comharradh a' ghaisgich romansaich. Ach bha brìgh chuiltearach nan dàn a' fàs aig an aon àm 's a bha firinneachd nan 'eadar-theangachaidhean' ga cur gu dùbhlan. Thàinig a' chiad dhùbhlan 's am fear a bu chudromaiche bho chìrean cròin ud nan litreachan sa chuid mu dheireadh den ochdamh ceud deug, Somhairle MacIain (1709–1784).[7] B' e MacIain a' chiad duine a thug seachad am beachd, ann an 1775, gur ann breugach a bha na dàintean 's nach robh annta ach rannaigheachd a chaidh a chur ri chèile ann an 'stoidhle' an duain-eachdraidh chlasaigich. Chan e *Fragments of Ancient Poetry* bu choireach ris an dùbhlan seo uiread ri *Fingal* agus *Temora*. Bha MacMhuirich air a chur air adhart gun robh an dà obair a b' anmoiche seo 'nan dàintean iomlan a 'lorg' e ann an Gaidhealtachd na h-Alba agus a 'dh'eadar-theangaich' e dìreach bhon Ghàidhlig. Theagamh gun robh MacIain deònach aideachadh gun deachaidh *Fragments of Ancient Poetry* a chruinneachadh bho thaghaidhean de bhàrdachd sgrìobhte 's de bheul-aithris a bha ri fhaotainn ann an Gàidhlig, ach dhiùlt e a chreidsinn gun robh làn duain-eachdraidh ri fhaotainn ann an riochd air an robh barantas pàipeir. Bha an ionnsaigh a thug e air MacMhuirich cho borb ge-tà 's gun do dh'iarr MacMhuirich 'riarachadh na còmhraig dhithist' air. Bha de ghliocas aig MacMhuirich 's gun tug e an dùbhlan seo do bhodach aost' a bha crùbach bho rugadh e, a bha ann an galar air choreigin daonnan, a bha bodhar san dàrna cluais 's a bha cam. Mar a bha nàdarra gu leòr cha do ghabh MacIain ris an dùbhlan agus chaill an eachdraidh a cothrom air bìdeag dràma bhith aice, èibhinn neo dubhach 's gum bitheadh e, a dh'innseadh sgeulachd Oiseineach tur eadar-dhealaichte.[8] Air a shon sin, rud a mheudaich amharas an luchd litreachais b' e nach robh MacMhuirich deònach, neo comasach, na làmh-sgrìobhainnean tùsail a nochdadh.

Anns an t-suidheachadh seo cha robh MacIain leis fhèin 'na mhì-chinnt a thaobh ùghdarrasachd nan 'eadar-theangachaidhean' aig MacMhuirich, ged a bha guthan gan togail air dà thaobh na h-argamaid. Chaidh a' chonnspaid gu ìre, sna bliadhnachan an dèidh bàs MhicMhuirich ann an 1796, 's gun do dh'òrdaich Comann na Gaidhealtachd an Dùn Èideann *Report on Ossian* a bha air a dheilbh gu fìrinneachd nan tobraichean aig MacMhuirich a chur gu deuchainn. Cha do rinn na co-dhùnaidhean aige – gur e bàrdachd Ghàidhlig a bh' ann an Dàin 'Oisein', ach anns an

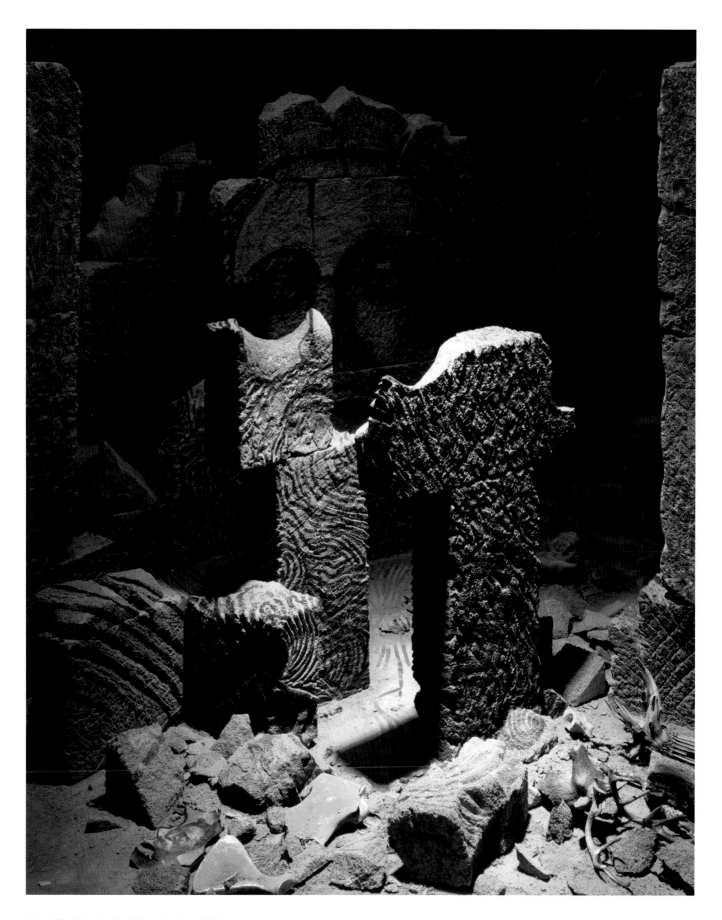

Cat.5 **Blind Ossian V** · Clàr 5 **Oisein Dall V**

Ossian was Gaelic verse, but only in the loosest and most cryptic sense of the term, did little to enhance Macpherson's reputation. This growing uncertainty concerning the credibility of Macpherson's claims was increased in 1805 when Malcolm Laing (1762–1818) published *The Poems of Ossian*, an annotated edition of the poems that highlighted the spectacular parallels with classical literature, Shakespeare, Milton, and the Bible. Indeed, the controversy spills over into contemporary times for Hugh Trevor-Roper has proclaimed that Macpherson 'created an indigenous literature for Celtic Scotland and, as a necessary support to it, a new history. Both this literature and this history, in so far as they had any connection with reality, had been stolen from the Irish.'[9] The view persists, then, that the epic of Ossian was a fraud; a constructed translation, without any meaningful source in Gaelic culture, and consequently a wholly manufactured history and poetry.

A body of modern scholarship, however, has sought to rehabilitate Macpherson, or, at least, come to a fuller understanding of the nature of his ambitious project. As early as 1952, the Gaelic scholar, Derick S. Thomson, published *The Gaelic Sources of Macpherson's 'Ossian'* and identified many of the key texts and fragments upon which the epic was founded. Later, Fiona Stafford's *The Sublime Savage: A Study of James Macpherson and the Poems of Ossian*, published in 1988, recovered the author from the pit of disdain and offered an important re-evaluation of the poems. More recently, Howard Gaskill's edited collection *Ossian Revisited*, published in 1991, has advanced scholarly study to new levels of sophistication and critical appraisal.

To some degree this reassessment must be set against the backdrop of the revival in national consciousness and of the political debate concerning Scottish devolution and independence. Macpherson, and the drama of Ossian's reception, highlights a host of issues moulded into the culture of nationhood. In fact, the defence of Macpherson has focused attention on the history of Scotland in respect of its association with its southern neighbour. Robert Crawford has noted how 'the Ossianic fragments are part of the aftermath of Culloden'.[10] More colourfully, William

t-seagh as laige 's as dìomhaire aig na faclan – a bheag gu cliù MhicMhuirich àrdachadh. Chaidh an teagamh seo mun ìre chun an gabhadh tagraidhean MhicMhuirich a chreidsinn – teagamh a bha a' sìor èirigh – a mheudachadh ann an 1805 an uair a dh'fhoillsich Maol-Chaluim Laing (1762–1818) *The Poems of Ossian*, anns an tug e seachad na dàintean còmhla ri notaichean a shoillsich gun robh iad iongantach coltach ann an àiteachan ri litreachas na Grèige 's na Ròimhe, ri Shakespeare, ri Milton 's ris a' Bhìoball. Gu dearbh, tha a' chonnspaid a' cur thairis don linn againn fhìn, oir tha Ùistean Trevor-Roper air a chur an cèill gun do 'chruthaich MacMhuirich litreachas dùthchasach do dh'Alba nan Ceilteach agus, mar thaice riatanach ris a-sin, eachdraidh ùr. Bha an litreachas agus an eachdraidh seo, chun na h-ìre 's gun robh ceangal sam bith aca ris an fhìrinn, air an goid bho na h-Èireannaich.'[9] Tha a' bharail ann fhathast, ma-thà, nach robh ann an duan-eachdraidh Oisein ach foill: eadar-theangachadh togte, gun fhìor thobar sam bith ann an dualchas na Gàidhlig, agus mar sin 'na eachdraidh agus 'na bhàrdachd a chaidh a chur ri chèile a dh'aona ghnothach.

Rinn meall de sgoilearachd an latha againn fhìn, ge-tà, oidhirp air cliù MhicMhuirich aiseag thuige, no co-dhiù oidhirp air tighinn gu tuigse nas iomlaine air nàdar a' phròiseict mhòir aige. Cho tràth ri 1952 dh'fhoillsich an sgoilear Gàidhlig Ruaraidh MacThòmais *The Gaelic Sources of Macpherson's 'Ossian'* agus chuir e a chorrag air mòran de na prìomh theacsachan 's bhloighean air an deach an duan-eachdraidh a stèidheachadh. Nas anmoiche, tharraing *The Sublime Savage: A Study of James Macpherson and the Poems of Ossian*, a dh'fhoillsicheadh ann an 1988, MacMhuirich a-mach á sloc an dìmeas agus thug e ath-luachadh cudromach air na dàintean. A-rithist, bhrùth *Ossian Revisited*, an co-chruinneachadh deasaichte aig Howard Gaskill a dh'fhoillsicheadh ann an 1991, sgoilearachd a' chuspair a-mach gu crìochan ùra de shùbailteachd 's de luachadh sgrùdach.

Gu ìre, bu chòir an t-ath-luachadh seo a chur fa chomhair ath-bheothachadh an fhèin-aithneachaidh nàiseanta agus fa chomhair na deasbaid phoileataigich mu dheidhinn fèin-riaghladh agus neo-eisimeileachd na h-Alba. Tha MacMhuirich – agus dràma na fàilte a thugadh do dh'*Oisein* – a' cur solas air meall cheistean a tha 'nam pàirt de chuiltear na nàiseantachd. Gu dearbh, tharraing an dìon a fhuair MacMhuirich aire dhaoine gu eachdraidh na h-Alba 's a cuid cheanglaichean ri a nàbaidh mu dheas. Thug Raibeart Crawford fa-near mar tha 'na bloighean Oiseineach 'nam pàirt de na lean Cùil Lodair'.[10] 'S e a' cleachdadh barrachd dhathan, tha Uilleam MacFhearghais a' cumail a-mach gun robh 'an t-uabhas bròin agus mì-chinnt an lùib briseadh an t-seann t-saoghail

Ferguson argues that 'with the break-up of the old Highland society there was much misery and uncertainty, and something of the period's melancholic sense of decline and fall pervaded Macpherson's thoughts'.[11] In essence, it is suggested that Macpherson's revival of a heroic Highland tradition was a response to the incorporation of Scotland into Great Britain, and the tragic history of the Highland clans in the period after the Jacobite rebellions. Ossian, then, was a salve created to heal the wounds of defeat, displacement, disillusion and decay. More than this, it reasserted national identity in a period of rapid change, and established a sense of a virtuous and vigorous tradition at the point when custom and culture were in turmoil.

It is at this point that the parallels between Macpherson and Colvin become evident. Macpherson, it now seems clear, gathered together some fragments of Highland and Irish verse and utilised these as the basis of his Ossianic ballads. He was a 'translator' of these tales in the specifically eighteenth-century sense that he firstly borrowed, then adapted, amended and embroidered the sparse originals. He did this as a Romantic poet responding to the social, political and cultural upheaval that had traumatised Scotland. He was in every sense – as a writer, poet and adventurer – completely in thrall to his age. Colvin, in a similar way, has come to explore the cultural ambiguity, intellectual ambivalence, and moral relativism of the modern world. His images, 'translated' from everyday items, synthesised from high and low art, glossed with the icons of the Scottish cultural tradition, are a fantastic kaleidoscopic mirror of contemporary life.

II

In Scotland, and beyond, the 'Celtomania' that flowed from Macpherson's Ossian was expressed in every variety of art. In the visual arts, alongside its pervasiveness in France, Germany, and Scandinavia, there existed a strong Ossianic influence in the work of several eminent Scottish painters. The most significant of these was Alexander Runciman (1736–1785). Runciman had initially trained as a decorative artist in Edinburgh, but travelled to Rome in

Ghaidhealaich', agus gun robh 'an snighe tùrsach sin a bhuineadh ri linn a' ghrodaidh 's a' chnàimh' a' drùdhadh air smaointean MhicMhuirich.[11] Gu bunaiteach, thathar a' cur an cèill gun robh an aiseirigh a thug MacMhuirich air dualchas gaisgeach Gaidhealach 'na freagairt ri filleadh na h-Alba ann am 'Breatainn Mhòr', agus cuideachd 'na freagairt ri eachdraidh dhubh nan Gaidheal anns an linn a lean na h-iomairtean Seumasach. Bha *Oisein*, ma-tà, 'na ìocshlaint a chaidh ullachadh gu leigheas a thoirt air na creuchdan a chaidh fhosgladh le ruaig, le fuadachd, le mealladh dùil 's le cnàmh. A thuilleadh air seo, chuir e fèin-aithneachadh nàiseanta an cèill as ùr ri linn 's gun robh nithean ag atharrachadh gu luath, agus stèidhich e eòlas air dualchas a bha beusach agus beòthail aig àm a bha gnàthachadh agus cuiltear air a dhol tro chèile.

Is ann aig an ìre seo a tha na coimeasan eadar MacMhuirich agus Colvin a' tighinn am follais. Tha e coltach gu bheil e soilleir a-nis gun do chruinnich MacMhuirich bloighean de bhàrdachd 's de dhàintean Gàidhlig 's gun do dh'ùisnich e iad seo mar bhonn-stèidh nan laoidhean Oiseineach aige. Rinn e 'eadar-theangachadh' air na sgeulachdan seo ann an seagh a bhuineas ris an ochdamh ceud deug a-mhàin – an toiseach thruis e tùsan a bha car gann, agus an uair sin rinn e an atharrachadh, an càradh 's an sgeadachadh. Rinn e seo mar bhàrd Romansach a bha a' freagairt ris an aimhreit shòisealta, phoileataigich agus chuiltearaich a bha air Alba a shlaiseadh. Bha e anns gach seagh – mar sgrìobhaiche, mar bhàrd, mar fhear-dàna – buileach fo smachd an linn anns an robh e beò. Air dòigh gu math coltach theann Colvin ri sgrùdadh a thoirt air dà-sheaghachd chuiltearach, mì-chinnt inntinne agus dàimhealachas moralta an latha againn fhìn. 'Eadar-theangaichte' mar a tha iad bho rudan a chì sinn uile-thimcheall oirnn, 's iad air an co-chur bho ealain àrd agus ìosal 's air am mìneachadh le suaicheantais dualchas cuiltearach na h-Alba, tha a chuid ìomhaighean 'nan sgàthan iongantach sìor-atharrachail air saoghal an latha an-diugh.

II

Ann an Alba 's thall thairis bha an Ceilteachas faoin a shruth bho *Oisein* MhicMhuirich air a chur an cèill ann an ealain de gach seòrsa. Sna h-ealain lèirsinneach, a thuilleadh air cho drùidhteach 's a bha i anns an Fhraing, anns a' Ghearmailt 's ann an Lochlainn bha buaidh làidir Oiseineach anns an obair aig grunnan pheantairean cliùiteach Albannach. B' e am fear a bu chudromaiche dhiubh seo Alastair Runciman (1736–1785). Fhuair Runciman oileanachadh bho thùs mar ealainiche sgeadachaidh ann an Dùn Èideann, ach ann an 1767 chaidh

1767 where he garnered the lessons of neoclassical and Italian art. On returning to Scotland in 1772, he was commissioned to paint decorative murals at Penicuik House. He chose the then fashionable theme of Ossian. Though these murals were destroyed in a fire of 1899, some drawings and etchings remain, among them images of *Ossian Singing*, *Fingal and Coban-cargla*, and *The Death of Oscar*. Accompanying these is one of the most prized etchings of the blind bard Ossian, pictured dreaming on the deeds of his kinsfolk.[12] This etching, by Runciman, was used as the frontispiece for The Highland Society of London's *Poems of Ossian* published in 1807, but it is also the spectre that inhabits the desolate and ruined landscape of Calum Colvin's *Blind Ossian* cycle (fig.1).

This central group of nine images, titled *Blind Ossian* (cats.1–9), sits at the heart of Colvin's recent work and is remarkable for the depth of its melancholy. Remarkable, for Colvin is often viewed as an artist who embraces the comic. Indeed, his images have often been joyous, endlessly decorated with kitsch symbolism, and replete with ribald humour. But these are surface attributes. In fact, there has consistently been a dark core to Colvin's photography. It has, almost unfailingly, described landscapes in decay, a world littered with ambiguity, and a humanity sated by doubt and uncertainty. The Ossian images are, perhaps, the starkest testimony of this vision.

Formally, the nine photographs of the *Blind Ossian* cycle mark a significant development in the artist's oeuvre. While depicting an architecture in ruins – the broken and fragmented temple of the Romantic landscape – they are pre-eminently concerned with light. Each image is shaped, and redefined, by the lighting. In some, darkness pervades and details within the ruins are obscured and lost; in others, the light opens out hidden areas, flooding a detail and focusing on a minute incident. In others again the light is filtered, becoming a darkened blue or an umber. These subtle tonal gradations enhance the mood of despondency that creeps through these spaces. Overall, there is a sense that the ruined landscape has a temporal or historical presence. Each shift in lighting unveils a different moment in time and reveals the gradual, insidious, disintegration of the

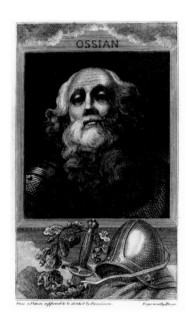

Fig.1 · Alexander Runciman, frontispiece from *The Poems of Ossian*, 1807
The Trustees of the National Museums of Scotland

Fig.1 · Alastair Runciman, tùs-dhealbh bho *The Poems of Ossian*, 1807
Urrasairean Taighean-Tasgaidh Nàiseanta na h-Alba

e don Ròimh far an do thruis e leasanan na h-ealain nuachlasaigich 's Eadailtich. Nuair a thill e a dh'Alba ann an 1772 chaidh a chomiseanadh gu dealbhan balla a pheantadh ann an Taigh Phenicuik. Mar chuspair thagh e Oisein a bha cho fasanta aig an àm. Ged a chaidh na dealbhan balla seo a sgrios ann an teine ann an 1899, tha corra sgeidse 's shnaidheadh ann fhathast; 'nam measg tha ìomhaighean *Oisein a' Seinn*, *Fionn agus Coban-Cargla* agus *Bàs Osgair*. Còmhla riutha seo tha fear de na snaidhidhean as motha prìs a th' againn an-diugh de dh'Oisein am bàrd dall, 's e air a shealltainn a' bruadar air gnìomhan a luchd-dàimh.[12] Chaidh an snaidheadh seo a chleachdadh mar thùs-dhealbh *Poems of Ossian* a dh'fhoillsich Comann Gaidhealtachd Lunnainn ann an 1807, ach tha e cuideachd air a dhol 'na thaibhse tha tathaich dùthaich nan tobhtaichean fàs a gheibhear sa chuairt *Oisein Dall* aig Calum Colvin (fig.1).

Tha an sreath bunaiteach seo de naoi ìomhaighean (clàir 1–9) aig cridhe na rinn Colvin bho chionn ghoirid. Tha e iongantach airson doimhneachd a bhròin, oir tha Colvin ga fhaicinn tric mar ealainiche a bhios a' cleachdadh feala-dhà. Gu dearbh, is tric a bha na h-ìomhaighean aige sunndach, air an sgeadachadh fad an t-siubhail le samhlachas gach cruth-ealain as suaraiche 's a' cur thairis le àbhachdas abaich. Ach tha na feartan seo air an uachdar a-mhàin, oir bha cridhe dubh riamh aig fotosgrìobhadh Cholvin. Thug e cunntas gu math cunbhalach air dùthchannan fàs, air saoghal truaillte le dà-sheaghachd, air clann-daoine làn teagaimh agus mì-chinnt. Dh'fhaoidte gur iad na h-ìomhaighean Oiseineach an teisteanas as duirche don t-sealladh seo.

Gu foirmeil, tha na naoi dealbhan camara sa chuairt *Oisein Dall* a' nochdadh leasachadh cudromach ann an obair an ealainiche. Ged a tha iad a' sealltainn ailtireachd air a sgrios – sprùilleach an teampaill bhriste ann an dùthaich Romansach – 's e am fìor chuspair an solas. Tha an solasachadh a' deilbh gach ìomhaigh 's an uair sin ga h-ath-tarraing. Ann an cuid dhiubh tha an dorchadas drùidhteach agus tha rudan beaga am broinn nan tobhtaichean ann an duathar no air an call; ann an cuid eile tha an solas a' fosgladh a-mach bheàrnan falaichte, a' bogadh rud meanbh air choreigin 's a' cur tachartas beag beag fo sgrùdadh; ann an cuid eile a-rithist tha an solas air a chriathradh 'na dhubhghorm no 'na dhubhdhonn. Tha na h-atharraichean sùbailte dath tha seo a' daingneachadh an dubh-bhròin a tha ag èaladh tro na beàrnan. Uile gu lèir thathar a' faireachdainn gu bheil làthaireachd thimeil no eachdraidheil aig an dùthaich sgriosta. Tha gach diofar sholas a' nochdadh uair eile ann an tìm agus a' leigeil fhaicinn mar a tha an sealladh ga shìor shlaodadh ás a-chèile. Tha sgleò de bhagarrachd 's de dh'iargaltas air

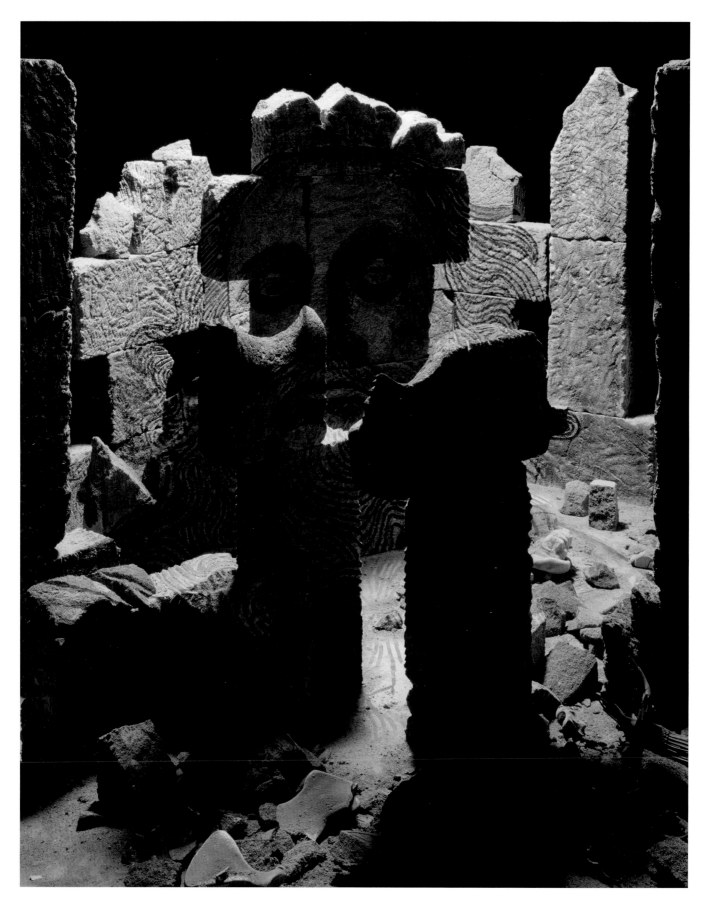

Cat.6 **Blind Ossian VI** · Clàr 6 **Oisein Dall VI**

scene. There is, throughout, a sinister and menacing feel to these images, a sense of inevitable decay and melancholic regret.

Closer examination releases those spectral presences that help mark the tragic sentiment at the heart of these photographs. In each, the ghost of Runciman's etching of Ossian is present. In more than half of the nine works, the head of the blind bard is clearly seen: a totemic, omniscient figure brooding in the ruined landscape. The flowing hair and beard of the bard falls into a pattern of loops and curls. This pattern becomes mapped on the broken stone of the temple architecture, a fractured tracery recalling the interlace of Celtic design. In the debris a few iconic images are just visible. At the bottom left of these photographs there sits the partly scorched image of an aboriginal head, a tattooed Maori (fig.2). The rhythmical facial tattoos mirror the Celtic tracery in Ossian. More subtly, this juxtaposition recalls that fatal conceit in Macpherson's creation myth of the Scottish people, the suggestion that the Scots were not an Irish tribe, but a native and indigenous Celtic people who colonised Ireland.[13] Colvin introduces the Maori, in part, as an ironic leitmotif representing the fallibility of history and the problem, even the absurdity, of those narratives that search for essences, particularly racial essences.

At the right side, of each of the nine images in the cycle, there is a more straightforward symbolism. Amongst the broken stones there sits the head and antlers of a porcelain stag. The stag appears as an emblem that references the Clearances of the Highlands in the period after the Jacobite rebellions.[14] Following the defeat of the Stuarts, the clan system began to disintegrate and the Highlands were gradually 'cleared' of its native populace and given over to more profitable sheep and deer. The extraordinary savagery and brutality of the Clearances, resulting ultimately in Highland depopulation and emigration to the New World, remains an open wound in the history of the Highlands to this day. Indeed, in some degree it was these very processes that Macpherson was responding to in Ossian. Hence the decapitated stag is omnipresent in this series as a memory of these events, a counterpoint perhaps to Edwin

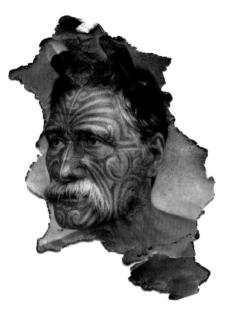

Fig.2 · Maori Head · Ceann Maori

feadh nan ìomhaighean seo air fad 's iad a' toirt thugainn smaointean air crìonadh do-sheachanta 's air aithreachas truagh.

Tha sgrùdadh nas dlùithe a' fuasgladh nan làthaireachdan taibhseach a tha a' cuideachadh gus aithne a thoirt don àmhghar a tha aig cridhe nan dealbhan camara seo. Tha taibhse an t-snaidhidh a rinn Runciman de dh'Oisein an làthair anns gach gin. Ann an còrr agus leth de na naoi obraichean chithear ceann a' bhàird dhoill gu soilleir: pearsa samhlachail uilfhiosrach 'na smaointean trom san dùthaich sgriosta. Tha fhalt fada 's fheusag shruthach a' dol 'nam pàtran camalùbach casurlach. Tha am pàtran seo a' dol an uair sin 'na mhap' air clach bhriste ailtireachd an teampaill – dealbhachd phronn a tha a' toirt gu cuimhne eadar-shnaoimean na h-ealain Cheiltich. Am measg an sprùillich tha grunnan ìomhaighean suaicheanta ri fhaicinn, ged as ann air èiginn. Air taobh ìochdrach clì nam fotosgrìobhaidhean seo chithear ìomhaigh phàirt-dhòite de cheann tùsanach, Maori tatuaichte (fig.2). Tha na tatuaichean ruitheamach air 'aodann 'nan sgàthan air an dealbhachd Cheiltich ann an Oisein. Nas sùbailte, tha an còmhghar seo a' toirt gu cuimhne an car mì-shealbhach sin ann an uirsgeul-cruthachaidh MhicMhuirich mu shluagh na h-Alba, an nòisean nach e treubh Èireannach a bh' anns na Sgotaich idir ach sluagh dualchasach dùthchasach Ceilteach a chaidh a dh'fhuireach a dh'Èirinn.[13] Tha Colvin a' toirt thugainn a' Mhaori, gu ìre, mar *leitmotif* ìoranach a tha a' sealltainn mar dh'fhaodas eachdraidh a bhith fàillingeach agus duilgheadas, seadh amaideas, nan aithrisean sin a bhios an tòir air brìghean, gu sònraichte brìghean cinne.

Air taobh deas gach ìomhaigh sa chuairt tha samhlachas nas sìmplidhe. Am measg nan clachan briste tha an ceann cabrach aig damh porsalain. Tha an damh mar shuaicheantas a' toirt tarraing air Fuadachd nan Gaidheal sna bliadhnachan a lean Cùil Lodair.[14] Chaill na Stiùbhartaich am blàr, thòisich saoghal nan Gaidheal a' crìonadh, agus beag air bheag chaidh na Gaidhil fhògradh 's am fearann a thoirt do chaoraich 's do dh'fhèidh a dhèanadh tuilleadh airgid. Tha buirbe 's brùidealachd iongantach nam Fuadaichean, a chrìochnaich sa cheann thall ann am fàsachadh na Gaidhealtachd 's ann an eilthireachd an t-sluaigh don t-Saoghal Ùr, 'nan creuchd fhosgailt' ann an eachdraidh na Gaidhealtachd gus an latha an-diugh. Gu dearbh, 's ann ris na h-atharraichean seo gu ìre a bha MacMhuirich a' freagairt ann an *Oisein*. Mar sin tha an damh dìcheannach an làthair air feadh an t-sreath mar chuimhne air na tachartasan, 'na chontrapuing 's dòcha ris a' pheantadh bhuadhach shuaicheanta aig Edwin Landseer, *The Monarch of the Glen*.

Air a shon seo, tha àileadh *Oisein Dall* nas doimhne 's

22

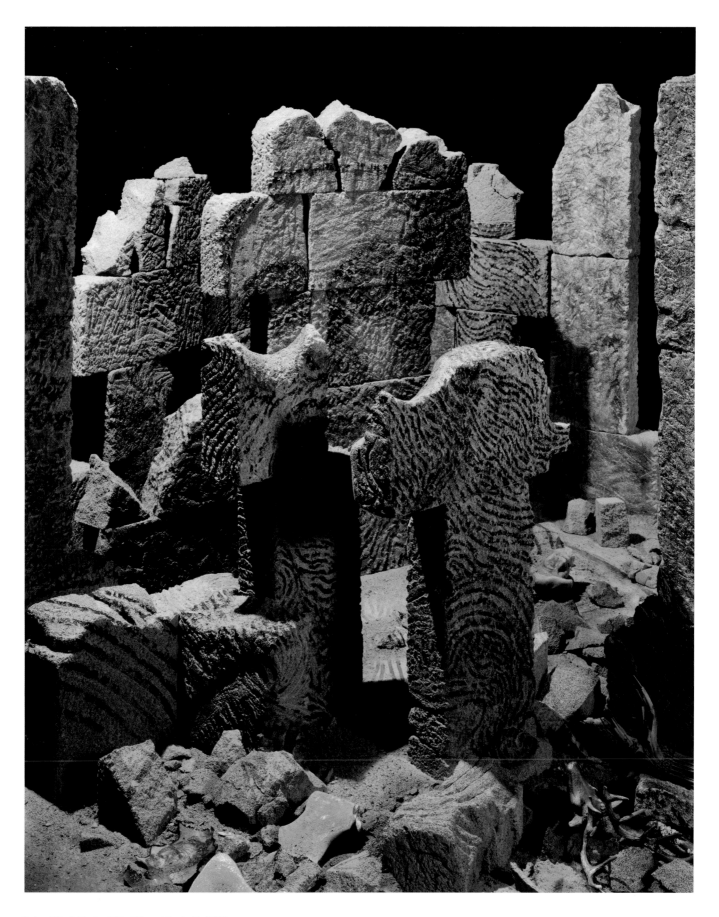

Cat.7 **Blind Ossian VII** · Clàr 7 **Oisein Dall VII**

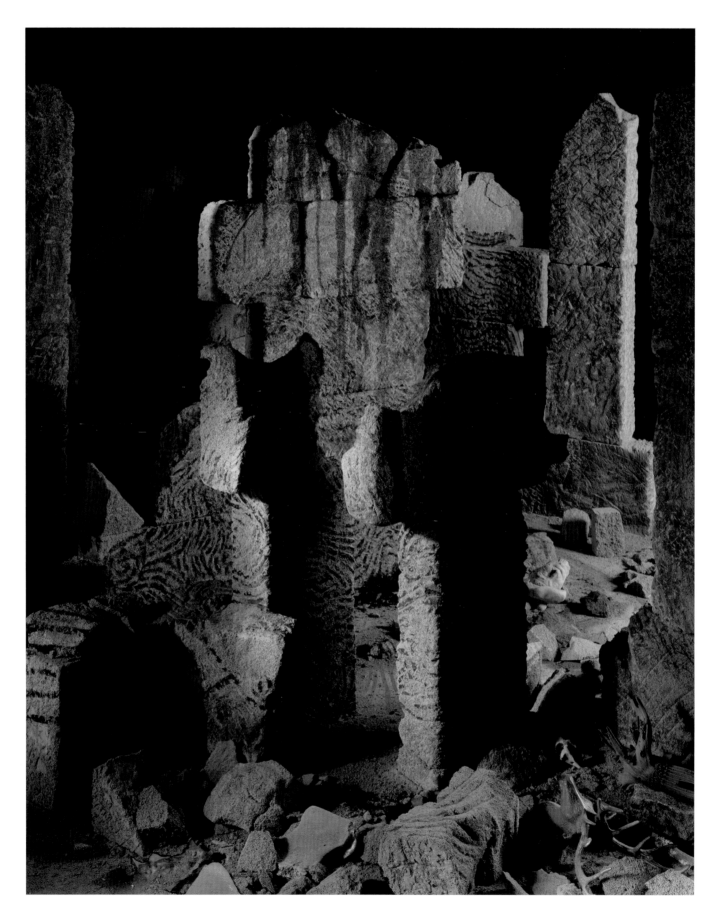

Cat.8 **Blind Ossian VIII** · Clàr 8 **Oisein Dall VIII**

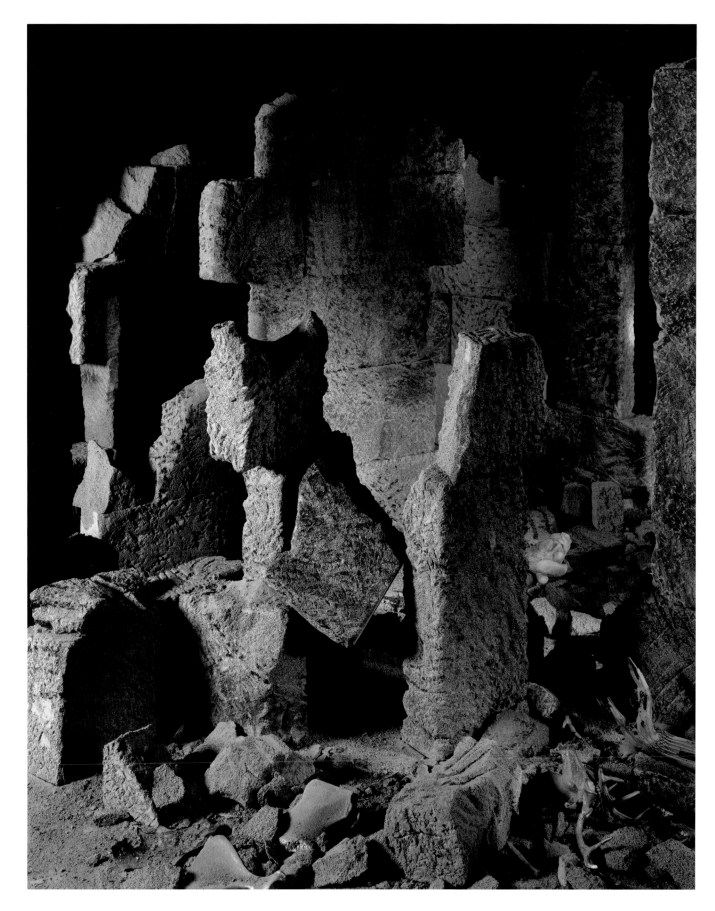

Cat.9 **Blind Ossian IX** · Clàr 9 **Oisein Dall IX**

Landseer's triumphant and iconic painting, *The Monarch of the Glen.*

For all this, the atmosphere of the *Blind Ossian* series is deeper and darker than the sum of its parts. Throughout it there is a measured disintegration. By the ninth and final image, reference to Ossian has faded, the 'Maori' doppelgänger has been seared, and the ruined landscape has reached a final collapse. Colvin's tragic world has become a nightmare landscape, an apocalyptic vision of destruction and devastation. Here again the references are layered. At some level, Colvin is reflecting on the sense of loss and regret that exists at the core of Macpherson's project. He is reprising the romantic idea that a world can be vanished yet remain known as a shadow of itself, the romance of the 'ruin'. Equally, he is reproducing the kind of devastated landscape that has become a recognisable feature of our contemporary world – the bombed and battle-scarred landscapes of newsreel footage. Yet Colvin's mind is constantly alive to more obtuse associations and relationships. In this case, he has created a subtle congress between two poems; Macpherson's *Ossian* and *The City of Dreadful Night*, an extraordinary poem completed over a century later by the Scottish poet, James Thomson (1834–1882).

The ruins of the *Blind Ossian* cycle may easily be read as a shattered and nightmarish cityscape. Overall, there is a surreal quality to the images for they show a dream world at once despairing and terrifying. It was this nightmare world that Thomson described in what was one of his most celebrated and febrile works.[15] Thomson's numbingly pessimistic poem records a night spent wandering in a modern city. The scenes he records are both gruesome and horrifying, the product of a manic imagination. Throughout the poem there is a sense of unremitting despair: 'The City is of Night; / perchance of Death, / But certainly of Night'.[16] Interestingly, the topography of this city is mirrored in Colvin's *Blind Ossian* cycle where we see 'Great ruins of an unremembered past' and 'worn faces that look deaf and blind / Like tragic masks of stone'.[17] In fact, the very ghost of Ossian appears in Thomson's city:

nas duirche na suim a phàirtean. Tha crìonadh cunbhalach air fheadh. Mun ruig sinn an naoidheamh ìomhaigh 's an tè mu dheireadh chaill sinn lorg air Oisein, chaidh an co-choisiche Maori a lèigh-losgadh, agus ràinig an dùthaich sgriosta a leagadh deireannach. Chaidh an saoghal truagh aig Colvin 'na dhùthaich throm-ligheach 's 'na roi-shealladh air latha mòr a' bhròin, a' mhillidh 's an lèirsgrios. An-seo a-rithist tha reifreansan air muin a-chèile. Aig ìre air choreigin tha Colvin a' meòrachadh air a' chall 's an truas aig cridhe pròiseact MhicMhuirich. Tha e a' toirt gu cuimhne prionnsabal nan Romansach gum faod eòlas a bhith aig daoine air saoghal a dh'fhalbh mar fhaileas dheth fhèin, ròlaist an 'tobhta'. Aig an aon àm tha e a' nochdadh an t-seòrsa de dhùthaich sgriosta a chaidh 'na pàirt aithnichte den t-saoghal anns a bheil sinn beò – na raointean bomaichte blàrloisgte a chì sinn air aithrisean filmichte naidheachdan. Ach tha inntinn Cholvin fosgailte daonnan ri ceanglaichean agus buintealasan nas maoile. Anns an eisimpleir seo chruthaich e còmhail shùbailte eadar dà bhàrdachd, *Oisein* MhicMhuirich agus *The City of Dreadful Night*, dàn iongantach a chaidh a chrìoch-nachadh còrr agus ceud bliadhna na b' anmoiche leis a' bhàrd Albannach Seumas MacThòmais (1834–1882).

Tha e furasta tobhtaichean *Oisein Dall* a leughadh 'nan dealbh de bhaile mòr fo lèirsgrios trom-ligheach. Air feadh gach nì tha coltas os-fìor aig na h-ìomhaighean, oir tha iad a' sealltainn saoghal-aislinge eagallach, neo-dhòchasach. Thug MacThòmais cunntas air an t-saoghal uabhasach seo san dàn a tha air fear de na h-obraichean as ainmeile 's as fhiabhraich' aige, dàn a làthas an fhuil le eudòchas.[15] Tha e mu dheidhinn màirnealachd oidhche mu bhaile mòr san latha aige fhèin. Tha na seallaidhean air a bheil e toirt iomradh an dà chuid gairisinneach agus uabhasach, an toradh aig mac-meanmna air bhoil. Air feadh an dàin tha sinn mothachail do dh'eudòchas gun abhsadh: 'The City is of Night; / perchance of Death, / But certainly of Night'.[16] Tha e ùidheil gu bheil dreach a' bhaile seo air a thoirt beò a-rithist ann an *Oisein Dall* aig Colvin far a bheil sinn a' faicinn 'Great ruins of an unremembered past' agus 'worn faces that look deaf and blind / Like tragic masks of stone'.[17] Gu dearbh, tha taibhse Oisein fhèin ri fhaicinn am baile MhicThòmais:

Some say that phantoms haunt those shadowy streets,
And mingle freely there with sparse mankind;
And tell of ancient woes and black defeats,
And murmur mysteries in the grave enshrined.[18]

Chuir Colvin a chorrag, ma-thà, air mar a thàinig sean agus ùr còmhla an-seo, agus tha e a' liùgachadh nan cuspairean sa a-staigh do na dealbhan camara aige. Ach 's e

Some say that phantoms haunt those
  shadowy streets,
And mingle freely there with sparse mankind;
And tell of ancient woes and black defeats,
And murmur mysteries in the grave enshrined:[18]

Colvin, then, has identified this confluence of the historical and the modern and insinuates these themes into his photographs. Yet it is, unnervingly, the mood of these diverse poetical works that is reprised with startling clarity in Colvin's disturbing images. Both Macpherson and Thomson were seduced by the poetic force of melancholy. Scholars have consistently remarked how Macpherson's work was attractive to his contemporaries because its audience was 'captivated by the concepts of "mourning", "melancholy", and "reflection"'.[19] This melancholia is almost always foreshadowed by a sense of loss. In *Fragments of Ancient Poetry* it is usually loss occasioned by heroic death, hence the refrain 'Sad are my thoughts alone'.[20] In Thomson's poem there is a deeper sense of loss, a pure alienation or a raw anomie, and so:

I spoke, perplexed by something in the signs
Of desolation I had seen and heard
In this drear pilgrimage to ruined shrines:
When Faith and Love and Hope are dead indeed,
Can life still live? By what doth it proceed?[21]

Melancholy, loss, and hopelessness saturate the *Blind Ossian* cycle. It is these feelings that define the photographs. Moreover, it is this 'mood' that is transformed into the accompanying array of related images.

In the closing passages of Thomson's *The City of Dreadful Night*, the troubled night walker comes upon 'The bronze colossus of a winged Woman'.[22] This sculpture, described by the Scottish poet, Edwin Morgan, as 'the presiding deity or patron saint of the night city',[23] is clearly based on Albrecht Dürer's famous engraving of 1514, *Melencolia I* (fig.3). Thomson is careful to note 'the instruments of carpentry and science / Scattered about her feet' and to enumerate the 'Scales, hour-glass, bell, and magic square above'.[24] This is a none too subtle itinerary of Dürer's loaded iconography, and there can be little doubt that Thomson wrote these closing stanzas with a

an rud a chuireas brisg fon t-sùil cho iongantach soilleir 's a tha ìomhaighean bruailleanach Colvin ag ùrachadh càil nan diofar obraichean bàrdail seo. Chaidh an dà chuid MacMhuirich agus MacThòmais a bhuaireadh le neart bàrdail a' bhròin. Chuir sgoilearan an cèill uair agus uair cho tarraingeach 's a bha obair MhicMhuirich do a cho-aoisean air sgàth 's gun robh a luchd-leughaidh 'air am beò-ghlacadh leis na coincheapan "caoidh", "bròn" agus "smaointean"'.[19] Tha am bròn seo air a roi-shealladh cha mhòr daonnan le mothachadh a' challa. Ann am *Fragments of Ancient Poetry* tha an call a' tighinn mar as trice bho bàs gaisgeil. 'S ann bhuaithe sin a tha an t-sèis 'Sad are my thoughts alone'.[20] San dàn aig MacThòmais tha mothachadh a' challa a' dol nas doimhne gu bhith 'na dhealachadh glan neo 'na eudòchas amh a thig bho ainriaghailt shaoghalta, agus mar sin:

I spoke, perplexed by something in the signs
Of desolation I had seen and heard
In this drear pilgrimage to ruined shrines:
When Faith and Love and Hope are dead indeed,
Can life still live? By what doth it proceed?[21]

Tha *Oisein Dall* air a bhogadh am bròn, an call 's an eudòchas. 'S iad na faireachdainnean seo a tha a' toirt ciall do na dealbhan camara. 'S e an 't-àileadh' seo cuideachd a tha air a chruth-atharrachadh a-staigh don t-sreath ìomhaighean dàimheach a tha còmhla ris.

Anns na h-earrainnean mu dheireadh den *City of Dreadful Night* tha coisiche dubhach na h-oidhche a' tighinn thairis air 'The bronze colossus of a winged Woman'.[22] Tha an obair-shnàidhte seo, air an tug am bàrd Albannach Edwin Morgan 'dia riaghlaidh no pàtran naomh baile na h-oidhche',[23] air a stèidheachadh gu follaiseach air snaidheadh ainmeil a rinn Albrecht Dürer ann an 1514, *Melencolia I* (fig.3). Tha MacThòmais cho faiceallach 's gu bheil e ag ainmeachadh 'the instruments of carpentry and science / Scattered about her feet' agus a' clàradh gach 'Scales, hour-glass, bell, and magic square above'.[24] Seo cairt-thurais gu math neo-shùbailte don ìoconosgrìobhadh luchdaichte aig Dürer, agus faodar a bhith cinnteach gun do sgrìobh MacThòmais na rannan mu dheireadh tha seo le lethbhreac de shnaidheadh Dürer ri thaobh. Bha mar amas aige 'The sense that every struggle brings defeat … That all is vanity and nothingness' a chur an cèill, sealladh neonitheach a tha gar toirt gu fhacail mu dheireadh, 'confirmation of the old despair'.[25] 'S ann air an 'old despair' tha seo, a th' air a chur an cèill gu samhlachail san t-sàr obair thòimhseachanaich ud aig Dürer 's a chithear ann am bàsmhorachd Cheilteach *Oisein* MhicMhuirich, a tha MacThòmais a' toirt tarraing

copy of Dürer's etching at his side. His aim was to give expression to 'The sense that every struggle brings defeat … That all is vanity and nothingness', a nihilistic vision that would lead to his final statement, the 'confirmation of the old despair'.[25] It is this 'old despair', mirrored in the Celtic fatalism of Macpherson's Ossian, that is explicitly referenced in Thomson's *The City of Dreadful Night*, and symbolically presented in Dürer's puzzling masterwork. It was inevitable, then, that Colvin should prepare his own meditation on this theme, as seen in his work, *Scota 01* (cat.10).

Albrecht Dürer (1471–1528) created in *Melencolia I* one of the most intriguing images in the history of art.[26] Erwin Panofsky and Fritz Saxl published the classic iconographic study of this image in 1923.[27] Here, the symbolism of the piece was opened out. Broadly, the authors identified two competing intellectual systems in the engraving. On the one hand there existed a series of references related to astrological theory in the Middle Ages. Within this frame, the temperament of melancholy is governed by planetary action and is symbolised in specific ciphers. Hence, the rainbow and comet in the background to the piece represent dominant planetary phenomena. The bat moving within the arc of the rainbow symbolises darkness, with an accompanying sense of menace. The keys and purse on the winged figure of melancholy allude to wealth and power, while the laurel wreath on her crown represents fame. Other symbols, like the 'magic square' above the figure's head can be related to numerology and related mystical systems. Finally, the companion dog mirrors the melancholy of the central figure.

This medieval symbolism in the engraving is balanced by a series of references that lock the image into the Neo-Platonic idealism of Renaissance scholarship. Here Panofsky and Saxl identified a number of features promoting rationalist principles, particularly an interest in the sciences and mathematics. In this case, the scales come to signify a sense of justice and order, while the book in the lap of the central figure embodies logic and reason. By extension the 'magic square' presents issues in mathematical reasoning, and the sphere and polyhedron accompany this as models of abstract

cho follaiseach anns an *City of Dreadful Night*. Bha e do-sheachanta, ma-thà, gun ullaicheadh Colvin a smaointean fhèin mun chuspair, mar chithear 'na obair *Scota 01* (clàr 10).

Ann am *Melencolia I* chruthaich Dürer (1471–1528) tè de na h-ìomhaighean as tòimhseachanaiche ann an eachdraidh na h-ealain.[26] Ann an 1923 dh'fhoillsich Erwin Panofsky agus Fritz Saxl stuidear clasaigeach ìocono-sgrìobhach na h-ìomhaighe seo anns an deachaidh samhlachas a' phìos fhosgladh a-mach.[27] San fharsaingeachd chuir na h-ùghdairean an corrag air dà sheòrsa feallsanachd a bha an co-fharpais ri chèile san t-snaidheadh. Air an dàrna làimh tha sreath reifreansan ann ceangailte ri draoidheachd nan reul sna Meadhoin Aoisean. Am broinn na beairte seo tha nàdar a' bhròin air a riaghladh le gnìomharran nam planaidean agus air a shamhlachadh ann an codaichean sònraichte. Mar sin, tha am bogha froise agus an reul seachrain ann an cùl a' phìos a' riochdachadh sìontan riaghlaidh nam planaidean. Tha an ialtag a tha a' gluasad am broinn stuadh a' bhogha froise a' samhlachadh dorchadas agus maoidheadh. Tha na h-iuchraichean 's an sporan air pearsa sgiathach a' bhròin ag innse mun chumhachd 's mun bheairteas, agus tha fleasg an labhrais air a crùn a' riochdachadh cliù. Faodar samhlaidhean eile, leithid 'ceàrnag dhraoidheach' thar

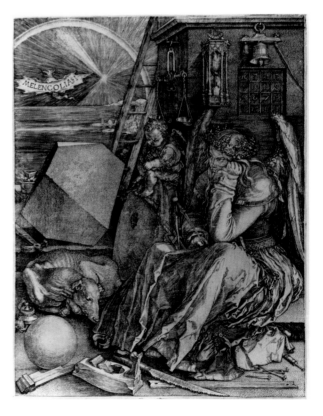

Fig.3 · Albrecht Dürer, *Melencolia I*
National Gallery of Scotland · Galaraidh Nàiseanta na h-Alba

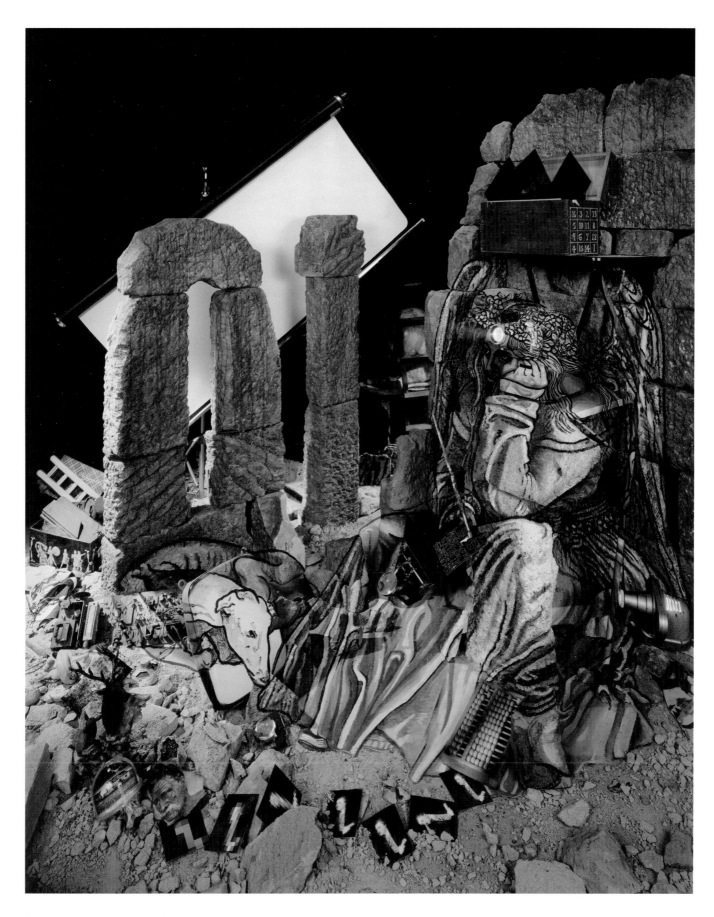

Cat.10 **Scota 01** · Clàr 10 **Scota 01**

thought. The tools and paraphernalia surrounding the winged figure are evidently instruments of creative thought, while the ladder represents some sense of aspiration and ambition.

Dürer's *Melencolia I*, however, is so richly-layered and fundamentally esoteric that a host of alternative theories can be offered concerning its symbolism. They range from alchemy through astrology to occult numerology. What remains significant is the core idea of melancholy, and its broad reference to unfulfilled creative endeavour. Panofsky and Saxl viewed *Melencolia I* as a thinly disguised allegory on the creative artist, and indeed as a deliberately ambiguous self-portrait by Dürer. The central figure, the winged woman, is slouched and defeated. Her face is darkened and rests on her clenched fist. This gesture is emblematic of breakdown and failure, hence 'the clenched fist, hitherto a mere symptom of disease, now symbolises the fanatical concentration of the mind which has truly grasped a problem, but which at the same moment feels itself incapable either of solving or of dismissing it'.[28] In this respect the surrounding paraphernalia become the symbols of that spectacular loss. The discarded tools and scientific instruments represent the means to creative fulfilment, now recognised as mere props. The ladder is unused, the sphere ignored, the polyhedron a heavy symbol of creative 'block' rather than a challenging mathematical problem. By a cruel irony the 'putto', to the left of the central figure, labours intensively writing in a book and signifies 'the careless equanimity of a being that has only just learnt the contentment of activity, even when unproductive, and does not yet know the torment of thought'.[29]

Melencolia I, then, with her stilled wings, bedraggled laurel wreath of fame, her weighty symbols of power and wealth, and posture of defeat, is a loaded vision of grief, fatigue and creative failure. This is the root of a philosophical, indeed existential, melancholy. Colvin has visited this idea before, most notably in his series *The Seven Deadly Sins and the Four Last Things*, 1993, where the winged 'action men' and skeletal figures representing the sin of sloth embody the idea of creative frustration. Now, Melencolia has fallen into the landscape of

ceann na pearsa, a cheangal ri draoidheòlas àireamhan agus ri siostaman dìomhair a th' ann an dàimh ris. Mu dheireadh, tha an companach coin 'na sgàthan air bròn na pearsa sa mheadhoin.

Tha an samhlachas meadhoin-aoiseach san t-snaidheadh air a chothromachadh le sreath reifreansan a tha a' glasadh na h-ìomhaigh a-staigh don fhoirfeachd Nuaphlatonaich aig sgoilearachd an Athbheothachaidh. An-seo chuir Panofsky agus Saxl an corrag air grunnan nithean a tha a' cur air adhart prionnsabalan na reusantachd, gu sònraichte ùidh anns na saidheansan 's ann am matamataig. A rèir seo thig na meidhean gu bhith a' ciallachadh smaointean mu òrdan 's mu cheartas, agus tha an leabhar an uchd na pearsa sa mheadhoin a' riochdachadh ciall agus reusan. Tha 'a' cheàrnag dhraoidheach' cuideachd a' cur air adhart ceistean ann an reusanachadh matamataigeach, agus tha an cruinne 's an t-iomataobhach a' tighinn còmhla rithe mar mholltairean do smaointean eascruthach. Tha e follaiseach gu bheil an acainn agus nithean eile timcheall na pearsa sgiathaich 'nan ionnsramaidean do smaointean cruthachail, agus tha am fàradh a' riochdachadh tomhas de dhùil 's de dhòchas.

Tha *Melencolia I* aig Dürer, ge-tà, cho làn ìrean eadar-dhealaichte agus cho buileach dìomhair 's gun gabh iomadh barail eile a chur air adhart a thaobh a shamhlachais, bhon ailcheime tro dhraoidheachd nan reul gu draoidheòlas dìomhair àireamhan. Na nithean a tha a' fuireach cudromach 's iad am bròn a tha 'na chridhe agus an tarraing fharsaing a tha i a' toirt air strì chruthachail gun choileanadh. Bha Panofsky agus Saxl a' faicinn *Melencolia I* mar shamhla (fo bhreug-riochd tana) don ealainiche chruthachail, agus gu dearbh mar dhealbh Dürer fhèin a tha a dh'aona ghnothach dà-sheaghach. Tha a' phearsa sa mheadhoin, am boireannach sgiathach, 'na crùban claoidhte. Tha a h-aodann dorchnaichte an taice snaoim teann a dùirn. Tha an cruth-bodhaig seo samhlachail do bhriseadh 's do dh'fhàilling, agus mar sin 'tha snaoim an dùirn, nach robh roimhe ach 'na chomharradh euslainte, a-nis a' samhlachadh dlùthachadh eudmhorach na h-inntinn a tha gu fìrinneach air imcheist a ghreimeachadh, ach a tha aig an aon àm ga faireachdainn fhèin eucomasach air an dàrna cuid a fuasgladh neo a fuadachadh'.[28] A rèir seo tha na nithean a tha timcheall oirre a' dol 'nan samhlaidhean don chall thaisbeanach seo. Tha an acainn chaithte agus na h-ionnsramaidean saidheansach a' riochdachadh an rathaid gu coileanadh cruthachail, ach tha iad a-nis air an aithneachadh mar chonbhallas lom. Chan eil am fàradh ga chleachdadh, tha an cruinne gun ùisneachadh, tha an t-iomataobhach 'na shamhla trom don 'bhloc' chruthachail seach 'na cheist dhùbhlanach mhatamataigeach. Le ìoranas mì-chneasta,

Ossian. Here she is a cipher for fatalism and defeat, a metaphor for the aspirational artist brought low by the forces of the world. And, in Colvin's scheme, a symbolic sister not only to Ossian but to the aesthetic of photography.

It is characteristic of Colvin's practice that ideas overlap, are cross-referenced, and are freely associated with contrasting themes. His kaleidoscopic mind insists that a subject, far from being self-contained, will constantly metamorphose into loosely related hypotheses. Hence, the landscape of the *Blind Ossian* cycle remains as a residue in his reworking of Dürer while the associations multiply and change shape. In this event Colvin's title for his reworking of *Melencolia I* is *Scota 01*, a subtle word-play that denotes a complex of issues relating to identity and modernity. The substance of the Dürer piece remains, however, showing the winged figure seated with head collapsed into her clenched hand. The ruins of the Ossianic scene open around her and in this space a symbolic world lies scattered. It is the iconography of this debris that exposes the changing meanings within the image. Some of these references are straightforward. Colvin includes, to the left of the image, a box of tools topped by a small ladder, mirroring, comically, the tools and implements in Dürer's original. Likewise, in the background, a ladder is propped against a plastic globe and this reprises Dürer's interest in the folly of worldly ambition. More obviously, the magic square is repeated in the exact position it occupies in Dürer's engraving, here printed on the side of a wooden box filled with nineteenth-century glass-plate negatives discovered by Colvin in an Edinburgh junkshop. This find is significant for it sets the leitmotif for his reworking of Dürer's image.

At the foot of Melencolia, or Scota as she has become, lies a series of photographs. These are computer manipulated images of a version of the *Portrait of James Macpherson*, painted by Sir Joshua Reynolds (1723–1792) in 1761. The series of seven photographs moves from an analogue representation to a heavily pixillated digitised image. At this point, Colvin has created a kind of visual pun, as the manipulation of Macpherson's image echoes the 'manipulated' verse of Ossian. More fundamentally, this

tha an gille òg sgiathach air taobh clì na pearsa sa mheadhoin gu dìcheallach an sàs a' sgrìobhadh ann an leabhar; tha esan a' ciallachadh 'inntinn shocair an duine a dh'ùr-ionnsaich toileachas na gnìomhachd – ged nach bi toradh ann – agus nach do dh'fhiosraich fhathast àmhghar na smuainte'.[29]

Tha *Melencolia I*, ma-tà, 's a sgiathan 'nan tàmh, le fleasg-labhrais luidreach a' chliù aice, le samhlaidhean troma a' chumhachd 's a' bheairtis aice, agus a cainnt-bhodhaig chlaoidhte, 'na shealladh luchdaichte de sgìths, de bhròn 's de dh'fhàilling chruthachail. Seo freumh a' bhròin a tha feallsanach, fiùs bithealach. Thadhail Colvin air an smuain seo roimhe, gu seachd sònraichte 'na shreath *Na Seachd Peacainnean Bàsmhor 's na Ceithir Nithean Deireannach*, 1993, far a bheil na 'fir ghnìomha' sgiathach agus na figearan cnàmhach a tha a' riochdachadh peacadh na leisg a' toirt leotha nòisean a' bhacaidh chruthachail. A-nise thuit Melencolia a-staigh do dhùthaich Oisein. An-seo tha i 'na samhla do bhàsmhorachd 's do chlaoidh, 'na meatafor don ealainiche mhiannach a chaidh ìsleachadh le cumhachdan an t-saoghail – agus, a rèir sgeama Cholvin, 'na piuthar shamhlachail chan ann do dh'Oisein a-mhàin ach do bhòidhcheòlas an fhotosgrìobhaidh.

A rèir a' ghnàiths aig Colvin, tha beachd-smuaintean a' dol thar a-chèile le croisreifreansan agus tha iad air an ceangal gu saor ri cuspairean tur eadar-dhealaichte. Tha an inntinn iongantach ghrad-atharrachail aige a' toirt air cuspair sam bith, fada bho bhith neo-eisimeileach, a bhith a' sìor dhol 'na thràchdasan aig a bheil dàimh las air choireigin ris. Mar sin anns an ath-obrachadh a thug e air Dürer tha dùthaich *Oisein Dall* a' fuireach 'na fuigheall ged a bhios na ceanglaichean a' meudachadh 's ag atharrachadh cruth. Anns an eisimpleir seo 's e an tiotal a th' aig Colvin don ath-obrachadh aige air *Melencolia I* ach *Scota 01*, cluiche shùbailte fhacal a tha a' toirt tarraing air meall cheistean ceangailte ri dearbh-aithne 's ris an linn anns a bheil sinne beò. Tha brìgh a' phìos aig Dürer ann fhathast, ge-tà, a' sealltainn na pearsa sgiathaich 'na suidhe 's a ceann aomt' ann an snaoim a dùirn. Tha tobhtaichean an t-seallaidh Oiseinich a' fosgladh mun cuairt oirre agus anns a' bheàrn seo tha saoghal samhlachail 'na laighe sgapte. Tha ìoconosgrìobhadh an sprùillich seo a' nochdadh nan ciall atharrachail am broinn na h-ìomhaigh. Tha cuid de na reifreansan seo sìmplidh. Air taobh clì na h-ìomhaighe tha Colvin a' cur bogs' acainn le fàradh beag air a bhàrr, a' cuimhneachadh le feala-dhà na h-acainn 's nan inneal san dealbh thùsach aig Dürer. Anns a' chùl tha fàradh an taice ri cruinne plastaig, agus tha seo a' toirt 'nar cuimhne an ùidh a bh' aig Dürer ann an amaideas gach miann shaoghalta. Nas follaisiche, tha a' cheàrnag dhraoidheach ga toirt dhuinn a-rithist anns an dearbh àite

opposition between the analogue and the digital opens the picture to a discussion of creative photography as an art form. It is evident that the trail of Macpherson's changing image leads to a computer motherboard, which is, in fact, a discreet reference to Ossian's harp. To the right of Scota, and indeed incorporated into her forehead is a slide projector. The blank projection screen has taken the place of the polyhedron in Colvin's picture. In the lap of the central figure, replacing the closed book of the original, is another computer motherboard and broken computer parts can be seen among the debris.

Among other things this image is a meditation on the changing nature of contemporary photography, but it is also an ethical discourse. In the right hand of the central figure is a paintbrush, which rests on a computer part. This opposition establishes a dialectic that runs throughout the image: the glass-plate negative is contrasted with the slide, the analogue photograph with the digitised image, the paintbrush with the computer. In each case some notion of creative choice is presented, but crucially these choices are set in a landscape of despair. Here is a world in ruins, in which the savage and the sophisticated share a desolate stage. Within this frame Dürer's Melencolia is mirrored in the melancholy of the photographer who recognises the failure of photography to reveal 'truth', and who also considers the failure of civilisation and modernity to realise enlightenment. Here is the apotheosis of melancholy, and Colvin has transformed the Ossian legend into a parable for our times.

Two details in this photograph, *Scota 01*, lead to a further development in Colvin's Ossian project. Scota refers to the old tradition that an Egyptian princess of that name was 'the progenitor of the race of the Gaels or Scots'[30] and, once again, highlights an interest in creation myths. More particularly, it foregrounds Colvin's determination to locate his free associations on the Ossian theme within the problematic issue of Scottish identity. In fact this idea is further developed in the triptych titled *Cruthni* which includes stylised fingerprints and DNA molecular strands as the ironic imprint of 'identity' and origin.[31] The other relevant symbol is that

sa bheil i anns an t-snaidheadh aig Dürer, 's i air a clò-bhualadh an-seo air taobh bogsa fiodha a th' air a lìonadh le clàir-àichidh phlàta-ghloine bhon naoidheamh ceud deug a lorg Colvin ann am bùth threalaich an Dùn Èideann. Tha an fhaodail seo cudromach oir tha i a' stèidheachadh an *leitmotif* airson an ath-obrachaidh aige den ìomhaigh aig Dürer.

Mu chasan Melencolia – neo Scota, oir 's i sin a th' innte a-nis – tha sreath de dhealbhan camara. 'S iad seo ìomhaighean compiutar-làimhsichte de bhreacadh den *Phortrait of James Macpherson* a pheant Sir Joshua Reynolds (1723–1792) ann an 1761. Tha an sreath de sheachd dealbhan camara a' gluasad bho riochdachadh analog gu ìomhaigh mheuraichte throm-phigsilichte. Aig an ìre seo chruthaich Colvin seòrsa de chluich-fhaclan lèirsinneach, oir tha làimhseachadh na h-ìomhaigh aig MacMhuirich ag atharrais air bàrdachd 'làimhsichte' Oisein. Nas bunaitiche, tha an spàirn seo eadar an t-analog agus am meurach a' fosgladh an deilbh gu deasbaireachd mun fhotosgrìobhadh chruthachail mar ghnè ealain. Tha e follaiseach gu bheil ceum na h-ìomhaigh atharrachail aig MacMhuirich a' treòrachadh gu bòrd-màthar compiutair a tha, ann an da-rìribh, 'na reifreans socair ri clàrsach Oisein. Air taobh deas Scota, agus gu dearbh mar phàirt d'a bathais, tha pròiseactar shleamhnan. Ghabh an sgrìne-chaithimh bhàn àite an iomataobhaich ann an dealbh Cholvin. Ann an uchd na pearsa sa mheadhoin tha bòrd-màthar compiutair eile a' gabhail àite an leabhair dhùinte san dealbh thùsail, agus chithear pàirtean briste compiutair am measg an sprùillich.

Am measg nithean eile tha an ìomhaigh seo 'na meòrachadh air nàdar atharrachail fotosgrìobhadh an latha an-diugh, ach tha i cuideachd 'na conaltradh beuseòlach. Ann an làmh dheas na pearsa sa mheadhoin tha bruis-pheanta a' suathadh ri pàirt chompiutair. Tha a' chòmhstri seo a' stèidheachadh deasbaireachd a tha a' ruith tron ìomhaigh gu lèir: tha an clàr-àichidh plàta-ghloine air a chur ris an t-sleamhnan, an dealbh-camara analog ris an ìomhaigh mheuraichte, a' bhruis-pheanta ris a' chompiutar. Anns gach caigeann tha nòisean air choreigin de roghainn chruthachail air a chur air adhart ach, nì a tha glè chudromach, tha na roghainnean seo air an cur ann an dùthaich an eudòchais. Seo saoghal air a sgrios, anns a bheil brùidealachd agus suairceas air an aon àrd-ùrlar uaigneach còmhla. Am broinn na beairte seo tha Melencolia aig Dürer air a shealltainn ann am bròn an fhotosgrìobhadair a tha ag aithneachadh nach eil am fotosgrìobhadh a' deargadh air 'fìrinn' a nochdadh, agus a tha cuideachd a' beachdachadh nach eil an t-sìobhaltachd agus an ùr-nodhachd a' deargadh air soillseachadh a thoirt gu bith. Seo a-nis mullach a' bhròin, agus tha Colvin air

curious 'translation' from Dürer's image, the curled and reclining figure of the dog. In the symbolic world of Dürer's engraving the dog is usually viewed as a mirror of human emotions. In which case the dog can be seen to share the melancholic nature of the central figure. And yet, it is this same dog that will stand up in the shattered landscape of the melancholic artist and stroll off into the comic scenery of Robert Burns's Scotland. In making this short journey it will open out yet another vista in Colvin's search for Ossian's legacy.

Robert Burns was a contemporary and an admirer of Macpherson and the poems of Ossian. In writing to Agnes McLehose, his sometime muse 'Clarinda', he speaks of 'Ossian, prince of Poets'.[32] While in a letter to the Edinburgh bookseller, Peter Hill, in which he discusses James Cririe's poem *Address to Loch Lomond*, he compliments Cririe's description of landscape by claiming it 'truly Ossianic'.[33] His discreet respect for Macpherson, however, is evidenced in the poem that occupies the opening pages of the 1786 Kilmarnock edition of his verse, the tale of *The Twa Dogs*. This 'tale', consisting of a dialogue between two dogs, one 'o' high degree' and the other 'a ploughman's collie',[34] concerns issues of class and virtue in human society. It typifies Burns's fascination with the comic, the vernacular, and with the subjects of social justice and human folly. The dogs are named Caesar and Luath. Caesar represented the classical world and was palpably 'nane o' Scotland's dogs'. Luath, on the other hand, was named 'After some dog in Highland sang, / Was made lang syne, lord knows how lang'. In fact, this was a reference to Cuchullin's dog in Macpherson's *Fingal*. It was, moreover, the name that Burns gave to his own favourite collie, and his respect for Macpherson's invention was at least evidenced in this homage.

Colvin takes these associations as a starting point for his *Twa Dogs* (cat.11), but reinvents the idea in terms of a more contemporary dualism. At the most obvious level Colvin's *Twa Dogs* represents the unresolved conflict between Celtic and British identity in modern Scotland. In this respect the image connects with the duality of Highland and Lowland culture and the two languages of Scotland,

sgeul Oisein ath-chruthachadh 'na pharabal do ar linn.

Tha dà rud bheag anns an dealbh chamara seo *Scota 01* a' treòrachadh gu leasachadh eile sa phròiseact Oiseineach aig Colvin. Tha Scota a' toirt tarraing air seanchas nan Gaidheal gum b' i banaphrionnsa Èipheiteach den ainm sin 'prìomh shinnsir cinneadh nan Gaidheal no nan Sgotach'[30] agus tha sin aon uair a-rithist a' cur solas air ùidh ann an uirsgeulan cruthachaidh. Nas sònraichte, tha e a' cur ann an uinneag na bùtha cho leagte 's a tha Colvin gun suidhich e na ceanglaichean saora aige air cuspair Oisein am broinn ceist thoinnte na h-ionannachd Albannaich. Gu dearbh tha an smuain seo air a leasachadh nas fhaide san dealbh-fa-thrì ris an canar *Cruithnich* anns a bheil, am measg eile, lorgan-meòir stoidhlichte agus snàithleinean moiligealach DNA mar chlò ìoranach 'ionannachd' agus fhreumh.[31] 'S e an samhla iomchaidh eile an 't-eadar-theangachadh' neònach ud bhon ìomhaigh aig Dürer, an cù sìnte 'na chuaichein. Ann an saoghal samhlachail snaidheadh Dürer tha an cù mar as trice air fhaicinn mar sgàthan nam faireachdainnean aig clann daoine. A rèir seo chithear an cù a' compàirteachadh ann an nàdar brònach na pearsa sa mheadhoin. Ge-tà 's e an aona chù seo a tha dol a sheasamh ann an dùthaich sgriosta an ealaniche bhrònaich a ghabhail cuairt a-staigh do sheallaidhean èibhinn na h-Alba aig Raibeart Burns. Ann a bhith a' gabhail na cuairt bhig tha seo fosglaidh e a-mach fàire eile san turas rannsachaidh aig Colvin a dh'ionnsaigh dìleab Oisein.

Bha Raibeart Burns 'na cho-aoiseach aig MacMhuirich 's aig 'dàin Oisein' agus bha e measail orra. 'S e a' sgrìobhadh gu Agnes NicilleThòmhais, a bha uaireigin 'na miùs 'Clarinda' dha, tha e a' bruidhinn air 'Oisein, prionnsa nam Bàrd'.[32] Ann an litir gu ceannaiche leabhraichean ann an Dùn Èideann, Pàdraig Hill, anns a bheil e a' seanchas mun dàn aig Seumas Cririe, *Address to Loch Lomond*, tha e a' moladh an deilbh-fhaclan a tha Cririe a' peantadh den dùthaich le bhith a' cumail a-mach gu bheil e 'fìor Oiseineach'.[33] Tha an spèis shocair a tha e a' toirt do MhacMhuirich, ge-tà, air a shealltainn san dàn ann an duilleagan-toisich an leabhair bhàrdachd aige a thàinig a-mach an Cille Mheàrnaig ann an 1786, sgeul an *Dà Chù*. Tha an 'sgeul' seo, a tha 'na chòmhradh eadar dà chù, fear 'o' high degree' agus fear eile 'na 'ploughman's collie',[34] mu dheidhinn ceistean a bhuineas ri inbhe agus beusan am measg clann daoine. Tha e a' suimeachadh an tarraing do Bhurns a bha aig àbhachdas, aig cainnt nan daoine, agus aig cuspairean a' cheartais shòisealta agus an amaideis dhaonna. 'S iad ainmean nan con Caesar agus Luath. Bha Caesar a' riochdachadh saoghal na Grèige 's na Ròimhe, 'nane o' Scotland's dogs' gu follaiseach. Bha Luath air ainmeachadh, air an làimh eile, 'After some dog in

Gaelic and Scots. By extension a further series of dualisms are exposed, most notably the notion of corporate competitiveness symbolised in the Nike and Adidas training shoes that hang on each side of the domestic fireplace. These sports shoes lead to the core conflict in the photograph, the near primordial hostility between Rangers and Celtic football clubs. In consequence Burns's two dogs, those articulate commentators on the absurdity of social class, have become representatives of tribal factionalism. Luath signifies the Celtic contingent while Caesar, here renamed Kaiser,[35] is firmly planted on Rangers' divide.

The scene itself is created around a modern domestic hearth. In fact the stonework is reclaimed from the ruins of Ossian's world, and the carved stones from the Ossianic landscape have been reconstructed for this tableau. On the ashen floor two rugs mark the territory of the duelling identities; one is blue and emblazoned with the logo of Glasgow Rangers, the other green and inscribed with the insignia of Celtic Football Club. The feeding bowls of each are filled with the syndicated confections of the other.

Surrounding the dogs are the emblems of folly and conflict: an empty 'Gale's' honey jar on the coffee table, and the orange sugar-balls in the Rangers jar by the fireplace. The decorative fan is a pun on rival supporters and 'fanatics'. Just behind this is a paperback of the appropriately titled *Scotch on the Rocks*,[36] and, nearer the foreground lies an equally appropriate miniature 'Celtic' whisky bottle. The theme of music proliferates partly reprising Ossian's role as a bardic singer, but also referencing the power of the sectarian song. Consequently an ancient record player sits with a rock atop the turntable. The rock presents a multiple symbolism. It is a leaden weight like the polyhedron in Dürer's *Melencolia I* and, therefore, a block to creative action. Equally it is a presentation of Scotland's Highland landscape, represented more straightforwardly in the inset photograph to the left of the record player. It is perhaps the 'rock' of 'rock 'n' roll' ironically juxtaposed against the album cover advertising the more bucolic pleasures of *Scotlands Own Tartan Lads*. This musical theme is completed with a wooden recorder, deftly painted as a

Highland sang, / Was made lang syne, lord knows how lang'. Ann an da-rìribh, bha seo a' toirt tarraing air madadh Chu-Chulainn ann am *Fingal* aig MacMhuirich. B' e cuideachd an t-ainm a thug Burns air a' chù chaorach a b' fheàrr leis fhèin, agus aig a' char as lugha bha an ùmhlachd seo 'na fianais air an spèis a bh' aige do dh'innleachd MhicMhuirich.

Tha Colvin a' gabhail nan ceanglaichean seo mar àite-tòiseachaidh don *Dà Chù* aigesan (clàr 11), ach tha e a' cruth-atharrachadh na smuain a rèir dùbailteachd a tha nas fhaisg' air an latha againn fhìn. Air an ìr' as follaisiche tha an *Dà Chù* aig Colvin a' riochdachadh na còmhstri neo-fhuasgailte eadar ionannachd Cheilteach agus Bhreatannach ann an Alba an-diugh. A thaobh seo tha an ìomhaigh a' buntainn ri dùbailteachd cuiltear nan Gaidheal 's nan Gall agus ri dà chànan na h-Alba, a' Ghàidhlig 's a' Bheurla. Bhuaithe seo tha sreath dhùbailteachdan eile a' nochdadh, gu sònraichte nòisean na co-fharpaiseachd chorpaichte a tha air a shamhlachadh anns na brògan-trèanaidh Nike agus Adidas a tha a' crochadh ri dà thaobh an teallaich. Tha na brògan spòrs seo a' treòrachadh don chòmhstri aig cridhe an deilbh chamara, an gamhlas cha mhòr tùsail eadar clubaichean ball-coise Rangers agus Celtic. Mar thoradh air seo tha an dà chù aig Burns, an luchd-seanchais deas-bhriathrach sin air amaideas na h-inbhe shòisealta, air a dhol 'nan riochdairean aig pàirtealas a' chinnidh. Tha Luath a' riochdachadh muinntir Celtic agus tha Caesar, air ath-ainmeachadh Kaiser an-seo,[35] air a chur gu daingeann air taobh Rangers na còmhstri.

Tha an sealladh fhèin air a chruthachadh timcheall air teallach taighe bhon latha an-diugh. Ann an da-rìribh chaidh a' chlachaireachd a thoirt air ais bho thobhtaichean saoghal Oisein, agus chaidh clachan snàidhte dùthaich Oisein a thogail as ùr airson a' chlàir-dheilbh seo. Air an ùrlar luaithre tha dà ruga a' comharradh crìochan na dà ionannachd chòmhstrithich: fear dhiubh gorm, sgeadaichte le suaicheantas Rangers Ghlaschu, am fear eile uaine le suaicheantas Club Ball-Coise Celtic. Tha bobhla biadhaidh gach coin air a lìonadh le suiteas oifigeil a' choin eile.

Timcheall nan con tha samhlaidhean an amaideis agus na còmhstri: crogan falamh meala 'Gale's' air a' bhòrd chofaidh, agus na buill-shiùcair orains ann an crogan Rangers an cois an teallaich. Tha 'm fan-gaoithe maiseach 'na chluiche-facail air luchd-taice còmhstritheach 's air 'fanatics'. Bìdeag air chùl seo tha còmhdach bog fon tiotal iomchaidh *Scotch on the Rocks*,[36] agus nas fhaisg' air a' bheulaibh tha botal beag uisge-beatha 'Celtic' a tha cheart cho iomchaidh. Tha cuspair a' chiùil air fheadh, gu ìre a' cuimhneachadh dreuchd Oisein mar sheinneadair bàrdail,

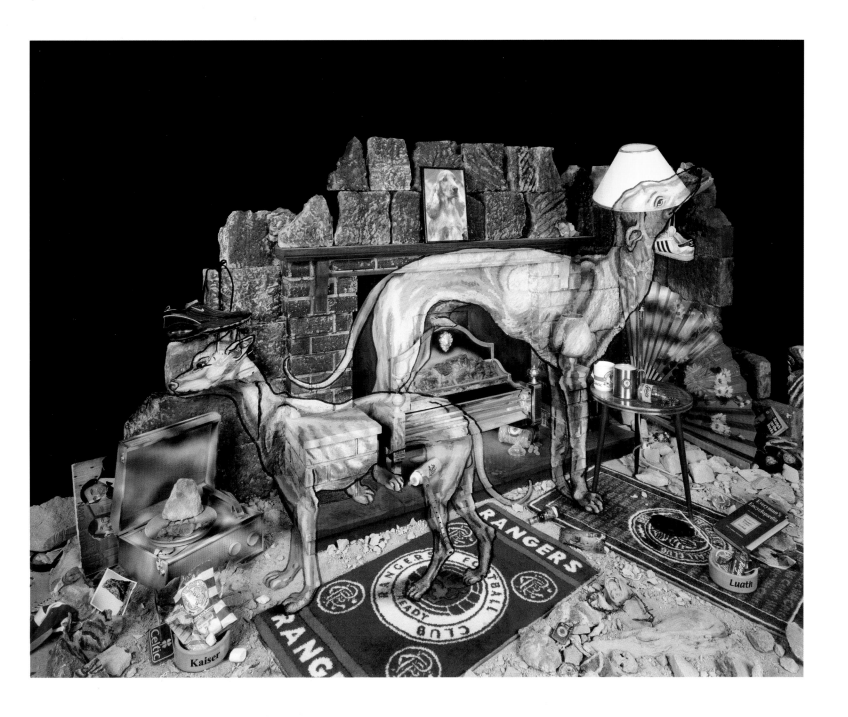

Cat.11 **Twa Dogs** · Clàr 11 **Dà Chù**

bone in the leg of Kaiser, and representing the flute of the sectarian marching bands.

In the *Twa Dogs* Colvin has created a complex dialectic with thesis and antithesis competing against one another, but each united in a common paradigm. Something of this interdependence is indicated in the copy of *Everyman's Encyclopaedia* that lies to the right of the tableau. It is the edition detailing the index D to F, specifically the concepts 'Dramatic Unities to Football'. This is typical of Colvin's penetrating humour; that juxtaposition of Aristotle's theory on the three rules of dramatic construction set against the world of football, and the irony of 'dramatic unities' folding into the divisive tribal loyalties of the football supporter. In this clash high and low culture, the classical and the modern world, the sublime and the ridiculous, are engaged in a fantasy duel. In turn this becomes a saga of perpetual discord with Catholic and Protestant, the Highlander and the Lowlander, the Celtic Scot and the 'North Briton', competing over a contested and unattainable 'identity'. Tragically, in some measure, Colvin presents a world wherein these two dogs will be locked in vicious and pointless combat for evermore. This, then, is the wretched bequest of Ossian's dream, a world of unresolved conflict and perpetual despair.

III

Nevertheless, inside this darkness Colvin has searched for light and hope. If his *Twa Dogs* represents the least attractive dimension of Scotland's culture then the portrait studies that accompany this series provide its glorious apotheosis, not least the *Portrait of Robert Burns* (cat.12). Burns was, of course, the author of *The Twa Dogs* who on observing human society finally declaimed 'When up they gat, an' shook their lugs, / Rejoic'd they were na men, but dogs'. This concord, and the poet's own role as humanist and freethinker, made him a natural subject for this project. More importantly, perhaps, was the idea that Scotland's national bard of modern times should be presented in order to create a link with the ancestral bard, Ossian. In the event, Colvin created an iconic image of Burns, replete with

ach cuideachd a' toirt tarraing air cumhachd an òrain bhuidhnich. Mar sin tha seann ghramafon 'na shuidhe le creag air a chlàr-thionndaidh. Tha a' chreag a' cur an cèill samhlachas iomadaidh. Tha i 'na cudrom luaidhe coltach ris an iomataobhach ann am *Melencolia I* aig Dürer agus mar sin tha i 'na bacadh ri gnìomh cruthachail. Aig an aon àm tha i a' cur an cèill dùthaich na Gaidhealtachd, a tha air a riochdachadh nas sìmplidhe san dealbh chamara a tha air a chur a-staigh air taobh clì a' ghramafon. 'S i 's dòcha an 'rock' ann an 'rock 'n' roll' 's i air a cur gu h-ìoranach ri taobh a' chòmhdaich album a tha a' foillseachadh nan toileachas as tuataidh a gheibhear bho *Scotlands Own Tartan Lads*. Tha cuspair a' chiùil a tha seo air a choileanadh le recòrdar fiodha, a tha air a pheantadh gu sgileil mar chnàimh ann an lurgainn Khaiser, a' riochdachadh cuisle-chiùil nan còmhlan-caismeachd buidhneach.

Anns an *Dà Chù* chruthaich Colvin deasbaireachd thoinnte anns a bheil tràchdas agus anatràchdas a' còmhstri ri chèile ged a tha iad aonaichte san aon chliath-cheangal. Tha rudeigin den eadar-eisimeileachd seo air a chomharrachadh anns an lethbhreac de *Everyman's Encyclopaedia* a tha air taobh deas a' chlàir-dheilbh. Chì sinn bhon chòmhdach gur e seo an leabhar anns a bheil a' mhòrchuid de na litrichean D gu F – *Dramatic Unities* ('Aontaidhean Dràma') gu *Football* ('Ball-Coise'). Tha seo 'na eisimpleir mhath den fheala-dhà dhrùidhteach aig Colvin: mar a tha e a' cur beachd-smuain Aristotle air trì riaghailtean structair an dràma ri taobh saoghal ball-coise, agus an t-ìoranas gu bheil 'aontaidhean dràma' a' filleadh ann an dìlseachd sgàineach chinneadail luchd-taice ball-coise. Anns a' chòmhstri seo tha cuiltear àrd agus ìseal, saoghal na Grèige, na Ròimhe 's an latha 'n-diugh, 's an glic 's an gòrach, uile an sàs ann an sabaid masa-fìor. Tha seo a' dol an uair sin 'na sgeul fada aimhreiteach gun chrìoch le Caitligeach agus Pròstanach, Gaidheal agus Gall, Sgotach Ceilteach agus 'Breatannach fa Thuath' a' còmhstri thairis air 'ionannachd' a tha connspaideach agus do-ruigsinn. Gu dòlasach, gu ìre bhig, tha Colvin a' cur an cèill saoghal far am bi an dà chù seo glaiste gu bràth tuilleadh ann an còmhstri mhì-chneasta gun stàth. Seo, ma-tà, tiomnadh truagh aisling Oisein, saoghal anns a bheil còmhstri gun cheann agus eudòchas buan.

III

Am broinn an dorchadais seo, ge-tà, bha Colvin an tòir air solas agus dòchas. Ma tha an *Da Chù* aige a' riochdachadh an taobh as gràinde de chuiltear na h-Alba, tha na dealbhan daoine an cois an t-sreath seo a' nochdadh a mhullaich àghmhoir, gu sònraichte 's dòcha an *Dealbh de*

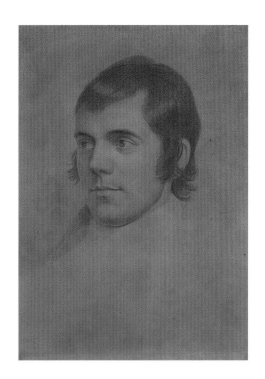

symbolic references to his finest poems and
intimately linked to the fragmented world of
the Ossianic landscape.

Interestingly, in selecting a model for Burns,
Colvin turned away from the famous portrait
by Alexander Nasmyth (1758–1840), painted in
1787, and looked to the delicate drawing of the
poet by Archibald Skirving (fig.4). Skirving
(1749–1819) found his living as a portraitist,
though he worked principally in the medium
of chalk. His red-chalk study of Burns was,
itself, based on the Nasmyth portrait and so the
sense of 'translation' from Nasmyth through
Skirving into Colvin's image echoes the
'translation' of Ossian's poetry through
Macpherson. In the event, Colvin's photograph
resonates with the subtlety and grace of
Skirving's drawing, but also provides a context
that marries the image to the broader theme of
Ossian and Scottish identity.

It is evident that the head of Burns is
painted onto the fractured landscape already
witnessed in the photographs of *Blind Ossian*
and *Scota 01*. The carved and broken stone is
set down on a foreground of scattered rock,
distressed totems, and charred bone. Incorporated into this ruin is a bookcase, which is the
frame for the painted head of Burns, and also a
pillar. The bookcase, a natural choice of
backdrop for an image of a poet, contains three

Raibeart Burns (clàr 12). Tha fios gum b' e Burns ùghdar an
Dà Chù a bha a' toirt sùil air comann chlann daoine 's a
thuirt mu dheireadh: 'When up they gat, an' shook their
lugs, / Rejoic'd they were na men, but dogs'. Dh'fhàg an co-
aonta seo (agus dreuchd a' bhàird fhèin mar dhaonnaire 's
mar smaoineadair saor) Burns 'na chuspair nàdarra don
phròiseact seo. Na bu chudromaiche fhèin 's dòcha bha an
smuain gum bu chòir bàrd nàiseanta na h-Alba san linn
againn fhìn a chur an cèill gus ceangal a chruthachadh ris
a' bhàrd shinnsreil, Oisein. Mar a thachair, chruthaich
Colvin ìomhaigh shuaicheantail de Bhurns, làn reifreansan
samhlachail ris na dàin as fheàrr aige agus air a dlùth
cheangal ri saoghal pronn dùthaich Oisein.

Gu h-ùidheil, ann a bhith a' taghadh molltair do
Bhurns, chuir Colvin a chùl ris an dealbh ainmeil le
Alastair Nasmyth (1758–1840), peantaichte ann an 1787,
agus choimhead e ris an tarraing fhìnealta den bhàrd le
Gilleasbaig Skirving (fig.4). Thug Skirving (1749–1819) a
chosnadh á dealbhan daoine, ged a bha e ag obair mar bu
trice tro mheadhoin na cailce. Rinn e stuidear cailc-ruadh
de Bhurns a bha e fhèin stèidhicht' air an dealbh le
Nasmyth, agus mar sin tha nòisean an 'eadar-theangach-
aidh' bho Nasmyth tro Skirving don ìomhaigh aig Colvin
ag atharrais air 'eadar-theangachadh' bàrdachd Oisein tro
MhacMhuirich. Mar a thachair, tha an dealbh camara aig
Colvin a' toirt gu cuimhne sùbailteachd agus gràs na sgeids
aig Skirving, ach tha e cuideachd a' cur air dòigh
coitheacsa a tha a' pòsadh na h-ìomhaighe ris a' chuspair
as farsainge, Oisein agus ionannachd na h-Alba.

Tha e follaiseach gu bheil ceann Bhurns air a pheantadh
air an dùthaich phronn a chunnacas a-cheana sna
dealbhan camara ann an *Oisein Dall* 's ann an *Scota 01*. Tha
a' chlach shnàidhte bhriste air a cur sìos air ùrlar beòil air a
bheil creag sgapte, samhlaidhean àmhgharach agus
cnàmhan loisgte. Mar phàirt den lèirsgrios seo tha cèis-
leabhraichean – a tha 'na frèam timcheall air ceann
peantaichte Bhurns – agus colbh. Anns a' chèis-
leabhraichean, roghainn nàdarra cùirteir-chùil do
dh'ìomhaigh bàird, tha trì leabhraichean. Tha iad seo 'nam
breacaidhean den chlàr-mholltair ud de dh'iomairt an
t-Soillseachaidh, an *Encyclopaedia Britannica*. Chaidh gach
leabhar fhosgladh gu faiceallach aig reifrens air leth: 's e
sin, *Rhythm* ('Ruitheam'), *Typography* ('Clòdhaireachd')
agus *Art Treasures* ('Ulaidhean Ealain'). Tha fios gur e
reifreansan luchdaichte samhlachail tha seo. Tha
'Ruitheam' ceangailte ri loidhneachan stuadhach falt agus
feusag Oisein, a' chamalag shlais-chuipe a dh'ath-
chruthaicheadh gu tatuaichean baroque ceann a' Mhaori, a
tha ag atharrais air stoidhle shnaoimeach loidhneach nan
làmh-sgrìobhainnean Ceilteach. Tha 'Clòdhaireachd' a'
ceangal ri smaointean teacsaichean, agus cuideachd ri

books. These are editions of that template of Enlightenment enterprise, the *Encyclopaedia Britannica*. Each book has been carefully opened at a particular reference: specifically 'Rhythm', 'Typography', and 'Art Treasures'. Naturally, these are loaded and symbolic references. 'Rhythm' relates to the arcing lines of Ossian's hair and beard, the whiplash curl that was transformed into the baroque tattoos of the Maori head, an echo of the ornate linear style of Celtic manuscript. 'Typography' keys into notions of text, and by extension to the theme of printing. Printing is, of course, the working method of the etching and the photograph, and so recalls the processes that are interrelated in this project as a whole. Finally, 'Art Treasures' is evidently an ironic reference to the products on display. Here the precious world of fine art is strewn across a battered wasteland and the icons of cultural excellence are set against a catastrophic wilderness.

Yet the emblems of cultural achievement are everywhere in this portrait. Atop the pillar, to the left of the poet, is a bouquet of flowers complete with a resplendent red rose. The rose rests on a book, poetry most likely but just possibly a Bible. Both would suit this spectral image of the national bard for his quarrels with the Kirk are well documented while these differences were almost always occasioned by his roving eye. The 'red, red rose' then needs no explanation. Neither, for that matter, do the green rushes piled at the back of the poet's head. These references to Burns's most famous songs, with melodies adapted from established Gaelic airs, signal the highpoint of his achievement. However, more obtuse emblems are scattered throughout the photograph. In the lower right corner a saltire is folded across a pen, a succinct note on the idea of a Scottish national bard. Beyond this a stag's head rests against a swollen hot-water bottle; this novelty item is coloured bright red and shaped in the manner of a heart. Clearly Colvin is referring to Burns's sentimental air *My Heart's in the Highlands* the first two lines of which run 'My heart's in the Highlands, my heart is not here, / My heart's in the Highlands a-chasing the deer'.[37] Moreover this symbol reprises the image of the deer and its associated corre-

cuspair a' chlò-bhualaidh. Tha fios gur e an clò-bhualadh dòigh obrach an dealbhsgrìobhaidh 's an fhotosgrìobhaidh, agus mar sin tha e a' toirt gu cuimhne nan dòighean obrach a tha eadar-dhàimhichte sa phròiseact seo san fharsaingeachd. Mu dheireadh, tha 'Ulaidhean Ealain' a rèir choltais a' toirt tarraing air an t-seòrsa toraidh a tha air a chur m'ar coinneamh. An-seo tha saoghal prìseil na h-àrd ealain sgapte tarsainn air dùthaich leadairte lom agus tha suaicheantais an fheabhais chuiltearail air an cur an aghaidh fàsach rùisgt' an lèirsgrios.

Air a shon sin tha suaicheantais a' choileanaidh chuiltearail air feadh an deilbh-dhuine seo. Air bàrr a' chuilbh, air taobh clì a' bhàird, tha badan fhlùraichean le ròs brèagha dearg 'nam measg. Tha an ròs sìnte air leabhar bàrdachd, a rèir coltais, ach dh'fhaodadh e bhith 'na Bhìoball, oir thigeadh gin seach gin ris an ìomhaigh thaibhsich seo den bhàrd nàiseanta – tha pàipear gu leòr air a chuid chonnspaidean ris an Eaglais, agus mar bu trice b' i a shùil shiùbhlach a bu choireach ris na h-eas-aontaidhean seo. Mar sin cha leigear a leas an 'ròs dearg dearg' no an luachair uaine a th' air a càrnadh air chùl ceann a' bhàird a mhìneachadh. Tha na reifreansan seo ris na h-òrain as ainmeile aig Burns, air fuinn òrain aithnichte Ghàidhlig, a' comharradh mullach a shoirbheachais. Ge-tà, tha suaicheantais nas doilleire air an sgapadh air feadh an deilbh chamara. San oisinn ìochdraich dheis tha crann na h-Alba air a phasgadh tarsainn air peann, nota soilleir air nòisean a' bhàird nàiseanta Albannaich. Taobh thall seo tha ceann daimh an taice ri botal-uisge-teth tòcte; tha an t-annas seo air a dhathadh làn dearg 's air chumadh cridhe. Tha e follaiseach gu bheil Colvin a' toirt tarraing air an òran tiamhaidh ud aig Burns *My Heart's in the Highlands*, far a bheil a' chiad dà shreath a' ruith 'My heart's in the Highlands, my heart is not here, / My heart's in the Highlands a-chasing the deer'.[37] Tha an samhla seo a' toirt gu cuimhne ìomhaigh an fhèidh cuideachd, agus tha an co-bhuintealas aige ri Fuadachd nan Gaidheal follaiseach san t-sreath *Oisein Dall*. A' crìochnachadh an t-samhlachais eapaigreamaich san oisinn ìochdraich dheis seo den *Dealbh de Raibeart Burns* tha cruinne brùite plastaig le farchan 'na shuidhe air a mhullach. Tha am farchan a' toirt tarraing air ciùird a' chlachaire agus cuideachd air an Òrd Chlachaireach, comann cruinneach anns an robh dreuchd fhosgarra aig a' bhàrd.

Tha an *Dealbh de Raibeart Burns* tha seo, ma-thà, 'na thòimhseachan dìomhair loma-làn tabhainn, còmhdach-aidh shocair agus cheanglaichean eadhoin nas saoire. Anns an oisinn ìochdraich chlì tha ceann a' Mhaori a' nochdadh a-rithist, ach an turas seo tha gnùis a' bhàird a' sgaoileadh thairis. Gu ìre bhig tha seo ag aithneachadh mar a thug Burns thuige fhèin a' phearsantachd aig sluagh

spondence with the Highland Clearances is evident in the *Blind Ossian* series. Completing the epigrammatic symbolism in this lower right hand corner of the *Portrait of Robert Burns* is a crushed plastic globe on top of which sits a mallet. The mallet is an allusion to the mason's trade and by extension to the Masonic Order, a worldwide organisation in which the national bard played a four-square role.

This *Portrait of Robert Burns*, then, is a cryptic puzzle full of suggestion, discreet quotation and even freer association. In the bottom left corner the Maori head reappears, but this time it has been overlain with the features of the poet. To some extent this recognises the sense in which Burns took the character of a 'native' people, the Scottish peasantry, as his subject and muse. In respect of this the two black candles to the right of the poet's head allude to the idea of an altar, and specifically to the devil-worship that was the core of the epic tale *Tam o' Shanter*. A more obtuse notion is presented in the centre foreground where there is a smashed portrait of Elvis Presley. Elvis is an established theme in Colvin's work, most notably canonised in his project *The Two Ways of Life* from 1991, and symbolising an omnipresent secular deity. Within this portrait, and strictly in the Scottish context, Elvis has been subject to an iconoclastic destruction and replaced with the figure of Burns. All in all here is a Burns for the modern age, a beautiful apparition set upon a shattered landscape filled with the scorched and random symbols of a postmodern culture. And, through all this, the still serene face of the poet contemplates a distant prospect.

With this work Colvin has created a portrait worthy of the tradition it represents. His *Portrait of Robert Burns* stands in the lineage of Nasmyth and Skirving, respectful of its ancestry yet reflecting present circumstance. In all this *Burns* is a dignified and decorous homage to human and humane sentiment – a worthy endowment to the democratic and celebratory tradition of Scottish portraiture. However, a darker mood returns to Colvin's work in his portrait study of Sir Walter Scott. In part this is occasioned by the selection of Bertel Thorvaldsen's marble bust of the writer as the

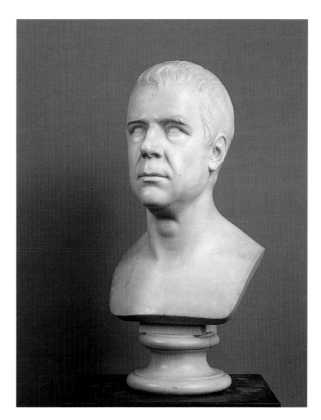

Fig.5 · Bertel Thorvaldsen, *Sir Walter Scott*
Scottish National Portrait Gallery

Fig.5 · Bertel Thorvaldsen, *Sir Bhàtar Scott*
Galaraidh Nàiseanta Albannach nan Dealbhan Daoine

'dùthchasach' – tuath na h-Alba – mar chuspair 's mar cheòlraidh. A rèir seo tha an dà choinnil dhuibh air taobh deas ceann a' bhàird a' bruidhinn air nòisean na h-altrach, 's gu sònraichte air an adhradh-dheamhan aig cridhe an duain-eachdraidh *Tam o' Shanter*. Tha nòisean nas doilleire air a chur an cèill ann am meadhoin an ùrlair-bheòil far a bheil dealbh Elvis Presley 'na spealgan. Tha Elvis 'na chuspair cunbhalach an obair Cholvin. Tha e air a naomhachadh air leth 'na phròiseact *An Dà Dhòigh Bheatha* bho 1991, 's e a' samhlachadh dia saoghalta uile-làthaireach. Am broinn an deilbh-dhuine seo, agus buileach anns a' choitheacsa Albannach, dh'fhuiling Elvis sgrios ìoconobhristeach agus chaidh pearsa Bhurns a chur 'na àite. Uile gu lèir, seo Burns do shaoghal an latha an-diugh, tanasg bòidheach air a chur air dùthaich bhriste bhrùite a tha air a lìonadh air thuaiream le samhlaidhean loisgte a' chuilteir iar-nodha. Throimhe seo air fad tha gnùis a' bhàird, socair sèimh fhathast, a' coimhead fada bhuaithe.

Anns an obair seo chruthaich Colvin dealbh duine as fiù an dualchas a tha e a' riochdachadh. Tha an *Dealbh de Raibeart Burns* aige a' seasamh ann an sloinntireachd Nasmyth agus Skirving, measail air a shinnsreachd ach 'na

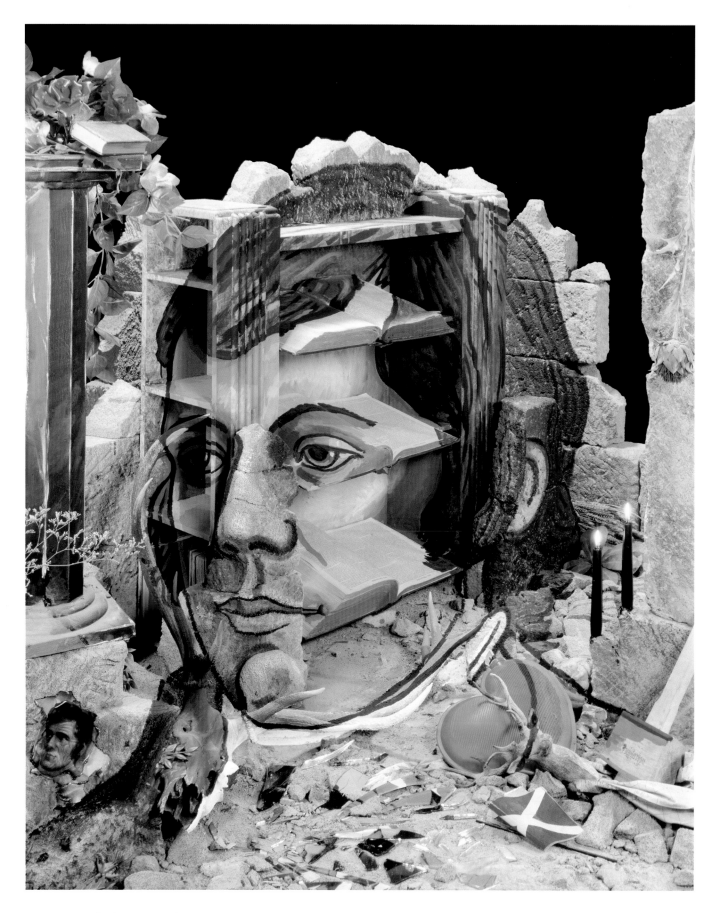

Cat.12 **Portrait of Robert Burns** · Clàr 12 **Dealbh de Raibeart Burns**

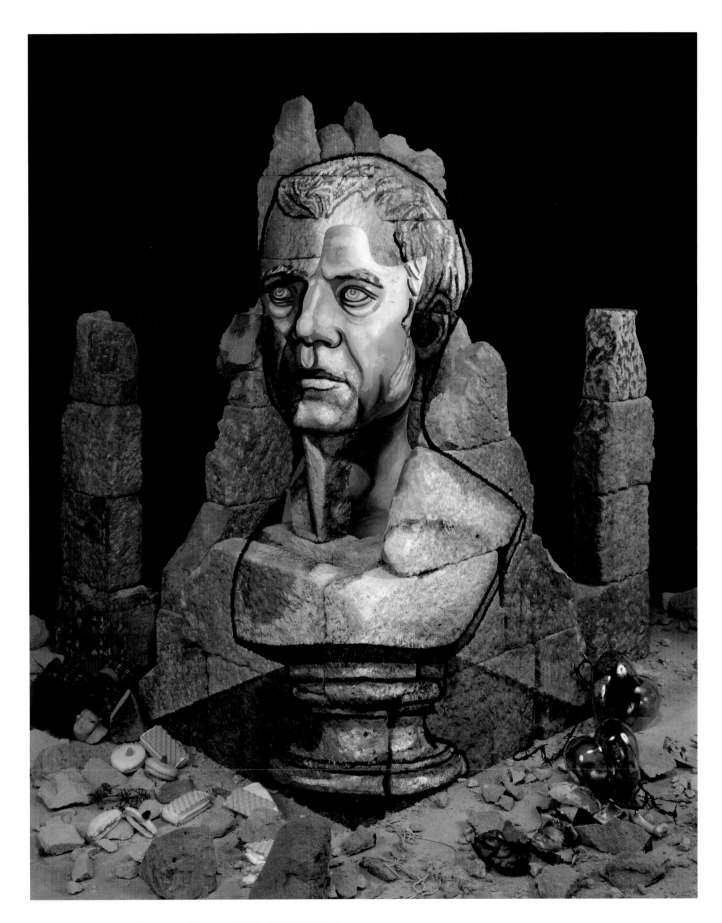

Cat.13 **Portrait of Sir Walter Scott** · Clàr 13 **Dealbh de Shir Bhàtar Scott**

model for his image (fig.5). Thorvaldsen (1770–1844) was a Danish neoclassical sculptor and sometime associate of the influential Antonio Canova (1757–1822) in Rome. His bust of Scott which is a cold, somewhat imperious, likeness of his subject was completed in 1834, two years after the writer's death. But, consequent to this, the dark tragedy of this image returns the project to the overwhelming melancholy of the *Blind Ossian* images.

Sir Walter Scott emerges, naturally, in this pantheon of Scottish bards as heir to the tradition of the Border ballads, the esteemed author of those Romantic novels often celebrating Scottish and Highland history, and as a progenitor of Scottish kitsch. His reputation, in the nineteenth century, attained the level of an international cult and eclipsed that of any other Scot. His longer poems, like *The Lay of the Last Minstrel*, 1805 and *The Lady of the Lake*, 1810, established a predilection for the Romanticism that would spread throughout Europe after 1815. Likewise, his novels created a mood for historical epics with a sentimental ambience and virtuous manner that chimed with public taste. Those set in Scotland, like *Waverley*, 1814, *Rob Roy*, 1818, and the exceptional *The Heart of Midlothian* of the same year, broadly provided a sense of Scottish history and Highland life that readers found compatible with a post-Union Britain. However, despite the Ossianic feel of some of Scott's verse, notably the descriptions of Highland landscape in *The Lady of the Lake*, and indeed the epic battle scenes in a number of the novels, Scott's relationship with Macpherson's 'Ossian' was equivocal. In part this was occasioned by Scott's personal friendship with Malcolm Laing, the historian, who did much to undermine Macpherson's account of Celtic history in his introduction to *The Poems of Ossian*, 1805.[38] More pertinent, perhaps, was his innate conservatism and pro-Union sympathy, a condition that allows William Ferguson to claim that 'Scott went with the tide, keen not to strike an anti-English or anti-unionist note'.[39]

Whatever the subtleties of Scott's relation to Macpherson's oeuvre he is presented here in the lineage of Scotland's bards. For all that he would be cruelly decried as 'a sham bard of a sham nation'[40] Scott remains a monumental

sgàthan air cor an t-saoghail an-diugh. A thaobh seo air fad tha *Burns* 'na ùmhlachd uasal stuama do dh'fhaireachdainnean cneasta chlann daoine – tiodhlac fiachail do dhualchas fàilteach sluafhlaitheach nan dealbhan-daoine Albannach. Ge-tà tha faireachdainn nas duirche a' tilleadh gu obair Cholvin 'na stuidear dealbhach de Shir Bhàtar Scott. Gu ìre 's e as coireach ri seo gun do thagh e mar mholltair an ceann màrmoir a rinn Bertel Thorvaldsen den sgrìobhaiche (fig.5). Bha Thorvaldsen (1770–1844) 'na shnaidheadair nuachlasaigeach ás an Danmhairg a bha uaireigin 'na chompanach don t-snaidheadair phrionnsail sin Antonio Canova (1757–1822) anns an Ròimh. Chrìochnaich e ceann Scott, a tha 'na choltas fuar, car ìmpireil, den chuspair, ann an 1834, dà bhliadhna as dèidh bàs an sgrìobhaiche. Mar thoradh, tha bròn-chluich dhubh na h-ìomhaighe seo a' tilleadh a' phròiseict gu bròn uabhasach *Oisein Dall*.

Tha fios gu bheil Sir Bhàtar Scott a' seasamh a-mach am measg bàird mhòra na h-Alba mar oighre dualchas laoidhean nan Crìochan, mar ùghdar urramach nan nobhailean Romansach sin a tha cho tric a' toirt gu cuimhne eachdraidh na h-Alba 's nan Gaidheal, agus mar chiad shinnsir ealain-shuarach neo *kitsch* na h-Alba. Dh'èirich a chliù anns an naoidheamh ceud deug gu ìre creideamh brèige eadar-nàiseanta agus chuir e gach Albannach eile san dubhar. Chuir a dhàintean as fhaide, leithid *The Lay of the Last Minstrel*, 1805, agus *The Lady of the Lake*, 1810, air chois tlachd anns an Romansachd a sgaoil air feadh na Roinn Eòrpa as dèidh 1815. Air an aon dòigh, chruthaich na nobhailean aige blas do dh'eapaigean eachdraidheil anns an robh àrainneachd fhaireachdainneach agus stoidhle bheusach a chòrd ri blas an t-sluaigh. Anns an fharsaingeachd chuir an fheadhainn a bh' air am planndachadh an Albainn – leithid *Waverley*, 1814, *Rob Roy*, 1818, agus an sàr *Heart of Midlothian* bhon aon bhliadhna – air tairgse dealbh de dh'eachdraidh na h-Alba 's de shaoghal nan Gaidheal a thàinig gu comhartail an inntinn an luchd-leughaidh ri Breatainn as dèidh an Aonaidh. Ge-tà, a dh'ainneoin a' bhlais Oiseinich a bh' air cuid de bhàrdachd Scott, gu sònraichte na cunntaisean air dùthaich na Gaidhealtachd ann an *The Lady of the Lake*, agus gu dearbh na seallaidhean mòrdhalach catha ann am feadhainn de na nobhailean, 's ann dà-ghuthach a bha buintealas Scott ri 'Oisein' MhicMhuirich. Gu ìre b' e càirdeas pearsanta Scott ri Maol-Chaluim Laing (an t-eachdraiche a rinn mòran gu cunntas MhicMhuirich air eachdraidh nan Ceilteach a spreadhadh 'na roi-ràdha do *The Poems of Ossian*, 1805) a bu choireach.[38] Na bu dlùithe do chnag na cùise, 's dòcha, bha an glèidhteachas a bu dual dha agus an taice a bha e a' toirt don Aonadh, nithean a leig le Uilleam MacFhearghais

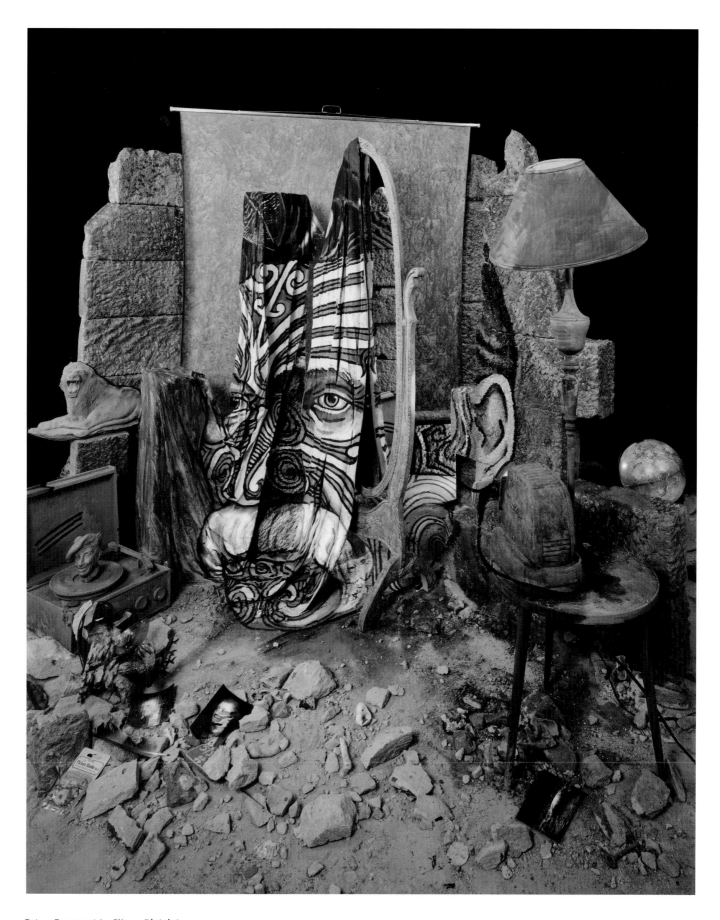

Cat.14 **Fragment I** · Clàr 14 **Bloigh I**

figure in Scottish culture. Within Colvin's pantheon he is represented austerely. His image, *Portrait of Sir Walter Scott* (cat.13), is that of a marble bust, complete with pedestal. The features follow the hard and cool aloofness of Thorvaldsen's original, and there is certainly none of the warmth and vitality of David Wilkie's famous representation of Scott in his *Abbotsford Family* portrait of 1817. The background for the Colvin portrait is a ruined tower complete with broken buttresses. The architecture of this set, while it recollects the ruins of *Blind Ossian*, recalls also the Gothic Revival spire of the Scott Monument in Edinburgh. Recessed in the architecture, in Colvin's work, is a naked female torso, an ironic 'canvas' for the reserved features of the writer. Certainly this is a dark and ascetic image, but it is leavened by the detritus at the base of Scott's 'plinth'. This includes a selection of cakes and biscuits, a reference to Scotland as 'the land o' cakes',[41] not to mention the notorious national diet. And, in the foreground to the right of Scott's pedestal, the omnipresent 'Maori' head that is repeated, along with Scott's own, in two blue plastic heart-shaped moulds; a cold refrain of the passionate red heart presented in the portrait of Robert Burns.

One further symbol creeps into the *Portrait of Sir Walter Scott*. At the left of the photograph, part hidden in the debris and rocks, is that sardonic emblem of modern Scottish identity, the 'Jimmy' hat. This headgear, tartan cap complete with fake orange hair, has become an ironic reference to cultural and national independence. The humour in this is caricature, and the defiance deferential and apolitical. In this sense it echoes the fatal legacy of Scott's achievement. In 1822, on the occasion of George IV's state visit to Scotland, it was Scott who choreographed the pageantry and festival. In some degree the whole paraphernalia of kitsch tartanry can be traced to this event. Herein Highland culture and history became picturesque entertainment and the dissenting aspects of the Celtic world, with Ossian as its most pertinent representative, became a tourist's trinket. In some degree the coldness of this portrait is traceable to this history. Colvin, however, can be seen to be compiling a gallery of portrait heads that meditate on the theme of

a bhith cumail a-mach gun deachaidh Scott 'leis an làn, 's e cùramach nach buaileadh e pong an aghaidh Shasainn no an Aonaidh'.[39]

Ga brith dè cho sùbailte 's a bha, no nach robh, buintealas Scott ri obair MhicMhuirich, seo e am measg bàird na h-Alba. Ged a chaidh aoireadh gu dubh mar 'bhàrd masa-fìor aig nàisean masa-fìor'[40] tha Scott fhathast 'na phearsa uabhasach mòr ann an cuiltear na h-Alba. Ann an comann-diathan Cholvin tha e air a chur an cèill le cruadal. Tha 'ìomhaigh, *Dealbh de Shir Bhàtar Scott* (clàr 13), 'na cheann màrmoir, seadh 's le bonn. Tha a ghnùis a' leantainn uabhar cruaidh fionnar a' chinn a rinn Thorvaldsen, agus chan eil sgeul air a' bhlàths no air a' bheòthalachd a ghlac Dàibhidh Wilkie nuair a nochd e Scott 'na dhealbh *Abbotsford Family* ann an 1817. 'S e ùrlar-cùil an deilbh-dhuine aig Colvin tùr pronn le conbhallais bhriste. Tha ailtireachd an t-seata seo a' toirt gu cuimhne tobhtaichean *Oisein Dall* agus binnean nuaghothach Carragh Scott ann an Dùn Èideann. Domhainn san ailtireachd an obair Cholvin tha brollach rùisgte boireannaich, 'canbhas' ìoranach do ghnùis stuama an sgrìobhaiche. Tha fios gur e ìomhaigh dhorcha chruaidh-chràbhach tha seo, ach tha i air a h-aotromachadh leis an sprùilleach aig bonn 'clach-stèidhidh' Scott. 'Nam measg seo tha taghadh de chèicean 's de bhriosgaidean, a tha a' toirt tarraing air Alba 'na 'tìr bhonnach',[41] gun luaidh air diathad nàiseanta na mollachd. Anns an ùrlar-bheòil air taobh deas a' bhuinn aig Scott tha ceann uile-làthaireach a' Mhaori, a tha air atharrais, còmhla ri ceann Scott fhèin, ann an dà mholltair phlastaig air chumadh cridhe: sèist fhuar air a' chridhe phaiseanta dhearg a fhuair sinn san dealbh de Raibeart Burns.

Tha aon samhla eile ag èaladh a-staigh do *Dhealbh Shir Bhàtair Scott*. Air taobh clì an deilbh chamara, leth-fhalaichte am measg an sprùillich 's nan creag, tha an suaicheantas sardònach sin de dh'ionannachd na h-Alba an-diugh, an ad 'Jimmy'. Tha a' cheannabheart seo, anns a bheil bonaid thartain còmhla ri leadan de ghruag ruadh masa-fìor, air a dhol 'na reifreans ìoranach ri neo-eisimeileachd chuilteireil agus nàiseanta. 'S e mag-dhealbh a th' anns an fheala-dhà an-seo, agus tha an dùbhlan a tha i toirt seachad ùmhail agus neo-phoileataigeach. A thaobh seo tha e toirt gu cuimhne an dìleab bhàsmhor aig na rinn Scott. Ann an 1822, nuair a thug Deòrsa IV cuairt stàite air Alba, b' e Scott a chuir air dòigh an taisbeanachd 's an fhèis. Gu ìre bhig faodar a h-uile rud a bhuineas ri trealaich shuarach an tartain a shloinneadh suas chun an tachartais seo. 'S ann ri linn a chaidh dualchas agus eachdraidh nan Gaidheal 'nan dibhearsain àlainn 's a chaidh na nithean a b' easaontaile ann an saoghal nan Ceilteach, aig nach robh riochdaire na b' iomchaidhe na

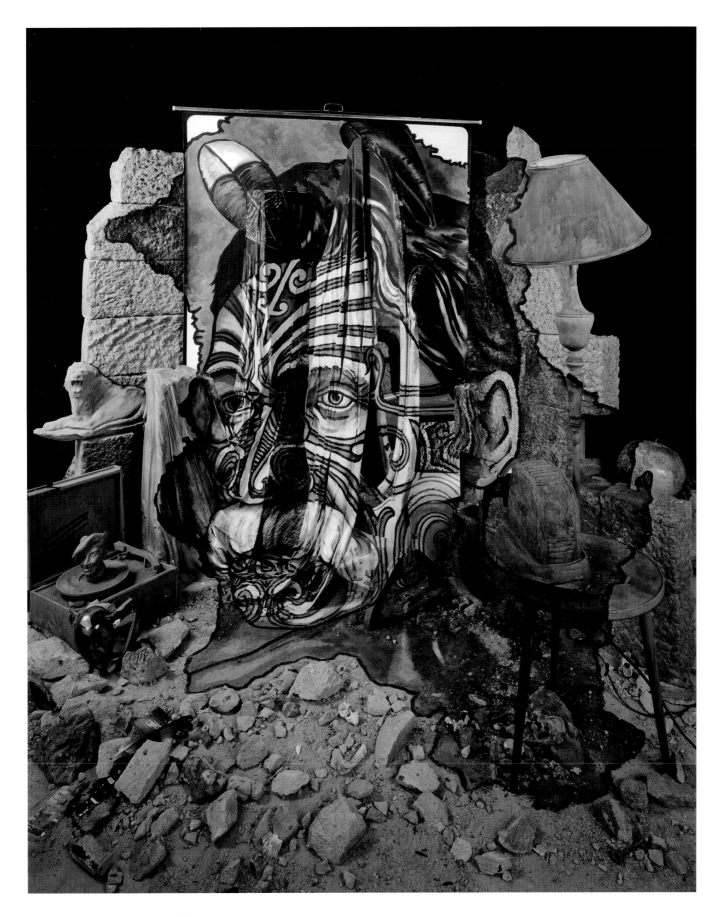

Cat.15 **Fragment II** · Clàr 15 **Bloigh II**

'identity' in Scotland. In completing the project he has constructed a further series of nine images, collectively titled *Fragments* (cats.14–22), that echoes the introductory sequence on *Blind Ossian*. He has, in fact, taken two generic, but emblematic, figures to create this coda and has concluded his meditation with a 'forged' portrait of James Macpherson himself.

In *Fragment II* is a full-sized portrait of the 'Maori' head that has featured in all the photographs within the project. This pastiche of an anthropological illustration functions as a doppelgänger for Ossian, a mirror to the unknowable 'primitive' poet. The idea that Macpherson had discovered a 'noble savage' in Ossian was absolutely contemporary with his era. Jean-Jacques Rousseau (1712–1778), the political philosopher and originator of the theory of 'the noble savage', was a personal friend of the Enlightenment philosopher, David Hume (1711–1776), and the subject of an exceptional portrait by Allan Ramsay.[42] Rousseau, who famously declaimed that 'man is born free, and everywhere he is in chains', created in his major work of political philosophy *The Social Contract*, 1762, a myth of the 'savage' as an unsullied child of nature. By extension it was assumed that the responses of the 'savage', to nature and to others, were intuitive, sublime and poetic. Consequently Ossian was viewed as the representative of a largely benign 'savage' culture. To this extent James Boswell chose to call Macpherson 'The Sublime Savage',[43] while John Dwyer in his essay on Ossian titles him 'The Melancholy Savage'.[44] The 'Maori' head, then, is a reflection of Ossian, a mirror that unites the Celtic bard with his primal kin.

In the photograph, *Fragment III* (cat.16), the image of the Maori has been greatly enlarged and set against a viewing screen. In front of the screen is a slide projector complete with discreet images from the film *Brigadoon*. In some degree the subject of photography, as a means of recording 'truth', is reprised in this work. Throughout the series the Maori has been transformed into Ossian and vice versa. Equally, the tattoos emblazoned on the Maori head constantly metamorphose into the Celtic patterns of Ossian's world. In which case the sense of an 'authentic' or 'original' being is

Oisein, 'nan seudan siùbhlaiche. 'S i an eachdraidh sa gu ìre a tha a' mìneachadh fuarachd an deilbh seo. Chithear ge-tà gu bheil Colvin a' cruinneachadh galaraidh de dhealbhan cinn a tha a' cnuasachadh cuspair na 'h-ionannachd' ann an Albainn. Ann a bhith a' toirt a' phròiseict gu buil thog e sreath eile de naoi ìomhaighean, air a bheil an tiotal trusaidh *Bloighean* (clàir 14–22), a tha a' toirt gu cuimhne an t-sreath *Oisein Dall* a bh' aig toiseach ghnothaichean. Gu dearbh, thug e thuige dà phearsa a bha gnèitheach ach suaicheantail gus an coda seo a chruthachadh, agus chrìochnaich e a chnuasachd le ìomhaigh 'fheall-dheilbhte' de Sheumas Bàn MacMhuirich fhèin.

Ann am *Bloigh II* tha dealbh làn-mheudachd den aona cheann 'Maori' a nochd sna dealbhan camara gu lèir anns a' phròiseact. Tha an colmadh seo de dh'fhigear daoineòlach a' frithealadh mar cho-choisiche do dh'Oisein, mar sgàthan don bhàrd 'phrìomhadail' nach gabh eòlas a chur air. Bha an smuain gun do lorg MacMhuirich 'samhanach uasal' ann an Oisein tur co-aoiseach ris an linn anns an robh e beò. Bha Jean-Jacques Rousseau (1712–1778), am feallsanach poileataigeach a thug nòisean an 't-samhanaich uasail' gu bith 's a thuirt gu h-ainmeil gun do 'rugadh mac an duine ann an saorsa' agus gu bheil e 'anns gach àit' ann an slabhraidhean', 'na charaid pearsanta don fheallsanach Shoillseachaidh Dàibhidh Hume (1711–1776) agus 'na chuspair do dhealbh-duine suaicheanta a rinn Ailean Ramsay.[42] 'Na shàr obair feallsanachd phoileataigeach *An Cùmhnant Sòisealta*, 1762, chruthaich Rousseau uirsgeul den 't-samhanach' mar phàiste neo-thruaillte nàdair. Bha ri thuigsinn bhuaithe sin gur ann imfhiosach, òirdheirc, bàrdail a bha freagairtean an 't-samhanaich' ri nàdar agus ri càch. Mar sin bha Oisein ga fhaicinn mar riochdaire aig cuiltear 'borb' a bha, anns a' mhòrchuid, suairc. Gus an ìre seo roghnaich Seumas Boisil 'An Samhanach Òirdheirc' a ràdh ri MacMhuirich,[43] agus 'na aiste air Oisein tha Iain Dwyer ag ràdh 'An Samhanach Brònach' ris.[44] 'S e Oisein fhèin, ma-tà, a tha ceann a' Mhaori a' toirt m'ar coinneamh, cleas sgàthan a tha ag aontachadh a' bhàird Cheiltich ri a phrìomh luchd-cinnidh.

Anns an dealbh chamara *Bloigh III* (clàr 16) chaidh ìomhaigh a' Mhaori a mheudachadh gu mòr 's a chur ri sgrìne choimhid. Air beulaibh na sgrìne tha pròiseactar shleamhnan còmhla ri ìomhaighean socair bhon fhilm *Brigadoon*. Gu ìre bhig tha cuspair an fhotosgrìobhaidh, mar mheadhoin air 'fìrinn' a chlàradh, air a thoirt gu cuimhne san obair seo. Air feadh an t-sreath bha am Maori air a dhol 'na Oisein 's Oisein air a dhol 'na Mhaori. Gus an aon ìre, tha na tatuaichean air ceann a' Mhaori ag atharrachadh a-rithist 's a-rithist gu pàtrain Cheilteach

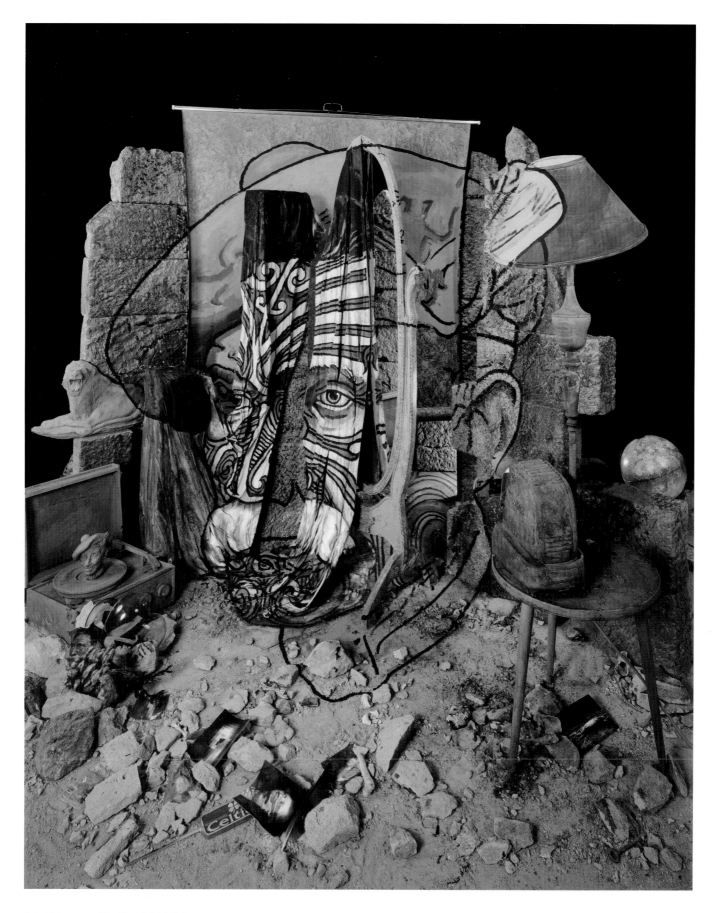

Cat.16 **Fragment III** · Clàr 16 **Bloigh II**

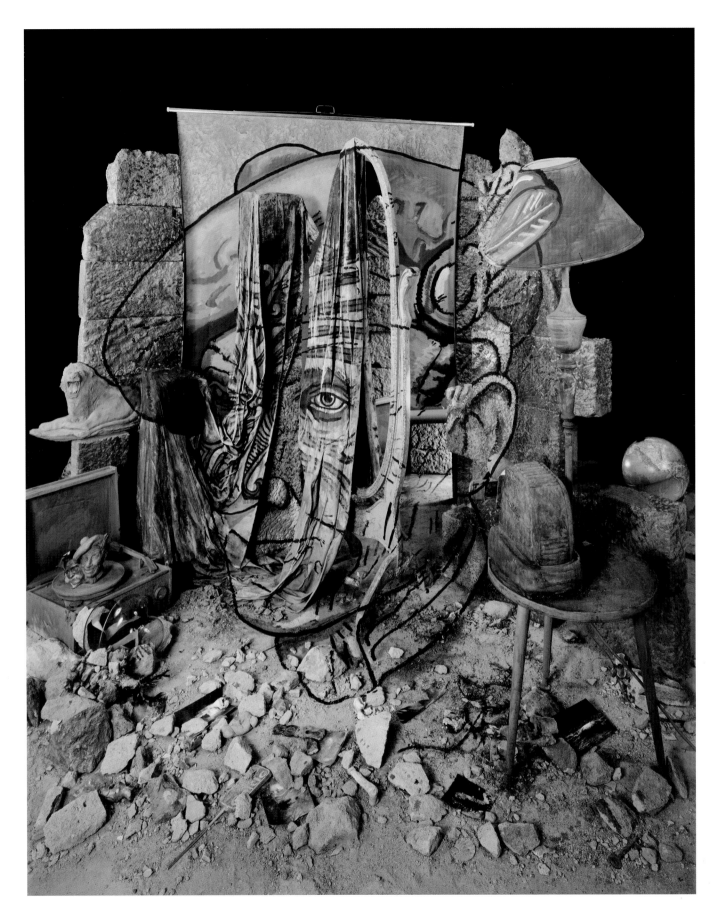

Cat.17 **Fragment IV** · Clàr 17 **Bloigh IV**

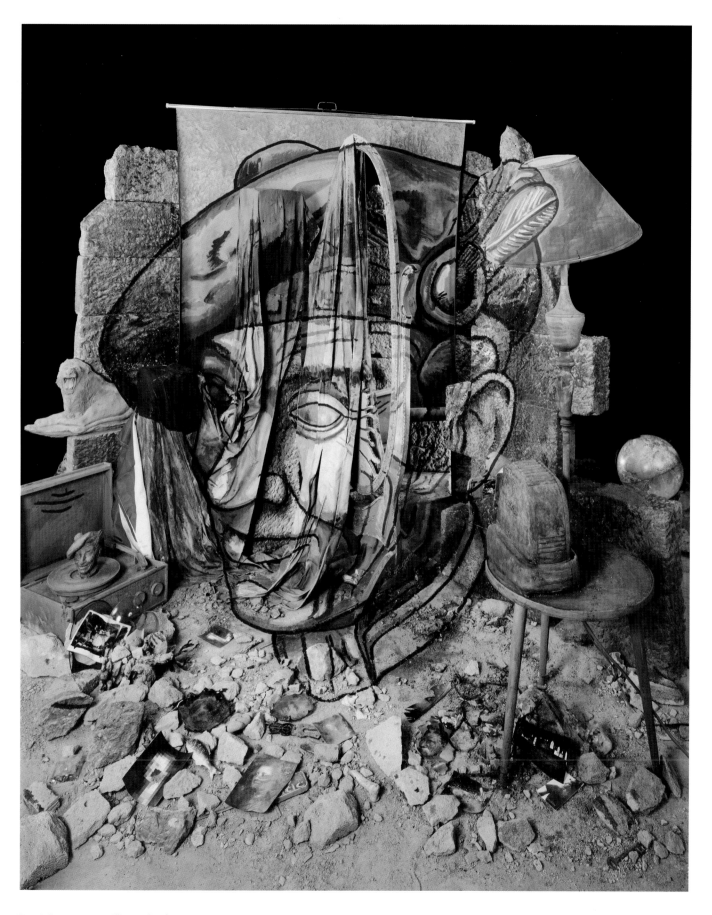

Cat.18 **Fragment V** · Clàr 18 **Bloigh V**

constantly questioned. Simultaneously the materials within the set raise further questions concerning origins and authenticity. The globe to the right side of the photograph asserts a notion of racial interdependence rather than ethnic division. In the bottom left hand corner of the image there is the singed remains of a packet labelled 'Picture Hooks', partly obscured so as to read the word 'Pict'. This is set against a Celtic Football Club confection, again with lettering masked so it reads 'Celt'. Hence, the duality of Celt and Pict is subtly presented as a discourse on the problematic of ancestral roots. All of this is placed, once again, in an apocalyptic wilderness as if to emphasise the fragile and potentially morbid nature of these debates on origins and identity.

At this point Colvin looks to complicate further his gallery of symbolic portraits. To the left of the 'Maori' figure Colvin has placed an aged record player, the echoing chorus of Ossian's song. On the turntable he has balanced a plaster head. Parenthetically, this same head has featured in the landscape of the *Blind Ossian* series and in the photograph titled the *Twa Dogs*. It is a kitsch ornament, a junk-shop cast off comically representing the archetypal 'Highland Laddie', perhaps loosely modelled on the music-hall entertainer Harry Lauder (fig.6). This grinning, inebriated caricature is the subject of Colvin's finale to the Ossian series. Conceived as the antithesis to the blind Ossian figure, this distant relative of the bard is represented in a sequence of photographs showing his transforming and fading features, a series of images tentatively sub-titled 'Blind Harry'.[45]

In the *Fragments* series the set of the Maori portrait gradually disintegrates and the head itself is replaced by the image of the cartoon Highlander. These are sequential 'wasteland' images in which Colvin has reprised the core elements of projector, screen and record player. He also includes the now scorched digital and analogue photographs of James Macpherson himself. With these photographs Colvin has affected a full transformation. Here, he has turned his kaleidoscope of forms and figures such that the various personas of cultural identity meld and mutate. Simultaneously the symbols of national character and

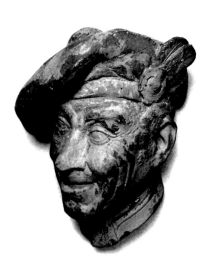

Fig.6 · *Head of a Scotsman*
Ceann Albannaich (Harry Lauder?)

saoghal Oisein. A rèir seo tha nòisean a' bhith 'ùghdarrasaich' neo 'thùsail' ga shìor cheasnachadh. Aig an aon àm tha na nithean am broinn an t-seata a' togail cheistean eile mu dheidhinn fhreumhan agus ùghdarrasachd. Tha an cruinne air taobh deas an deilbh chamara a' cur air adhart nòisean de dh'eadar-eisimeileachd chinealta seach sgaradh nan cinneadh. Ann an oisinn ìochdrach chlì na h-ìomhaighe tha fuighleach dòite pacaid air a bheil *Picture Hooks* ('Dubhain Deilbh'), 's pàirt dheth air a dhubhadh ach gun leughar am facal *Pict* ('Cruithneach'). Tha seo air a chur mu choinneamh suiteas Club Ball-Coise Celtic, a-rithist le litrichean an dubhar ach gun leughar *Celt* ('Ceilteach'). Mar sin tha dùbailteachd a' Cheiltich 's a' Chruithnich air a cur f'ar comhair mar aithris air imcheist nam freumhan sinnsreil. Tha seo uile air a chur, uair eile, ann am fàsach an lèirsgrios mar gun robh e a' cur cudrom air nàdar bristeach ('s ma dh'fhaoidte mì-fhallain) nan deasbadan seo mu fhreumhan 's mu ionannachd.

Aig an ìre seo tha Colvin a' tòiseachadh air corra char eile a chur 'na ghalaraidh de dhealbhan samhlachail dhaoine. Air taobh clì a' phearsa 'Maori' chuir e seann ghramafon, mac-talla sèist nan òran aig Oisein, agus chothromaich e ceann plàst air a' chlàr-thionndaidh. Nochd an aona cheann seo mar eadar-ràdh ann an dùthaich an t-sreath *Oisein Dall* agus anns an dealbh chamara air a bheil an *Dà Chù*. Tha e 'na bhall-maise ealain shuaraich, 'na fhuigheall á bùth sgudail a tha a' riochdachadh le feala-dhà a' 'Ghille Ghaidhealaich' phrìomh-shamhlachail, 's e a' las-atharrais gu ìre air glaoicire ud nan tallachan ciùil, Harry Lauder (fig.6). Tha am mag-dhealbh misgeach braoiseach seo 'na chuspair don t-soraidh slàn a tha Colvin a' fàgail aig sreath Oisein. 'S e air a chruthachadh mar anatràchdas pearsa Oisein Doill, tha am fear-cinnidh fad-ás seo aig a' bhàrd air a riochdachadh ann an sreath dhealbhan camara a tha a' nochdadh a ghnùis a' cruth-atharrachadh 's a' dol bhuaithe, sreath ìomhaighean air a bheil am fo-thiotal teagmhach 'Eanraig Dall'.[45]

Anns an t-sreath *Bloighean* tha seata dealbh a' Mhaori a' sìor thuiteam ás a-chèile 's tha ìomhaigh Gaidheal nan cartun a' gabhail àite a' chinn fhèin. 'S e ìomhaighean sreathail 'fàsaich' tha seo anns a bheil Colvin a' toirt gu cuimhne bun-eileamaidean a' phròiseactair, na sgrìne 's a' ghramafon, ach tha e a' cur riutha na dealbhan camara meurach agus analog de Sheumas Bàn fhèin 's iad a-nis dòite. Leis na dealbhan camara seo chuir Colvin làn chruth-atharrachadh an gnìomh. An-seo chuir e car d'a chalìodoscop de chruthan 's de phearsachan gu ìre 's gu bheil na diofar phearsantachdan de dh'ionannachd chuiltearail a' colmadh 's a' mùthadh. Aig an aon àm tha

50

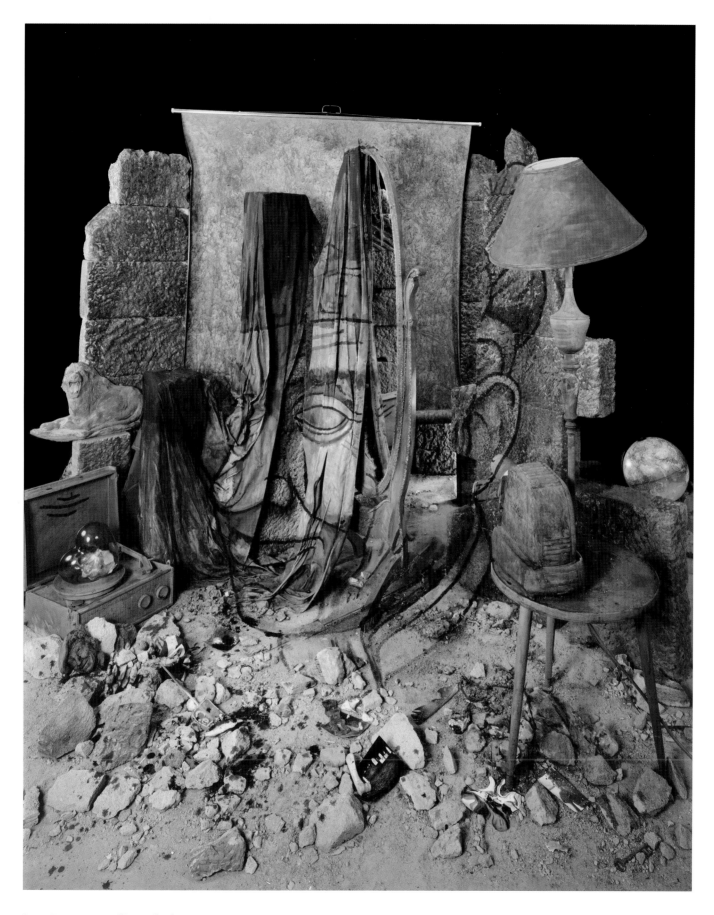

Cat.19 **Fragment VI** · Clàr 19 **Bloigh VI**

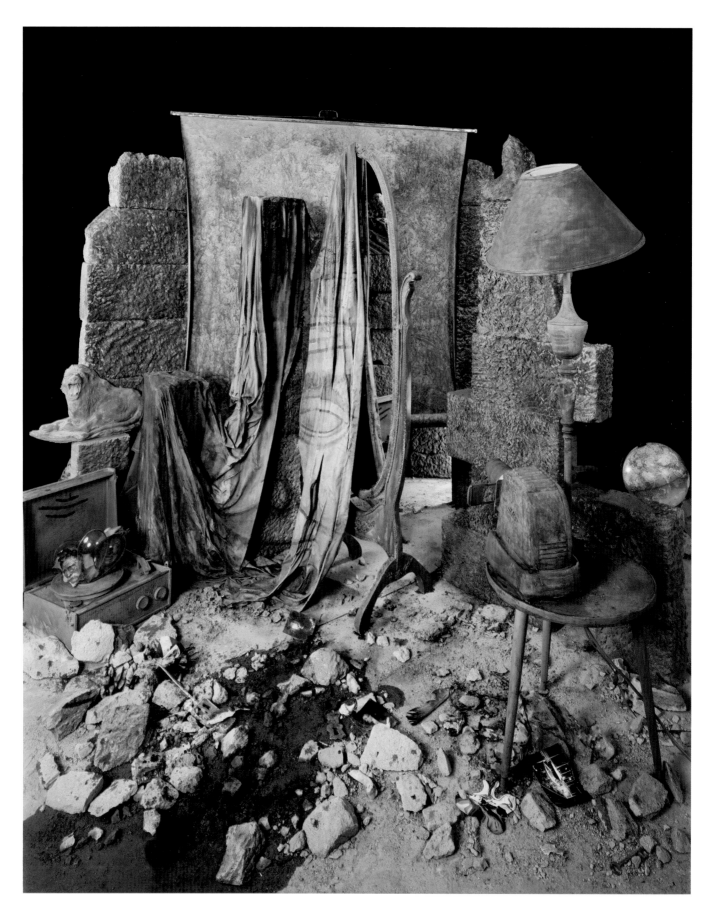

Cat.20 **Fragment VII** · Clàr 20 **Bloigh VII**

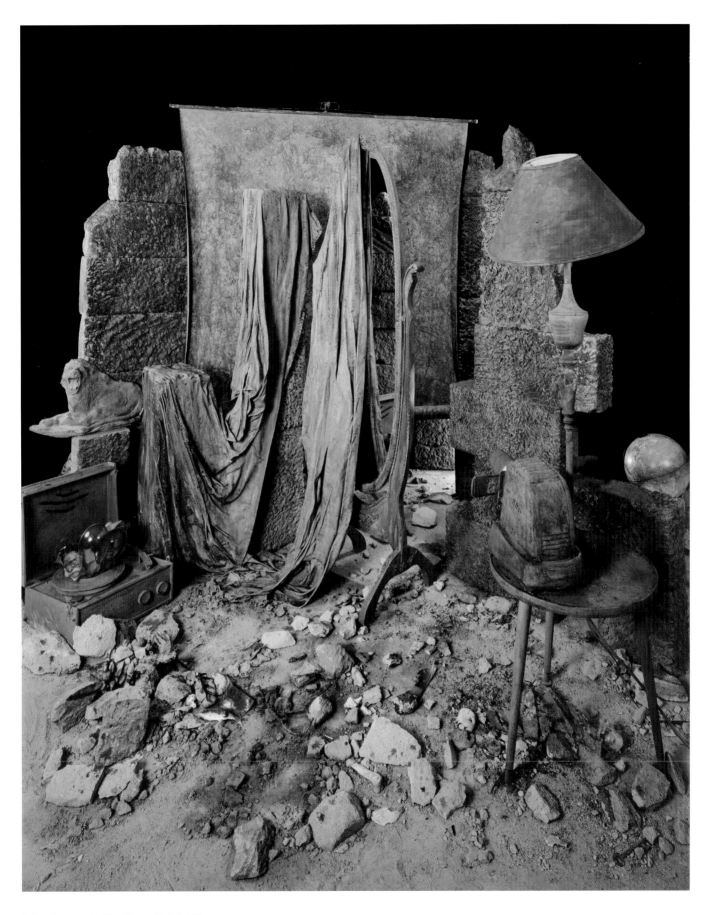

Cat.21 **Fragment VIII** · Clàr 21 **Bloigh VIII**

distinctiveness reveal both their diversity and their universality. Hence, the figure of 'savage' Ossian folds into the 'noble' Maori; Burns and Scott become twin to 'Blind Harry' who is now a composite poet, entertainer and cartoon. And all are kin and companion to the mysterious, controversial figure of James Macpherson.

It is Macpherson, himself, who acts as originator to this entire project and, rightly, Colvin has produced a portrait of the controversial poet as a grand finale. In a fitting manner he has created an image saturated in ambiguity, for this work is a kind of 'compound forgery'. The template for Colvin's constructed photograph of Macpherson is the portrait of the poet by an unknown artist after Sir Joshua Reynolds and currently held at the Scottish National Portrait Gallery (fig.7). The original painting is held in the Egremont Collection at Petworth House and the Scottish version is either a copy by Reynolds, or by some other hand.[46] There is, then, a delicious correspondence between Macpherson's disputed reputation as 'forger' and the authenticity of his official portrait in Scotland. Colvin compounds this by placing his image against the common backdrop of the 'Maori' and 'Blind Harry' sets. However, rather than paint the portrait onto the set, the technique of all the attendant pieces, he has used computer software to manoeuvre the head into the scene. More than this, he has taken the 'original' portrait and manipulated it so that it 'resembles' a painted work by Colvin, and then set it onto the stage. This is Colvin's 'forgery', created to reprise the spectacular, surreal, and infamous debate surrounding Macpherson's life and work.

With the *Fragments* cycle of transforming photographs of the 'Maori', 'Blind Harry', and finally 'Macpherson' himself (frontispiece), Colvin has completed his journey into Scottish life and character, a trail manifestly littered with heroes, apparitions and phantoms. For these works are surely the dreamscapes of a nation, as stable as phosphorus and as solid as air.

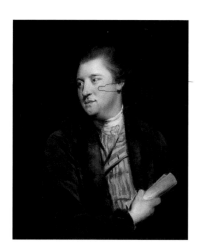

Fig.7 · Unknown artist after Sir Joshua Reynolds, *James Macpherson*
Scottish National Portrait Gallery

Fig.7 · Ealainiche gun urra air dhòigh Shir Joshua Reynolds, *Seumas MacMhuirich*
Galaraidh Nàiseanta Albannach nan Dealbhan Daoine

samhlaidhean na pearsantachd 's na suaicheantachd nàiseanta a' nochdadh an dà chuid an iomadaidheachd agus an coitcheannachd. Mar sin, tha pearsa an Oisein 'bhuirb' a' filleadh anns a' Mhaori 'uasal', agus tha Burns agus Scott a' dol 'nan leithein aig 'Eanraig Dall' a tha a-nis 'na cholmadh de bhàrd, de ghlaoicire 's de chartun. Agus tha iad uile 'nan càirdean 's 'nan companaich do phearsa dìomhair connspaideach Sheumais Bhàin MhicMhuirich.

'S e MacMhuirich fhèin as freumh don phròiseact seo air fad, agus chan eil e ach ceart gun do dheasaich Colvin dealbh den bhàrd chonnspaideach mar shoraidh mhòr slàn. Ann an dòigh iomchaidh chruthaich e ìomhaigh a th' air a bogadh ann an dà-sheaghachd, oir tha an obair seo 'na seòrsa de 'dh'ioma-mheallsgrìobhadh'. 'S e an cliath-chlàr don dealbh-chamara thogte a rinn Colvin de MhacMhuirich an dealbh den bhàrd a rinn ealainiche gun urra air dhòigh Shir Joshua Reynolds a tha ga chumail an-dràsta ann an Galaraidh Nàiseanta Albannach nan Dealbhan Daoine (fig.7). Tha an dealbh tùsach ann an Cruinneachadh Egremont aig Taigh Phetworth agus tha am breacadh Albannach 'na lethbhreac le Reynolds no le làmh air choreigin eile.[46] Mar sin tha co-fhreagairt bhlast' ann eadar cliù connspaideach MhicMhuirich mar 'mheallsgrìobhadair' agus ùghdarrasachd a dheilbh oifigeil an Alba. Tha Colvin a' dèanamh seo nas dorra le bhith a' cur na h-ìomhaigh aige an aghaidh cùirtear-cùil cumanta seataichean a' 'Mhaori' 's 'Eanraig Dhoill'. Ge-tà, seach an dealbh a pheantadh air an t-seata, an dòigh obrach a chleachd e sna pìosan a tha 'na chois, chleachd e bathar-bog compiutair gus an ceann a ghluasad a-staigh don t-sealladh. A bharrachd air seo, ghabh e an dealbh 'tùsail' agus làimhsich e e gus gu bheil e 'coltach' ri obair pheantaichte le Colvin, agus shuidhich e an uair sin air an àrd ùrlar e. Seo 'meallsgrìobhadh' Cholvin, a chruthaich e gus an deasbaireachd shuaicheanta, osfìrinneach, mhì-chliùiteach mu bheatha 's obair MhicMhuirich a thoirt gu cuimhne.

Le cuairt *Bloighean* nan dealbhan ath-chruthachail den 'Mhaori', de 'dh'Eanraig Dall', agus mu dheireadh de 'MhacMhuirich' fhèin (tùs-dhealbh), chrìochnaich Colvin a thuras a-staigh do bheatha 's do phearsantachd na h-Alba, rathad a tha gu follaiseach air a bhreacadh le gaisgich, le taibhsean 's le tanasgan. Oir 's e 's cinnteach na h-obraichean seo na tìrean aislinge a bhuineas do nàisean, cho daingeann ri fosfar 's cho cruaidh ris an eidhir.

IV

The leitmotif of this entire project has been Calum Colvin's fascination with the figure of Ossian. A spectral figure: part myth, part

IV

B' e *leitmotif* a' phròiseict seo gu lèir an tarraing a tha aig pearsa Oisein do Chalum Colvin. Pearsa taibhseil: pàirt uirsgeul, pàirt 'structar', pàirt 'làimhseachadh'. Ach tha

'construction', part 'manipulation'. But Ossian is real in the sense that his legend has become an intimate part of the national culture, identity, and even psyche. To some degree, then, it is through the mythology of Ossian that Scotland comes to recognise itself, and Colvin has sought to explore the indeterminate nature of this recognition.

Ossian, then, is a mirror image, but a mirror clouded with uncertainty, ambiguity, and fantasy. It is these half-seen features that Colvin has looked to examine – the shadowland between reality and illusion. In consequence, all of these photographs present a dark and mysterious landscape haunted by spectres. Each of the painted heads, and even the subject pictures, are 'translated' from established works of art or from junk-shop icons. Moreover they are reinterpreted in a phantom form, as they each appear as apparitions within the stony landscape. Through this device Colvin has sought to accent the contingent nature of these subjects. They are 'known' through a glass but darkly, they are the icons of cultural identity left open to translation, mediation, and manipulation. In this way, Colvin recognises the conditional, and indeed provisional, nature of culture: its dependence on history, on social needs, and on political circumstance.

As if to highlight this contingency Colvin creates, throughout these photographs, a series of competing dualisms. There are obvious contrasts between Celt and Pict, Highlander and Lowlander, nationalist and unionist, the 'Twa Dogs' of Celtic and Rangers football clubs, even the opposition of the passionate Burns to the austere Scott. But there are also subtler and less certain dualities hidden in these images. It is possible to sense the undercurrent of tension between the thistle and rose in these works, most notably in the portrait of Burns. Likewise there is a discreet dialogue between notions of 'enlightenment' and 'savagery' in almost all the photographs, a dialectic that ingeniously critiques the conceit of 'progress'. In respect of this there is a related contrast between ana-logue and digital technologies, and between old and new cultures. Throughout the series Colvin meditates upon how a thing is both itself and its other, and how culture is a constant search for meaningful synthesis.

Oisein fìor san t-seagh gun deach an sgeulachd aige 'na cuid bhunaiteach de chuiltear, de dh'ionannachd agus eadhoin de dh'aigne an nàisein. Gu ìre air choreigin, ma-thà, 's ann tro uirsgeulachd Oisein a thig Alba gu fèin-aithneachadh, agus dh'fheuch Colvin ri nàdar neo-chinnteach an aithneachaidh seo a rannsachadh.

Tha Oisein 'na ìomhaigh san sgàthan, ma-thà, ach air an sgàthan seo tha sgleò na mì-chinnt, na dà-sheaghachd 's na h-òrachd. Dh'fheuch Colvin ris na h-eileamaidean leth-fhaicsinneach seo – tìr nam faileas eadar fìrinn 's mac-meanmna – a sgrùdadh. Mar thoradh, tha na dealbhan camara sa air fad a' cur an cèill dùthaich dhìomhair dhorcha ga tathaich le taibhsean. Tha gach gin de na cinn pheantaichte, 's eadhoin na dealbhan cuspaireach, air an 'eadar-theangachadh' bho obraichean stèidhichte ealain neo bho shuaicheantais nam bùithtean sgudail. Cuideachd, tha iad air an ath-mhìneachadh ann an cruth taibhseil, 's iad uile a' nochdadh 'nan tanasgan air aghaidh chorrach na dùthcha. Tron innleachd seo dh'fheuch Colvin ri cudrom a chur air nàdar tubaisteach nan cuspairean sa. Chan eil iad air an 'aithneachadh' ach dorcha tro ghlainne, 's e th' annta ach suaicheantais na h-ionannachd chuiltearail a bh' air am fàgail fosgailte do dh'eadar-theangachadh, do dh'eadraiginn 's do làimhseachadh. Air an dòigh seo tha Colvin ag aithneachadh nàdar cùmhnantach, 's gu dearbh sealadach, a' chuilteir: cho eisimeileach 's a tha e air eachdraidh, air feuman sòisealta agus air cor poileataigs.

Mar gun robh e a' caitheamh solas air leth air an tubaisteachd seo tha Colvin a' cruthachadh, air feadh nam fotosgrìobhaidhean sa, sreath de dhùbailteachdan a tha an aghaidh a-chèile. Tha còmhstrithean follaiseach eadar Ceilteach agus Cruithneach, Gaidheal agus Gall, nàiseantach agus aonaidheach, an 'Dà Chù' aig clubaichean ball-coise Rangers agus Celtic, fiùs Burns a tha cho paiseanta fa chomhair Scott a tha cho cruaidh. Ach tha dùbailteachdan nas sùbailte 's nas mì-chinntiche am falach sna h-ìomhaighean seo cuideachd. Gabhaidh sruth aigeanta an teannachaidh eadar cluaran agus ròs aithneachadh annta, 's gu sònraichte ann an dealbh Burns. Air an aon dòigh tha còmhradh socair a' dol eadar smaointean 'soillseachaidh' agus 'buirbe' anns cha mhòr a h-uile gin de na fotosgrìobhaidhean, deasbaireachd a tha a' toirt beachd innleachdach air nòisean an 'adhartais'. A thaobh seo tha còmhstri dhàimheach ann eadar teicneòlasan analog agus meurach, agus eadar cuiltearan aosta 's ùr. Air feadh an t-sreath tha na smaointean aig Colvin gur e a tha ann an rud sam bith ach an rud fhèin agus an rud eil' aige, agus gur e th' ann an cuiltear ach sealg a' cho-chuir chiallaich.

Ge-tà, tha eudòchas neònach anns na h-ìomhaighean

However, there is a peculiar pessimism in these images. This is most obvious in the one barely changing feature of the set, the landscape of ruins and fragments. In part this echoes the romantic and sentimental nature of the cultural tradition, and especially its manifestation in the sense of loss that permeates Macpherson's *Ossian*. Nevertheless, a mood of melancholy disturbs the surface of these photographs, accented by the ghostly apparitions, and further stressed by the uncertainty of an intellectual resolution to the issues presented. There can be little doubt that in this Colvin is reflecting the ethos of the contemporary world. His study of this historical subject is, then, a critical commentary on the here and now, and a challenge to experiment.

It is this challenge to experiment that is the positive dimension of these extraordinary photographs. They are images replete with vigour and vitality, decorous charm and riotous wit, provocative argument and stimulating insight. Where Colvin suggests that the essence of culture and identity is unknowable, and ever changing, he offers a landscape of unending possibilities, open and inviting. It is surely this challenge that a modern Scotland will embrace.

seo. 'S ann as follaisiche a chithear seo san aon rud san t-seata as gann a dh'atharraicheas idir – an dùthaich loma-làn tobhtaichean agus sprùillich. Gu ìre tha seo a' toirt gu cuimhne nàdar romansach agus faireachdainneach an dualchais chuilteireil, agus gu sònraichte mar a tha e nochdadh san nòisean de chall a tha a' drùdhadh air 'Oisein' MhicMhuirich. A dh'ainneoin sin, tha ataireachd a' bhròin a' cur dragh air uachdar nam fotosgrìobhaidhean seo, 's i air a neartachadh le na tanasgan taibhseil 's air a daingneachadh nas fhaide le amharas nach eil fuasgladh sam bith ann ris na ceistean a chaidh a thogail. Faodar a bhith cinnteach a thaobh seo gu bheil ealain Cholvin 'na sgàthan air aigne an t-saoghail anns a bheil sinn beò. Mar sin tha an stuidear seo a rinn e air a' chuspair eachdraidheil sa 'na aithris bhreithneachail air na th' againn a-bhos an-dràst' agus 'na dhùbhlan gu bhith a' cur gu deuchainn.

'S e an dùbhlan seo gu bhith a' cur gu deuchainn an rud a tha adhartach mu na fotosgrìobhaidhean seo. Tha iad 'nan ìomhaighean loma-làn de spionnadh 's de bheathalachd, de tharraing shuairc 's de dh'àbhachdas aimhreiteach, de dh'argamaid bhuaireasach 's de gheur-bheachd brosnachail. Far a bheil Colvin a' cur air thuaiream gu bheil brìgh a' chuilteir 's na h-ionannachd an dà chuid do-aithnichte 's a' sìor mhùthadh, tha e a' tabhann dùthaich loma-làn de na dh'fhaodas a bhith ann gu bràth tuilleadh, 's i fosgailte, fiathachail. Is cinnteach gun gabh Alba an latha an-diugh ris an dùbhlan seo.

1 The notion of Ossian as a 'Celtic Homer' was first popularised by the Revd John Macpherson, no relation, who proposed the idea in his *Critical Dissertation* on Ossian. Robert Crawford has noted that Thomas Jefferson 'said that Ossian was better than Homer', see Crawford 1996.

2 The full title was *Fragments of Ancient Poetry, collected in the Highlands of Scotland, and translated from the Gaelic, or Erse Language*, Edinburgh 1760.

3 Fully, *Fingal, an Ancient Epic Poem, in six Books; Together with several other Poems, composed by Ossian, the son of Fingal: translated from the Galic language*, and, *Temora, an Epic in Eight Books.*

4 For a discussion of eighteenth-century moral codes in Macpherson's epics see John Dwyer 'The Melancholy Savage: Text and Context in the Poems of Ossian' in Gaskill 1991.

5 The best discussion of Macpherson's Ossian and its influence remains Fiona Stafford in Stafford 1988. See also Gaskill 1991, and MacLachlan 1998, the special edition on Ossian. For a discussion of the influence of Ossian on the visual arts, see Okun 1967.

6 For a discussion of Wordsworth's problematic relationship with Macpherson's Ossian, see Fiona Stafford '"Dangerous Success": Ossian, Wordsworth, and English Romantic Literature' in Gaskill 1991.

7 Johnson's most significant published attack came in his *Journey to the Western Islands of Scotland*, 1775.

8 The subject of Johnson's attack on Macpherson is properly explored in Stafford 1988. For a fascinating discussion of Johnson's attack on Macpherson, one that links it to a recurring 'Scottophobia' in eighteenth-century England, see the chapter titled 'James Macpherson and "The Invention of Ossian"' in Ferguson 1998.

9 Hugh Trevor-Roper 1983, p.17.

10 Crawford 1996.

11 Ferguson 1998, p.232.

12 For some discussion of Ossianic art in Scotland see Hugh Cheape 'The Culture and Material Culture of Ossian 1760–1900' in MacLachlan 1998, and see Macmillan 1986, and Macdonald 2000. It should also be noted that this particular etching of *Blind Ossian* is created 'From a Picture supposed to be sketched by Runciman'. A condition that makes it doubly apposite to Colvin's project.

13 Macpherson proposed this contentious revision in *An Introduction to the History of Great Britain and Ireland* in 1771. It was to become a further aspect in the dispute concerning the veracity of his records thereafter.

14 The Clearances of Highland people from ancestral lands can be traced from the 1740s, with an acceleration of these events in the 1770s and 1780s. The process continued in the nineteenth century with instances still reported in the 1840s.

15 James Thomson who was described by his biographer Bertram Dobell as the 'laureate of pessimism', was a Glasgow born poet who lived in London. He completed *The City of Dreadful Night* between 1870 and 1874.

16 Thomson 1998, p.29.

17 Thomson 1998, p.30.

18 Thomson 1998, p.43.

19 John Dwyer in Gaskill 1991.

20 Macpherson, *Fragments of Ancient Poetry* in Crawford and Imlah 2000, p.267. Colvin, himself, prepared for the making of these photographs by referencing Gaskill 1996.

21 Thomson 1998, p.33.

22 Thomson 1998, p.69.

23 Thomson 1998, p.22.

24 Thomson 1998, p.69.

25 Thomson 1998, p.71.

26 In classical mythology Melencolia was a daughter of Saturn. She represented one of the Four Temperaments: melancholic, phlegmatic, choleri and sanguine. These temperaments were bound to the Four Humours: black bile, phlegm, yellow bile and blood. Melancholy being conditioned by the over representation of black bile.

27 For some considerable time this study was out of print, and plans for its re-publication were upset during the Second World War. The work was eventually incorporated in the expanded thesis by Klibansky, Panofsky and Saxl 1964.

28 Klibansky, Panofsky and Saxl 1964, p.319.

29 Ibid. p.321.

30 Ferguson 1998, p.9, and *passim* for further discussion of this myth.

31 Cruthni was one (obscure) name for the Pictish tribes of Dalriada, and it is this cryptic note on racial origins that Colvin conjures with in this triptych of photographs.

32 Ferguson and Roy, vol.1 (1780–1789) 1985, p.265.

33 Ferguson and Roy, vol.1 (1780–1789) 1985, p.327.

34 These, and subsequent quotations from *The Twa Dogs* are from Burns 2001.

35 Colvin renamed Caesar, Kaiser, on learning that the nickname of Celtic Football Club's eminent alumnus Billy McNeill was 'Caesar', a coincidence that would not chime with the designations in the photograph.

36 *Scotch on the Rocks* by Douglas Hurd and Andrew Osmond, London 1971, is a fiction concerning terrorism in Scotland.

37 Significantly Burns's note on this song remarked that 'The first half stanza is old – the rest is mine', and he set the song to the Gaelic tune, *Fàilte na Misg*. In which case we see Macpherson's method is mirrored in Burns.

38 For an account of this see Ferguson 1998, pp.261–5.

39 Ferguson 1998, p.313.

40 This is the import of writer and poet Edwin Muir's thesis in *Scott and Scotland*, first published in 1936 and presenting a highly controversial view of Scott and of Scottish writing.

41 This phrase, as an idiosyncratic description of Scotland, has a long lineage. Apart from its use as a comment on the preponderance of oatcakes in the diet of Scottish peoples, it was quoted by the vernacular poet Robert Fergusson (1750–1774) in his poem *The King's Birthday in Edinburgh*, and by Burns in *On the Late Captain Grose's Peregrinations Thro' Scotland*. It was also incorporated into a speech given by George IV on the occasion of his visit to Edinburgh in 1822.

42 Ramsay painted Rousseau in 1766 following a request by Hume. The relationship between the two philosophers was fractious and ended in bitter recriminations.

43 In his *London Journal* of 1762–1763 Boswell noted 'I dined with Dempster, having engaged to meet Dr Blair and Mr Macpherson at his house. The Sublime Savage (as I call Macpherson) was very outrageous today, throwing out wild sallies against all established opinions.' Cited in Stafford 1988.

44 See endnote no.4.

45 *Blind Harry* resurrects both the association with blind Ossian, and the link to Harry Lauder. Just as importantly it recalls another significant Scottish poet the eponymous Blind Harry (*c*.1450–1493), author of the epic on William Wallace *The Actis and Deidis of the Illustere and Vailyeand Campioun Schir William Wallace, Knicht of Ellerslie*.

46 The history of this image is even more complicated. There is a good provenance for the portrait at Petworth which is certainly by Reynolds. Copies of the painting are held at the National Portrait Gallery in London, NPG 983, and the Scottish version in Edinburgh, PG 1439. A further copy was recently sold at Sothebys.

1 Chaidh cliù Oisein mar 'Hòmar Ceilteach' a sgaoileadh bho thùs leis an Urr. Iain MacMhuirich ás an Eilean Sgitheanach, a chuir an smuain sin air adhart 'na *Critical Dissertation* air Oisein. Thug Raibeart Crawford an aire gun tuirt Tòmas Jefferson 'gun robh Oisein na b' fheàrr na Hòmar', faic Crawford 1996.

2 B' e an làn tiotal *Fragments of Ancient Poetry, collected in the Highlands of Scotland, and translated from the Gaelic, or Erse Language*, Dùn Èideann 1760.

3 Gu h-iomlan, *Fingal, an Ancient Epic Poem, in six Books; Together with several other Poems, composed by Ossian, the son of Fingal: translated from the Galic language*, agus *Temora, an Epic in Eight Books*.

4 Airson beachdachadh mu chodaichean moralta san ochdamh ceud deug sna duaineachdraidh aig MacMhuirich faic John Dwyer 'The Melancholy Savage: Text and Context in the Poems of Ossian' ann an Gaskill 1991.

5 'S e am beachdachadh as fheàrr fhathast air 'Oisein' MhicMhuirich agus a bhuil ach Fiona Stafford ann an Stafford 1988. Faic cuideachd Gaskill 1991 agus MacLachlan 1998. Airson beachdachadh air buaidh 'Oisein' air na h-ealain lèirsinneach faic Okun 1967.

6 Airson beachdachadh air buintealas imcheisteach Wordsworth ri Oisein faic Fiona Stafford '"Dangerous Success": Ossian, Wordsworth, and English Romantic Literature' ann an Gaskill 1991.

7 Thàinig an ionnsaigh fhoillsichte as cudromaiche aig MacIain 'na *Journey to the Western Islands of Scotland*, 1775.

8 Tha cuspair na h-ionnsaigh aig MacIain air MacMhuirich air a sgrùdadh ceart ann an Stafford 1988. Airson beachdachadh uabhasach tarraingeach air ionnsaigh MhicIain air MacMhuirich, a tha an t-ùghdar a' ceangal ri gràin phillteach do dh'Alba ann an Sasainn san ochdamh ceud deug, faic an caibideal air a bheil 'James Macpherson and "The Invention of Ossian"' ann am Ferguson 1998.

9 Hugh Trevor-Roper 1983, td.17.

10 Crawford 1996.

11 Ferguson 1998, td.232.

12 Airson beagan beachdachaidh air ealain Oiseineach ann an Alba faic Hugh Cheape 'The Culture and Material Culture of Ossian 1760–1900' ann am MacLachlan 1998, Macmillan 1986, agus Macdonald 2000. Bu chòir a thoirt an aire cuideachd gun deach an snaidheadh àraidh seo de dh'*Oisein Dall* a dhèanamh 'Bho Dhealbh a tha an Ainm a bhith air a sgeidseadh le Runciman' – cor a tha ga fhàgail air leth iomchaidh do phròiseact Cholvin.

13 Chuir MacMhuirich air adhart am beachd ùr connspaideach seo 'na *Introduction to the History of Great Britain and Ireland* ann an 1771. Bha e a-rithist ri dhol 'na eileamaid eile san deasbaireachd mu dheidhinn cho fìrinneach 's a bha na tobraichean aige.

14 Gabhaidh fuadaichean nan Gaidheal bho fhearann an sinnsrean a lorg bho na 1740an. Thog iad astar anns na 1770an agus na 1780an agus lean iad anns an naoidheamh ceud deug, le eisimpleirean a' tachairt fhathast anns na 1840an.

15 Rugadh Seumas MacThòmais (mu'n tuirt am fear a sgrìobh eachdraidh a bheatha, Bertram Dobell, gur e bh' ann ach 'bàrd mòr an eudòchais') ann an Glaschu agus chaidh e a dh'fhuireach a Lunnainn. Chrìochnaich e *The City of Dreadful Night* eadar 1870 agus 1874.

16 Thomson 1998, td.29.

17 Thomson 1998, td.30.

18 Thomson 1998, td.43.

19 John Dwyer ann an Gaskill 1991.

20 Macpherson, *Fragments of Ancient Poetry* ann an Crawford agus Imlah 2000, td.267. Dheasaich Colvin fhèin ris na dealbhan camara seo a dhèanamh le tarraing a thoirt air Gaskill 1996.

21 Thomson 1998, td.33.

22 Thomson 1998, td.69.

23 Thomson 1998, td.22.

24 Thomson 1998, td.69.

25 Thomson 1998, td.71.

26 Ann an uirsgeulachd na Grèige 's na Ròimhe bha Melencolia 'na nighean aig Satharna. Bha i a' riochdachadh tè de na Ceithir Càilean: dubh, trom, feargach agus dòchasach. Bha na càilean seo ceangailte ris na Ceithir Lionnan: lionn dubh, lionn trom, lionn ruadh (neo fionn) agus fuil (neo lionn dearg). Bha bròn air adhbhrachadh le cus lionn duibh.

27 Bha an stuidear seo greis mhath a-mach á clò, agus bha planaichean airson 'ath-fhoillseachaidh air an cur tro-chèile ri linn an Dàrna Cogaidh Mhòir. Mu dheireadh chaidh an obair fhilleadh anns an tràchdas leasaichte le Klibansky, Panofsky agus Saxl 1964.

28 Klibansky, Panofsky agus Saxl 1964, td.319.

29 *Ibid.*, td.321.

30 Ferguson 1998, td.9, agus *passim* airson tuilleadh beachdachaidh air an uirsgeul seo.

31 Tha Cruthni 'na ainm (dubharach) aig luchd Beurla do threubhan Cruithneach Dhail Riada a-mhàin, agus 's e am pong dubharach sa a chluicheas Colvin an-seo 'na dhealbh-fa-thrì de dhealbhan camara.

32 Ferguson agus Roy, lr.1 (1780–1789), 1985, td.265.

33 Ferguson agus Roy 1985, td.327.

34 Tha na còmhdachaidhean seo, agus an fheadhainn a leanas, bhon *Dà Chù* air an toirt á Burns 2001.

35 Dh'ath-ainmich Colvin Caesar mar Kaiser nuair fhuair e mach gum b' e Caesar am farainm aig Bilidh MacNèill, a bha uaireigin 'na sgiobair 's 'na mhanaidsear aig Club Ball-Coise Celtic – co-thuiteamas nach tigeadh ris na h-ainmean san dealbh chamara.

36 'S e tha ann an *Scotch on the Rocks* le Douglas Hurd agus Andrew Osmond, Lunnainn 1971, ach ficsean mu oillteachas an Albainn.

37 A rèir nota cudromach a sgrìobh Burns mun òran seo 'Tha a' chiad leathrann aost' – is leamsa an còrr', agus rinn e an t-òran air fonn *Fàilte na Misg*. Mar sin tha dòigh obrach Burns ag atharrais air dòigh obrach MhicMhuirich.

38 Airson cunntais air seo faic Ferguson 1998, tdd.261–5.

39 Ferguson 1998, td.313.

40 Seo brìgh an tràchdais aig Edwin Muir, bàrd agus sgrìobhadair, ann an *Scott and Scotland*, a dh'fhoillsicheadh an toiseach ann an 1936 agus a chuir an cèill beachd a bha fìor chonnspaideach air Scott 's air sgrìobhadh Albannach.

41 Tha sloinntireachd fhada aig an abairt seo mar chunntas car annasach air Alba. Bhite ga cleachdadh mar bheachd air cho cumanta 's a bha bonnaich coirc ann an diathad muinntir na h-Alba. Chaidh a còmhdachadh le bàrd an t-sluaigh, Raibeart MacFhearghais (1750–1774), 'na dhàn *The King's Birthday in Edinburgh*, agus le Burns ann an *On the Late Captain Grose's Peregrinations Thro' Scotland*. Agus chaidh a filleadh ann an òraid a thug Deòrsa IV an uair a thug e cuairt air Dùn Èideann ann an 1822.

42 Pheant Ramsay Rousseau ann an 1766 air iarrtas Hume. Bha an dàimh eadar an dà fheallsanach gu math aimhreiteach agus chrìochnaich i ann an coireachadh searbh.

43 'Na *London Journal* 1762–1763 tha Boisil a' sgrìobhadh 'Ghabh mi biadh còmhla ri Dempster, an dèidh dhomh aontachadh coinneachadh ri Dr Blair agus Mgr MacMhuirich san taigh aige. Bha an Samhanach Òirdheirc (mar chanas mi ri MacMhuirich) buileach riaslach an-diugh, 's e a' toirt beumannan fiadhaich an aghaidh a h-uile beachd stèidhte.' Air a chòmhdachadh ann an Stafford 1988.

44 Faic nota-deiridh 4.

45 Tha *Eanraig Dall* a' toirt gu cuimhne an dà chuid a' bhuintealais ri Oisein dall 's a' cheangail ri Harry (neo Eanraig) Lauder. A-cheart cho cudromach, tha e a' toirt gu cuimhne bàrd mòr Albannach eile, Eanraig Dall (*c*.1450–1493), ùghdar an duain-eachdraidh air Uilleam Uallas *The Actis and Deidis of the Illustere and Vailyeand Campioun Schir William Wallace, Knicht of Ellerslie*, a thug 'ainm don dealbh.

46 Tha eachdraidh na h-ìomhaigh seo eadhoin nas toinnte. Tha eachdraidh earbsach air cùl an deilbh ann am Petworth, a tha gu cinnteach le Reynolds. Tha lethbhric den pheantadh air an glèidheadh ann an Galaraidh Nàiseanta nan Dealbhan Daoine ann an Lunnainn, NPG 983, 's tha am breacadh Albannach ann an Dùn Èideann, PG 1439. Chaidh lethbhreac a bharrachd a reic bho chionn ghoirid aig Sothebys.

SELECT BIBLIOGRAPHY

BURNS 1938
Robert Burns, *Complete Poetical Works*, Glasgow, 1938

BURNS 2001
Robert Burns, *Selected Poems*, Edinburgh, 2001

CRAWFORD 1996
Robert Crawford, 'Post-Cullodenism: The Poems of Ossian and Related Works', *London Review of Books*, 3 October, 1996

CRAWFORD AND IMLAH 2000
R. Crawford & M. Imlah, *Scottish Verse*, London, 2000

FERGUSON 1998
William Ferguson, *The Identity of the Scottish Nation*, Edinburgh, 1998

FERGUSON AND ROY 1985
J. De Lancey Ferguson & G. Ross Roy, *The Letters of Robert Burns*, 2 vols., Oxford, 1985

GASKILL 1991
Howard Gaskill (ed.), *Ossian Revisited*, Edinburgh, 1991

GASKILL 1996
Howard Gaskill (ed.), *The Poems of Ossian and Related Works*, Edinburgh, 1996

KLIBANSKY, PANOFSKY AND SAXL 1964
R. Klibansky, E. Panofsky & F. Saxl, *Saturn and Melancholy*, London, 1964

MACDONALD 2000
Murdo Macdonald, *Scottish Art*, London, 2000

MACLACHLAN 1998
Christopher MacLachlan (ed.), *Scotlands 4.1*, Edinburgh, 1997

MACMILLAN 1986
Duncan Macmillan, *Painting in Scotland: The Golden Age*, Oxford, 1986

MUIR 1982
Edwin Muir, *Scott and Scotland*, introduction by Allan Massie, Edinburgh, 1982

OKUN 1967
Henry Okun, 'Ossian in Painting', *Journal of the Warburg and Courtauld Institutes 30*, 1967

PITTOCK 1997
Murray Pittock, *Inventing and Resisting Britain: Cultural Identities in Britain and Ireland, 1685–1789*, London, 1997

STAFFORD 1988
Fiona Stafford, *The Sublime Savage: A Study of James Macpherson and the Poems of Ossian*, Edinburgh, 1988

THOMSON 1952
Derick S. Thomson, *The Gaelic Sources of Macpherson's 'Ossian'*, Edinburgh, 1952

THOMSON 1998
James Thomson, *The City of Dreadful Night*, introduction by Edwin Morgan, Edinburgh, 1998

TREVOR-ROPER 1983
Hugh Trevor-Roper, 'The Invention of Tradition: the Highland Tradition of Scotland', in *The Invention of Tradition*, Eric Hobsbawm & Terence Ranger (eds.), Cambridge, 1983

TAGHADH LEABHRAICHEAN

BURNS 1938
Robert Burns, *Complete Poetical Works*, Glaschu, 1938

BURNS 2001
Robert Burns, *Selected Poems*, Dùn Èideann, 2001

CRAWFORD 1996
Robert Crawford, 'Post-Cullodenism: The Poems of Ossian and Related Works', *London Review of Books*, 3 Dàmhair, 1996

CRAWFORD AGUS IMLAH 2000
R. Crawford & M. Imlah, *Scottish Verse*, Lunnainn, 2000

FERGUSON 1998
William Ferguson, *The Identity of the Scottish Nation*, Dùn Èideann, 1998

FERGUSON AGUS ROY 1985
J. De Lancey Ferguson & G. Ross Roy, *The Letters of Robert Burns*, 2 lr., Àth nan Damh, 1985

GASKILL 1991
Howard Gaskill (deas.), *Ossian Revisited*, Dùn Èideann, 1991

GASKILL 1996
Howard Gaskill (deas.), *The Poems of Ossian and Related Works*, Dùn Èideann, 1996

KLIBANSKY, PANOFSKY AGUS SAXL 1964
R. Klibansky, E. Panofsky & F. Saxl, *Saturn and Melancholy*, Lunnainn, 1964

MACDONALD 2000
Murdo Macdonald, *Scottish Art*, Lunnainn, 2000

MACLACHLAN 1998
Christopher MacLachlan (deas.), *Scotlands 4.1*, Dùn Èideann, 1997

MACMILLAN 1986
Duncan Macmillan, *Painting in Scotland: The Golden Age*, Àth nan Damh, 1986

MUIR 1982
Edwin Muir, *Scott and Scotland*, roi-ràdha le Allan Massie, Dùn Èideann, 1982

OKUN 1967
Henry Okun, 'Ossian in Painting', *Journal of the Warburg and Courtauld Institutes 30*, 1967

PITTOCK 1997
Murray Pittock, *Inventing and Resisting Britain: Cultural Identities in Britain and Ireland, 1685–1789*, Lunnainn, 1997

STAFFORD 1988
Fiona Stafford, *The Sublime Savage: A Study of James Macpherson and the Poems of Ossian*, Dùn Èideann, 1988

THOMSON 1952
Derick S. Thomson, *The Gaelic Sources of Macpherson's 'Ossian'*, Dùn Èideann, 1952

THOMSON 1998
James Thomson, *The City of Dreadful Night*, roi-ràdha le Edwin Morgan, Dùn Èideann, 1998

TREVOR-ROPER 1983
Hugh Trevor-Roper, 'The Invention of Tradition: the Highland Tradition of Scotland', ann an *The Invention of Tradition*, Eric Hobsbawm & Terence Ranger (deas.), Drochaid a' Chaim, 1983

BIOGRAPHY
BEATHA

1961
Born in Glasgow

1979–83
Diploma in Sculpture, Duncan of Jordanstone College of Art, Dundee

1983–5
MA in Photography, Royal College of Art, London

1983
SED Travelling Fellowship

1986
Prize-winner, 'Young European Photographer of the Year Award'

1987
The Photographers Gallery 'Brandt Award'

1989
Royal Photographic Society Gold Medal

1997
The 13th Higashikawa Overseas Photographer Prize

2000
Scottish Arts Council / National Lottery Creative Scotland Award
Leverhulme Trust Research Fellowship

2001
Awarded OBE for contribution to the Visual Arts

2002
Carnegie Trust Award
Currently Professor of Fine Art Photography, University of Dundee

SELECTED INDIVIDUAL EXHIBITIONS
TAISBEANAIDHEAN TAGHTE AON-DUINE

1986–8
Constructed Narratives (with Ron O'Donnell): Photographers' Gallery, London; Arts Centre, Plymouth; Stills Gallery, Edinburgh; Axiom Centre for the Arts, Cheltenham; Watershed, Bristol; Taideteollisuumuseo, Helsinki; Glasgow Arts Centre; Stirling Smith Art Gallery; Premises Art Centre, Norwich

1987–90
Calum Colvin: Riverside Studios, London; Kathleen Ewing Gallery, Washington DC; Sander Gallery, New York; Friedman-Guinness Gallery, Heidelberg; Torch Gallery, Amsterdam; Richard Pomoroy Gallery, London; Seagate Gallery, Dundee; Salama Caro Gallery, London; Galeria 57, Madrid; Glenn/Dash Gallery, Los Angeles; California State University, Long Beach; Friedman-Guinness Gallery, Frankfurt; Pier Arts Centre, Stromness; Harris Museum and Art Gallery, Preston; Portfolio Gallery, Edinburgh

1990
Brief Encounter: Fruitmarket Gallery, Edinburgh; Aberdeen Art Gallery
Calum Colvin: Post Modern Photography: Haggerty Museum of Art, Milwaukee, Wisconsin

1991
The Two Ways of Life: Art Institute of Chicago; San Francisco Museum of Modern Art; Nickle Arts Museum, Calgary; Winnipeg Art Gallery; Badischer Kunstverein, Karlsruhe

1993–2000
The Seven Deadly Sins and the Four Last Things: Portfolio Gallery, Edinburgh; Photographers Gallery, London; Photosynkyria, Thessalonki, Greece; Norwich Arts Centre; Banco Central Art Gallery, Quenca, Ecuador; British Council, Quito, Ecuador; Royal Photographic Society, Bath; Fotomuseum, Stadtmuseum, Munich; Seagate Gallery, Dundee; Photography Centre of Athens; Forum Gallery, Zagreb, Croatia; Varazdin Town Museum, Croatia; BM Contemporary Art Centre, Istanbul; Izfas Art Gallery, Ismir; State Fine Arts Gallery, Ankara; Encontros da Imagem, Braga, Portugal; Kawasaki City Museum, Japan; The Meffan Institute, Forfar

1995
Unlikely Stories: Kulturhuset, Stockholm; Photographic Museum of Finland, Helsinki

1996
Ornithology: Jason and Rhodes Gallery, London

1996–2000
Pseudologica Fantastica: Impressions Gallery, York; Focal Point Gallery, Southend-on-Sea; Portfolio Gallery, Edinburgh; Theatr Clwyd, Mold, Wales; Fundacio Cultural Caixa de Terassa, Barcelona; University of Salamanca; Centro de Arte Contemporaneo, Seville; Viewpoint Gallery, Salford, Manchester; Leeds Metropolitan University Gallery; Piece Hall Gallery, Halifax

1998
Sacred and Profane: Scottish National Gallery of Modern Art, Edinburgh; National Machado de Castro Museum, Coimbra, Portugal; Martha Schneider Gallery, Chicago

1985
The 85 Degree Show: Serpentine Gallery, London

1986
Recontres Internationales De La Photographie:
Arles
2D–3D: Laing Art Gallery, Newcastle

1987
Towards a Bigger Picture: Victoria & Albert
Museum, London
True Stories and Photofictions: Ffotogallery,
Cardiff; Camerawork, London; Collins Gallery,
Glasgow
The Vigorous Imagination: New Scottish Art:
Scottish National Gallery of Modern Art,
Edinburgh

1988
Foco 88: British Council tour throughout Spain,
inaugurated at Circulo de Bellas Artes, Madrid

1989
*Through the Looking Glass: Photographic Art in
Britain 1945–89*: Barbican Art Gallery, London
Machine Dreams: Photographers' Gallery, London
Das Konstruierte Bild: Kunstverein, Munich
Scottish Art Since 1900: Scottish National Gallery
of Modern Art, Edinburgh; Barbican Art Gallery,
London

1990
New Scottish Photography: Fotofest, Houston;
Scottish National Portrait Gallery, Edinburgh;
Centro Cultural Conde Duque, Madrid; Fundacio
Cultural de la Caixa de Terressa, Barcelona
Photography on Site (with Ron O'Donnell):
California State University
Scotland Creates: 5000 Years of Art and Design:
McLellan Galleries, Glasgow

1991
De Composition: Chapter Arts Centre, Cardiff;
Museu de Arte de Sao Paulo; Escola de Artes
Visualis do Parque Lage, Rio de Janeiro;
Sociedade Brasileira de Cultura Inglesa, Salvador,
Brazil; Centro Cultural Recoleta, Buenos Aires;
Chilean-British Institute, Santiago, Chile;
J. Harriman Gallery of the ACPP, Lima, Peru;
Museo de Arte Moderno, Quenca, Ecuador;
Museo de Arte Moderno, Bogota, Colombia;
Museo de Artes Visuales Alejandro Otero,
Caracas, Venezuela; Pepperdine Center for the
Arts, Pepperdine University, Malibu, USA;
National Gallery, Kingston, Jamaica

1992
Addressing the Forbidden: Art Gallery, Brighton
Polytechnic; Stills Gallery, Edinburgh
La Photographie Britannique: Arles
International Photo Triennale, Esslingen,
Germany

1994
Elvis + Marilyn 2 x Immortal: Institute of
Contemporary Art, Boston; Contemporary Arts
Museum, Houston, Texas; New York Historical
Society; Columbus Museum of Art, Ohio; The
Philbrook Museum of Art, Tulsa; Daimaru
Museum, Umeda-Osaka; Takamatsu City
Museum of Art, Japan
Revisions: Kulturreferat Der Landeshaupstradt,
Munich

1995
Light from the Dark Room: Royal Scottish
Academy, Edinburgh
An American Passion: Royal College of Art,
London; McLellan Galleries, Glasgow

1996
Photography after Photography: Aktionsforum
Praterinsel, Munich; Kunsthalle, Krems; Erlangen
Municipal Gallery; Brandenburgishe
Kunstsammlungen, Cottbus; Museet for
Fotokunst, Odense; Fotomuseum, Winterthur;
Finlands Fotografiska Museum, Helsinki;
Institute of Contemporary Art, Philadelphia,
USA; Adelaide Festival 1998, Australia
A Collection for the Future: Ferens Art Gallery,
Hull

1997
Body Politic: Wolverhampton Art Gallery and
Derby Art Gallery
History: the Mag Collection: Ferens Art Gallery,
Hull; Fruitmarket Gallery, Edinburgh
*On The Bright Side of Life – Contemporary British
Photography*: NGBK, Berlin; Badischer
Kunstverein, Karlsruhe; Kunstverein
Ludwigshafen am Rhein, Germany
Northern Exposure: Harris Museum and Art
Gallery, Preston
Cyberealismo: Galleria Photology, Milan

1999
Scotland's Art: City Art Centre, Edinburgh

2000
Expressions: Scottish Art 1976–1989: Aberdeen Art
Gallery; Dundee Contemporary Arts/Dundee
City Museum
100 Years of Scottish Prints: Edinburgh
Printmakers
*Optical Delusions: Jokes, Puns, and Sleights-of-
Hand in Photography*: Art Institute of Chicago
Writers of Our Time: Scottish National Portrait
Gallery, Edinburgh

2001
Narcissus – 20th Century Self Portraits: Scottish
National Portrait Gallery, Edinburgh
*Still Lifes and Portraits from the Manfred Heiting
Collection*: Rijksmuseum, Amsterdam

True Fictions: Bad Arolsen, nr Kassel, Germany;
Ludwig Forum für Internationale Kunst, Aachen;
Kunst Haus Dresden; Kunstverein, Lingen
Can You Judge a Book by its Cover?: Scottish
National Gallery of Modern Art, Edinburgh
The Fine Art of Photography: Scottish National
Portrait Gallery, Edinburgh

2002
*Scotland Calls – 20th Century Scottish
Photography*: Boston Public Library
Seeing Things: Photographing Objects 1850–2001:
Canon Photography Gallery, Victoria & Albert
Museum, London

SELECTED BIBLIOGRAPHY
LEABHRAICHEAN TAGHTE

Mattie Boom, *Still Lifes & Portraits*, Rijksmuseum, Amsterdam, 2001

David Brittain, *Constructed Narratives: Photographs by Calum Colvin and Ron O'Donnell*, exhibition catalogue, Photographers' Gallery, London, 1986

David Brittain and Sara Stevenson, *New Scottish Photography*, exhibition catalogue, Scottish National Portrait Gallery, Edinburgh, 1990

Bill Hare, *Scottish Painting*, exhibition catalogue, Talbot Rice Gallery, Edinburgh, 1993

Keith Hartley, *Scottish Art Since 1900*, exhibition catalogue, Scottish National Gallery of Modern Art, Edinburgh, 1989

Keith Hartley *et al.*, *The Vigorous Imagination: New Scottish Art*, exhibition catalogue, Scottish National Gallery of Modern Art, Edinburgh, 1987

Mark Haworth-Booth *et al.*, *British Photography, Towards a Bigger Picture*, New York, 1988

James Holloway *et al.*, *A Companion Guide to the Scottish National Portrait Gallery*, Edinburgh, 1999

Sarah Kent, *Through the Looking Glass*, exhibition catalogue, Barbican Art Gallery, London, 1989

Michael Langford, *Story of Photography*, London, 1997

James Lawson, *Sacred and Profane*, exhibition catalogue, Scottish National Gallery of Modern Art, Edinburgh, 1998

Murdo Macdonald, *History of Scottish Art*, London, 2000

Brian McGeoch and Steven Porch, *Looking at Scottish Art*, East Sussex, 1996

Duncan Macmillan, *Scottish Art 1460–1990* (revised edition), Edinburgh, 2000

David Alan Mellor, *Calum Colvin*, exhibition catalogue, Fruitmarket Gallery, Edinburgh, 1990

David Alan Mellor, *On the Bright Side of Life: Zeitgenossiche Britische Fotografie*, Berlin, 1997

David Alan Mellor, *Portfolio no.24*, Portfolio Gallery, Edinburgh, 1996

Tom Normand, *The Seven Deadly Sins and the Four Last Things*, exhibition catalogue, Portfolio Gallery, Edinburgh, 1993

Ulrich Pohlmann *et al.*, *Revisions*, Munich, 1994

Florian Rötzer *et al.*, *Photography after Photography*, Munich, 1996

Sara Stevenson *et al.*, *Light from the Dark Room*, exhibition catalogue, Royal Scottish Academy, Edinburgh, 1995

Sara Stevenson and Duncan Forbes, *A Companion Guide to Photography in the National Galleries of Scotland*, Edinburgh, 2001

Studies in Photography, Scottish Society for the History of Photography, 1998

Dr Andreas Vowinckel, *The Two Ways of Life and Other Photographic Works*, exhibition catalogue, Badischer Kunstverein, Karlsruhe, 1993

Colin Westerbeck and David Alan Mellor, *The Two Ways of Life*, exhibition catalogue, Art Institute of Chicago, 1991

WEBSITE
LÀRACH-LÌN

www.calumcolvin.com

COLLECTIONS
CRUINNEACHAIDHEAN

Aberdeen Art Gallery

Arnolfini Collection Trust, Bristol

Art Institute of Chicago

Boswell Collection, University of St Andrews

The British Council, London

City Art Centre, Edinburgh

Columbus University, Georgia

Ferens Art Gallery, Hull

Gallery of Modern Art, Glasgow

Metropolitan Museum of Art, New York

Museum of Fine Arts, Houston

Royal Photographic Society, London

Scottish National Gallery of Modern Art, Edinburgh

Scottish National Portrait Gallery, Edinburgh

Victoria & Albert Museum, London